# TARGET ORGAN TOXICOLOGY SERIES

# CARDIOVASCULAR TOXICOLOGY

## THIRD EDITION

# TARGET ORGAN TOXICOLOGY SERIES

Series Editors

A. Wallace Hayes, John A. Thomas, and Donald E. Gardner

TOXICOLOGY OF SKIN
*Howard I. Maibach, editor, 558 pp., 2000*

TOXICOLOGY OF THE LUNG, THIRD EDITION
*Donald E. Gardner, James D. Crapo, and Roger O. McClellan, editors, 668 pp., 1999*

NEUROTOXICOLOGY, SECOND EDITION
*Hugh A. Tilson and G. Jean Harry, editors, 386 pp., 1999*

TOXICANT–RECEPTOR INTERACTIONS: MODULATION OF SIGNAL
TRANSDUCTIONS AND GENE EXPRESSION
*Michael S. Denison and William G. Helferich, editors, 256 pp., 1998*

TOXICOLOGY OF THE LIVER, SECOND EDITION
*Gabriel L. Plaa and William R. Hewitt, editors, 444 pp., 1997*

FREE RADICAL TOXICOLOGY
*Kendall B. Wallace, editor, 454 pp., 1997*

ENDOCRINE TOXICOLOGY, SECOND EDITION
*Raphael J. Witorsch, editor, 336 pp., 1995*

CARCINOGENESIS
*Michael P. Waalkes and Jerrold M. Ward, editors, 496 pp., 1994*

DEVELOPMENTAL TOXICOLOGY, SECOND EDITION
*Carole A. Kimmel and Judy Buelke-Sam, editors, 496 pp., 1994*

IMMUNOTOXICOLOGY AND IMMUNOPHARMACOLOGY, SECOND EDITION
*Jack H. Dean, Michael I. Luster, Albert E. Munson, and Ian Kimber, editors, 784 pp., 1994*

NUTRITIONAL TOXICOLOGY
*Frank N. Kotsonis, Maureen A. Mackey, and Jerry J. Hjelle, editors, 336 pp., 1994*

TOXICOLOGY OF THE KIDNEY, SECOND EDITION
*Jerry B. Hook and Robin J. Goldstein, editors, 576 pp., 1993*

OPHTHALMIC TOXICOLOGY
*George C. Y. Chiou, editor, 352 pp., 1992*

TOXICOLOGY OF THE BLOOD AND BONE MARROW
*Richard D. Irons, editor, 192 pp., 1985*

TOXICOLOGY OF THE EYE, EAR, AND OTHER SPECIAL SENSES
*A. Wallace Hayes, editor, 264 pp., 1985*

CUTANEOUS TOXICITY
*Victor A. Drill and Paul Lazar, editors, 288 pp., 1984*

TARGET ORGAN TOXICOLOGY SERIES

# CARDIOVASCULAR TOXICOLOGY

## Third Edition

Edited by

# Daniel Acosta, Jr.

College of Pharmacy
University of Cincinnati
Cincinnati, Ohio
USA

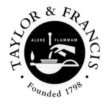

London and New York

Third edition published 2001
by Taylor & Francis
11 New Fetter Lane, London EC4P 4EE

Simultaneously published in the USA and Canada
by Taylor & Francis
29 West 35th Street, New York, NY 10001

*Taylor & Francis is an imprint of the Taylor & Francis Group*

© 2001 Taylor & Francis

Second edition published 1992 by Raven Press Ltd., New York.

Typeset in Times by
Prepress Projects Ltd, Perth, Scotland
Printed and bound in Great Britain by
St Edmundsbury Press, Bury St Edmunds, Suffolk

Every effort has been made to ensure that the advice and information in
this book is true and accurate at the time of going to press. However,
neither the publisher nor the authors can accept any legal responsibility
or liability for any errors or omissions that may be made. In the case of
drug administration, any medical procedure or the use of technical
equipment mentioned within this book, you are strongly advised to
consult the manufacturer's guidelines.

*British Library Cataloguing in Publication Data*
A catalogue record for this book is available
from the British Library

*Library of Congress Cataloging in Publication Data*
Cardiovascular toxicology/edited by Daniel Acosta, Jr. – 3rd ed.
p.cm – (Target organ toxicology series)
Includes bibliographical references and index.
1. Cardiovascular Diseases. I. Acosta, Daniel, 1945– II. Series.
[DNLM: 1. Cardiovascular Diseases – chemically induced. 2.
Cardiovascular System – drug effects. WG 100 C267 2001]
RC677 .C37 2001
616.1′07–dc21    00-037720

ISBN 0-415-24869-8

# CONTENTS

*List of contributors*                                                      xi
*Series preface*                                                           xiv
*Preface*                                                                    xv


**PART I**
**Introduction**                                                             **1**


**1    Cardiovascular toxicology: introductory notes**                       **3**
RUSSELL B. MELCHERT, CAI YUAN, AND DANIEL ACOSTA, JR.

*Introductory remarks  3*
*Cardiac myocyte growth and programmed death: emerging areas*
*    for research in cardiovascular toxicology  4*
*In* vitro *model systems for studying cardiac myocyte hypertrophic*
*    growth and apoptotic death  4*
*Cardiac myocyte growth  7*
*Hypertrophic growth  14*
*Cardiac myocyte apoptosis  16*
*Conclusions  22*


**PART II**
**Methods**                                                                 **31**


**2    Acute and chronic evaluation of the cardiovascular toxicity**
**     of drugs: an industrial perspective**                                **33**
SHAYNE C. GAD

*Pharmacologic profiling  34*
*In* vivo *parameter evaluations in standard studies  35*
*Clinical pathology  41*
*Pathology  46*

CONTENTS

*Animal models  51*
In vitro *models and their use  51*
*Summary  56*

**3   Evaluation of *in vitro* cytotoxicity modeling**                     **59**
ENRIQUE CHACON, JOHN M. BOND, AND JOHN J. LEMASTERS

*Overview  59*
*Primary heart cell cultures for cytotoxicity screening  65*
*Cytotoxicity assessment  67*
*Summary and conclusions  73*

**4   Monitoring of cardiovascular dynamics in conscious animals**         **79**
STEPHEN F. VATNER, THOMAS A. PATRICK, AMELIA B. KUDEJ, YOU-TANG SHEN,
AND KUNIYA ASAI

*Large animal techniques for measurement of*
*    cardiovascular parameters  80*
*Instrumentation for smaller animals  90*
*Summary  95*

**PART III**
**Principles of myocardial cell injury**                                   **103**

**5   Cell injury and cell death: apoptosis, oncosis, and necrosis**       **105**
BENJAMIN F. TRUMP, SEUNG H. CHANG, PATRICIA C. PHELPS,
AND RAYMOND T. JONES

*Characteristics of cellular response*
*    following a lethal injury  105*
*Oncosis  107*
*Principal mechanisms of oncosis  112*
*Energy metabolism  122*
*Altered gene expression  123*
*Hypothesis of [Ca$^{2+}$] and oncosis  127*
*Apoptosis  133*
*Principal proposed mechanisms of apoptosis  140*
*What determines whether an injury leads to*
*    apoptosis or oncosis  146*
*Cell death  148*
*Necrosis  149*
*Other terms and concepts used in reference to cell death  152*
*Conclusions  154*

**6    Pathobiology of myocardial ischemic injury**                164
L. MAXIMILIAN BUJA

*Introduction  164*
*Role of coronary alterations in myocardial ischemia  164*
*Mechanisms of myocardial ischemic injury  167*
*Evolution of myocardial infarction  173*
*Modulation of myocardial ischemic injury  176*


**PART IV**
**Cardiotoxicity**                                                185

**7    Cardiovascular toxicity of antibacterial antibiotics**     187
J. KEVIN KERZEE, KENNETH S. RAMOS, JANET L. PARKER, AND
H. RICHARD ADAMS

*Introduction  187*
*Clinical reports  188*
*Respiratory depressant actions: link*
*    to cardiovascular function  191*
*Autonomic effects  193*
*Cardiovascular effects  194*
*Summary  208*

**8    Bacterial lipopolysaccharide (endotoxin) and**
**    myocardial dysfunction**                                    222
LEONA J. RUBIN, JANET L. PARKER, AND H. RICHARD ADAMS

*Introduction  222*
*Cardiac dysfunction in clinical LPS and sepsis syndromes  223*
*Cardiac dysfunction in experimental LPS and sepsis models: in vivo*
*    studies  226*
*Cardiac dysfunction in experimental*
*    LPS and sepsis models  231*
*Mediators of myocardial toxicity of LPS and sepsis  241*
*Conclusion and implications  250*

**9    Catecholamine-induced cardiomyopathy**                     269
NARANJAN S. DHALLA, HIDEKI SASAKI, SEIBU MOCHIZUKI, KEN S. DHALLA,
XUELIANG LIU, AND VIJAYAN ELIMBAN

*Introduction  269*
*Cardiotoxicity of catecholamines  270*

*Characteristics of catecholamine-induced cardiomyopathy 271*
*Interventions on catecholamine-induced cardiomyopathy 281*
*Mechanisms of catecholamine-induced cardiomyopathy 287*
*Summary and conclusions 301*

**10 Cardiovascular effects of centrally acting drugs**      **319**
KENNETH A. SKAU AND GARY GUDELSKY

*Antidepressant agents 319*
*Antipsychotic agents 320*
*Stimulants 320*
*Depressants 323*
*Anticonvulsants 323*

**11 Toxins that affect ion channels, pumps, and exchangers**      **328**
N. SPERELAKIS, M. SUNAGAWA, M. NAKAMURA, H. YOKOSHIKI, AND T. SEKI

*Introduction 328*
*Target ion channels 328*
*Target pumps and exchangers 349*
*Summary 358*

**12 Cardiotoxicity of anthracyclines and other antineoplastic agents**      **374**
JANE PRUEMER

*Anthracyclines 374*
*Cardioprotectants 379*
*Other anti-tumor agents 385*
*Biologics 389*
*Summary 390*

**13 Passive smoking causes heart disease**      **402**
STANTON A. GLANTZ AND WILLIAM W. PARMLEY

*Effects of second-hand smoke on oxygen delivery, processing, and exercise 403*
*Platelets 404*
*Endothelial function 406*
*Atherosclerosis 406*
*Free radicals in second-hand smoke and ischemic damage 410*
*Myocardial infarction 411*

*Epidemiologic studies 411*
*Conclusion 416*


**14    Cardiovascular effects of steroidal agents**                                    **425**
RUSSELL B. MELCHERT, RICHARD H. KENNEDY, AND DANIEL ACOSTA, JR.

*Introduction 425*
*Vascular effects of steroidal agents 432*
*Cardiac effects of steroidal agents 450*
*Further considerations regarding steroidal agents and cardiovascular*
*    function 461*
*Conclusions: cardiovascular toxicology*
*    and steroidal agents 463*


**PART V**
**Vascular toxicity**                                                                    **477**

**15    Vascular toxicology: a cellular and molecular perspective**                       **479**
KENNETH S. RAMOS, J. KEVIN KERZEE, NAPOLEON F. ALEJANDRO,
AND KIM P. LU

*Introduction 479*
*Structural and functional characteristics*
*    of the blood vessel wall 479*
*Vascular cell biology 481*
*Principles of vasculotoxic specificity 484*
*Selected vascular toxins 488*
*Concluding remarks 507*

**16    Pathobiology of the vascular response to injury**                                 **525**
PETER G. ANDERSON, ZADOK RUBEN, AND BERNARD M. WAGNER

*Introduction 525*
*Regulation of normal vascular structure and function 525*
*Vascular injury 527*
*Nitric oxide and peroxynitrite in vascular disease 529*
*Pathology of vascular interventions 530*
*Mechanical vascular injury: experimental models*
*    and study paradigms 531*
*Animal models in the study of vascular interventions 533*
*Morphometric techniques in studies of restenosis 547*
*Concluding remarks 550*

**17    The arterial media as a target of injury by chemicals**          **557**

PAUL J. BOOR

*Introduction  557*
*Vasoactive chemicals  558*
*Lesions secondary to endothelial injury  563*
*Structural injury to the media: lathyrism  566*
*Nutritional deficiencies; genetic errors  573*
*Conclusions  575*

*Index*          583

# CONTRIBUTORS

**Daniel Acosta, Jr.** is Dean and Professor of the University of Cincinnati, College of Pharmacy, 3223 Eden Avenue, ML 0004, Cincinnati, OH 45267-0004, USA.

**H. Richard Adams** is Dean and Professor at the Department of Veterinary Physiology and Pharmacology, College of Veterinary Medicine, Texas A & M University, College Station, TX 77843-4461, USA.

**Napoleon F. Alejandro** is at the Department of Physiology and Pharmacology, College of Veterinary Medicine, Texas A & M University, College Station, TX 77843-4466, USA.

**Peter G. Anderson** is at the University of Alabama at Birmingham, Birmingham, AL, USA.

**Kuniya Asai** is at the Cardiovascular Research Institute, UMDNJ, New Jersey Medical School, Hackensack University Medical Center, 30 Prospect Avenue, Hackensack, NJ 07601, USA.

**John M. Bond** is at the Riverside Veterinary Hospital, Rocky Mount, NC, USA.

**Paul J. Boor** is at the Department of Pathology, University of Texas Medical Branch, Galveston, TX 77555-0609, USA

**L. Maximilian Buja** is Dean and Professor at the Department of Pathology and Laboratory Medicine, The University of Texas-Houston Medical School, USA.

**Enrique Chacon** is at the CEDRA Corporation, Austin, TX 78754, USA.

**Seung H. Chang** is at the Department of Pathology, University of Maryland School of Medicine, Baltimore, MD 21210, USA.

**Ken S. Dhalla** is at the Institute of Cardiovascular Sciences, St. Boniface General Hospital Research Centre, and Department of Physiology, Faculty of Medicine, University of Manitoba, Winnipeg, Canada.

**Naranjan S. Dhalla** is at the Institute of Cardiovascular Sciences, St. Boniface General Hospital Research Centre, and Department of Physiology, Faculty of Medicine, University of Manitoba, Winnipeg, Canada.

**Vijayan Elimban** is at the Institute of Cardiovascular Sciences, St. Boniface General Hospital Research Centre, and Department of Physiology, Faculty of Medicine, University of Manitoba, Winnipeg, Canada.

**Shayne C. Gad** is at Gad Consulting Services, Cary, NC 27511, USA.

**Stanton A. Glantz** is at the  Division of Cardiology, Department of Medicine, Cardiovascular Research Institute, University of California, San Francisco, CA 94143, USA.

**Gary Gudelsky** is at the University of Cincinnati College of Pharmacy, 3223 Eden Avenue, Cincinnati, OH 45267, USA.

**Raymond T. Jones** is at Department of Pathology, University of Maryland School of Medicine, Baltimore, MD 21210, USA.

**Richard H. Kennedy** is Professor and Chair at the Department of Pharmaceutical Sciences, University of Arkansas for Medical Sciences, College of Pharmacy, 4301 W. Markham St., Slot 522, Little Rock, AR 72205, USA.

**J. Kevin Kerzee** is at the Department of Physiology and Pharmacology, College of Veterinary Medicine, Texas A & M University, College Station, TX 77843-4466, USA.

**Amelia B. Kudej** is at the Cardiovascular Research Institute, UMDNJ, New Jersey Medical School, Hackensack University Medical Center, 30 Prospect Avenue, Hackensack, NJ 07601, USA.

**John J. Lemasters** is at the Department of Cell Biology and Anatomy, Curriculum in Toxicology, School of Medicine, University of North Carolina at Chapel Hill, Chapel Hill, NC 27599-7090, USA.

**Xueliang Liu** is at the Institute of Cardiovascular Sciences, St. Boniface General Hospital Research Centre, and Department of Physiology, Faculty of Medicine, University of Manitoba, Winnipeg, Canada.

**Kim P. Lu** is at the Department of Physiology and Pharmacology, College of Veterinary Medicine, Texas A & M University, College Station, TX 77843-4466, USA.

**Russell B. Melchert** is Assistant Professor at the Department of Pharmaceutical Sciences, University of Arkansas for Medical Sciences, College of Pharmacy, 4301 W. Markham St., Slot 522, Little Rock, AR 72205, USA.

**Seibu Mochizuki** is at the Department of Internal Medicine, Jikei University School of Medicine, Tokyo, Japan.

**M. Nakamura** is at the Department of Molecular and Cellular Physiology, College of Medicine, University of Cincinnati, 231 Bethesda Avenue, PO Box 67057, Cincinnati, OH 45267-0576, USA

**Janet L. Parker** is at the Department of Medical Physiology, College of Medicine, Texas A & M University, College Station, TX 77843-4461, USA.

**William W. Parmley** is at the Division of Cardiology, Department of Medicine, Cardiovascular Research Institute, University of California, San Francisco, CA 94143, USA.

**Thomas A. Patrick** is at the Cardiovascular Research Institute, UMDNJ, New Jersey Medical School, Hackensack University Medical Center, 30 Prospect Avenue, Hackensack, NJ 07601, USA.

**Patricia C. Phelps** is at the Department of Pathology, University of Maryland School of Medicine, Baltimore, MD 21210, USA.

**Jane Pruemer** is at the Department of Pharmacy Services, The University Hospital, Health Alliance of Greater Cincinnati, Cincinnati, OH, USA.

**Kenneth S. Ramos** is at the Department of Physiology and Pharmacology, College of Veterinary Medicine, Texas A & M University, College Station, TX 77843-4461, USA.

**Zadok Ruben** is at Patoximed Consultants, Westfield, NJ, USA.

**Leona J. Rubin** is at the Department of Veterinary Biomedical Sciences, College of Veterinary Medicine, University of Missouri – Columbia, Columbia, MO 65211, USA.

**Hideki Sasaki** is at the Institute of Cardiovascular Sciences, St. Boniface General Hospital Research Centre, and Department of Physiology, Faculty of Medicine, University of Manitoba, Winnipeg, Canada.

**T. Seki** is at the Department of Molecular and Cellular Physiology, College of Medicine, University of Cincinnati, 231 Bethesda Avenue, PO Box 67057, Cincinnati, OH 45267-0576, USA.

**You-Tang Shen** is at the Cardiovascular Research Institute, UMDNJ, New Jersey Medical School, Hackensack University Medical Center, 30 Prospect Avenue, Hackensack, NJ 07601, USA.

**Kenneth A. Skau** is at the University of Cincinnati College of Pharmacy, 3223 Eden Avenue, Cincinnati, OH 45267, USA.

**N. Sperelakis** is at the Department of Molecular and Cellular Physiology, College of Medicine, University of Cincinnati, 231 Bethesda Avenue, PO Box 67057, Cincinnati, OH 45267-0576, USA.

**M. Sunagawa** is at the Department of Molecular and Cellular Physiology, College of Medicine, University of Cincinnati, 231 Bethesda Avenue, PO Box 67057, Cincinnati, OH 45267-0576, USA.

**Benjamin F. Trump** is at the Warwick Research Institute, Baltimore, MD 21210, and AMC Cancer Research Center, Denver, CO 88214, USA.

**Stephen F. Vatner** is at the Cardiovascular Research Institute, UMDNJ, New Jersey Medical School, Hackensack University Medical Center, 30 Prospect Avenue, Hackensack, NJ 07601, USA.

**Bernard M. Wagner** is at Short Hills, NJ, USA.

**H. Yokoshiki** is at the Department of Molecular and Cellular Physiology, College of Medicine, University of Cincinnati, 231 Bethesda Avenue, PO Box 67057, Cincinnati, OH 45267-0576, USA.

**Cai Yuan** is at St. Elizabeth's Medical Center of Boston, Tufts University School of Medicine Teaching Affiliate, Department of Psychiatry, 736 Cambridge Street, Boston, MA 02135-2997, USA.

# SERIES PREFACE

## Target Organ Toxicology Series

The concept of a Target Organ Toxicology Series began nearly two decades ago with the late Dr. Robert L. Dixon. His early vision provided the initial stimulus and the guidance for the early years of the series. The series began at a time when technical achievements in the field of toxicology were undergoing rapid growth leading to a vast accumulation of scientific information, m uch of which was focused on identifying the mechanisms associated with the biological action of chemicals on various physiological systems. emerging knowledge enhanced the understanding of the hazards of environmental contaminants, and the resulatant basic assessment led to the formation of a number of federal and state policies promulgating the protection of the public from exposure to chemicals in the environment. The rapid growth of toxicology created a need to address critical issues and recent advances in the assessment of the mechanism of chemically induced toxicity in various target organs. The Target Organ Toxicology Series set out to meet this challenge and has become internationally recognized as a successful series of monographs devoted to the careful and articulate review of critical areas in toxicology and environmental health and also as a major influence affecting future trends in the field of toxicology.

The objectives and goals of the series have always been to highlight a particular organ system and to present a comprhensive and critical synthesis of advances leading to a better understanding of the toxicology of that organ system.

The series is written for a broad scientific audience yet provides comprehensive coverage of dpecific areas of toxicology. The authors focus their presentation so that the information can be used not only to gain a general understanding of the principles of toxocology but also to be resource guide directing readers who want a deeper understanding regarding mechanisms of response of a specific substance on a specific target organ.

Beyond being a basic refernce resource, the series serves readers with more focused needs. For researchers who are interested in comparing target organ responses between and among species, the series provides a timely source useful in guiding future research. for educors, the series is a basic reference source as well as a directory to other related toxological literature. For reguatory scientists, it is a repository of comprehensive information useful in making and suppoting regulatory dedisions with a toxicological database that may not be available in other individual publications.

The series comprises monographs edited by leading, internationally recognized scientists with expertise in toxicology and the environmental sciences. The contributors of the various monographs are drawn from a diverse multidisciplinary background and represent industrial, government, academic, and research establishments but are always experts on the advances, issues, and concepts of the chapter's topic area. While for each of the topic areas coverage may appear too be highly specialized, together the complete series represents a unique overview of an interdisciplinary approach to evaluate target organ toxicity.

The series editors recognize that the field of toxicology continues to change rapidly, and that new and important advances will be forthcoming. As the needs arise and new knowledge is gained in the field of toxicolgy, the Target Organ Toxicology Series will provide timely new topics written by intenational experts.

# PREFACE

The first edition of *Cardiovascular Toxicology*, edited by Ethard W. Van Stee, was published in 1982, and Daniel Acosta, Jr. edited the second edition in 1992. The major objective of these two editions was to provide a comprehensive overview of the toxicology of drugs and chemicals to the myocardium and the vascular system. The second edition included more information on the vascular system and its response to toxic agents. These two editions have provided a wealth of information on cardiovascular toxicology to clinicians, public health officers, industrial and experimental toxicologists, and other interested professionals.

The third edition continues this tradition of highlighting major advances in the field of cardiovascular toxicology. The monograph follows the same format that was first developed in the second edition: an introductory section followed by four sections in the areas of Methods, Principles of Cell Injury, Cardiotoxicity, and Vascular Toxicity. All of the chapters have been updated, and in many cases have been significantly revised. In addition, some new chapters have been included in this edition: one on *in vitro* methods of assessing cardiotoxicity; one on the cardiotoxicity of steroidal agents; and another one on medial injury of large and elastic blood vessels. Many of the chapters have included information on the molecular aspects of toxicity to the cardiovascular system, including genomics information where appropriate.

We hope that the third edition fulfills our goal of providing state-of-the-art toxicologic insight into mechanisms of injury to the cardiovascular system by chemical agents. This edition should be of interest to graduate students thinking of a career in cardiovascular toxicology and to the many health professionals involved in the assessment of toxicity of drugs and chemicals to the heart and vascular system.

Daniel Acosta, Jr.
April 2001

# Part I

# INTRODUCTION

# 1

# CARDIOVASCULAR TOXICOLOGY

## Introductory notes

*Russell B. Melchert,\* Cai Yuan,† and Daniel Acosta, Jr.‡*

*\*Department of Pharmaceutical Sciences, University of Arkansas for Medical Sciences, Little Rock, AR, USA; †St. Elizabeth's Medical Center of Boston, Tufts University School of Medicine Teaching Affiliate, Department of Psychiatry, Boston, MA, USA; and ‡University of Cincinnati, College of Pharmacy, Cincinnati, OH, USA*

### Introductory remarks

The discipline of cardiovascular toxicology is concerned with the adverse effects of xenobiotics on the heart and circulatory system of living organisms. By its very nature and by being ubiquitous in the body, it is not surprising that the introduction of chemicals into the body may involve some interaction with the heart and vascular system. To understand better the potentially damaging effects of xenobiotics on the cardiovascular system, this volume focuses on four major areas: (1) methods to assess cardiovascular function and toxicity, (2) general principles of myocardial cell injury, (3) toxicity of chemical agents to the heart, and (4) vascular toxicity of chemical agents. The intent of this monograph is to provide a mechanistic understanding of the cell injury process induced in the heart and vascular system by chemical agents and other injurious stimuli such as ischemia and hypoxia. These introductory notes briefly summarize the interest of many investigators on the biologic roles of hypertrophy and apoptosis in the physiology and pathophysiology of cardiac function. Molecular and cellular mechanisms are stressed to stimulate future studies of cardiac myocyte hypertrophy and apoptosis and their relationship to toxic cardiovascular agents. The other chapters in this new edition provide additional insights into other biologic mechanisms involved in the cardiovascular toxicity of chemicals and other injurious stimuli.

# Cardiac myocyte growth and programmed death: emerging areas for research in cardiovascular toxicology

## *Overview*

Cardiac hypertrophy and programmed death (apoptosis) have been the focus of many investigations in recent years. Molecular and cellular mechanisms responsible for these physiologic and/or pathophysiologic processes are unfolding. The importance of understanding mechanisms responsible for growth and death of cardiac myocytes is best exemplified by the realization that cardiac injury induced by ischemia ensues via necrosis and apoptosis, and subsequent ventricular remodeling includes reactive hypertrophy of remaining myocytes. Furthermore, the acute inflammatory response is now known to contribute to injury and remodeling following myocardial infarction, and increasing evidence demonstrates that cytokines and growth factors elicit significant direct effects on cardiac myocytes. Several important reviews elegantly summarize the current understanding of stimuli, receptors, and signaling pathways responsible for cardiac myocyte hypertrophic growth (Morgan and Baker, 1991; Chien *et al.*, 1993; Komuro and Yazaki, 1993; MacLellan *et al.*, 1993; Hefti *et al.*, 1997; Schaub *et al.*, 1997) and cardiac myocyte apoptotic death (Davies, 1997; James, 1997; MacLellan and Schneider, 1997; Narula *et al.*, 1997; Pulkki, 1997). Therefore, the purpose of this chapter is not to provide an additional detailed review of apoptotic and hypertrophic stimuli, receptors, and signaling pathways. Rather, the introductory chapter is intended to (1) identify useful *in vitro* model systems for studies of cardiac myocyte hypertrophy and apoptosis and (2) incite thought and hypotheses by suggesting where future research could identify major cardiac myocyte hypertrophic and apoptotic stimuli and pathways vulnerable to disruption by xenobiotics.

Before proceeding with the discussion, however, one must immediately throw out any preconceived notion that all cardiac hypertrophic or apoptotic responses are inherently detrimental to cardiac function. Hypertrophic growth of the myocardium is a normal process throughout development and in response to increased workload (Chien *et al.*, 1993; Komuro and Yazaki, 1993). By the same token, apoptotic death in the myocardium is most likely a normal process during development of the heart when thinning of the right ventricular wall occurs (James, 1997). Of course, the largely unanswered questions are: when do these apparently normal physiologic responses become pathologic processes, and what stimuli and signaling pathways are responsible for converting a hypertrophied heart to a failing heart? An appropriate time is approaching for these questions to be considered within the context of cardiovascular toxicology.

## *In vitro* model systems for studying cardiac myocyte hypertrophic growth and apoptotic death

Neonatal and adult rat cardiac myocyte cultures have long been important models to study mechanisms of chemical- or drug-induced cardiotoxicity (Acosta and Ramos, 1984; Acosta *et al.*, 1985; Chacon and Acosta, 1991; Welder *et al.*, 1991; Melchert *et al.*, 1996; Yuan and Acosta, 1996). For nearly as long, neonatal rat cardiac myocyte cultures have been used for investigation of cellular and molecular mechanisms of cardiac hypertrophy (Simpson *et al.*, 1982; Simpson, 1983, 1985). The majority of research into signaling pathways of cardiac myocyte hypertrophic growth has utilized the neonatal model (Hefti *et al.*, 1997), and increasing studies are reporting use of this model for examining signaling pathways of cardiac myocyte apoptotic death. However, persistent concern regarding relevance of neonatal cardiac myocyte hypertrophic growth *in vitro* to adult cardiac hypertrophy *in vivo* has led to increasing interest in the adult model. Concerns exist regarding the adult model as well, but these two *in vitro* models are the best available systems for examining individual stimuli and cellular signaling pathways in controlled environments devoid of systemic intervention.

### Neonatal rat cardiac myocyte cultures

A brief overview of methodology used for isolation and culture of neonatal rat cardiac myocytes is provided here. Detailed methodology can be found in the review provided by Welder and Acosta (1993). Neonatal rat heart cells are isolated by trypsin or collagenase digest of tissue surgically dissected from post-natal rats aged 1–5 days. Worthy of note here is the fact that the majority of studies using this model for investigation of hypertrophic signaling pathways have limited the age of rats to less than 2 days. Differential plating separates the non-muscle cells (mostly fibroblasts) from myocytes, because the non-muscle cells attach earlier (< 3 h) to culture substrates than do the myocytes. Conveniently, neonatal cardiac myocytes easily attach to a variety of growth surfaces, and within 24–48 h a spontaneously contracting monolayer of relatively pure myocytes (usually > 95 percent) will have formed. Culture purity is maintained throughout the culture period by addition of DNA synthesis inhibitors such as bromodeoxyuridine. For toxicity studies, neonatal rat cardiac myocytes have routinely been grown in culture medium supplemented with newborn calf serum. In contrast, the strong growth-promoting properties of serum forced hypertrophy investigators to modify culture conditions in which myocytes are grown initially overnight in serum-containing medium, then the medium is replaced with serum-free medium supplemented with insulin, transferrin, and selenium (Simpson *et al.*, 1982; Simpson, 1983, 1985).

The neonatal rat cardiac myocyte culture model currently receives heavy use for research into signaling mechanisms of cardiac hypertrophy because neonatal cardiac myocytes are relatively easy to isolate, grow in culture, and transfect, thus providing elegant means to assess molecular mechanisms. Some disadvantages to using neonatal cardiac myocyte cultures for study of hypertrophic growth or apoptotic death deserve attention. For example, readily apparent in the wealth of data reported in hypertrophy-related papers (many referenced in this chapter) is the observation that cardiac myocytes undergo only modest increases in total cellular protein content normalized to DNA content upon exposure to hypertrophic stimuli. In addition, it is clear that with serum-free culture medium insulin, transferrin, and selenium supplementation provides growth stimulation for control cells, although less of a response is observed in these cells than in cells exposed to serum (Simpson et al., 1982; Simpson, 1983, 1985). Therefore, a true steady state in protein synthesis is difficult to reach as control cells continue to grow, and the alternative is unacceptable because cardiac myocytes deprived of serum and supplements will undergo apoptosis (Sheng et al., 1997). In summary, there are some problems with the neonatal rat cardiac myocyte culture model, but this model has contributed significantly to our understanding of signaling pathways responsible for cardiac hypertrophy, and continued research is beginning to identify signaling pathways responsible for cardiac apoptosis.

### Adult rat cardiac myocyte cultures

Detailed reviews of isolation and culture of adult rat cardiac myocytes can be found in the articles by Welder et al. (1991) and Mitcheson et al. (1998). In short, adult rat myocytes are isolated by initial perfusion of surgically removed hearts with collagenase in very low calcium buffer (Welder et al., 1991). Following perfusion periods of 10–20 min, ventricles are dissected and subsequently further digested mechanically and/or enzymatically in a shaking water bath. The goal of isolation is to obtain the greatest number of rod-shaped myocytes as possible because these cells are viable and will attach to a culture substrate (Mitcheson et al., 1998). Unlike neonatal myocytes, adult myocytes are more frequently plated on culture substrates that have been coated with attachment factors such as laminin. Much like the neonatal myocyte culture model, adult myocyte cultures used for toxicity studies are frequently grown in culture medium supplemented with fetal calf serum, and useful serum-free media are now frequently used. As such, there are two basic culturing methods for adult rat cardiac myocytes: (1) serum-supplemented "redifferentiating" cultures in which myocytes become rounded after isolation, have delayed attachment, and then the cells attach and spread on the culture substrate and may spontaneously contract and remain viable for extended periods (in excess of 2 weeks); and (2) serum-free "differentiated" cultures in which myocytes maintain rod-shaped morphology, rapidly attach, do not spontaneously contract, and remain viable for only short periods (Mitcheson et al., 1998).

Freshly isolated adult rat ventricular myocytes, obtained by the aforementioned techniques with some variations, have been used extensively for electrophysiologic studies (Liu et al., 1997; Mitcheson et al., 1998). Given the disadvantages of neonatal rat cardiac myocyte cultures for examination of hypertrophic signaling pathways, interest in the adult model has increased. However, some disadvantages of the adult model deserve attention. For example, adult cardiac myocytes are generally more difficult to isolate, grow in culture, and transfect than the neonatal cells, and difficulty is encountered when trying to determine which of the two culture methods for adult cells is most appropriate for the study of interest. Hypertrophy studies using serum-free (rapidly attaching) cultures are complicated by the limited period of viability (generally less than 1 week). Liu *et al.* (1998) used the serum-free, rapidly attaching adult rat cardiac myocyte cultures for examining angiotensin II hypertrophy. However, they found that the control myocytes (isolated from normal animals) were shrinking with time over the culture period, and angiotensin II merely prevented cell shrinkage (Liu *et al.*, 1998). Whether this response to angiotensin II represents hypertrophic growth is certainly questionable. Ironically, the rapidly attaching, serum-free adult cardiac myocyte cultures elicit a problematic response that is exactly opposite to that in the neonatal model, i.e. adult control myocytes shrink and neonatal control myocytes continue to grow larger. In summary, there are some problems with the adult rat cardiac myocyte culture model, and current use of this model for examining signaling pathways of cardiac hypertrophy is complicated. Indeed, it is extremely desirable to use adult cardiac myocytes for growth and death investigations because the human population most susceptible to alterations in cardiac myoycte growth and death includes primarily mature individuals. Further research is particularly needed that compares the response to known hypertrophic and apoptotic stimuli both in rapidly attaching, serum-free cultures and in redifferentiating cultures to determine the most appropriate adult myocyte culture methods for these types of investigations.

## Cardiac myocyte growth

Cardiac myocyte hypertrophy refers to an increase in cell size in the absence of an increase in cell number. Use of neonatal rat cardiac myocyte cultures for the study of hypertrophy began when Simpson *et al.* (1982) found that norepinephrine stimulated hypertrophic but not hyperplastic growth of cardiac myocytes, including increased protein synthesis in the absence of DNA replication. Since then, the model has been used extensively under the rationale that neonatal rat cardiac myocytes undergo a switch from an "adult" cardiac phenotype to a "fetal" cardiac phenotype similar to mature cardiac tissue during hypertrophy *in vivo* (Bishopric *et al.*, 1987; Paradis *et al.*, 1996; Vandenburgh *et al.*, 1996). The switch from "adult" to "fetal" phenotype (commonly referred to as reinduction of the fetal program) includes up-regulation of "fetal" skeletal $\alpha$-actin, $\beta$-myosin heavy chain, and atrial natriuretic factor with down-regulation of "adult" cardiac $\alpha$-actin (Bishopric *et al.*, 1987; Paradis *et al.*, 1996). Using the neonatal rat cardiac myocyte culture model, previous investigations have identified $\alpha_1$-adrenergic, angiotensin II, and other receptors as important mediators of cardiac hypertrophy.

### *Defining cardiac myocyte hypertrophy* in vitro

More recent findings suggest that the increase in protein synthesis accompanying hypertrophic growth is not necessarily coupled to reinduction of the fetal program (Sadoshima and Izumo, 1995; Boluyt *et al.*, 1997; Hefti *et al.*, 1997). For example, the macrolide immunosuppressant rapamycin inhibits p70 S6 kinase and protein synthesis in phenylephrine- and angiotensin II-induced hypertrophic growth of neonatal cardiac myocyte cultures but does not inhibit phenylephrine- or angiotensin II-induced up-regulation of the fetal program (Sadoshima and Izumo, 1995; Boluyt *et al.*, 1997). Similarly, interleukin-1β induces cardiac myocyte hypertrophic growth, as defined by increased protein content, but it does not up-regulate the fetal program and actually inhibits phenylephrine induction of the fetal program (Palmer *et al.*, 1995; Patten *et al.*, 1996). Coupled with the extensive research in hypertrophic signal transduction pathways, these findings have led to the conclusion that "there is no such thing as a general type of hypertrophic reaction" (Hefti *et al.*, 1997). Therefore, defining cardiac myocyte hypertrophy *in vitro* must include (1) increased total cellular protein content and/or protein synthesis, and might include (2) activation of one or more hypertrophic signal transduction pathways, and/or (3) increased transcription of one or more "immediate–early" genes and other late genes associated with the hypertrophic phenotype.

### *Hypertrophic stimuli*

Known hypertrophic stimuli (Table 1.1) identified in cardiac myocyte cultures and some limited *in vivo* studies include (1) $\alpha_1$-adrenergic agonists such as epinephrine, norepinephrine, and phenylephrine (Simpson *et al.*, 1982; Simpson, 1983, 1985; Fuller *et al.*, 1990); (2) mechanical load or stretch (Kent and McDermott, 1996; Komuro *et al.*, 1996; Miyata *et al.*, 1996; Slinker *et al.*, 1996); (3) contraction (McDermott and Morgan, 1989; McDermott *et al.*, 1989; Wada *et al.*, 1996); (4) growth factors such as angiotensin II (Miyata and Haneda, 1994; Susic *et al.*, 1996), endothelin-1 (Yamazaki *et al.*, 1996), transforming growth factor-β (MacLellan *et al.*, 1993), and insulin-like growth factor-I (Foncea *et al.*, 1997); (5) cytokines such as leukemia inhibitory factor (Kunisada *et al.*, 1996), interleukin-1β (Palmer *et al.*, 1995), cardiotrophin-1 (Wollert *et al.*, 1996), and tumor necrosis factor-α (Nakamura *et al.*, 1998); (6) hormones such as aldosterone in the presence of high glucose (Sato and Funder, 1996), testosterone (Marsh *et al.*, 1998), and thyroid hormone (Morgan and Baker, 1991; Gosteli-Peter *et al.*, 1996); and (7) other substances such as prostaglandin $F_{2\alpha}$ (Lai *et al.*, 1996). Importantly, considerable overlap in signal transduction mechanisms coupling these stimuli to the hypertrophic response exists, and overlap may begin at the level of stimulation. For example, mechanical load or stretch may stimulate the secretion of growth factors such as angiotensin II and transforming growth factor-β from cardiac myocyte cultures (Sadoshima and Izumo, 1993a; MacLellan *et al.*, 1994; Miyata *et al.*, 1996). Likewise, $\alpha_1$-adrenergic stimulation and angiotensin II may induce the myocardial production of transforming growth factor-β (Paradis *et al.*, 1996). Moreover, local cardiac angiotensin II production may stimulate

8

*Table 1.1* Stimuli of cardiac myocyte hypertrophic growth

α-Adrenergic agents
    Epinephrine
    Norepinephrine
    Phenylephrine

Cytokines
    Cardiotrophin-1
    Interleukin-1β
    Leukemia inhibitory factor
    Tumor necrosis factor-α

Growth factors
    Angiotensin II
    Endothelin-1
    Transforming growth factor-β

Hormones
    Aldosterone
    Testosterone
    Thyroid hormone

Other substances
    Prostaglandin $F_2$

Physical stimuli
    Contraction
    Mechanical load or stretch

norepinephrine release from sympathetic nerve terminals (Kent and McDermott, 1996). Therefore, a reasonable assumption is that at least part of the hypertrophic response involves myocardial secretion of growth factors which then act as hypertrophic stimuli in an autocrine or paracrine fashion (MacLellan *et al.*, 1993; Sadoshima and Izumo, 1993a). Overall, multiple stimuli for the hypertrophic response of cardiac myocytes exist, and it is highly likely that many other growth factors, hormones, or drugs may also serve as hypertrophic stimuli. So, the question now arises whether cardiotoxic agents may either serve as hypertrophic stimuli or alter levels of endogenous hypertrophic stimuli.

### *Hypertrophic signaling pathways*

Following interactions of hypertrophic stimuli with receptors, a multitude of enzyme systems and second messengers are activated (Figure 1.1): phospholipases $A_2$, C, and D (PLA$_2$, PLC, and PLD), protein kinase C (PKC), three subfamilies of mitogen-activated protein kinases (MAPKs) [extracellular signal-regulated kinases (ERK 1/2), c-*jun* NH$_2$-terminal kinase/stress-activated protein kinases (JNK/SAPKs), and p38 reactivating kinase (p38 RK)], receptor tyrosine kinases

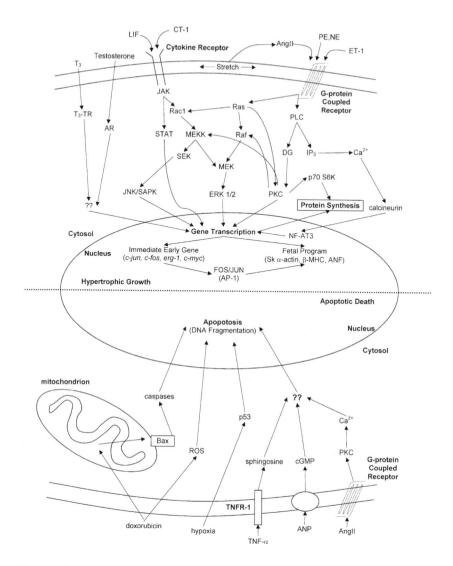

*Figure 1.1* Signaling pathways of cardiac myocyte hypertrophic growth and apoptotic death. The pathways presented here are from the literature referenced throughout the text, and only those pathways for which evidence has demonstrated their presence in cardiac myocytes or heart tissue are presented. Arrows represent activation or increases in second messengers, and opposing pathways are not shown. Question marks represent additional steps leading to responses that have not been identified. *Abbreviations for stimuli*: AngII, angiotensin II; ANP, atrial natriuretic peptide; CT-1, cardiotrophin 1; ET-1, endothelin-1; LIF, leukemia inhibitor factor; NE, norepinephrine; PE, phenylephrine; $T_3$, thyroid hormone; and TNF-α, tumor necrosis factor-α. *Abbreviations for hypertrophic growth pathways*: AR, androgen receptor; $Ca^{2+}$, intracellular free calcium; DG, diacylglycerol; ERK 1/2, extracellular signal-regulated kinases 1 and 2; $IP_3$, inositol-1,4,5-trisphosphate; JAK, janus kinase; JNK/SAPK, c-Jun N-terminal kinase/stress-activated protein kinase;

(RTKs), S6 kinases, increases in intracellular free calcium ($[Ca^{2+}]_i$), and calcineurin (Sadoshima and Izumo, 1993a; Komuro *et al.*, 1996; Rabkin, 1996; Touyz *et al.*, 1996; Hefti *et al.*, 1997; Molkentin *et al.*, 1998). Importantly, considerable "cross-talk" between these general pathways exists (Hefti *et al.*, 1997). For example, increases in PLC and PLD activity stimulate increases in PKC activity and $[Ca^{2+}]_i$ through increased formation of diacylglycerol (DG) and inositol triphosphate ($IP_3$) (Sadoshima and Izumo, 1993a; Sprenkle *et al.*, 1995; Touyz *et al.*, 1996). Receptor tyrosine kinases may activate PLC, PKC, and MAPKs (Sadoshima and Izumo, 1993a). In addition, PKC activates MAPKs and may activate JNK/SAPKs in cardiac myocyte cultures exposed to mechanical stretch (Komuro *et al.*, 1996). The common downstream effectors in these "cross-talk" schemes seem to be PKC, ERK 1/2, and JNK/SAPKs, and in cardiac myocyte cultures various hypertrophic stimuli are coupled to these enzyme systems.

## *PKC pathway (PLC/PLD→DG→PKC)*

Agonists of the $\alpha_1$-adrenergic receptor (Henrich and Simpson, 1988), angiotensin II (Sadoshima and Izumo, 1993b; Miyata and Haneda, 1994), and mechanical stretch (Sadoshima and Izumo, 1993a) have been shown to activate PKC in cardiac myocytes, suggesting that PKC plays a critical role in hypertrophic growth for a number of stimuli. In addition, elevated PKC activity was required for glucose-dependent, aldosterone-induced cardiac myocyte hypertrophic growth mediated by mineralocorticoid receptors, and PKC is known to be involved in the regulation of steroid receptor-mediated actions (Sato and Funder, 1996). Although under developmental regulation, neonatal rat cardiac myocytes grown in culture express at least four of the known isoforms of PKC ($\alpha$, $\delta$, $\epsilon$, $\zeta$) (Puceat *et al.*, 1994; Rybin and Steinberg, 1994). The calcium-dependent isoform (PKC-$\alpha$) does not appear to be activated by $\alpha_1$-adrenergic agonists or endothelin, but phenylephrine (PE) did activate calcium-independent PKC-$\delta$ and PKC-$\epsilon$ in neonatal cardiac myocytes (Puceat *et al.*, 1994), suggesting a role for these isoforms in PE-induced hypertrophy. The role of PKC-$\zeta$ (calcium and phorbol ester independent) in cardiac myocyte growth is largely unknown (Puceat *et al.*, 1994; Rybin and Steinberg, 1994).

MEK, mitogen-activated protein kinase effector kinase; MEKK, MEK kinase; p70 S6K, ribosomal S6 kinase; PKC, protein kinase C; PLC, phospholipase C; Rac, a member of the Ras superfamily; Raf, a mitogen-activated protein kinase kinase kinase; Ras, a GTPase; SEK, SAPK effector kinase; STAT, signal transducer and activator of transcription; TR, thyroid hormone receptor. *Abbreviations for nuclear components*: ANF, atrial natriuretic factor; AP-1, heterodimeric transcription factor consisting of FOS and JUN; $\beta$-MHC, $\beta$-myosin heavy chain; JUN, protein product of c-*jun*; FOS, protein product of c-*fos*; NF-AT3, nuclear factor and activator of T cells 3; Sk $\alpha$-actin, skeletal $\alpha$-actin. *Abbreviations for apoptotic death pathways*: Bax, homolog of Bcl-2, a protein originally identified in B-cell lymphoma; $Ca^{2+}$, intracellular free calcium; cGMP, cyclic guanosine monophosphate; p53, 53-kDa tumor-suppressor protein; PKC, protein kinase C; ROS, reactive oxygen species; TNFR-1, tumor necrosis factor receptor-type 1.

## MAPK pathways

Mechanical stretch (Sadoshima and Izumo, 1993a; Komuro *et al.*, 1996), angiotensin II (Yamazaki *et al.*, 1996), endothelin-1 (Yamazaki *et al.*, 1996), leukemia inhibitory factor (Kunisada *et al.*, 1996), and phenylephrine (Post *et al.*, 1996) activate the Ras→Raf→MEK (MAPK/ERK kinase)→ERK 1/2 pathway in neonatal cardiac myocyte cultures. In addition, mechanical stretch (Komuro *et al.*, 1996) and angiotensin II (Kudoh *et al.*, 1997) activate the Ras/Rac-1→MEKK (MEK kinase)→SEK (SAPK kinase)→JNK/SAPK pathway in cardiac myocyte cultures. It is interesting to note that although the ERK and JNK/SAPK pathways may have opposing effects in other cell types, inducing proliferation or growth arrest respectively (Coroneos *et al.*, 1996), cardiac myocytes may utilize both of these pathways during the hypertrophic response. In addition, "cross-talk" between pathways may result in simultaneous activation of ERKs and JNK/SAPK through, for example, Ras activating Rac-1, Raf, or MEKK (Hefti *et al.*, 1997). Finally, a suggestion for a role of the Ras/Rac-1→?→RKK (RK kinase)→p38 RK (a MAPK) pathway in cardiac myocyte hypertrophy has been made; however, stimuli and pathways leading to its activation are, as yet, poorly defined (Heft *et al.*, 1997). Interestingly, activation of different isoforms of p38 RK may result in either hypertrophic growth (p38$\beta$) or apoptotic death (p38$\alpha$) of cardiac myocytes (Wang, Y. *et al.*, 1998).

## PLC/PLD→IP$_3$→Ca$^{2+}$

Intracellular free calcium ([Ca$^{2+}$]$_i$) homeostasis may be an important component in hypertrophic growth of cardiac myocytes (Touyz *et al.*, 1996). For example, in neonatal rat cardiac myocyte cultures, angiotensin II increased [Ca$^{2+}$]$_i$ and the amplitude and frequency of calcium transients (Touyz *et al.*, 1996). However, others have shown that calcium may play a permissive role in the mechanisms of cardiac hypertrophy and may not be a causative factor (Sadoshima and Izumo, 1993a; Miyata and Haneda, 1994). Overall, elevated [Ca$^{2+}$]$_i$ is a frequent finding during the hypertrophic response observed in cardiac myocyte cultures, but the significance of this effect was not clear until recently. Elevations in [Ca$^{2+}$]$_i$ may lead to activation of calcineurin and subsequent hypertrophic growth (Molkentin *et al.*, 1998), as discussed in the section on other signaling pathways.

## Other pathways

Other signal transduction pathways related to cardiac myocyte hypertrophic growth have been described, and the possibility that these pathways play major roles in the hypertrophic response certainly exists. For example, cytokines [leukemia inhibitory factor (LIF), cardiotrophin-1 (CT-1), and IL-1$\beta$] are known to activate the janus kinase (JAK)→stress-activated protein kinase (STAT) pathways (Hefti *et al.*, 1997), and in cardiac myocytes LIF activates JAK1, STAT3, and ERKs

(Kunisada *et al.*, 1996; Kodama *et al.*, 1997). Thus, "cross-talk" of the JAK→STAT pathway with the ERK pathway suggests that the MAPK (ERK and JNK) pathways are critical pathways leading to cardiac myocyte hypertrophy. Thyroid hormone induces cardiac hypertrophy; however, the signal transduction pathways involved are, as yet, not well defined (Hefti *et al.*, 1997). Also in the steroid superfamily, testosterone and dihydrotestosterone were recently shown to stimulate hypertrophic growth of neonatal rat cardiac myocyte cultures, a response that was blocked by androgen receptor antagonist (Marsh *et al.*, 1998). But again, the exact signaling pathways responsible for dihydrotestosterone- or testosterone-induced hypertrophic growth are not clear. Discussion on androgen-mediated cardiac hypertrophy is continued in Chapter 14, to which the reader is referred for further details. Most recently, an angiotensin II- and phenylephrine-activated calcineurin pathway leading to cardiac hypertrophy was identified in neonatal rat cardiac myocytes, and cyclosporine blocked and reduced angiotensin II- and phenylephrine-induced hypertrophic growth respectively (Molkentin *et al.*, 1998). The calcineurin pathway involved dephosphorylation and activation of the transcription factor, nuclear factor of activated T cells (NF-AT3), and its importance was verified in transgenic mice overexpressing active forms of calcineurin or NT-AT3 that developed cardiac hypertrophy (Molkentin *et al.*, 1998; Sussman *et al.*, 1998).

### *Gene expression during cardiac myocyte hypertrophy*

#### *Immediate–early gene expression*

Expression of immediate–early genes (c-*fos*, c-*jun*, *erg-1*, and c-*myc*) is increased during cardiac myocyte hypertrophy. Although the mediators of immediate–early gene expression are not entirely known, increased PKC activity from hypertrophic stimuli does stimulate c-*fos* expression in adult feline (Kent and McDermott, 1996) and neonatal rat cardiac myocyte cultures (Sadoshima and Izumo, 1993b). The induction of c-*fos* by hypertrophic stimuli is followed by increases in Fos protein, which, when coupled to Jun protein, forms the AP-1 transcription activator complex (Kent and McDermott, 1996). In contrast, the induction of c-*jun* expression following hypertrophic stimuli may occur through activation of SAPK, but c-*jun* is also expressed in unstimulated cardiac myocyte cultures (Komuro *et al.*, 1996), which suggests that c-*fos* expression may be the limiting factor in the formation of AP-1. Therefore, c-*fos* likely plays a pivotal role in the production of the hypertrophic response, and expression of Fos protein may represent the rate-limiting step in AP-1 formation during hypertrophy. Finally, the induction of c-*myc* expression during the hypertrophic response provides another point of overlap of signaling pathways leading to hypertrophic growth and apoptotic death.

*Late gene expression*

Increased expression of immediate–early genes may result in the production of transcription factors that directly enhance expression of late genes such as skeletal α-actin (Sk-αA), β-myosin heavy chain (β-MHC), and atrial natriuretic factor (i.e. the fetal program). For example, the AP-1 transcription activator complex has been shown to bind to the promoter region of the Sk-αA gene in cardiac myocytes, and it was suggested that the binding was directly related to the increase in Sk-αA in response to adrenergic stimuli (Bishopric *et al.*, 1992). Other accessory factors may also be involved (e.g. transcription-enhancing factor-1; TEF-1), which may be required for AP-1 interactions with the serum response element of the promoter (MacLellan *et al.*, 1994; Karns *et al.*, 1995). Noteworthy also is the possibility that PKC may directly interact with TEF-1 to increase expression of both Sk-αA and β-MHC (Karns *et al.*, 1995). Although the exact mechanisms involved may be debatable, it is clear that many hypertrophic stimuli reinduce expression of Sk-αA and β-MHC.

# Hypertrophic growth

In addition to changes in gene expression, a logical end-point for many investigations into mechanisms of cardiac hypertrophy has been total cellular protein content (Simpson *et al.*, 1982; Simpson, 1983, 1985; Miyata and Haneda, 1994; Miyata *et al.*, 1996). How the increase in protein synthesis actually occurs is not entirely clear, although decreased protein degradation is likely not involved (Meidell *et al.*, 1986). One explanation is that hypertrophic stimuli increase the rate of ribosomal RNA synthesis (McDermott *et al.*, 1989), thereby increasing the cellular capacity for protein synthesis (McDermott and Morgan, 1989). This could occur through an increase in ribosomal DNA transcription factor (UBF-1) content, as observed with $\alpha_1$-adrenergic stimulation or contraction (Hannan *et al.*, 1995, 1996a), or activity, as observed with endothelin-1 stimulation (Hannan *et al.*, 1996b).

As mentioned previously, evidence suggests that distinct signaling pathways exist for increased protein synthesis and expression of the fetal program genes. For example, angiotensin II increases protein synthesis by activating p70 S6 kinase, which phosphorylates the S6 protein of the 40S ribosomal subunit to increase specific mRNA translation (Sadoshima and Izumo, 1995; Paradis *et al.*, 1996). Rapamycin, an inhibitor of p70 S6 kinase, inhibits phenylephrine- and angiotensin II-induced protein synthesis of neonatal cardiac myocyte cultures, but does not inhibit phenylephrine-induced up-regulation of the fetal program or angiotensin II-induced activation of PKC, MAPK, and up-regulation of the immediate–early and fetal program genes (Sadoshima and Izumo, 1995; Boluyt *et al.*, 1997). Overall, these studies demonstrate that measuring hypertrophic growth *in vitro* must include multiple end-points rather than just one particular marker. Ideally, these experiments should include at least one more "functional" end-point, such as total protein content or rates of protein synthesis, and at least one marker of expression of fetal program genes, such as atrial natriuretic factor.

## *Possibilities for cardiac myocyte growth in response to toxicants or toxicant-induced injury*

Little is known regarding cardiac myocyte hypertrophic growth following exposure of the heart to exogenous substances, including xenobiotics. Indeed, nearly all of the hypertrophic stimuli identified to date are endogenous substances, including catecholamines, growth factors, cytokines, and hormones. The exception, of course, is phenylephrine, which has been demonstrated to induce hypertrophic growth of cardiac myocytes through $\alpha_1$-adrenergic receptor stimulation. A very interesting toxicologic consideration of the phenylephrine findings may apply to a similar compound, ephedrine. Largely unregulated nutritional supplements containing *Ephedra sinica* (ma huang) have been associated with numerous cardiovascular deaths, and "nutraceutical" products from health food stores were found to contain significant amounts of ephedrine (Gurley *et al.*, 1998). Furthermore, these same "nutraceutical" products were found to elicit significant cardiovascular responses in humans, including elevated heart rate (White *et al.*, 1997). Thus, an obvious question would be "does ephedrine induce hypertrophic growth of cardiac myocytes and/or cardiac hypertrophy in animals and humans?". Finally, other exogenous substances that are found to modulate similar signaling pathways in other cell types (e.g. PKC pathways) should be considered as potentially altering hypertrophic signaling pathways in cardiac myocytes. Research into these areas remains largely ignored.

As mentioned at the beginning of the chapter, myocardial injury is associated with subsequent ventricular remodeling, which includes reactive hypertrophy of remaining myocytes. Therefore, significant unanswered toxicologically oriented questions are not just "how does a toxicant induce injury?" (e.g. mechanism of toxicity), but "what happens to the remaining viable myocytes following toxic insult?". There is currently a significant amount of important work regarding repair mechanisms in renal proximal tubular cell cultures following toxic insult (Counts *et al.*, 1995; Kays and Schnellmann, 1995) and similar studies are being conducted in other cell types; however, little is known regarding "repair" mechanisms in non-proliferating cardiac myocyte cultures following toxic insult. At this point, it is tempting to speculate that classic cardiotoxicants such as doxorubicin or tricyclic antidepressants may kill a significant number of cardiac myocytes, leading to reactive hypertrophy of remaining myocytes, but few, if any, data exist to corroborate this supposition. If support were found for this hypothesis, classic cardiotoxicants would have to be considered as potentially altering hypertrophic signaling pathways indirectly. In addition, given the large number of cytokines implicated in hypertrophic growth of cardiac myocytes, toxicants that alter cytokine synthesis or release should be considered as potentially altering hypertrophic signaling pathways in an indirect fashion.

## *Summary*

All of the information regarding stimuli and signal transduction pathways of cardiac myocyte hypertrophy presented here should highlight that these signaling pathways are important for maintenance of appropriate cardiac myocyte growth. Thus, exogenous compounds that may alter any of these pathways should be questioned in terms of ability to alter the growth response. Many of these stimuli and signaling pathways have been identified in cultured cardiac myocytes and found to be important in cardiac hypertrophy *in vivo*. However, whether these stimuli and pathways are directly involved in the transition of hypertrophy to cardiac dysfunction and failure is still largely unknown. So, designing and implementing toxicology studies regarding hypertrophy is important, but these studies will likely be hampered by the same question posed before: if toxicant-induced changes in hypertrophic signaling pathways are found, do these alterations cause cardiac dysfunction?

# Cardiac myocyte apoptosis

Apoptosis, or programmed cell death, is a form of cell death by which animals eliminate extraneous or dangerous cells. Both proliferating and quiescent cells are capable of undergoing apoptosis in response to noxious or sublethal events (Wu *et al.*, 1997). During apoptosis, a number of consistent observations are reported: cells shrink and dissociate from surrounding cells; the organelles retain definition; and the nuclei display a distinctive pattern of heterochomatization and eventually become fragmented (Thompson, 1998a,b). As mentioned previously, several important reviews considering the topic of apoptosis in the heart have been published (Davies, 1997; James, 1997; MacLellan and Schneider, 1997; Narula *et al.*, 1997; Pulkki, 1997). Many of these reviews include excellent summaries of the plethora of investigations that have been published in recent years regarding apoptotic stimuli, receptors, and signaling pathways in cell types other than cardiac myocytes, and these reviews attempt to correlate those findings to emerging evidence in the heart. Indeed, it is highly likely that many of the receptors and signaling pathways for apoptosis identified in other tissues are also expressed in the heart, but clear identification of most of these receptors and pathways in cardiac myocytes is only beginning to surface. This section of the chapter will include some of those receptors and signaling pathways, but, in the interest of brevity, only a cursory review will be provided and focus will be on known stimuli of cardiac myocyte apoptosis.

For examining cellular and molecular mechanisms of apoptosis in the heart, *in vitro* models provide a well-controlled environment. To this end, many of the published data derive from either neonatal rat or adult rat cardiac myocyte cultures. Of interest is the fact that these models also provide controlled environments for the study of cellular and molecular mechanisms responsible for cardiac hypertrophy, as discussed previously. Numerous pathophysiologic conditions in the heart initiate apoptosis of cardiac cells with subsequent reactive hypertrophy of remaining myocytes. Therefore, the *in vitro* cardiac myocyte culture models offer the advantage of multiple studies in the same model system, perhaps simultaneously attempting to clarify the molecular mechanisms responsible for the dual events following cardiac injury. From such investigations, increasing evidence suggests that hypertrophic stimuli serve as antiapoptotic stimuli and *vice versa*. Furthermore, several investigations have identified either overlapping signaling pathways for cardiac myocyte hypertrophic growth and apoptotic death (Adams *et al.*, 1998) or divergent functions for different members of a family of closely related signaling kinases resulting in either hypertrophy or apoptosis (Wang, Y. *et al.*, 1998). Overall, these *in vitro* models are well suited for identifying toxicologic intervention in terms of stimuli, receptor function, signaling pathways, and the end-points of hypertrophic growth or apoptotic death in cardiac myocytes.

### *Cardiac myocyte apoptotic stimuli*

Apoptosis of mammalian cells can be initiated by intrinsic or extrinsic agents. The agents include cytokines (Barinaga, 1996), cytotoxic drugs (Fisher, 1994), radiation (Meyn *et al.*, 1996), glucocorticoids (Wyllie, 1980), bacterial toxins and oxidants (Susin *et al.*, 1998). However, when considering cardiac myocytes specifically, fewer apoptotic stimuli have been identified (Table 1.2). Given the extremely high interest concerning apoptosis in the heart, ongoing research will most definitely add a significant number of substances to the list of known apoptotic stimuli in cardiac myocytes.

Currently available data indicate that several peptides and cytokines directly activate programmed cell death of cardiac myocytes. For example, atrial natriuretic peptide (ANP) was shown to induce apoptosis of neonatal rat cardiac myocytes (Wu *et al.*, 1997), which is very interesting because myocytes undergoing hypertrophic growth synthesize and secrete ANP as discussed previously. Angiotensin II, although demonstrated by many laboratories to be a hypertrophic stimulus, has been shown, at least in two studies, to induce apoptosis of adult rat ventricular myocytes (Kajstura *et al.*, 1997) and neonatal rat cardiac myocytes (Cigola *et al.*, 1997). Other factors, perhaps developmental or environmental, most likely determine exactly how a myocyte will respond to angiotensin II. Also in the category of protein stimuli of cardiac myocyte apoptosis is tumor necrosis factor-$\alpha$ (TNF-$\alpha$). Although TNF-$\alpha$ is known to induce apoptosis in a variety of cell types, and the signaling pathways for TNF-$\alpha$-induced apoptosis are fairly well understood, similar knowledge regarding effects in cardiac myocytes is only beginning to unfold. In adult rat ventricular myocytes, for example, TNF-$\alpha$ was shown to induce apoptosis (Krown *et al.*, 1996), but similar effects were not observed in neonatal cardiac myocytes (Krown *et al.*, 1996). Furthermore, one investigation demonstrated that TNF-$\alpha$ stimulated hypertrophic growth of the neonatal cells (Nakamura *et al.*, 1998). Possible explanations for these disparate findings include different developmental stages and, as suggested, a potential for

*Table 1.2* Stimuli of cardiac myocyte apoptotic death

---

Drugs
    *cis*-Platinum
    Daunorubicin
    Doxorubicin
    Isoproterenol

Other chemical compounds
    Ceramide
    Saturated fatty acids
    Staurosporine

Peptides and cytokines
    Angiotensin II
    Atrial natriuretic peptide
    Tumor necrosis factor-$\alpha$

Properties of the culture medium
    Prolonged hypoxia (> 48 h)
    Serum deprivation

---

deficient expression of TNF-$\alpha$ receptors in neonatal cells (Krown *et al.*, 1996). Other peptides and cytokines will likely be identified in the near future, and many other substances in this peptide/cytokine class exert antiapoptotic effects in cardiac myocytes such as cardiotrophin-1 (Sheng *et al.*, 1997).

Other chemicals and endogenous compounds have been shown to induce apoptosis of cardiac myocytes. In neonatal rat cardiac myocytes, staurosporine, ceramide, and saturated fatty acids have been demonstrated to induce apoptosis (Umansky *et al.*, 1997; de Vries *et al.*, 1997). Also of major toxicologic interest is the fact that numerous drugs serve as cardiac apoptotic stimuli. These include the anthracyclines daunorubicin (Sawyer *et al.*, 1999) and doxorubicin (Umansky *et al.*, 1997), which induce neonatal cardiac myocyte apoptosis. Furthermore, administration of isoproterenol to rats resulted in significant cardiac myocyte apoptosis (Shizukuda *et al.*, 1998). The possibility seems likely that numerous other xenobiotics serve as apoptotic stimuli.

Alterations in culture medium content complete the list of currently known apoptotic stimuli of cardiac myocytes. For example, short periods (24 h) of serum and supplement deprivation induced neonatal rat cardiac myocyte apoptosis (Sheng *et al.*, 1997; Umansky *et al.*, 1997). In addition, prolonged periods (48 h) of hypoxia resulted in apoptosis of neonatal myocytes (Long *et al.*, 1997), demonstrating an *in vitro* model for examination of molecular mechanisms responsible for apoptosis during pathophysiologic events such as ischemia and myocardial infarction. Lastly, it is worth revisiting the investigation demonstrating that saturated fatty acids induce apoptosis of cardiac myocytes (de Vries *et al.*, 1997). An importance of this finding is that close attention must be given to the exact contents of the culture medium, particularly in the case of supplementation of media or isolation buffers with bovine serum albumin as it serves as a carrier protein for a variety of fatty acids.

In summary, identification of cardiac apoptotic stimuli is increasing rapidly. Cultures of rat cardiac myocytes have facilitated this research and provided model systems for cellular and molecular studies of pathophysiologic events that occur *in vivo* and result in apoptosis and reactive hypertrophy. However, caution regarding culture conditions is in order as components found in culture media or supplements may interfere with apoptotic or hypertrophic responses. Given the increasing identification of drugs and chemicals which may induce apoptosis in the heart, future research should consider re-evaluation of the mechanisms of toxicity of some compounds previously evaluated in these culture models, such as cocaine and tricyclic antidepressants, because these substances may also induce cardiac myocyte apoptosis.

### *Targets for apoptosis*

The aforementioned stimuli may act on various targets in the heart to initiate apoptosis. However, the vast majority of information identifying specific targets stems from investigations in other tissues. As such, the assumption is that many of these targets are similar in cardiac myocytes. Targets for apoptosis are frequently found on the cell surface and are often called "death receptors." The death receptors have been recently identified as subgroups of the tumor necrosis factor (TNF) receptor superfamily, including TNF receptor-1, CD95 (Fas/APO-1), TNF-receptor-related apoptosis-mediated protein (TRAMP) and TNF-related apoptosis-inducing ligand (TRAIL) receptor-1 and -2. Several receptors are able to transmit cytotoxic signals into the cytoplasm. In addition to a role in apoptosis, these receptors also have other functions, such as cell differentiation and proliferation (Schulze-Osthoff *et al.*, 1998). As mentioned previously, Krown *et al.* (1996) found that TNF-$\alpha$ induced apoptosis of adult rat cardiac myocytes. They further demonstrated that the effect was dependent upon TNF receptors, and that receptor stimulation resulted in increases in sphingosine (Krown *et al.*, 1996). Therefore, evidence for functional death receptors on the surface of cardiac myocytes already exists, and future studies should clarify signaling pathways of TNF receptors as well as attempt to locate other death receptors on these cells.

Cell-surface apoptotic targets are known to exist in cardiac myocytes, and these targets are coupled to a variety of intracellular second messenger systems such as cyclic nucleotides and intracellular calcium homeostasis. For example, when atrial natriuretic peptide was found to induce apoptosis of neonatal rat cardiac myocyte cultures, an associated and likely causative increase in cyclic guanosine monophosphate (GMP) was found (Wu *et al.*, 1997). Furthermore, angiotensin II-induced apoptosis of neonatal and adult rat cardiac myocytes was associated with increases in intracellular calcium (Cigola *et al.*, 1997; Kajstura *et al.*, 1997), and in the neonatal myocytes the increased calcium was presumably a secondary effect of activation of protein kinase C (Kajstura *et al.*, 1997).

Targets for apoptosis are also frequently found in the cytoplasm of a variety of cell types. Recently, a key role for mitochondria in apoptosis has become clear. At least two mitochondrial proteins, cytochrome $c$ and apoptosis-inducing factor, have been identified as key signaling molecules of apoptosis (Cai *et al.*, 1998). Importantly, cytochrome $c$ is essential to activate the protease caspase-3 (Liu *et al.*, 1996). Numerous studies have demonstrated that a variety of apoptotic stimuli, including ionizing irradiation, peroxides, and etoposide, all promote release of cytochrome $c$ which further activates caspase-3 and leads to apoptosis (Cai *et al.*, 1998). Furthermore, mitochondrial disruption is a frequently found event accompanying a variety of cardiotoxic agents such as doxorubicin (Chacon and Acosta, 1991). These previous findings may very well have been serendipitously at the forefront of identifying initial signs of imminent cardiac myocyte apoptosis.

The nucleus is the other target of apoptotic stimuli. It has been well established that most cytotoxic chemotherapeutic agents induce killing of tumor cells through apoptotic mechanisms (Hannun, 1997), and apoptosis is becoming a widely accepted mechanism of cytotoxic agents. Drug-induced DNA lesions are believed to be the initiating event and apoptosis ensues via the p53 pathway (Zunino *et al.*, 1997). Therefore, chemicals that damage DNA may trigger apoptosis, and special consideration should be given to agents such as anthracyclines for which generation of reactive oxygen species and possibly DNA damage may initiate apoptosis in cardiac myocytes (Sawyer *et al.*, 1999).

### *Apoptotic signaling pathways*

Cellular response to apoptotic stimuli varies with cell type, differentiation state, characteristic gene expression, phase of the cell cycle, and severity of the insult (Wertz and Hanley, 1996). Apoptosis is controlled and modulated by a large number of oncogene and suppressor gene products. The most important proapoptotic modulators include the Bcl-2 family (Bcl-xs, Bax, Bak, and Bad), p53 and c-Myc. The other Bcl-2 family members, such as Bcl-2, Bcl-xl, A1, and Mcl-1, along with Bag1 and Abl are antiapoptotic modulators (Zunino *et al.*, 1997). Currently, very little is known about the signaling pathways for cardiac myocyte apoptosis, and, again, the assumption is that these pathways will be relatively conserved among the various mammalian cells. Figure 1.1 provides a summary of known apoptotic signaling pathways in cardiac myocytes.

### *Bcl-2 family*

Bcl-2 is considered to be a downstream regulator of apoptosis. It is largely localized on the outer membrane of mitochondria (Hockenbery *et al.*, 1993; Jong *et al.*, 1994; Lithgow *et al.*, 1994). The observation that overexpression of Bcl-2 and Bcl-xl prevent the release of cytochrome $c$ into the cytosol provides an important insight into a gatekeeping mechanism (Kluck *et al.*, 1997). In addition, a further downstream antiapoptotic effect of Bcl-2 has also been shown after cytochrome $c$

is released or when cytochrome *c* is microinjected into cells (Li *et al.*, 1997). Bcl-2 homologs interact closely in the regulation of apoptosis. The Bcl-2/Bax ratio is the critical determinant for the induction or inhibition of apoptosis. When Bcl-2 is present in excess, apoptosis is inhibited; when Bax is overexpressed, apoptosis is stimulated (Staunton and Gaffney, 1998).

## *p53*

It has become increasingly clear that the tumor-suppressor protein p53 can induce apoptosis. p53-dependent apoptosis can be triggered by a variety of signals, including DNA damage and hypoxia (Clarke *et al.*, 1993). In cells lacking functional p53, there is reduced susceptibility to apoptosis induced by radiation and cytotoxic drugs (Lowe *et al.*, 1993). Transcription-dependent mechanisms of p53 have been implicated. Furthermore, Bax has been shown to play a role in p53-mediated apoptosis (McCurrach *et al.*, 1997). Induction of Bax depends on functional p53, and Bax has been suggested to be a p53 target gene (Selvakumaran *et al.*, 1994). There is a line of evidence showing that p53 highly induces some genes, including *p21* and *PIG1-13*, many of which encode proteins involved in the response to oxidative stress. This fact leads to a speculation that p53 may induce apoptosis by stimulating the production of reactive oxygen species that in turn damage mitochondria and cause mitochondrial permeability transition (Polyak *et al.*, 1997). This possible mechanism is supported by the finding that inhibition of reactive oxygen species generation and the mitochondrial permeability transition blocks p53-induced apoptosis (Polyak *et al.*, 1997). Moreover, p53-mediated apoptosis also leads to activation of caspase-3, although the precise pathway is not clear (Fuchs *et al.*, 1997). Finally, p53 has been shown to be involved in cardiac apoptosis. For example, in neonatal rat cardiac myocytes, prolonged hypoxia (48 h) resulted in elevated p53 and apoptosis (Long *et al.*, 1997).

## *c-Myc*

c-Myc is the protein encoded by the c-*myc* oncogene. Interestingly, c-Myc is involved in apoptosis in at least two ways – preventing or inducing apoptosis (Thompson, 1998b). Both glucocorticoids (Wood *et al.*, 1994) and TGF-β (Fischer *et al.*, 1994) cause a decrease in c-*myc* expression, leading to apoptosis. A fall in c-Myc precedes cell death by several hours, suggesting that c-Myc involvement is early in the pathways leading to programmed cell death (Wood *et al.*, 1994). In contrast, elevated c-*myc* expression may also lead to apoptosis (Packham and Cleveland, 1995). Cells with transgenic expression of c-*myc* showed signs of increased apoptosis (Scott *et al.*, 1996). Furthermore, it has been suggested that p53 is associated with c-Myc-evoked apoptosis (Hermeking and Eick, 1994). Max also appears to be necessary for apoptosis following inappropriate c-Myc expression (Amati *et al.*, 1993). Two hypotheses have been advanced to explain the dual functions of c-Myc in apoptosis. One hypothesis proposes that cells respond via apoptosis to the multiple signals stemming from increased c-*myc* expression. The other suggests that a natural consequence of increased c-*myc* expression is generation of dual signals leading to cell growth and death (Thompson, 1998b).

### *Effectors of apoptosis*

Apoptosis is an event that requires disassembly of the cellular scaffolding, and proteolysis is necessary for this to occur (Kinloch *et al.*, 1999). It has become clear that the final stage of apoptosis occurs through the activation of caspases, aspartic acid-specific cysteine proteases (Green, 1998). These caspases reside in the cytosol (Green, 1998), but a sizeable fraction of caspase-3 is also localized in the mitochondria (Samali *et al.*, 1998). It is thought that caspases are capable of producing some of the biochemical markers of apoptosis such as DNA fragmentation, chromatin condensation, membrane blebbing, cell shrinkage and formation of apoptotic bodies (Thornberry and Lazebnik, 1998). However, the overall picture of caspase contribution to apoptosis is not fully understood. A number of proteins, including poly-(ADP ribose) polymerase, lamin B1, spectrin and β-actin, have been reported to be proteolysed at the beginning of apoptosis (Kinloch *et al.*, 1999). The activation of the caspases has been linked to signal transduction via cell-surface death receptors related to the TNF family (Hsu *et al.*, 1996). In addition, p53-mediated apoptosis leads to activation of caspases (Chandler *et al.*, 1997). Overall, caspases serve as one of the major effectors of apoptosis, but little is known about the involvement of caspases in cardiac apoptosis.

### *Toxicant-induced cardiac myocyte apoptosis*

Apoptosis in cardiac muscle has been recently recognized as a consequence of toxic insult by xenobiotics. Doxorubicin, a well-known cardiotoxic agent, causes DNA fragmentation in cardiac myocytes, and it appears that doxorubicin-induced apoptosis is associated with an increased levels of Bax and activation of caspase-3 (Wang, L. *et al.*, 1998). Interestingly, cocaine has recently been reported to induce apoptosis in cardiac tissues *in vivo* (Devi and Chan, 1999). Although the precise mechanism is not known, cocaine-induced oxidative stress may play a critical role in apoptosis (Devi and Chan, 1999). Other classic cardiotoxic agents (e.g. tricyclic antidepressants) should be evaluated for ability to induce apoptosis of cardiac myocytes.

## Conclusions

Study of the stimuli, receptors, and signaling pathways responsible for cardiac hypertrophy and apoptosis is an extremely important and challenging field. Physiologic and pathophysiologic importance of growth and death in the myocardium is well established. Stimuli and pathways for hypertrophic growth in the myocardium are becoming fairly well understood, and, although less is known about apoptotic death in the myocardium, newer information suggests a considerable overlap in stimuli and pathways leading to either growth or death. As increasing evidence demonstrates that toxicants may interfere with the complex regulatory mechanisms controlling cardiac myocyte growth and death, future research into xenobiotic-induced alterations in these two diverse cardiac responses is of the utmost importance.

## Acknowledgment

The authors would like to thank Dr. Mark S. Luer for his help with the artwork presented in this chapter.

## References

Acosta, D. and Ramos, K. 1984. Cardiotoxicity of tricyclic antidepressants in primary cultures of rat myocardial cells. *Journal of Toxicology and Environmental Health* 14: 137–143.

Acosta, D., Sorensen, E.M., Anuforo, D.C., Mitchell, D.B., Ramos, K., Santone, K.S., and Smith, M.A. 1985. An in vitro approach to the study of target organ toxicity of drugs and chemicals. *In Vitro Cellular and Developmental Biology* 21: 495–504.

Adams, J.W., Sakata, Y., Davis, M.G., Sah, V.P., Wang, Y., Liggett, S.B., Chien, K.R., Brown, J.H., and Dorn, G.W. 1998. Enhanced G$\alpha$q signaling: a common pathway mediates cardiac hypertrophy and apoptotic failure. *Proceedings of the National Academy of Sciences of the United States of America* 95: 10140–10145.

Amati, B., Littlewood, T.D., Evan, G.I., and Land, H. 1993. The c-Myc protein induces cell cycle progression and apoptosis through dimerization with Max. *EMBO Journal* 12: 5083–5087.

Barinaga, M. 1996. Forging a path to cell death. *Science* 273: 735–737.

Bishopric, N.H., Simpson, P.C., and Ordahl, C.P. 1987. Induction of the skeletal $\alpha$-actin gene in $\alpha_1$-adrenoceptor-mediated hypertrophy of rat cardiac myocytes. *Journal of Clinical Investigation* 80: 1194–1199.

Bishopric, N.H., Jayasena, V., and Webster, K.A. 1992. Positive regulation of the skeletal $\alpha$-actin gene by Fos and Jun in cardiac myocytes. *The Journal of Biological Chemistry* 267: 25535–25540.

Boluyt, M.O., Zheng, J.-S., Younes, A., Long, X., O'Neill, L., Silverman, H., Lakatta, E.G., and Crow, M.T. 1997. Rapamycin inhibits $\alpha_1$-adrenergic receptor-stimulated cardiac myocyte hypertrophy but not activation of hypertrophy-associated genes. Evidence for involvement of p70 S6 kinase. *Circulation Research* 81: 176–186.

Cai, J., Yang, J., and Jones, D.P. 1998. Mitochondrial control of apoptosis: the role of cytochrome c. *Biochimica et Biophysica Acta* 1366: 139–149.

Chacon, E. and Acosta, D. 1991. Mitochondrial regulation of superoxide by $Ca^{2+}$: an alternative mechanism for the cardiotoxicity of doxorubicin. *Toxicology and Applied Pharmacology* 107: 117–128.

Chandler, J.M., Alnemri, E.S., Cohen, G.M., and MacFarlane, M. 1997. Activation of CPP32 and Mch3 alpha in wild-type p53-induced apoptosis. *Biochemical Journal* 322: 19–23.

Chien, K.R., Zhu, H., Knowlton, K.U., Miller-Hance, W., van-Bilsen, M., O'Brien, T.X., and Evans, S.M. 1993. Transcriptional regulation during cardiac growth and development. *Annual Review of Physiology* 55: 77–95.

Cigola, E., Kajstura, J., Li, B., Meggs, L.G., and Anversa, P. 1997. Angiotensin II activates programmed myocyte cell death in vitro. *Experimental Cell Research* 231: 363–371.

Clarke, A.R.C.A., Purdie, D.J., Harrison, D.J., Morris, R.G., Bird, C.C., Hooper, M.L., and Wyllie, A.H. 1993. Thymocyte apoptosis induced by p53-dependent and independent pathways. *Nature* 362: 849–852.

Coroneos, E., Wang, Y., Panuska, J.R., Templeton, D.J., and Kester, M. 1996. Sphingolipid metabolites differentially regulate extracellular signal-regulated kinase and stress-activated protein kinase cascades. *Biochemical Journal* 316: 13–17.

Counts, R.S., Nowak, G., Wyatt, R.D., and Schnellmann, R.G. 1995. Nephrotoxicant inhibition of renal proximal tubule cell regeneration. *American Journal of Physiology* 269: F274–F281.

Davies, M.J. 1997. Apoptosis in cardiovascular disease. *Heart* 77: 498–501.

Devi, B.G. and Chan, A.W.K. 1999. Effect of cocaine on cardiac biochemical functions. *Journal of Cardiovascular Pharmacology* 33: 1–6.

Fischer, G., Kent, S.C., Joseph, L., Green, D.R., and Scott, D.W. 1994. Lymphoma models for B cell activation and tolerance. X. Anti-m-mediated growth arrest and apoptosis of murine B cell lymphomas are prevented by the stabilization of myc. *Journal of Experimental Medicine* 179: 221–228.

Fisher, D.E. 1994. Apoptosis in cancer therapy: crossing the threshold. *Cell* 78: 539–542.

Foncea, R., Andersson, M., Ketterman, A., Blakesley, V., Sapag-Hagar, M., Sugden, P.H., LeRoith, D., and Lavandero, S. 1997. Insulin-like growth factor-I rapidly activates multiple signal transduction pathways in cultured rat cardiac myocytes. *The Journal of Biological Chemistry* 272: 19115–19124.

Fuchs, E.J., McKenna, K.A., and Bedi, A. 1997. p53-dependent DNA damage-induced apoptosis requires Fas/APO-1-independent activation of CPP32b. *Cancer Research* 57: 2550–2554.

Fuller, S.J., Gaitanaki, C.J., and Sugden, P.H. 1990. Effects of catecholamines on protein synthesis in cardiac myocytes and perfused hearts isolated from adult rats. *Biochemical Journal* 266: 727–736.

Gosteli-Peter, M.A., Harder, B.A., Eppenberger, H.M., Zapf, J., and Schaub, M.C. 1996. Triiodothyronine induces over expression of alpha-smooth muscle actin, restricts myofibrillar expansion and is permissive for the action of basic fibroblast growth factor and insulin-like growth factor I in adult rat cardiomyocytes. *Journal of Clinical Investigation* 98: 1737–1744.

Green, D. 1998. Apoptotic pathways: the roads to ruin. *Cell* 94: 695–698.

Gurley, B.J., Gardner, S.F., White, L.M., and Wang, P.L. 1998. Ephedrine pharmacokinetics after the ingestion of nutritional supplements containing Ephedra sinica (ma huang). *Therapeutic Drug Monitoring* 20: 439–445.

Hannan, R.D., Luyken, J., and Rothblum, L.I. 1995. Regulation of rDNA transcription factors during cardiomyocyte hypertrophy induced by adrenergic agents. *The Journal of Biological Chemistry* 270: 8290–8297.

Hannan, R.D., Luyken, J., and Rothblum, L.I. 1996a. Regulation of ribosomal DNA transcription during contraction-induced hypertrophy of neonatal cardiomyocytes. *The Journal of Biological Chemistry* 271: 3213–3220.

Hannan, R.D, Stefanovsky, V., Taylor, L., Moss, T., and Rothblum, L.I. 1996b. Overexpression of the transcription factor UBF1 is sufficient to increase ribosomal DNA transcription in neonatal cardiomyocytes: implications for cardiac hypertrophy. *Proceedings of the National Academy of Sciences of the United States of America* 93: 8750–8755.

Hannun, Y.A. 1997. Apoptosis and the dilemma of cancer chemotherapy. *Blood* 89: 1845–1853.

Hefti, M.A., Harder, B.A., Eppenberger, H.M., and Schaub, M.C. 1997. Signaling pathways in cardiac myocyte hypertrophy. *Journal of Molecular and Cellular Cardiology* 29: 2873–2892.

Henrich, C.J. and Simpson, P.C. 1988. Differential acute and chronic response of protein kinase C in cultured neonatal rat heart myocytes to alpha1-adrenergic and phorbol ester stimulation. *Journal of Molecular and Cellular Cardiology* 20: 1081–1085.

Hermeking, H. and Eick, D. 1994. Mediation of *c-myc*-induced apoptosis by p53. *Science* 265: 2091–2093.

Hockenbery, D.M., Oltvai, Z.N., Yin, X.M., Milliman, C.L., and Korsmeyer, S.J. 1993. Bcl-2 functions in an antioxidant pathway to prevent apoptosis. *Cell* 75: 241–251.

Hsu, H., Shu, H., Pan, M., and Goeddel, D.V. 1996. TRADD–TRAF2 and TRADD–FADD interactions define two distinct TNF receptor 1 signal transduction pathways. *Cell* 84: 299–308.

James, T.N. 1997. Apoptosis in congenital heart disease. *Coronary Artery Disease* 8: 599–616.

Jong D.D., Prins, F.A., Mason, D.Y., Reed, J.C., Ommen, G.B.V., and Kluin, P.M. 1994. Subcellular localization of the bcl-2 protein in malignant and normal lymphoid cells. *Cancer Research* 54: 256–260.

Kajstura, J., Cigola, E., Malhotra, A., Li, P., Cheng, W., Meggs, L.G., and Anversa, P. 1997. Angiotensin II induces apoptosis of adult ventricular myocytes in vitro. *Journal of Molecular and Cellular Cardiology* 29: 859–870.

Karns, L.R., Kariya, K., and Simpson, P.C. 1995. M-CAT, CArG, and Sp1 elements are required for $\alpha_1$-adrenergic induction of the skeletal $\alpha$-actin promoter during cardiac myocyte hypertrophy. *The Journal of Biological Chemistry* 270: 410–417.

Kays, S.E. and Schnellmann, R.G. 1995. Regeneration of renal proximal tubule cells in primary culture following toxicant injury: response to growth factors. *Toxicology and Applied Pharmacology* 132: 273–280.

Kent, R.L. and McDermott, P.J. 1996. Passive load and angiotensin II evoke differential responses of gene expression and protein synthesis in cardiac myocytes. *Circulation Research* 78: 829–838.

Kinloch, R.A., Treherne, J.M., Furness, L.M., and Hajimohamadreza, I. 1999. The pharmacology of apoptosis. *Trends in Pharmacological Sciences* 20: 35–42.

Kluck, R.M., Bossy-Wetzel, E., Green, D.R., and Newmeyer, D.D. 1997. The release of cytochrome c from mitochondria: a primary site for Bcl-2 regulation of apoptosis. *Science* 275: 1132–1136.

Kodama, H., Fukuda, K., Pan, J., Makino, S., Baba, A., Hori, S., and Ogawa, S. 1997. Leukemia inhibitory factor, a potent cardiac hypertrophic cytokine, activates the JAK/STAT pathway in rat cardiac myocytes. *Circulation Research* 81: 656–663.

Komuro, I. and Yazaki, Y. 1993. Control of cardiac gene expression by mechanical stress. *Annual Review of Physiology* 55: 55–75.

Komuro, I., Kudo, S., Yamazaki, T., Zou, Y., Shiojima, I., and Yazaki, Y. 1996. Mechanical stretch activates the stress-activated protein kinases in cardiac myocytes. *FASEB Journal* 10: 631–636.

Krown, K.A., Page, M.T., Nguyen, C., Zechner, D., Gutierrez, V., Comstock, K.L., Glembotski, C.C., Quintana, P.J.E., and Sabbadini, R.A. 1996. Tumor necrosis factor alpha-induced apoptosis in cardiac myocytes. Involvement of the sphingolipid signaling cascade in cardiac cell death. *Journal of Clinical Investigation* 98: 2854–2865.

Kudoh, S., Komuro, I., Mizuno, T., Yamazaki, T., Younzeng, Z., Shiojima, I., Takekoshi, N., and Yazaki, Y. 1997. Angiotensin II stimulates c-jun $NH_2$-terminal kinase in cultured cardiac myocytes of neonatal rats. *Circulation Research* 80: 139–146.

Kunisada, K., Hirota, H., Fujio, Y., Matsui, H., Tani, Y., Yamauchi-Takihara, K., and Kishimoto, T. 1996. Activation of JAK-STAT and MAP kinases by leukemia inhibitory factor through gp130 in cardiac myocytes. *Circulation* 94: 2626–2632.

Lai, J., Jin, H., Yang, R., Winer, J., Li, W., Yen, R., King, K.L., Zeigler, F., Ko, A., Cheng, J., Bunting, S., and Paoni, N.F. 1996. Prostaglandin $F_{2\alpha}$ induces cardiac myocyte hypertrophy in vitro and cardiac growth in vivo. *American Journal of Physiology* 271: H2197–H2208.

Li, F., Srinivasan, A., Wang, Y., Armstrong, R.C., Tomaselli, K.J., Fritz, L.C. 1997. Cell-specific induction of apoptosis by microinjection of cytochrome c. *The Journal of Biological Chemistry* 272: 30299–30305.

Lithgow, T., Driel, R.C., Bertram, J.F., and Stasser, A. 1994. The protein product of the oncogene *bcl-2* is a component of the nuclear envelope, the endoplasmic reticulum, and the outer mitochondrial membrane. *Cell Growth and Differentiation* 5: 411–417.

Liu, S., Melchert, R.B., and Kennedy, R.H. 1997. Inhibition of L-type calcium current in rat ventricular myocytes by terfenadine. *Circulation Research* 81: 202–210.

Liu, X., Kim, C.N., Yang, J., Jemmerson, R., and Wang, X. 1996. Induction of apoptotic program in cell-free extraction: requirement for dATP and cytochrome c. *Cell* 86: 147–157.

Liu, Y., Leri, A., Li, B., Wang, X., Cheng, W., Kajstura, J., and Anversa, P. 1998. Angiotensin II stimulation in vitro induces hypertrophy of normal and postinfarcted ventricular myocytes. *Circulation Research* 82: 1145–1159.

Long, X., Boluyt, M.O., Hipolito, M.L., Lundberg, M.S., Zheng, J.-S., O'Neill, L., Cirielli, C., Lakatta, E.G., and Crow, M.T. 1997. p53 and the hypoxia-induced apoptosis of cultured neonatal rat cardiac myocytes. *Journal of Clinical Investigation* 99: 2635–2643.

Lowe, S.W., Ruley, H.E., Jacks, T., and Housman, D.E. 1993. p53-independent apoptosis modulates the cytotoxicity of anti-cancer agents. *Cell* 74: 957–967.

McCurrach, M.E., Connor, T.M.F., Knudson, C.M., Korsmeyer, S.J., and Lowe, S.W. 1997. bax-deficiency promotes drug resistance and oncogenic transformation by attenuating p53-dependent apoptosis. *Proceedings of the National Academy of Sciences of the United States of America* 94: 2345–2349.

McDermott, P.J. and Morgan, H.E. 1989. Contraction modulates the capacity for protein synthesis during growth of neonatal heart cells in culture. *Circulation Research* 64: 542–553.

McDermott, P.J., Rothblum, L.I., Smith, S.D., and Morgan, H.E. 1989. Accelerated rates of ribosomal RNA synthesis during growth of contracting heart cells in culture. *The Journal of Biological Chemistry* 264: 18220–18227.

MacLellan, W.R. and Schneider, M.D. 1997. Death by design. Programmed cell death in cardiovascular biology and disease. *Circulation Research* 81: 137–144.

MacLellan, W.R., Brand, T., and Schneider M.D. 1993. Transforming growth factor-$\beta$ in cardiac ontogeny and adaptation. *Circulation Research* 73: 783–791.

MacLellan, W.R., Lee, T.-C., Schwartz, R.J., and Schneider, M.D. 1994. Transforming growth factor-$\beta$ response elements of the skeletal $\alpha$-actin gene. *The Journal of Biological Chemistry* 269: 16754–16760.

Marsh, J.D., Lehmann, M.H., Ritchie, R.H., Gwathmey, J.K., Green, G.E., and Schiebinger, R.J. 1998. Androgen receptors mediate hypertrophy in cardiac myocytes. *Circulation* 98: 256–261.

Meidell, R.S., Sen, A., Henderson, S.A., Slahetka, M.F., and Chien, K.R. 1986. $\alpha_1$-Adrenergic stimulation of rat myocardial cells increases protein synthesis. *American Journal of Physiology* 251: H1076–H1084.

Melchert, R.B., Levin, P.S., and Acosta, D. 1996. Cardiotoxicity of nonsedating antihistamines in vitro. *In Vitro Toxicology* 9: 431–440.

Meyn, R.E., Stephens, L.C., and Milas, L. 1996. Programmed cell death and radioresistance. *Cancer and Metastasis Reviews* 15: 119–131.

Mitcheson, J.S., Hancox, J.C., and Levi, A.J. 1998. Cultured adult cardiac myocytes: future applications, culture methods, morphological and electrophysiological properties. *Cardiovascular Research* 39: 280–300.

Miyata, S. and Haneda, T. 1994. Hypertrophic growth of cultured neonatal rat heart cells mediated by type 1 angiotensin II receptor. *American Journal of Physiology* 266: H2443–H2451.

Miyata, S., Haneda, T., Osaki, J., and Kikuchi, K. 1996. Renin-angiotensin system in stretch-induced hypertrophy of cultured neonatal rat heart cells. *European Journal of Pharmacology* 307: 81–88.

Molkentin, J.D., Lu, J.-R., Antos, C.L., Markham, B., Richardson, J., Robbins, J., Grant, S.R., and Olson, E.N. 1998. A calcineurin-dependent transcriptional pathway for cardiac hypertrophy. *Cell* 93: 215–228.

Morgan, H.E. and Baker, K.M. 1991. Cardiac hypertrophy. Mechanical, neural, and endocrine dependence. *Circulation* 83: 13–25.

Nakamura, K., Fushimi, K., Kouchi, H., Mihara, K., Miyazaki, M., Ohe, T., and Namba, M. 1998. Inhibitory effects of antioxidants on neonatal rat cardiac myocyte hypertrophy induced by tumor necrosis factor-$\alpha$ and angiotensin II. *Circulation* 98: 794–799.

Narula J., Kharbanda, S., and Khaw, B.-A. 1997. Apoptosis and the heart. *Chest* 112: 1358–1362.

Packham, G. and Cleveland, J.L. 1995. c-Myc and apoptosis. *Biochimica et Biophysica Acta* 1242: 11–28.

Palmer, J.N., Hartogensis, W.E., Patten, M., Fortuin, F.D., and Long, C.S. 1995. Interleukin-1 beta induces cardiac myocyte growth but inhibits cardiac fibroblast proliferation in culture. *Journal of Clinical Investigation* 95: 2555–2564.

Paradis, P., MacLellan, W.R., Belaguli, N.S., Schwartz, R.J., and Schneider, M.D. 1996. Serum response factor mediates AP-1-dependent induction of the skeletal $\alpha$-actin promoter in ventricular myocytes. *The Journal of Biological Chemistry* 271: 10827–10833.

Patten, M., Hartogensis, W.E., and Long, C.S. 1996. Interleukin-1$\beta$ is a negative transcriptional regulator of $\alpha$1-adrenergic induced gene expression in cultured cardiac myocytes. *The Journal of Biological Chemistry* 271: 21134–21141.

Polyak, K., Xia, Y., Zweier, J.L., Kinzler, K.W., and Vogelstein, B. 1997. A model for p53-induced apoptosis. *Nature* 389: 300–305.

Post, G.R., Goldstein, D., Thuerauf, D.J., Glembotski, C.C., and Brown, J.H. 1996. Dissociation of p44 and p42 mitogen-activated protein kinase activation from receptor-induced hypertrophy in neonatal rat ventricular myocytes. *The Journal of Biological Chemistry* 271: 8452–8457.

Puceat, M., Hilal-Dandan, R., Strulovici, B., Brunton, L.L., and Brown, J.H. 1994. Differential regulation of protein kinase C isoforms in isolated neonatal and adult rat cardiomyocytes. *The Journal of Biological Chemistry* 269: 16938–16944.

Pulkki, K.J. 1997. Cytokines and cardiomyocyte death. *Annals of Medicine* 29: 339–343.

Rabkin, S.W. 1996. The angiotensin II subtype 2 (AT$_2$) receptor is linked to protein kinase C but not cAMP-dependent pathways in the cardiomyocyte. *Canadian Journal of Physiology and Pharmacology* 74: 125–131.

Rybin, V.O. and Steinberg, S.F. 1994. Protein kinase C isoform expression and regulation in the developing rat heart. *Circulation Research* 74: 299–309.

Sadoshima, J.-I. and Izumo, S. 1993a. Mechanical stretch rapidly activates multiple signal transduction pathways in cardiac myocytes: potential involvement of an autocrine/paracrine mechanism. *EMBO Journal* 12: 1681–1692.

Sadoshima, J.-I. and Izumo, S. 1993b. Signal transduction pathways of angiotensin II-induced *c-fos* gene expression in cardiac myocytes in vitro. Roles of phospholipid-derived second messengers. *Circulation Research* 73: 424–438.

Sadoshima, J. and Izumo, S. 1995. Rapamycin selectively inhibits angiotensin II-induced increase in protein synthesis in cardiac myocytes in vitro. Potential role of 70-kD S6 kinase in angiotensin II-induced cardiac hypertrophy. *Circulation Research* 77: 1040–1052.

Samali, A., Zhivotovsky, B., Jones, D., and Orrenius, S. 1998. Detection of pro-caspase-3 in cytosol and mitochondria of carious tissues. *FEBS Letters* 431: 167–169.

Sato, A. and Funder, J.W. 1996. High glucose stimulates aldosterone-induced hypertrophy via type I mineralocorticoid receptors in neonatal rat cardiomyocytes. *Endocrinology* 137: 4145–4153.

Sawyer, D.B., Fukazawa, R., Arstall, M.A., and Kelly, R.A. 1999. Daunorubicin-induced apoptosis in rat cardiac myocytes is inhibited by dexrazoxane. *Circulation Research* 84: 257–265.

Schaub, M.C., Hefti, M.A., Harder, B.A., and Eppenberger, H.M. 1997. *Journal of Molecular Medicine* 75: 901–920.

Schulze-Osthoff, K., Ferrari, D., Los, M., Wesselborg, S., and Peter, M.E. 1998. Apoptosis signaling by death receptors. *European Journal of Biochemistry* 254: 439–459.

Scott, D.W., Lamers, M., Kohler, G., Sidman, C.L., Maddox, B., and Carsetti, R. 1996. Role of *c-myc* and CD45 in spontaneous and anti-receptor-induced apoptosis in adult murine B cells. *International Immunology* 8: 1375–1385.

Selvakumaran, M., Lin, H.K., Miyashita, T., Wang, H.G., Krajewski, S., Reed, J.C., Hoffman, B., and Liebermann, D. 1994. Immediate early up-regulation of bax expression by p53 but not TGF beta1: a paradigm for distinct apoptotic pathway. *Oncogene* 9: 1791–1798.

Sheng, Z., Knowlton, K., Chen, J., Hoshijima, M., Brown, J.H., and Chien, K.R. 1997. Cardiotrophin 1 (CT-1) inhibition of cardiac myocyte apoptosis via a mitogen-activated protein kinase-dependent pathway. *The Journal of Biological Chemistry* 272: 5783–5791.

Shizukuda, Y., Buttrick, P.M., Geenen, D.L., Borczuk, A.C., Kitsis, R.N., Sonnenblick, E.H. 1998. Beta-adrenergic stimulation causes cardiocyte apoptosis: influence of tachycardia and hypertrophy. *American Journal of Physiology* 275: H961–H968.

Simpson, P.C. 1983. Norepinephrine-stimulated hypertrophy of cultured rat myocardial cells is an alpha$_1$ adrenergic response. *Journal of Clinical Investigation* 72: 732–738.

Simpson, P. 1985. Stimulation of hypertrophy of cultured neonatal rat heart cells through an $\alpha_1$-adrenergic receptor and induction of beating through an $\alpha_1$- and $\beta_1$-adrenergic receptor interaction. Evidence for independent regulation of growth and beating. *Circulation Research* 56: 884–894.

Simpson, P., McGrath, A., and Savion, S. 1982. Myocyte hypertrophy in neonatal rat heart cultures and its regulation by serum and catecholamines. *Circulation Research* 51: 787–801.

Slinker, B.K., Stephens, R.L., Fisher, S.A., and Yang, Q. 1996. Immediate–early gene responses to different cardiac loads in the ejecting rabbit left ventricle. *Journal of Molecular and Cellular Cardiology* 28: 1565–1574.

Sprenkle, A.B., Murray, S.F., and Glembotski, C.C. 1995. Involvement of multiple *cis* elements in basal- and $\alpha$-adrenergic-inducible atrial natriuretic factor transcription. Roles for serum response elements and an SP-1-like element. *Circulation Research* 77: 1060–1069.

Staunton, M.J. and Gaffney, E.F. 1998. Apoptosis: basic concepts and potential significance in human cancer. *Archives of Pathology and Laboratory Medicine* 122: 310–319.

Susic, D., Nunez, E., Frohlich, E.D., and Prakash, O. 1996. Angiotensin II increases left ventricular mass without affecting myosin isoform mRNAs. *Hypertension* 28: 265–268.

Susin, S.A., Zamzami, N., and Kroemer, G. 1998. Mitochondria as regulators of apoptosis: doubt no more. *Biochimica et Biophysica Acta* 1366: 151–165.

Sussman, M.A., Lim, H.W., Gude, N., Taigen, T., Olson, E.N., Robbins, J., Colbert, M.C., Gualberto, A., Wieczorek, D.F., and Molkentin, J.D. 1998. Prevention of cardiac hypertrophy in mice by calcineurin inhibition. *Science* 281: 1690–1693.

Thompson, E.B. 1998a. Special topic: apoptosis. *Annual Review of Physiology* 60: 525–532.

Thompson, E.B. 1998b. The many roles of c-Myc in apoptosis. *Annual Review of Physiology* 60: 575–600.

Thornberry, N.A. and Lazebnik, Y. 1998. Caspases: enemies within. *Science* 281: 1312–1316.

Touyz, R.M., Sventek, P., Lariviere, R., Thibault, G., Farch, J., Reudelhuber, T., and Schiffrin, E.L. 1996. Cytosolic calcium changes induced by angiotensin II in neonatal rat atrial and ventricular cardiomyocytes are mediated via angiotensin II subtype 1 receptors. *Hypertension* 27: 1090–1096.

Umansky, S.R., Shapiro, J.P., Cuenco, G.M., Foehr, M.W., Bathurst, I.C., and Tomei, L.D. 1997. Prevention of rat neonatal cardiomyocyte apoptosis induced by simulated *in vitro* ischemia and reperfusion. *Cell Growth and Differentiation* 4: 608–616.

Vandenburgh, H.H., Solerssi, R., Shansky, J., Adams, J.W., and Henderson, S.A. 1996. Mechanical stimulation of organogenic cardiomyocyte growth in vitro. *American Journal of Physiology* 270: C1284–C1292.

de Vries J.E., Vork, M.M., Roemen, T.H.M., de Jong, Y.F., Cleutjens, J.P.M., van der Vusse, G.J., and van Bilsen, M. 1997. Saturated but not mono-unsaturated fatty acids induce apoptotic cell death in neonatal rat ventricular myocytes. *Journal of Lipid Research* 38: 1384–1394.

Wada, H., Zile, M.R., Ivester, C.T., Cooper, G., and McDermott, P.J. 1996. Comparative effects of contraction and angiotensin II on growth of adult feline cardiocytes in primary culture. *American Journal of Physiology* 271: H29–H37.

Wang, L., Ma, W., Markovich, R., Chen, J.W., and Wang, P.H. 1998. Regulation of cardiomyocyte apoptotic signaling by insulin-like growth factor I. *Circulation Research* 83: 516–522.

Wang, Y., Huang, S., Sah, V.P., Ross, J., Brown, J.H., Han, J., and Chien, K.R. 1998. Cardiac muscle cell hypertrophy and apoptosis induced by distinct members of the p38 mitogen-activated protein kinase family. *The Journal of Biological Chemistry* 273: 2161–2168.

Welder, A.A. and Acosta, D. 1993. Preparation of primary cultures of postnatal rat myocardial cells for toxicological studies. In *Methods in Toxicology*, Vol. 1A. Tyson, C.A. and Frazier, J.M. (eds), pp. 147–158. Academic Press, San Diego, CA.

Welder, A.A., Grant, R., Bradlaw, J., and Acosta, D. 1991. A primary culture system of adult rat heart cells for the study of toxicologic agents. *In Vitro Cellular and Developmental Biology* 27A: 921–926.

Wertz, I.E. and Hanley, M.R. 1996. Diverse molecular provocation of programmed cell death. *Trends in Biochemical Sciences* 21: 359–364.

White, L.M., Gardner, S.F., Gurley, B.J., Marx, M.A., Wang, P.L., and Estes, M. 1997. Pharmacokinetics and cardiovascular effects of ma-huang (Ephedra sinica) in normotensive adults. *Journal of Clinical Pharmacology* 37: 116–122.

Wollert, K.C., Taga, T., Saito, M., Narazaki, M., Kishimoto, T., Glembotski, C.C., Vernallis, A.B., Health, J.K., Pennica, D., Wood, W.I., and Chien, K.R. 1996. Cardiotrophin-1 activates a distinct form of cardiac muscle cell hypertrophy. Assembly of sarcomeric units in series via gp130/leukemia inhibitory factor receptor-dependent pathways. *The Journal of Biological Chemistry* 271: 9535–9545.

Wood, A.C., Waters, C.M., Garner, A., and Hickman, J.A. 1994. Changes in *c-myc* expression and the kinetics of dexamethasone-induced programmed cell death (apoptosis) in human lymphoid leukaemia cells. *British Journal of Cancer* 69: 663–669.

Wu, C.-F., Bishopric, N.H., and Pratt, R.E. 1997. Atrial natriuretic peptide induces apoptosis in neonatal rat cardiac myocytes. *The Journal of Biological Chemistry* 272: 14860–14866.

Wyllie, A.H. 1980. Glucocorticoid-induced thymocyte apoptosis is associated with endogenous endonuclease activation. *Nature* 284: 555–556.

Yamazaki, T., Komuro, I., Kudoh, S., Zou, Y., Shiojima, I., Hiroi, Y., Mizuno, T., Maemura, K., Kurihara, H., Aikawa, R., Takano, H., and Yazaki, Y. 1996. Endothelin-1 is involved in mechanical stress-induced cardiomyocyte hypertrophy. *The Journal of Biological Chemistry* 271: 3221–3228.

Yuan, C. and Acosta, D. 1996. Cocaine-induced mitochondrial dysfunction in primary cultures of rat cardiomyocytes. *Toxicology* 112: 1–10.

Zunino, F., Perego, P., Pilotti, S., Pratesi, G., Supino, R., and Arcamone, F. 1997. Role of apoptotic response in cellular resistance to cytotoxic agents. *Pharmacology and Therapeutics* 76: 177–185.

# Part II

# METHODS

# 2

# ACUTE AND CHRONIC EVALUATION OF THE CARDIOVASCULAR TOXICITY OF DRUGS

## An industrial perspective

*Shayne C. Gad*

*Gad Consulting Services, Cary, NC, USA*

Industrial toxicologists have as their prime responsibility the identification of any or all adverse effects associated with compounds or mixtures that their employers intend to commercialize. In almost all cases, toxicologists in industry (although they may possess an individual expertise in one or more target organ systems) must perform as generalists, evaluating a compound for a broad range of adverse effects. Many of the standardized experimental designs that serve for detecting whether such effects are present are subject to regulatory mandate. This fact and the usual restraints of timing and cost have limited and guided what is done to identify cardiotoxic agents, including the determination that an effect exists, at what dose levels, and occasionally to determine whether the effect is reversible. As experience dictates, changes can be made in the collection or analysis of data to address concerns about specific concerns that arise, such as the exposure of the potential for induction of valvular heart disease by fenfluramine,[1] but such changes are limited in nature to either conducting additional studies or adding measures or means of analysis to existing study designs.

Compounds with therapeutic potential are the particular domain of interest of the pharmaceutical toxicologist. In this arena, the task becomes considerably more challenging. The challenge occurs because pharmaceutical agents are intended to be administered to a target species (usually humans, except for veterinary drugs) and are intended to have biologic effects. Occasionally, the commercial objective is an agent that alters the function of the cardiovascular system. To the pharmaceutical toxicologists, the task of evaluating cardiotoxicity frequently is expanded to identifying and understanding the mechanism of action, the relevance of findings to the target species, and quantitating the therapeutic dose (i.e. the separation between the dose with a desired effect and the higher dose that has an adverse effect). Indeed, the case of detecting cardiovascular toxicity is a function of the underlying mechanism of that toxicity; particularly if we are talking about individuals with pre-existing cardiovascular disease.

The basic principles of cardiovascular function and mechanisms of cardiovascular toxicity are presented elsewhere in this book, or in other reviews of cardiovascular toxicity[2-4] and are not addressed here.

Evaluations of cardiotoxicity, with the exception of one special case, tend to be performed by adding measurements and observations to existing "pivotal" test designs. These measures look at alterations in myocardial and vascular structure (pathology, clinical pathology) and function (electrocardiograms, clinical pathology, and clinical observations). Tests focused on the cardiovascular system are designed and executed only if an indication of an effect is found. The special case exception are so-called safety pharmacology studies, which seek to look at exaggerated pharmacologic effects in rather focused target organ functional studies. Additionally, there are currently efforts by the Food and Drug Administration (FDA) and others to develop (or refine existing) tests to detect agents effecting valvular tissue better. Such development is complicated by the fact that pre-existing conditions (hypertension) predispose individuals for the adverse effects.

## Pharmacologic profiling

The profiling of the pharmacologic effects of a new drug on the cardiovascular system is an essential element in early evaluations and development. Broad assessments of the effects on critical target organ functions (cardiovascular, renal, pulmonary, immune, peripheral and central nervous system) for which no action is intended are often called "safety pharmacology," although other purposes (such as the serendipitous discovery of additional desirable pharmacologic activities – i.e. new therapeutic opportunities) are also served. These assessments are carried out in the therapeutic to near-therapeutic dosage range, e.g. from the projected human $ED_{50}$ to perhaps the projected $ED_{90}$. Such evaluations can reveal other actions that were unintended and undesirable (side-effects), or extensions/ exaggerations of the intended pharmacology, which are either unacceptable or essential for interpreting results in actual toxicology studies. The regulatory guidelines for such "secondary" pharmacologic evaluations currently vary among the USA, the UK, and Europe (Table 2.1).

Such interpretations are more difficult, of course, when the agent is intended to have therapeutic cardiovascular effects. Brunner and Gross[5] and Gilman et al.[6] should be reviewed by anyone undertaking such an effort to ensure familiarity with basic cardiovascular pharmacology.

Focusing on cardiovascular effects, the concerns are both direct (on the heart and vasculature) and indirect (such as on adrenal release) effects in the short term. Accordingly, these studies look at function in the short term (hours to perhaps 3 days). The dog and the rat are generally the model species (although mice and primates may also be used), with parameters being evaluated including the following:

*Table 2.1* Safety pharmacologic evaluation of new chemical entities (NCEs)

| UK and Europe | USA |
|---|---|
| Central nervous system | Neuropharmacology |
| Autonomic system | Cardiovascular/respiratory |
| Cardiovascular system | Gastrointestinal |
| Respiratory system | Genitourinary |
| Gastrointestinal system | Endocrine |
| Other systems where relevant | Anti-inflammatory |
| | Immunoactive |
| | Chemotherapeutic |
| | Enzyme effects |
| | Other |

Note
These lists and terminologies are derived from the recommendations of the respective regulatory authorities, as laid out in the *EEC Notice to Applicants*, ISBN 92-825-9503 X, and in the *Guideline for the Format and Content of the Nonclinical Pharmacology/Toxicology Section of an Application*, Center for Drug Evaluation and Research, FDA, Washington, DC;1987.

- *Physiologic function*: systemic arterial blood pressure, heart rate, electrocardiogram (EKG), blood gases, blood flow.
- *Biochemistry*: enzyme release [lactate dehydrogenase (LDH), creatinine phosphokinase (CPK)], oxygen consumption, calcium transport, substrate utilization.

Several of these (EKG, LDH, and CPK) are also evaluated in traditional "pivotal" safety/toxicology studies at higher doses (up to 100 times the intended human dose) and are discussed in further detail here. Such studies also depend on extensive evaluation of clinical signs to indicate problems. By definition, the functional cardiovascular system is very dynamic. Accordingly, the times of measurement (sampling) must be carefully considered.

All of these could also be of concern for non-drug chemical entities but are generally only evaluated to the extent described later under pivotal studies (if at all).

## *In vivo* parameter evaluations in standard studies

For most new chemical entities, the primary screen for cardiotoxicity in industry consists of selected parameters incorporated into the "pivotal" or systemic toxicity studies of various lengths. These "shotgun" studies (so called because they attempt to collect as much data as possible to identify and crudely characterize toxicities associated with a drug or chemical) are exemplified by the 13-week study shown in Figure 2.1.

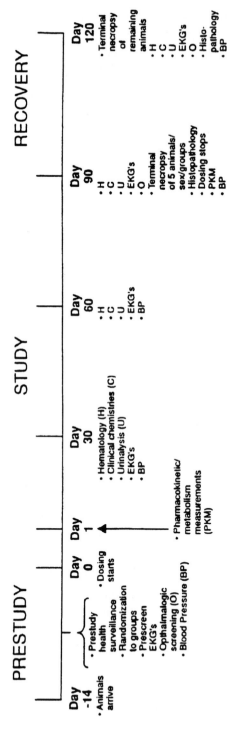

*Figure 2.1* Line chart for a standard or "pivotal" 13-week toxicity study. Four or more groups of sixteen (eight male and eight female) beagle dogs each; daily dosing (5 days per week for chemicals, 7 days per week for pharmaceuticals or food additives) at selected dose levels, with one group being controls and receiving only vehicle or sham exposure; mortality and morbidity checks twice per day, detailed clinical observations at least once per week; function observational battery (FOB[15]) on days 0, 4, 11, and 87; body weights of every animal on days −7, −1, 0, 4, 7, 11, and weekly thereafter; food consumption weekly. For the sake of illustration, what is shown is a dog study. The design is the same (except for numbers of animals) for studies conducted in other species (rats, primates, etc.). Dosing is by the appropriate route and frequency (usually, however, once daily in the morning).

As shown, a large number of variables are measured, with only a few of them either acting directly or indirectly as predictors of cardiovascular toxicity. These measures are taken at multiple time points and in aggregate compose a powerful tool set for identifying the existence of problems. Their sensitivity and value are limited, however, by several design features incorporated into the pivotal studies, i.e. those that use dogs, primates, etc., and the number of times that specific measurements are made. Both are limited by cost and logistics, and these limitations decrease the overall power of the study. The second feature is the complications inherent in dealing with background variability in many of these parameters. Although individual animals are typically screened prior to inclusion in a study to ensure that those with unacceptable baselines for parameters of interest (very typically EKGs, clinical chemistries, and hematologies) are eliminated, clearly some degree of variability must be accepted on grounds of economics or practicality. Proper analysis of the entire data set collected as an integrated whole is the key to minimizing these weaknesses.

### *Electrocardiograms*

Properly used and analyzed, electrocardiograms (EKGs) represent the most sensitive early indicator of cardiac toxicity or malfunction. Long before the other functional measures (blood pressure or clinical signs) or before the invasive measures (clinical chemistries or histopathology), the EKG should generally reveal that a problem exists.

Deceptively simple in form (for examples, see Figure 2.2), EKGs present a great deal of information.[7] Much of this information (amplitudes of the various waves, the lengths of intervals, and the frequency of events – i.e. heart rate) is quantitative in nature and can be analyzed by traditional statistical techniques. For this larger portion of the information in EKGs, the problems are that (1) baselines vary significantly from species to species (making interpretation of the relevance of changes seen in some models difficult) and (2) the task of actually collecting the EKGs and then extracting quantitative data from them is very labor intensive. There are now some computer-assisted analysis programs [such as that described in Watkinson *et al.*[8]] that perform the quantitative aspects of data extraction and analysis well.

There is also a significant amount of information in EKGs that is not quantitative, but rather more a pattern recognition nature. This requires a learned art and a great deal of experience for the more complex changes.

Interpretation of the underlying causes of changes in EKGs requires a knowledge of cardiac pathophysiology. Sodeman and Sodeman[9] present excellent overviews of this area, and Doherty and Cobbe[10] review the special cases of EKG changes in animal models.

Attention to technique is critical in the proper performance and interpretation of EKGs. Each species has different requirements for the placement and even the type of electrodes used.[11,12] In addition, there are differences in electrocardiographic

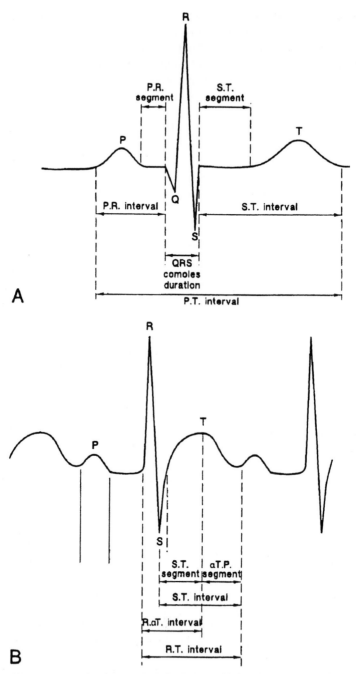

*Figure 2.2* Styled EKGs for humans (A) and adult rats (B). Although there are similarities between species, it is important to be aware of differences here and of differences that are dependent on age.

effects between sedated and non-sedated animals. Additionally, there are rather marked differences in EKGs between species, with the dog having a very labile T wave and the rat ST segment being short to non-existent (see Figure 2.2). In recent years, the QT interval (most often evaluated in the dog) has become of particular interest. Increases in QT-interval duration by a number of drugs have been associated with ventricular arrhythmias in humans.[13]

### *Blood pressure and heart rate*

These two traditional non-invasive measures of cardiovascular function have the advantages of being easy and inexpensive to perform. Their chief disadvantage is that they are subject to significant short-term variability, which significantly degrades their sensitivity and reliability. Techniques do exist for minimizing these disadvantages in various animal model species,[14,15] and careful attention to general animal husbandry and handling helps.

If EKGs are collected, then it is easy to extract the heart rate from the tracings. Most automated systems will, in fact, perform this calculation as a matter of course. Blood pressure, meanwhile, is attractive because it is a non-invasive measure of vascular function. Techniques for collecting it have improved significantly in recent years.

Neither of these measures is commonly collected in the pivotal or standard safety study, however. If clinical signs, particularly in larger (non-rodent) species, indicate that an effect is present, these should readily be added to a study.

### *Flow measurement techniques*

The major techniques (dye dilution, thermal dilution, and microspheres) are available to allow investigation of blood flow down to the capillary level, using the direct Flick technique as a calculation basis. This technique is based on a careful measurement of oxygen consumption of an individual and the determination of the amount of oxygen in the arterial and venous blood. By estimating the metabolic rate of the subject, one can determine the volume of blood that would be required to carry the volume of oxygen consumed in a set interval. This relationship yields the flow volume in milliliters per minute. The equation for calculating flow is as follows:

$$Q = q^2 / [O_2]_{pv} - [O_2]_{pa} \qquad (2.1)$$

where $Q$ is the cardiac output, $q^2$ is the oxygen consumption of the body, $[O_2]$ is the oxygen concentration, pv is the pulmonary vein, and pa is the pulmonary artery.

The direct Flick technique demands that stringent requirements are met to ensure accuracy of the flow measurements including (1) a stable metabolic rate over the sampling period, (2) the accurate determination of oxygen consumption and oxygen content in arterial and venous blood, (3) a representative venous blood sample or venous admixture, and (4) a valid method to determine metabolic rate. A cardinal rule for all of these techniques is that indicator is neither gained nor lost during the measurement period.

Indocyanine green has been used for many years for the determination of cardiac output using the Flick technique. A small amount of indocyanine green at a specific concentration is administered into the left side of the heart. Arterial blood then is sampled, preferably from the aorta, by constant withdrawal through an optical cuvette sensitive to the specific absorption spectrum of indocyanine green. The concentration of indocyanine green in the blood is automatically determined as the sample is withdrawn through the cuvette, plotted graphically, and described by a curve. By integrating the area under the curve and comparing this with a sample standard of known concentration, the average concentration of dye is calculated over the length of the sampling period. The volume of blood pumped per unit time then equals the cardiac output. A stringent requirement for this technique is that the withdrawal rate of blood through the cuvette must be constant and that the rate must be fast enough to obtain a representative sample of blood before recirculation of the dye begins. Also, the sampling catheter between the withdrawal pump and the animal must be kept as short as possible to reduce mixing of blood with dye and blood without dye.

Thermal dilution is a variation on the indicator dilution technique, which uses a bolus of cold, or room temperature, physiologic saline as the indicator and an intravascular thermocouple or thermistor as the detector. The bolus of cool saline is injected into the left side of the heart and the thermocouple is placed in the ascending aorta. The calculations of cardiac output with this technique are almost identical to those used for the indocyanine green determinations. The requirements for this technique are that a constant temperature of cold bolus must be injected and that no heat must be gained or lost by the blood as it circulates between the site of injection and the site of detection. Repetitive sampling is possible using this technique.

Microspheres are the third major indicator used for the determination of blood flow. Microspheres are small, carbonized spheres, usually 15 μm in diameter, that flow evenly distributed within the bloodstream and are trapped in the circulation at the arteriolar level. The microspheres can be used to determine qualitative flow by examining the organ for the presence of microspheres. As microspheres can be labeled with different radioactive tracers, tissue samples can be taken from the site in question to determine the radioactive level using a radioactive counting device (e.g. gamma counter). The total number of microspheres is proportional to the total number of counts recorded per unit time when compared with a standard dilution of such radiolabeled microspheres. To determine the effect of different interventions, different radiolabels can be used for each flow determination.

### *Magnetic resonance imaging*

Magnetic resonance imaging (MRI) relies mainly on the detection of hydrogen nuclei in water and fat to construct high-resolution images. The contrast in these images results from different $T_1$ and $T_2$ relaxation times for hydrogen nuclei in different tissue environments. MRI is based on the same principles as liquid-state nuclear magnetic resonance (NMR), i.e. the behavior of nuclei in a magnetic field under the influence of radiofrequency (RF) pulses, but the hardware, pulse sequences, and data processing are somewhat different. Improvements in electronics and computers since the mid-1990s have given MRI resolution capabilities in intact organisms down to ~ 3 mm, and therefore tremendous potential as a tool for studying mechanisms of toxicology.[16] MRI techniques provide detailed information on the response of specific organs to toxicants and can also be used to monitor xenobiotic metabolism *in vivo*. In addition, they could reduce the number of animals required for toxicology studies as a single animal could be followed over an extended period of time to monitor internal changes.

Angiography, utilizing X-rays to image coronary vasculature and blood flow in discrete regions during a study, has become a standard tool for evaluating effects on vascular function (including evaluating blockage, revascularization, and angiogenesis) when such are concerns or desired outcomes of treatment. Performance of such is usually restricted to use in dogs and swine, where it is a valuable tool for evaluating vascular/flow functional effects.[17]

### *Clinical signs/observations*

Clinical signs represent the oldest non-invasive assessment of general health and provide in animal studies a crude but broad and potentially very valuable screen for identifying adverse responses. Training, experience, and continuity of the observer are vitally important to these signs being both meaningful and reliable. A rigorous, regular, and formatted collection of such signs in an objective manner[18] provides an essential component of any systemic toxicity study.

A number of the observations collected in the standard clinical signs measurements either directly or indirectly address cardiovascular function. These include body temperature, the occurrence of cyanosis, flushing, weakness, pulse, and the results of careful palpitation of the cardiac region.

## Clinical pathology

Traditional systemic or "general" toxicology studies place their greatest reliance for detecting cardiotoxicity on the last two sets of tools presented here – clinical and anatomic pathology. Both of these are invasive and, therefore, entail either instilling at least some stress in test animals or killing the animals, but these studies are considered to be reasonably unequivocal in their interpretation. Also, both require a significant amount of experience/knowledge as to the normal characteristics of the model species.

Clinical pathology entails both hematology and clinical chemistry. Here, we are interested only in the latter because cardiovascular toxicity is not generally reflected in the hemogram. Urinalysis is likewise not a useful component of the clinical chemistry screen for detecting cardiotoxicity. Rather, serum levels of selected parameters are of primary interest. During actual myocardial infarction, there occurs a leakage of cellular constituents with rapid losses of ions and metabolites, resulting in transient increases in serum concentrations of these parameters. Later, there is a release of specific enzymes and proteins, which are in turn slowly cleared from the plasma. One can broadly classify the measurements made in serum as electrolytes, enzymes, proteins (other than enzymes), and lipids. Analysis of the findings as to their increases and decreases tends to be more powerful when it looks at patterns of changes across several end-points, such as increases in creatinine phosphokinase (CPK), γ-hydroxybutyrate dehydrogenase (γ-HBDH) and lactate dehydrogenase (LDH), and in serum glutamic–oxaloacetic transaminase (SGOT).

Although the most important parameters are generally considered to be CPK, γ-HBDH, LDH, and SGOT, each of which is primarily a muscle enzyme (and therefore increased levels of which may be indicative of either skeletal or cardiac muscle damage), it is appropriate to review the entire range of chemistry end-points.

### *Electrolytes*

Maintenance of the intracellular concentrations of cations (sodium, potassium, calcium, magnesium, and zinc) is essential for proper cardiovascular function. Alterations of the concentration of these cations may result in increased cardiac tissue sensitivity, arrhythmias, or significant adverse changes in vascular permeability. Concentrations of these cations are interrelated, making any significant disturbance of the ionic balance for one cation a consequence for the concentrations of the remaining ions. This interrelationship is observed with cardiac glycosides, which inhibit the sarcolemmal sodium pump $Na^+/K^+$-ATPase, causing increased intracellular sodium concentration, followed by increases of intracellular calcium and cardiac contractility. Where cardiac output is decreased, disturbances of plasma electrolytes may be the result of consequential alterations of renal function, e.g. reduced glomerular filtration rate (GFR). GFR may be evaluated by plasma creatinine and urea measurements. In addition, hypernatremia or hyponatremia may be observed in cardiac failure, depending on the volemic state of the animal.

When considering the effects of calcium and magnesium on cardiac function, the concentrations not bound to proteins (free) are more important than the total plasma concentration. Depending on the species, approximately 40 percent of the total plasma calcium and 30 percent of the plasma magnesium are bound to proteins. The need to consider plasma free-calcium concentration to protein-bound calcium concentration has been demonstrated by doxorubicin-induced cardiotoxicity in rabbits.[19] Hypercalcemia is not apparent when total plasma calcium is measured in doxorubicin-treated rabbits as there is a concomitant reduction of plasma albumin caused by renal toxicity. Increased plasma ionized calcium levels observed in these rabbits may therefore be partly due to the renal dysfunction. Excessive stress and use of restraining procedures during blood collection will markedly affect the potassium, calcium, and magnesium levels. In rodents, the sites used for blood collection and anesthetic techniques will also influence these plasma cation measurements.

Although changes of plasma anion concentrations often follow disturbances of cationic balance, these changes are of lesser significance for cardiac function. Plasma anions (chloride, bicarbonate, and inorganic phosphate) are poor markers of cardiotoxicity as their plasma concentrations may be altered for many reasons other than those associated with cardiac function.

### *Osmolality and acid–base balance*

Plasma osmolality determinations may be meaningful in conditions such as congestive cardiac failure, in which total body sodium concentration and extracellular fluid volume are increased but there is evidence of hyponatremia. Several formulas for the calculation of plasma osmolality from plasma concentrations of sodium, urea, and glucose have been used with humans but have limited applicability with other species, in which the component concentrations vary. Acid–base balance determinations can be used to monitor cardiotoxic effects on respiratory and metabolic functions, but the variability due to blood collection procedures on these determinations in small laboratory animals limits their regular use in toxicologic studies.

### *Enzymes*

Heart muscle tissue is rich in enzymes but only a few have proved to be useful markers of myocardial damage and congestive cardiac failure. A major limitation on use in animal studies is the relatively short half-life of these markers after damage has occurred. This makes the sampling design shown in Figure 2.1 very much a hit-or-miss proposition, particularly as different doses of the same compound will cause damage (and therefore evoke enzyme release) at different times. Additionally, it must be remembered that these enzymes are released by cells that are dead or dying. Damage that is functionally impairing to the organ or organism may not kill enough cells to be detected by this end-point.

There are also real limits on how many samples may be drawn from smaller animals, particularly when a large enough volume must be drawn for evaluation of all the clinical pathology parameters.

Plasma enzyme activity depends on the enzyme concentrations in different tissues, the mass of damaged tissue, the severity of damage, the molecular size of the enzyme, and the rate of clearance from the plasma. The distribution of enzymes in different tissues varies between species.[20,21] Differences between published data for tissue enzyme concentrations in the same species are in part due to the methods used for tissue preparation and sample collection (because of varying levels of physiologic stress), extraction of the enzyme, and enzyme measurement. The rate for enzyme removal from the intravascular space varies greatly for individual enzymes and species, as reflected by the differing relative half-lives of each enzyme.

For both CPK and LDH measurements, it is preferable to use plasma rather than serum, owing to the relatively high concentration of these enzymes in platelets and, hence, their release into serum during blood coagulation. Plasma samples with visible evidence of hemolysis should not be used because of the high enzyme concentrations in erythrocytes. Blood collection procedures may influence plasma enzyme values, particularly in rodents.

### *Creatine phosphokinase*

Creatine phosphokinase (CPK) has two subunits, B and M, which can form three cytosolic isoenzymes: the dimer consisting of two M (muscle) subunits (CPK-MM) is the "muscle-type" isoenzyme, the hybrid dimer (CPK-MB) is the "myocardial-type" isoenzyme, and the third dimer (CPK-BB) is the "brain-type" isoenzyme. A fourth isoenzyme ($CPK_M$) is located in the mitochondria of cardiac and other tissues.

Intramuscular injections cause increased plasma CPK activities: however, if blood samples are collected approximately 5 min after injection of an anesthetic agent sufficient to anesthetize rats fully, no effect on CPK is observed. The age of an animal may affect plasma CPK, with activities generally being higher in younger animals. Values also may be affected by stress and severe exercise.

### *Lactate dehydrogenase*

Lactate dehydrogenase (LDH) is a cytosolic tetrameric enzyme with five major isoenzymes consisting of M (muscle) and H (heart) subunits; a sixth isoenzyme of C subunits is found in some tissues. The five isoenzymes are numbered according to relative mobility during electrophoretic separation: $LDH_1$ consists of four H subunits; $LDH_5$ consists of four identical M units; and $LDH_2$, $LDH_3$, and $LDH_4$ are hybrid combinations of the two subunits (HHHM, HHMM, and HMMM respectively). The distribution of LDH in various tissues is often described as ubiquitous, and variations occur between species. For these reasons and because of the broad normal plasma LDH ranges often encountered in laboratory animals, the plasma total LDH values are often difficult to interpret; separation (and quantification) of plasma LDH isoenzymes therefore is helpful in cardiotoxicity studies.

Plasma α-hydroxybutyrate dehydrogenase (HBD) measurements reflect the activities of $LDH_1$ and $LDH_2$ isoenzymes. In seven of ten species examined, tissue HBD activities are highest in cardiac tissue. $LDH_5$ is the dominant isoenzyme in normal rat and dog plasma, whereas $LDH_1$ and $LDH_2$ are the dominant isoenzymes in plasma of several primates. Where $LDH_5$ is the major isoenzyme in the plasma, it may require a considerable increase of $LDH_1$ before total LDH values change significantly. Some drugs (such as streptokinase) modify the electrophoretic mobility of some LDH isoenzymes.

### Serum glutamic–oxaloacetic transaminase and serum glutamic–pyruvic transaminase

These two enzymes are commonly used as indicators of hepatotoxicity, but their plasma activities may also be altered following myocardial damage. Neither of these is tissue specific; in many laboratory animal species, cardiac tissue serum glutamic–oxaloacetic transaminase (SGOT) concentration is higher than in most other major tissues, whereas cardiac tissue serum glutamic–pyruvic transaminase (SGPT) concentrations vary between species. In the rat, dog, and mouse, hepatic tissue SGPT concentrations are generally higher than those in other major tissues, but hepatic and cardiac tissue concentrations are similar in several primate species. The plasma SGOT/SGPT ratio may be useful in detecting cardiac damage, but the ratios vary with species and often cannot be compared with published data because the ratios are dependent on methods.

There are two isoenzymes of SGOT – cytosolic and mitochondrial isoenzymes; SGPT also has cytosolic and mitochondrial isoenzymes, but SGPT often is commonly believed to be entirely cytosolic owing to the higher proportion of cytosolic to mitochondrial isoenzyme.

Table 2.2 broadly summarizes these patterns of change for the major classes of damage seen in or confused with cardiac toxicity.

*Table 2.2* Differentiation based on serum enzyme findings for major classes of cardiac damage and related/confounding events

| Condition | SGOT | SGPT | CPK | LDH |
|---|---|---|---|---|
| Myocardial cell death (infarct) | Increased | No change | Increased | Increased |
| Congestive heart failure (liver congestion) | Increased | Increased | No change | Increased |
| Muscle necrosis | Increased | No change | Increased | Increased |
| Lung embolism | No change | No change | Minimal increase | Increased |

Note
SGOT, serum glutamic–oxaloacetic transaminase; SGPT, serum glutamic–pyruvic transaminase; CPK, creatine phosphokinase; LDH, lactate dehydrogenase.

## Other proteins

Plasma albumin acts as a marker of plasma volume following cardiac damage; changes may simply reflect edema or plasma volume differences following congestive cardiac failure. Plasma albumin can be measured by dye-binding methods or more specific immunoassays. Plasma protein electrophoresis can confirm decreased plasma albumin levels and detect changes of other protein fractions. Serial plasma protein electrophoretic measurements may be useful in monitoring inflammatory processes, but changes are not specific for cardiac damage.

Plasma myoglobin can be used as a marker of myocardial damage, but the changes of plasma myoglobin occur more rapidly than those observed for plasma CPK. The myoglobin structure varies between different vertebrates, and the amino acid sequence imparts varying immunogenic properties, thus preventing the use of some latex agglutination and radioimmunoassay methods with certain species. Again, myoglobinemia may be caused by disease processes other than cardiovascular disorders.

Plasma fibrinogen is a useful measurement, particularly in the assessment of thrombolytic agents and episodic thrombolysis. Chromogenic substrates designed for human plasma fibrinogen assays do not react identically with samples from other species, and some assays for determining fibrin degradation products do not work with all species.

## Lipids

As markers of lipid metabolism, plasma lipids are indicators of potential risks for cardiotoxicity in contrast to some of the preceding markers, which directly or indirectly reflect cardiac tissue damage. In rabbits fed cholesterol-enriched vegetable oil, the relationship between hyperlipidemia and the resulting lesions of the aorta and coronary arteries were demonstrated over 70 years ago. Whereas hypolipidemic agents are designed to prevent atherosclerosis, some drugs may inadvertently moderate or modify metabolic pathways for lipid, lipoproteins, or apolipoproteins (through biliary secretion or lipid surface receptors). Adverse effects on lipid metabolism can be monitored by measuring plasma total cholesterol and triglycerides, with additional measurements of plasma lipoproteins, total lipids, phospholipids, apolipoproteins, and non-esterified fatty acids.

Plasma lipid patterns vary with age, sex, diet, and the period of food withdrawal prior to collection of blood samples. There are both qualitative and quantitative differences in the lipid metabolism of different laboratory animal species; these occur because of differences in the rates and routes of absorption, synthesis, metabolism, and excretion. In the rat, ferret, dog, mouse, rabbit, and guinea pig, the major plasma lipoprotein classes are the high-density lipoproteins, contrasting with old-world monkeys and humans, in which the low-density lipoproteins are the major lipoproteins in plasma.

For a more thorough review of the expected ranges for clinical chemistries in model species and their interpretation, one should consult Loeb and Quimby,[22] Evans,[23] Wallach,[24] or Mitruka and Rawnsley.[25]

## Pathology

As with plasma chemistries, major considerations in the use of anatomic pathology as a tool for detecting and evaluating cardiotoxicity are associated with sampling (i.e. how many sections are to be taken and from where). Histopathology is generally a terminal measure (the exception being the use of *in situ* biopsy techniques such as those proposed by Fenoglio and Wagner[26]), so the time point for study termination governs whether a lesion will have had time to develop and whether its interpretation will not be complicated by subsequent (after the injury of interest) events. Similarly, it is of concern how representative sections will be taken from collected tissues.

The heart shares a primary property with the nervous system, having cells with electrically excitable membranes, a potentially vulnerable target for toxins. These membranes are coupled to an intracellular contraction system and two properties, excitation and contraction, have high energy requirements. The heart has the highest energy demands on a weight basis of any organ in the body and requires a continued supply of oxygen to support aerobic metabolism. Oxygen supply and utilization are therefore another area of vulnerability. To clarify the basic principles of cardiac toxicology, the heart can simply be considered as an oxygen-dependent mass of contractile cells driven by excitable membranes that are subject to neurohumoral control. As a result, cardiotoxicity may be caused secondary to alterations in oxygen transport or neurohormonal release.

Cardiotoxicity is a relatively infrequent adverse observation in humans because of the "weeding" out of potential cardiotoxic materials during preclinical testing of drugs. However, a large number of compounds of potential therapeutic value in cardiovascular or neurologic disease are administered at high doses to animals in drug development studies and cardiotoxicity may frequently be encountered. The vast majority of effects are acute, transient functional responses, and are reversible if the animal does not die. These functional responses include bradycardia, tachycardia, and various forms of arrhythmia, and like their equivalents in the nervous system these "cardiotoxicities" are generally considered to be exaggerated pharmacologic effects.

In many of the best-studied cases of functional abnormalities, the mechanism is related to alterations in the ion shifts across the cell membrane (sarcolemma) that are used in the action potential. Digitalis and related cardiotonic chemicals are probably toxic by inhibiting membrane $Na^+/K^+/Ca^{2+}$-ATPase, which maintains the normal transcellular gradients of these ions. Other chemicals disturbing ion shifts across the cell membrane are tetrodotoxin, tetraethyl ammonium, and verapamil, which reduce the inflow of $Na^+$, $K^+$, and $Ca^{2+}$ respectively. Other toxins are thought to act on intracellular sites. Heavy metals alter mitochondrial function and may depress the energy production vital to excitation–contracting coupling. The depression of cardiac contractility by halothane may be related in part to inhibition of myosin ATPase activity. Thus, there are many potential intracellular mechanisms by which toxins may interfere with excitation–contraction coupling to produce functional abnormalities. Many cardiotoxic agents probably interfere with this process at several sites.

### Cardiomyopathy

In contrast to the frequent occurrence of functional effects, relatively few cardiotoxic agents cause structural changes in the heart. When effects are noted, they are usually characterized by degeneration followed by inflammation and repair. These lesions are designated cardiomyopathies. Myocardial (cardiac) necrosis is the most frequently studied cardiomyopathy. In principle, this can result indirectly by disturbance of the blood supply to the myocyte (hypoxic injury) or by direct chemical insult to the myocyte (cytotoxic injury) or by a combination of both effects. The end result, necrosis, is essentially the same, but the location of the lesion may differ. Hypoxic injury tends to affect fairly specific sites, whereas cytotoxic injury may be more widespread.

The classic cardiotoxic drugs which cumulatively cause congestive cardiomyopathy are the anthracycline anti-cancer/antibiotic drugs, exemplified by doxorubicin and daunomycin. For these, with continued dosing, there is widespread vacuolization of the intracellular membrane-bound compartments and mitochondrial degeneration occurring in a cumulative dose-responsive manner.[19]

Bronchodilators and vasodilators are the compounds classically producing site-specific necrosis. One or a few doses of isoproterenol produce acute cardiac necrosis in rat heart with a striking tendency for the subendocardial regions at the apex of the left ventricle. The vasodilator hydralazine acutely produces similar lesions; in beagles, the apex of the left ventricular papillary muscles is the favored site. Continued administration of hydralazine does not increase the incidence or severity of the lesions, and the initial acute lesions heal by fibrosis. Such acute cardiomyopathies could easily be missed in long-term studies, unless specific connective tissue stains (such as aniline black, Masson trichromal, van Gieson, or PTAH; for details, see Luna[27]) are used to highlight the fibrosis.

The pathogenetic mechanism of this site-specific necrosis is not totally understood, but myocardial hypoxia probably plays an important role. Vasodilation may lower coronary perfusion and tachycardia increases oxygen demand. As the capillary pressure is lowest subendocardially, this area is at most risk to oxygen deprivation. The papillary muscles supporting the forces on the valves have the greatest oxygen requirement and are similarly at risk. The sites of injury are thus consistent with the hypothesis of myocardial hypoxia. Acute cardiac necrosis produced by vasoactive drugs can be considered to be the result of an exaggerated pharmacologic effect.

Myocardial hypoxia depletes intracellular high-energy phosphate stores required to maintain membrane ion shifts. Disturbances of $Ca^{2+}$ transport lead to increased cytosolic $Ca^{2+}$, increasing the adenosine triphosphate (ATP) breakdown already initiated by hypoxia. Calcium overload ultimately leads to cell death. Histologically, the dead myofibers have homogeneous eosinophilic cytoplasm (hyaline necrosis) and shrunken or fragmented nuclei. The subsequent inflammatory infiltrate consists mainly of macrophages, with healing by fibrosis.

Cytotoxic injury is often chronic, in contrast to the acute lesion caused by vasodilators. The lesions resulting from antineoplastic anthracycline antibiotics such as daunorubicin and doxorubicin frequently appear several months after the start of therapy. The clinical picture is generally a chronic congestive cardiomyopathy. Morphologically, the two main features are cardiac dilatation and myofiber degeneration. The degeneration consists of myofibrillar loss, producing lightly stained cells, and vacuolation due to massive dilatation of the sarcoplasmic reticulum. At the ultrastructural level, many cellular components are affected. A similar chronic dose-related cardiomyopathy with congestive failure can be produced in animal models, and in rabbits the lesions tend to be distributed around blood vessels. The pathogenesis of the anthracycline cardiomyopathy is unclear.

Chronic cardiomyopathies can be produced by cobalt and brominated vegetable oils. Cobalt-induced cardiomyopathy was first discovered among heavy beer drinkers in Canada. Vacuolation, swelling, loss of myofibrils, and necrosis occur in experimentally poisoned rats and are found mainly in the left ventricle. Cobalt ions can complex with a variety of biologically important molecules and the potential sites for toxicity are numerous.

The cardiotoxicity of brominated vegetable oils is not characterized by necrosis, but by fat accumulation affecting the whole myocardium. Focal necrosis may occur in the more severely affected hearts. The hearts of rats treated with brominated cottonseed oil show a dose-related reduction in the ability to metabolize palmitic acid, probably accounting for the accumulation of lipid globules in the myofibers.

### *Cardiac hypertrophy*

An increase in the mass of heart muscle is occasionally found in toxicity studies. This is usually a compensatory response to an increase in workload of the heart, and in compound-related cases this is usually secondary to effects on the peripheral vasculature. Primary cardiac effects are rare, but can be produced by hormones such as growth hormones.

Pigment deposits in the heart are a common feature of aging animals. These aging pigments occur in lysosomes in the perinuclear regions of the sarcoplasm, and in extensive cases the heart appears brown at necropsy. This condition is known as brown atrophy. Food coloring pigment such as Brown FK may also accumulate in a similar manner and in routine hematoxylin and eosin (H&E) sections is impossible to differentiate from the lipofuscin of aging animals.

## Vasculature

Chemically induced lesions in blood vessels are uncommon except for local reactions to intravenous injections. Systemic effects generally affect the smaller muscular arteries and arterioles and the various lesions encountered are encompassed by the general diagnosis of arteriopathy.

There are several ways to produce arteriopathy, but the lesions generally follow a similar course. In acute lesions, the initial change is hyaline or fibrinoid degeneration of the intima and media. The increased eosinophilia seen histologically may be due to insudation of plasma proteins, necrosis of medial smooth muscle cells, or both. An inflammatory response often follows and the lesion may be described as an acute arteritis. Repair of the lesion is by proliferation of medial myofibroblasts extending into the intima.

The two best-known pathways of vascular injury are hemodynamic changes and immune complex deposition. Acute arterial injury can result from rapid marked hemodynamic changes produced by the exaggerated pharmacologic effects of high doses of vasoactive agents. The bronchodilators and vasodilators producing cardiac necrosis may also cause an arteritis in the dog heart, often in the right atrium. Agents producing vasoconstriction or hypertension such as norepinephrine or angiotensin infusion also produce lesions in small arteries in various regions of the body. Lesions also follow alternating doses of vasodilators and vasoconstrictors. The evidence suggests that a combination of plasma leakage due to physical effects on endothelial cells and acute functional demands on the smooth muscle cells plays an important role in the pathogenesis of these acute lesions.

Immune complex lesions such as vasculitis or hypersensitivity angitis have similar features to hemodynamic lesions, but tend to favor small vessels; therefore, fibrinoid change may be less conspicuous. In animals, immune complex lesions are produced most readily by repeated injection of foreign serum proteins.

Arteriopathies dominated by the proliferative component have been reported in women taking oral contraceptives. The lesions consist mainly of fibromuscular intimal thickenings with little or no necrosis or leukocyte infiltrations. Vascular lesions can also be produced in mice chronically dosed with steroid hormones.

## Hemorrhage

Blood may escape from vessels because of defects in clotting factors, platelets, or the vessel wall, either singly or in combination. Clotting factor and platelet defects lead to hemorrhage by preventing effective closure of an injured vessel. Hemorrhage due to direct injury of the vessel wall by chemicals is infrequent except as a local toxic effect. The most common form of chemically induced hemorrhage (purpura) is the widespread minor leakages that sometimes occur in the skin and mucous membranes in association with allergic vasculitis.

Hemorrhage is also a common artifact in animals that are dying (agonal artifact) or as a consequence of postmortem techniques. Hemorrhages in the germinal centers of the mandibular lymph node and thymic medulla are observed frequently in rats killed by intraperitoneal injection of barbiturates. These hemorrhages appear as red spots on the surface of the organ. Large areas of hemorrhage may occur in the lungs of rats killed by carbon dioxide inhalation, which may confound the interpretation of inhalation toxicity studies. Pulmonary hemorrhage may also occur in animals killed by physical means such as decapitation or cervical dislocation.

A much more complete discussion of the histopathology of drug and chemically induced cardiac disease can be found in Balazs and Ferrans[28] or Bristow.[29]

## Animal models

No review of the approaches used to identify and characterize cardiotoxic agents in industry would be complete without consideration of which animal models are used and what their strengths and weaknesses are.

Table 2.3 presents a summary of baseline values for the common parameters associated with cardiovascular toxicity in standard toxicity studies. These are presented for the species that see a degree of regular use in systemic toxicity studies (rat, mouse, dog, miniature swine, rabbit, guinea pig, ferrets, and two species of primates).

Major considerations in the use of the standard animal models to study cardiovascular toxicity are summarized as follows:[30]

| | |
|---|---|
| Rat | Very resistant to development of atherosclerosis; classic model for studying hypertension as some strains are easily induced. |
| Rabbit | Sensitive to microvascular constriction induced by release of epinephrine and norepinephrine. |
| Dog | Resistant to development of artherosclerosis. |
| Swine | Naturally developing high incidence of artherosclerosis; for this reason, a preferred model for study of the disease. |
| Primates | The rhesus is sensitive to the development of extensive artherosclerosis following consumption of high-cholesterol diets. |

More details on species, handling characteristics, and experimental techniques can be found in Gad and Chengelis.[31] There are also some special considerations when sudden cardiac death is a potential concern.[32]

## *In vitro* models and their use

*In vitro* models, at least as screening tests, have been with us in toxicology for some 20 years now. The last 5–10 years have brought a great upsurge in interest in such models. This increased interest is due to economic and animal welfare pressures, as well as technologic improvements. This is particularly true in industry, and cardiotoxicity is one area where *in vitro* systems have found particularly attractive applications.

Table 2.3 Baseline (normal) values for parameters potentially related to cardiac toxicity

| Species | HR (beats/min) | BP (systolic/diastolic) | CPK (±U l⁻¹) | SGOT (±U l⁻¹) | LDH (±U l⁻¹) | SGPT (±U l⁻¹) |
|---|---|---|---|---|---|---|
| Rat | 350–400 | 116/90 | $5.6 \pm 1.3$ | $200 \pm 152$ | $106 \pm 78$ | $42.2 \pm 3.0$ |
| Mouse | 300–750 | 113/81 | $3.7 \pm 1.5$ | $350 \pm 108$ | | $98 \pm 22$ |
| Dog (beagle) | 100–130 | 148/100 | $1.2 \pm 1.1$ | $31 \pm 7$ | $68 \pm 37.85$ | $21.7 \pm 8.4$ |
| Primate | 150–300 | 159/127 | 2.06–6.3 | $26.1 \pm 9.4$ | 100–446 | $14.5 \pm 8$ |
| (Cynomolgus rhesus) | | | 22–53 | $27 \pm 7$ | 43–426 | $42.1 \pm 21.2$ |
| Rabbit | 120–300 | 110/80 | 1.76 | $44 \pm 26$ | $104.8 \pm 30$ | $35 \pm 16$ |
| Ferret | 200–255 | 152/117 | | $95 \pm 52$ | $608 \pm 45.6$ | $208 \pm 217$ |
| Guinea pig | 260–400 | 77/47 | $0.95 \pm 0.2$ | $48 \pm 9.5$ | | $44.6 \pm 7.0$ |
| Swine | 58–86 | 128/95 | | $8.2 \pm 21.6$ | 96–160 | 9–17 |

Notes
Values are ± one standard deviation.
HR, heart rate; BP, blood pressure.
See references 28 and 29.

As predictive systems of the specific target organ toxicity case of cardiotoxicity, any *in vitro* system having the ability to identify those agents with a high potential to cause damage in a specific target organ at physiologic concentrations would be extremely valuable.

The second use of *in vitro* models is largely specific. This is to serve as tools to investigate, identify, and/or verify the mechanisms of action for selective target organ toxicities. Such mechanistic understandings then allow one to know whether such toxicities are relevant to humans (or to conditions of exposure to humans), to develop means either to predict such responses while they are still reversible or to form the means to intervene in such toxicosis (i.e. first aid or therapy), and finally potentially to modify molecules of interest to avoid unwanted effects while maintaining desired properties (particularly important in drug design). Such uses are not limited to studying chemicals, drugs, and manufactured agents; they can also be used in the study of such diverse things as plant, animal, and microbial toxins, which may have commercial, therapeutic, or military applications or implications[33] because of their cardiotoxicity.

There is currently much controversy over the use of *in vitro* test systems. Will they find acceptance as "definitive test systems," or will they only be used as preliminary screens for such final tests? Or, in the end, will they not be used at all? Almost certainly, all three of these cases will be true to some extent. Depending on how the data generated are to be used, the division between the first two is ill defined at best.

Before trying to answer these questions definitively in a global sense, each of the end-points for which *in vitro* systems are being considered should be overviewed and considered against the factors outlined up to this point.

Substantial potential advantages exist in using an *in vitro* system in toxicologic testing. These advantages include isolation of test cells or organ fragments from homeostatic and hormonal control, accurate dosing, and quantitation of results. It should be noted that, in addition to the potential advantages, *in vitro* systems *per se* also have a number of limitations that can contribute to their not being acceptable models. Findings from an *in vitro* system that either limit their use in predicting *in vivo* events or make them totally unsuitable for the task include wide differences in the doses needed to produce effects or differences in the effects elicited.

Tissue culture has the immediate potential to be used in two very different ways by industry. First, it has been used to examine a particular aspect of the toxicity of a compound in relation to its toxicity *in vivo* (i.e. mechanistic or explanatory studies). Second, it has been used as a form of rapid screening to compare the toxicity of a group of compounds for a particular form of response. Indeed, the pharmaceutical industry has used *in vitro* test systems in these two ways for years in the search for new potential drug entities: as screens and as mechanistic tools.

Mechanistic and explanatory studies are generally called for when a traditional test system gives a result that is either unclear or for which the relevance to the real life human exposure is doubted. *In vitro* systems are particularly attractive for such cases because they can focus on very defined single aspects of a problem or pathogenic response, free of the confounding influence of the multiple responses of an intact higher level organism. Note, however, that first one must know the nature (indeed the existence) of the questions to be addressed. It is then important to devise a suitable model system that is related to the mode of toxicity of the compound.

One must consider what forms of markers are to be used to evaluate the effect of interest. Initially, such markers have been exclusively morphologic (in that there is a change in microscopic structure), observational (is the cell/preparation dead or alive or has some gross characteristic changed), or functional (does the model still operate as it did before). Recently, it has become clear that more sensitive models do not just generate a single end-point type of data, but rather a multiple set of measures that, in aggregate, provide a much more powerful set of answers.

There are several approaches to *in vitro* cardiotoxicity models. The oldest is that of the isolated organ preparation. Perfused and superfused tissues and organs have been used in physiology and pharmacology since the late nineteenth century. There is a vast range of these available, and a number of them have been widely used in toxicology (Mehendale[34] presents an excellent overview). Almost any end-point can be evaluated, and these are the closest to the *in vivo* situation and therefore generally the easiest from which to extrapolate or conceptualize. Those things that can be measured or evaluated in the intact organism can largely also be evaluated in an isolated tissue or organ preparation. The drawbacks or limitations of this approach are also compelling, however.

An intact animal generally produces one tissue preparation. Such a preparation is viable generally for a day or less before it degrades to the point of being useless. As a result, such preparations are useful as screens only for agents that have rapidly reversible (generally pharmacologic or biochemical) mechanisms of action. They are superb for evaluating mechanisms of action at the organ level for agents that act rapidly – but not generally for cellular effects or for agents that act over the course of more than a day.

The second approach is to use tissue or organ culture. Such cultures are attractive because they maintain the ability for multiple cell types to interact in at least a near physiologic manner. They are generally not as complex as the perfused organs but are stable and useful over a longer period of time, increasing their utility as screens somewhat. They are truly a middle ground between the perfused organs and the cultured cells.

The third and most common approach is that of cultured cell models. These can be either primary or transformed (immortalized) cells, but the former have significant advantages in use as predictive target organ models.[35] Such cell culture systems can be utilized to identify and evaluate interactions at the cellular, subcellular, and molecular level on an organ- and species-specific basis.[35] The advantages of cell culture are that single organisms can generate multiple cultures, the cultures are stable and useful for protracted periods of time, and effects can be

*Table 2.4* Representative *in vitro* test systems for cardiovascular toxicity

| System[a] | End-point | Evaluation | Reference |
|---|---|---|---|
| Coronary artery smooth muscle cells (S) | Morphological evaluation: vacuole formation | Correlates with *in vivo* results | 36 |
| Isolated perfused rabbit or rat heart (M, S) | Functional: operation, electrophysiologic, biochemical, and metabolism | Long history of use in physiology and pharmacology | 34 |
| Isolated superfused atrial and heart preparations (S, M) | Functional: operational and biochemical | Correlation with *in vivo* findings for antioxidants | 37, 38 |
| Myocytes (S, M) | Functional and morphological | Correlates well with *in vivo* results on a local concentration basis | 39, 40 |

Note
a Letters in parentheses indicate primary employment of system: (S), screening system; (M), mechanistic tool.

studied very precisely at the cellular and molecular level. The disadvantages are that isolated cells cannot mimic the interactive architecture of the intact organ and will respond over time in a manner that becomes decreasingly representative of what happens *in vivo*. An additional concern is that, with the exception of hepatocyte cultures, the influence of systemic metabolism is not factored in unless extra steps are taken. Any such cellular systems would be more likely to be accurate and sensitive predictors of adverse effects if their function and integrity were evaluated while they were operational.

A wide range of target organ-specific models have already been developed and utilized. Their incorporation into a library-type approach requires that they be evaluated for reproducibility of response, ease of use, and predictive characteristics under the intended conditions of use. These evaluations are probably at least somewhat specific to any individual situation. Table 2.4 presents an overview of representative systems for cardiovascular toxicity. Not mentioned in this table are any of the new co-culture systems in which hepatocytes are "joined up" in culture with a target cell type to produce a metabolically competent cellular system.

## Summary

Presented here is an overview of current approaches and the state of the art for detecting and characterizing cardiotoxicity in industrial toxicology studies. This is a field that as yet, even in pharmaceutical companies, is not considered separate from the general case characterization of systemic toxicity. It depends on some very fixed tool sets to deal with both functional and structural toxicities. When the entire suite of methodology as presented here is used, it has performed very well (as judged by cardiotoxicity not being a frequent finding for products properly used and/or handled in humans). However, incremental improvements are under way in the field, utilizing some of the technologies presented elsewhere in this volume.

## References

1. Connolly HM, Crary JL, McGoon MD, Hensrud DD, Edwards BS, Edwards WD and Schaff HV. Valvular heart disease associated with fenfluramine-phentermine, *NEJM* 1997; 337: 581–588.
2. Van Stee EW. Cardiovascular toxicology: foundations and scope. In: Van Stee EW, ed. *Cardiovascular Toxicology*. New York: Raven Press, 1982; 1–34.
3. Balazs T, Hanig JP and Herman EH. Toxic responses of the cardiovascular system. In: Klaassen CD, Amdur MO and Doull J, eds. *Casarett and Doull's Toxicology: the Basic Science of Poisons*. New York: Macmillan, 1986; 387–411.
4. Smith TL, Koman LA and Mosberg AT. Cardiovascular physiology and methods for toxicology. In: Hayes AW, ed. *Principles and Methods in Toxicology*. New York: Raven Press, 1994; 917–935.

5. Brunner H and Gross F. Cardiovascular pharmacology. In: Zbinden G and Gross F, eds. *Pharmacologic Methods in Toxicology*. Oxford: Pergamon Press, 1979; 63–99.

6. Gilman AG, Rall JW, Nies AS and Taylor P. *The Pharmacological Basis of Therapeutics*. New York: Pergamon Press, 1990; 749–896.

7. Walker MJA and Pugsley MK. *Methods in Cardiac Electrophysiology*. Boca Raton, FL: CRC Press, 1998.

8. Watkinson WP, Brice MA and Robinson KS. A computer-assisted electrocardiographic analysis system: methodology and potential application to cardiovascular toxicology. *J Toxicol Environ Health* 1985; 15: 713–727.

9. Sodeman WA and Sodeman TM. *Pathologic Physiology*. Philadelphia: Saunders, 1979.

10. Doherty JD and Cobbe SM. Electrophysiological changes in an animal model of chronic cardiac failure. *Cardiovasc Res* 1990; 24: 309–316.

11. Atta AG and Vanace PW. Electrocardiographic studies in the *Macaca mulatta* monkey. *Ann NY Acad Sci* 1960; 85: 811–818.

12. Hamlin R. Extracting "more" from cardiopulmonary studies on beagle dogs. In: Gilman MR, ed. *The Canine as a Biomedical Model*. Bethesda, MD: American College of Toxicology and LRE, 1985; 9–15.

13. Goodman JS and Peter CT. Proarrhythmia: primum non nocere. In: Mandel WJ, ed. *Cardiac Arrhythmias: their Mechanisms, Diagnosis and Management*. Philadelphia: J.P. Lippincot Company, 1995; 173–179.

14. Vatner SF, Patrick TA and Murray PA. Monitoring of cardiovascular dynamics in conscious animals. In: Van Stee EW, ed. *Cardiovascular Toxicology*. New York: Raven Press, 1982; 35–55.

15. Garner D and Laks MM. New implanted chronic catheter device for determining blood pressure and cardiac output in the conscious dog. *Physiology* 1985; 363: H681–H685.

16. Webster JG. *Medical Instrumentation*. New York: John Wiley & Sons, 1998.

17. Riccardi MJ, Beohar N and Davidson CJ. Coronary catheterization and coronary angiography. In: Rosendorf C, ed. *Essential Cardiology*. Philadelphia: W.B. Saudners, 204–226.

18. Gad SC. A neuromuscular screen for use in industrial toxicology. *J Toxicol Environ Health* 1982; 9: 691–704.

19. Scheulen ME and Kappus H. Anthracyclines as model compounds for cardiac toxicity. In: Dehart W and Neumann HG, eds. *Tissue-specific Toxicity*. New York: Academic Press, 1992.

20. Clampitt RB and Hart RJ. The tissue activities of some diagnostic enzymes in ten mammalian species. *J Comp Pathol* 1978; 88: 607–621.

21. Lindena J, Sommerfeld U, Hopfel C and Traukschold I. Catalytic enzyme activity concentration in tissues of man, dog, rabbit, guinea pig, rat and mouse. *J Clin Chem Clin Biochem* 1986; 24: 35–47.

22. Loeb WF and Quimby FW. *The Clinical Chemistry of Laboratory Animals*. New York: Pergamon Press, 1989.

23. Evans GO. Biochemical assessment of cardiac function and damage in animal species. *J Appl Toxicol* 1991; 11: 15–22.

24. Wallach J. *Interpretation of Diagnostic Tests*. Boston: Little, Brown & Company, 1978.

25. Mitruka BM and Rawnsley HM. *Clinical Biochemical and Hematological Reference Values in Normal Experimental Animals.* New York: Masson, 1977.

26. Fenoglio JJ and Wagner BM. Endomyocardial biopsy approach to drug-related heart disease. In: Hayes AW, ed. *Principles and Methods of Toxicology.* New York: Raven Press, 1989; 649–658.

27. Luna L.G. *Manual of Histological Staining Methods of the Armed Forces Institute of Pathology.* New York: McGraw-Hill, 1968.

28. Balazs T and Ferrans JJ. Cardiac lesions induced by chemicals. *Environ Health Perspect* 1978; 26: 181–191.

29. Bristow MR. *Drug-induced Heart Disease.* New York: Elsevier, 1980.

30. Calabrese EJ. *Principles of Animal Extrapolation.* New York: Wiley, 1983.

31. Gad SC and Chengelis CP. *Animal Models in Toxicology.* New York: Marcel Dekker, 1991.

32. Chan PS and Cervoni P. Current concepts and animal models of sudden cardiac death for drug development. *Drug Dev Res* 1990; 19: 199–207.

33. Werdan K, Melnitzki SM, Pilz G and Kapsner T. The cultured rat heart cell: a model to study direct cardiotoxic effects of *Pseudomonas* endo- and exotoxins. In: *Second Vienna Shock Forum.* New York: Alan R Liss, 1989; 247–251.

34. Mehendale HM. Application of isolated organ techniques in toxicology. In: Hayes AW, ed. *Principles and Methods of Toxicology.* New York: Raven Press, 1989; 699–740.

35. Acosta D, Sorensen EMB, Anuforo DC, Mitchell DB, Ramos K, Santone KS and Smith MA. An in vitro approach to the study of target organ toxicity of drugs and chemicals. *In Vitro Cell Dev Biol* 1985; 21: 495–504.

36. Ruben Z, Fuller GC and Knodle SC. Disobutamide-induced cytoplasmic vacuoles in cultured dog coronary artery muscle cells. *Arch Toxicol* 1984; 55: 206–212.

37. Gad SC, Leslie SW, Brown RG and Smith RV. Inhibitory effects of dithiothreitol and sodium bisulfite on isolated rat ileum and atrium. *Life Sci* 1977; 20: 657–664.

38. Gad SC, Leslie SW and Acosta D. Inhibitory actions of butylated hydroxytoluene (BHT) on isolated rat ileal, atrial and perfused heart preparations. *Toxicol Appl Pharmacol* 1979; 48: 45–52.

39. Leslie SW, Gad SC and Acosta D. Cytotoxicity of butylated hydroxytoluene and butylated hydroxyanisole in cultured heart cells. *Toxicology* 1978; 10: 281–289.

40. Low-Friedrich I, Bredow F and Schoeppe W. *In vitro* studies on the cardiotoxicity of chemotherapeutics. *Exp Chemother* 1990; 36: 416–421.

# 3

# EVALUATION OF *IN VITRO* CYTOTOXICITY MODELING

*Enrique Chacon,\* John M. Bond,†*
*and John J. Lemasters‡*

*\*CEDRA Corporation, Austin, TX, USA; †Riverside*
*Veterinary Hospital, Rocky Mount, NC, USA; and*
*‡The Department of Cell Biology and Anatomy,*
*School of Medicine, University of North Carolina*
*at Chapel Hill, Chapel Hill, NC, USA*

## Overview

The ever-increasing number of chemical compounds synthesized by chemical and pharmaceutical industries has prompted the development of research methods for rapid cytotoxicity screening. In addition, public concern about pain and suffering to animals has encouraged toxicologists to develop substitute approaches for toxicity assessment. Present research efforts are directed at developing a series of *in vitro* assays that could serve as reliable, reproducible, and inexpensive alternatives to *in vivo* animal testing. In recent years, new approaches show promise for effective and inexpensive toxicity assessment that will minimize use of animals and that will increase the selection of lead candidate compounds. *In vitro* methods for toxicity assessment need to provide reproducible and informative data that are equivalent to accepted methods using live animals, such as the median lethal dose ($LD_{50}$). $LD_{50}$ testing is expensive, consumes large numbers of animals, and has been criticized as inhumane. Optional approaches have been suggested and are beginning to be adopted by manufacturers of pharmaceuticals, pesticides, cosmetics, and household products to reduce the number of animals used in toxicity screening. To validate the use of *in vitro* models for cytotoxicity assessments, attempts should be made to standardize methodology and, more importantly, to define criteria for lethality assessment. In this review, we present some new ideas and methodologies that may aid in increasing the effectiveness and efficiency of cytotoxicity assessments.

## *Credence of a model*

Validation of *in vitro* methods is needed to justify their use as *in vitro* alternatives to animal testing. Validation requires that assay results be reproducible between laboratories and that they provide informative data that are equivalent and similar to current accepted animal tests. The following criteria should be met: (1) the *in vitro* assay correlates well with the *in vivo* biologic response being modeled; (2) the *in vitro* assay has a biologic basis which links it to the cell injury process; and (3) the *in vitro* assay should be technically reliable and reasonably easy to conduct. Most methods currently under development meet some but not all of these criteria. The most promising models for *in vitro* toxicity studies are cells in culture. Numerous reports using cell culture models have shown relevance of cell culture models to *in vivo* toxicity.[1–10] Unfortunately, experimental design differences between laboratories hamper comparison of data, even for the same cell type and test agent. Here, we discuss ways to minimize the variability between laboratories. In addition, we present an alternative approach modeled after the progression of the cell injury process itself. In particular, we address issues of cardiotoxicology and the use of primary cultures of cardiac myocytes to investigate potential cardioactive agents. However, the same principles developed for heart cells may be applied to cells derived from other tissues.

### Problems in defining criteria for cytotoxicity assessment

Validation of cell culture systems as *in vitro* models for cytotoxicity assessment requires consensus as to criteria. These criteria are still being defined. As Cook and Mitchell[11] write: "The term 'cellular viability' and the diverse assays used to determine viability can strongly influence the interpretation of experimental results." In essence, different laboratories have a tendency to favor specific assay methods and express varying degrees of cytotoxicity using such terms as integrity, viability, cell survival, cell killing, irreversible cell injury, and cytotoxicity. The assignment of a particular end-point assay to the assessment of these terms is as varied as the terms themselves (Table 3.1). As we discuss below, an understanding of what cell death is helps to clarify the meaning of various assays of cell viability.

Viability assays have been referred to as permeability assays, functional assays, reproductive assays, and morphologic assays. Morphologic assays are usually limited to specific situations and, in general, have less utility than other assays. Permeability assays estimate failure of the plasma membrane permeability barrier that represents irreversible cell injury. Functional assays typically evaluate a state of impairment, be it reversible or not. The assumption is that cellular dysfunction may result in irreversible cell damage. Functional approaches may aid in identifying beneficial effects as well as toxic ones. Reproductive assays (usually colony-forming assays) estimate cellular proliferation. Because cardiac myocytes are generally not proliferating cells, increased cellular proliferation of cardiac cells would suggest potential for tumor formation by a xenobiotic. However, reproductive assays may be used to estimate toxicity to myocardial endothelial cells that normally do proliferate. In general, a reproductive assay may be considered a functional assay because cellular proliferation would be a characteristic function of a particular cell type.

*Table 3.1* Cytotoxicity assays

| Assays | Assessments | References |
|---|---|---|
| Permeability | | |
| Dye exclusion | Plasma membrane integrity | 2, 7, 12, 13 |
| Dye inclusion | Plasma membrane integrity | 2, 14 |
| LDH release | Plasma membrane integrity | 2, 3, 15–17 |
| [51]Cr release | Plasma membrane integrity | 18 |
| Functional | | |
| ATP, ADP, and AMP | Cellular energy capacity | 19–21 |
| Mitochondrial membrane potential | Cellular energy capacity | 2, 7, 13, 19, 22 |
| Succinate dehydrogenase activity (MTT assay) | Cellular energy capacity (mitochondrial integrity) | 2, 17, 19, 23–34 |
| Ion gradients | Ionic homeostasis | 2, 13, 19, 25–26 |
| Protein synthesis | Cellular synthesis capacity | 23 |
| DNA synthesis | Cellular synthesis capacity | 21 |
| Gene expression | Changes in signal transduction | 4, 27, 28 |
| Neutral red uptake | Lysosomal integrity | 2, 23 |
| Cardiac beating activity | Changes in electrical conductivity | 2, 6, 8, 29 |
| Colony formation | Infinite cell division capacity | 30, 31 |
| Growth rates | Cellular proliferation | 32 |
| Blebbing | Changes in plasma membrane structure | 2, 12, 17, 20 |
| Volume | Osmotic changes | 2, 9, 33 |

Assays for cytotoxicity assessment may be reduced to those that measure cellular functions and those that measure cell death. Functional assays typically evaluate reversible events. Conversely, cell death assays evaluate irreversible changes. Figure 3.1 illustrates a matrix of cellular events and respective assays that can be applied to assess cytotoxic responses. The complexity of interrelated cellular functions illustrated in this scheme emphasizes that functional assays reflect mechanisms of xenobiotic-induced cytotoxicity. Current approaches in cytotoxicity assessment often use narrowly focused end-points. Some authors have suggested that a battery of *in vitro* tests should be used to assess relative toxicity of potential toxicants.[23,34] The practical utility of a battery of assays becomes limited in high-volume screening comparisons. However, a clear understanding of cytotoxic mechanisms is important in the overall *in vitro* cytotoxicity profile of xenobiotics and may require specialized techniques and equipment not routinely available to all toxicologists.

### *Approaches for modeling cytotoxicity*

Cytotoxicity assessment should be based on events associated with the cell injury process itself. Ideal end-point parameters should evaluate a single common event.

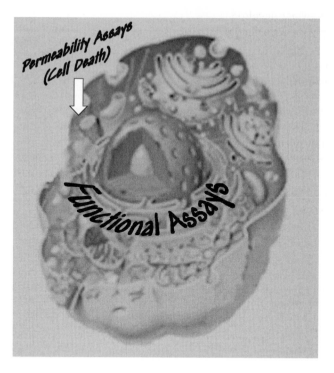

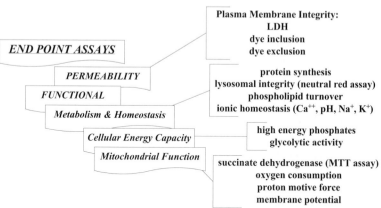

*Figure 3.1 In vitro* approaches for cytotoxicity assessment. Xenobiotic-induced toxic responses cause functional impairments leading to loss of cellular viability. Loss of cellular viability (cell death) is associated with breakdown of the plasma membrane. Functional impairments reflect alterations in cellular metabolism, homeostasis, and tissue-specific responses. Functional parameters associated with cellular homeostasis can be further divided to reflect sites of toxicant action. Functional assays may be too narrowly focused to make generalized cytotoxicity assessments. However, identification of xenobiotic-induced alterations in cell functions provide insights into the mechanisms underlying the cytotoxicity of toxicants.

Cell death (loss in cell viability) is a common irreversible event. By definition, viability is the state or quality of being alive. Importantly, the point at which cells lose viability should be defined, as events occurring after cell death are no longer relevant to the mechanisms critical to toxicity. Cell death is a rapid event, initiated by rupture of the plasma membrane and is coincident with the onset of irreversible injury.[13,35,36] Hence, cell death is an abrupt all-or-nothing event. Breakdown of the sarcolemma represents a permanent change in plasma membrane function and results in loss of cellular enzymes and ionic homeostasis such that normal physiology cannot be maintained.

The progression of irreversible injury and death of cells in a population is not synchronous; many minutes to hours may pass between the death of the first cell and the last one. This characteristic progression of cell death is observed *in vivo*, in isolated organs, and in cells in culture. Figure 3.2 illustrates the typical sigmoidal

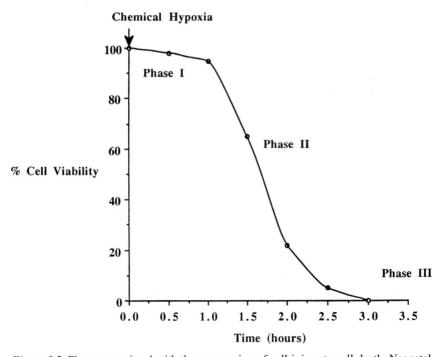

*Figure 3.2* Phases associated with the progression of cell injury to cell death. Neonatal rat cardiac myocytes were exposed to 2.5 mM NaCN (mitochondrial respiratory inhibitor) and 20 mM 2-deoxyglucose (glycolytic inhibitor) to mimic the ATP depletion and reductive stress associated with anoxia (chemical hypoxia). Cell death was monitored by increases in propidium iodide fluorescence measured with a multiwell fluorescence scanner. The progression of cell injury is represented by three separate phases. Phase I represents an initial lag phase in which the population of cells maintains plasma membrane integrity. Phase II represents the rate of cell killing. Phase III is the completion of phase II, where all cells have lost plasma membrane integrity.

progression of loss in cell viability in cultured neonatal rat cardiac cells exposed to toxic chemicals. Three distinct phases can be recognized. Phase I is an initial lag phase before any loss of viability occurs. Phase II starts as cells begin to lose viability. Phase III is the completion of phase II, indicating that all cells have lost viability. Alterations of functional parameters such as metabolism, ion homeostasis, membrane potentials, and so on that occur during the lag phase (phase I) may be critical to the mechanisms of toxic action. Onset of cell killing (phase II) following these functional impairments can suggest cause and effect relationships. By definition, cell death is an injury from which there is no recovery. Recently, techniques have become available to assess viability of cells cultured in multiwell plates, thus allowing a large number of samples to be screened.

The time-course of lethal cell injury can provide insights into mechanisms of cytotoxicity. Figure 3.3 illustrates killing curves for different toxicants that act by distinct mechanisms of action. Digitonin, a surfactant, causes rapid cell killing without a lag phase (curve A). NaCN and 2-deoxyglucose are respiratory and

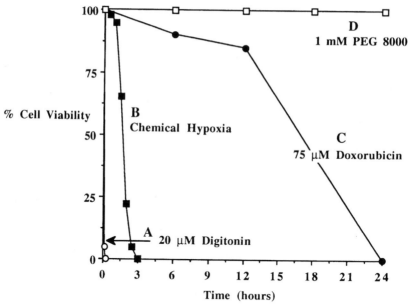

*Figure 3.3* Toxicity screening using multiple time point determinations. Cultured neonatal rat cardiac myocytes were exposed to different forms of insult and the rates of cell killing were estimated by monitoring the release of the cytosolic marker enzyme lactate dehydrogenase. Direct plasma membrane damage was accomplished using 20 μM digitonin (curve A). Chemical hypoxia causing ATP depletion was obtained using 2.5 mM NaCN with 20 mM 2-deoxyglucose (curve B). The cardioselective xenobiotic doxorubicin (75 μM) was used in curve C. Polyethylene glycol 8000 (1 mM) was used as a negative control (curve D). Note the differences in the lag phase before cell killing (phase I) and the rates of cell killing (phase II) for each agent.

glycolytic inhibitors that mimic the ATP depletion and reductive stress of anoxia ("chemical hypoxia"). Chemical hypoxia typically produces cell killing after a lag time of about an hour, and killing is complete after about 3 h (curve B). Doxorubicin is an anti-tumor agent that is cardiotoxic. Doxorubicin toxicity has a lag time of 12 h, but after 24 h virtually all cells have lost viability (curve C). Finally, curve D illustrates the response to the non-toxic agent PEG 8000. These curves illustrate that toxicants acting by different mechanisms have different characteristic killing curves. One cannot say that doxorubicin is less cytotoxic than digitonin or NaCN plus 2-deoxyglucose, because the different toxicants act by different mechanisms. Digitonin acts directly on the plasma membrane to initiate cell killing without any lag phase. NaCN plus 2-deoxyglucose initiate cell killing after a relatively short lag phase, whereas doxorubicin has a long lag phase. However, after 24 h, the toxic outcome is the same. These examples illustrate the importance of multiple time point readings in the assessment of potential toxicants. No single time point can adequately assess the pattern of cell killing caused by the various toxicants.

It is also insufficient to make measurements at a single concentration of test agent. Dose–response curves or a kill range of toxic activity are needed. Dose–response curves of well-characterized reference toxicants should be used as a basis for comparison with unknown test agents. This type of approach requires a high-volume/high-capacity assay for efficient screening. The use of 96-well plates and multiwell plate readers makes such an approach technically feasible. Further refinement of the test paradigm might include washout of the test substance after a short period of time (1–3 h) to mimic the *in vivo* transit time of a xenobiotic.

For reproducibility between laboratories, it is important that incubation buffers, oxygen and $CO_2$ concentrations, pH, and temperature be maintained relatively constant. pH of the incubation buffer is particularly important as even mild acidosis protects cells against many forms of chemical insult.[26,37–39] Accordingly, care must be taken when evaluating compounds with acid or basic salts. Cell culture medium containing serum may reduce cytotoxicity if the test agent binds to albumin or other serum proteins. However, some xenobiotics may require serum to gain access to the cell. Variability between laboratories probably cannot be avoided entirely. Thus, it is essential that laboratories make comparisons to well-characterized toxicants. In this way, relative toxicity of unknown agents can be determined without reference to reproducible standards.

## Primary heart cell cultures for cytotoxicity screening

Many investigators use cell cultures as *in vitro* models to evaluate the toxicity of xenobiotics.[40,41] The progression of injury in primary cell cultures is usually similar to *in vivo* models. The onset of irreversible injury *in vivo* or in cultured cell monolayers is a time-dependent event. In cell culture models, the time dependence of cell injury can be identified after both acute and chronic exposures. Cell culture systems permit assessment of cellular responses that are technically difficult *in vivo*. In particular, cardiac cell culture systems have served to further our understanding of the cellular and molecular basis of myocardial cell injury.[20,40] Several cell culture systems are available. Nearly all utilize hearts from the chick, rat, or rabbit as the source of tissue. Hearts are separated mechanically and enzymatically into a heterogeneous suspension of muscle and non-muscle cells. Separation of muscle from non-muscle cells is usually achieved by rate of attachment to cell culture dishes[42] or by centrifugal elutriation.[43] Non-muscle cell cultures are generally a mixture of endothelial cells and fibroblasts. It has been argued that cells in culture rely predominantly on glycolysis as their energy supply, a change from the β-oxidation characteristic of muscle cells *in vivo*. However, experiences from our laboratories with cultured heart cells indicate that mitochondrial metabolism is preserved in cultured myocytes and serves as a vital source of energy. In addition, cardiac cells in culture will utilize β-oxidation as a major energy source provided that appropriate substrates are present.[44,45] These characteristics make myocardial cell cultures appropriate models for cardiotoxicity assessment. Furthermore, myocardial cell cultures provide informative data with minimal investment of time and expense compared with models utilizing whole organs or live animals.

### Neonatal cardiac myocytes

Newborn rats aged 2–5 days are typically used as a source of cardiac myocytes. Neonatal cardiac myocytes are relatively easy to isolate and can be maintained for weeks in primary culture. To prevent overgrowth of fibroblasts and other cells, myocytes should be purified before culturing. Two methods are routinely used to obtain relatively pure myocyte preparations. The first method is based on the rapid rate of attachment of non-muscle cells to plastic culture dishes.[42] Enzymatic digests of whole hearts are placed in shallow plastic culture dishes. After 2–3 h of plating, more than 90 percent of non-muscle cells will have adhered to the dishes. Non-attached myocytes are then decanted into separate culture dishes. A second method of separating myocytes from non-muscle cells utilizes the technique of centrifugal elutriation.[43] Centrifugal elutriation separates cells based on size. Heart digests are infused into a rotating chamber in a direction against the centrifugal field. Cells remain trapped in the chamber until flow is increased or rotor speed decreased. As the force of flow begins to exceed the force of gravity, cells are eluted from the chamber, with the smallest cells being released first.

Purified neonatal cardiac myocytes are plated at 75 000 cells per well in 96-well plates or $10^6$ cells per 35-mm culture dish. After 3–4 days in culture, a nearly confluent monolayer of spontaneously contracting cells is obtained. Cells isolated by rate of attachment show significant contamination with fibroblasts after 5–6 days in culture. Cells isolated by elutriation show minimal contaminant cell growth, even after 30 days in culture. As metabolism of cultured cells may change over time, we typically use 5- to 8-day cultures of myocytes purified by centrifugal elutriation for cytotoxicity screening.

### Adult cardiac myocytes

In 1972, Chang and Cummings[46] described the cultivation of myocytes from human heart. Since larger and older animal hearts provide a terminally differentiated myocyte that more closely resembles adult human myocytes, much attention has been given to the development of adult cardiac myocyte cultures.[29,47-50] Adult cell isolations frequently demonstrate a "calcium intolerance" that causes isolated rod-shaped cells to hypercontract and lose viability when exposed to physiologic concentrations of calcium. Success in isolating adult cardiac myocytes is dependent on a number of variables. The quality of dissociative enzymes used in the cell isolation process is a major determinant for obtaining viable cells. Lot-to-lot variations of digestive enzyme seem particularly important and give rise to great variations of yield and viability. Other important variables include perfusion pressure, digestion time, temperature, electrolyte balance, and method of physical dispersion after perfusion. The difficulty of reliably obtaining large numbers of cardiac myocytes from adult sources has limited their use in cytotoxicity screening.

As in neonatal cell preparations, special attention must be given to the purity of myocardial cell cultures. Overgrowth of fibroblasts and other non-muscle cells can occur within 3–5 days in culture. Mitotic inhibitors, such as cytosine arabinoside, are frequently used to restrict contamination by fibroblasts and endothelial cells. Unlike neonatal cardiac myocytes, cultured adult cardiac myocytes do not spontaneously contract. However, the cells can be electrically stimulated to duplicate *in vivo* contractile activity. With the continued development of adult cardiac cell isolation techniques, investigators should be able to exploit the strengths of this model to evaluate the potential cardiotoxic effects of xenobiotics.

## Cytotoxicity assessment

### Sarcolemma breakdown

The basis of permeability assays is that bulky charged molecules normally cannot diffuse into and out of cells. Common cellular permeability assays are based on dye exclusion (uptake of trypan blue or propidium iodide), dye inclusion [retention of calcein or biscarboxyethyl-carboxyfluorescein (BCECF)], and leakage of cytoplasmic enzymes (lactate dehydrogenase).

### Dye exclusion assays

Various dye exclusion studies are used to assess plasma membrane integrity. The classic dye exclusion test utilizes trypan blue.[14] Cells are incubated with trypan blue, and blue nuclear staining is assessed by conventional optical microscopy. The trypan blue assay is reliable and relatively easy, but it is also time consuming and labor intensive. Thus, the trypan blue exclusion assay is not well suited to cytotoxicity screening. Fluorescent DNA-binding assays are an alternative to the trypan blue assay. Propidium iodide and ethidium bromide homodimer are fluorescent cationic compounds that are excluded from viable cells. After cell lysis of the plasma membrane, these dyes bind to double-stranded DNA of the nucleus. As they bind, the dyes exhibit a red shift and an increase in fluorescence emission, changes which can be used to quantitate loss of viability in large populations, as first shown in cell suspensions.[37] Fluorescent DNA-binding assays can also be applied to cells cultured in 96-well microtiter plates using a multiwell fluorescence scanner.[51-53] Advantages of DNA-binding assays are that measurements can be made continuously over time from the same cells in a non-destructive manner. With a multiwell fluorescence scanner, the assay has a high degree of statistical accuracy, is easy to perform, and can be used to screen large numbers of samples. Thus, these techniques are particularly well suited to cytotoxicity screening. However, as in any fluorescence assay, suitable controls must be performed to ensure that test agents are not fluorescent and do not cause other interferences with the fluorescence of propidium iodide or ethidium bromide.

### Cytosolic enzyme release

Release of lactate dehydrogenase is also commonly used to monitor loss of cell viability of cells in culture.[15,16,54,55] Enzyme activity is estimated from the conversion of NADH to NAD after pyruvate addition from the rate of decrease in 340-nm absorbance.[16] Lactate dehydrogenase can also be measured in 96-well microtiter plates using an enzyme-linked immunosorbent assay (ELISA) reader. This is particularly helpful for high-volume/high-capacity cytotoxicity screening.[56] Results can be expressed in international units of enzyme activity or percent of total releasable enzyme. Permeabilization with digitonin (20–30 µM) is a useful way to release total cellular content of lactate dehydrogenase that is more reliable and reproducible than cell scraping and sonication.[7,19,37] Utilizing an ELISA reader interfaced with a computer with kinetic software, large numbers of samples can be analyzed with minimal effort. As lactate dehydrogenase is a sulfhydryl-dependent enzyme, control experiments should ascertain that the test agent does not directly inhibit lactate dehydrogenase.

### Evaluation of data from permeability assays

To determine the concentration of toxicant that results in a specific response (e.g. 50 percent loss in cell viability; $V_{50}$), toxicologists rely on mathematical models to fit the data. Fitting of a line or curve to a set of data points is usually accomplished by some method of regression analysis. The simplest method is that of linear regression. However, dose–response curves rarely fit a linear model. Rather, dose–response curves are usually sigmoidal. Methods based upon logarithmic scales and probability (probit analysis) are commonly used to transform the data to log scales, which are then subjected to linear regression.[57]

The approach we use is based on logistic regression analysis (a form of probit analysis).[52,58,59] Logistic regression determines whether a subject is in one group or another. We are trying to estimate the probability that a given cell in a population of cells is either dead or alive. Thus, we use a dummy variable that takes on values of 0 (live) and 1 (dead) as the dependent variable. The probability of the event occurring is $P$, whereas the probability of the event not occurring is $1 - P$. The odds that an event will occur is:

$$O = P / 1 - P \qquad (3.1)$$

where $O$ is odds. In our case, $P$ equals the proportion of viable cells ($V$). Using a *logit* transformation:

$$\log O = \log(V / 1 - V) \qquad (3.2)$$

As $V$ is the average of a large population of cells, our dummy variable will have a binomial distribution with mean of $V$ and variance of $V(1 - V)$, provided that a cell can only be alive (0) or dead (1). Continuing the analysis, $\log(V / 1 - V)$ is plotted on the $y$-axis versus the log of the toxicant concentration along the $x$-axis. After fitting by linear regression, the $x$ intercept represents the concentration of toxicant causing 50 percent loss of cell viability ($V_{50}$). As illustrated in Figure 3.4 for cultured cardiac myocytes exposed to doxorubicin, $V_{50}$ was estimated in this way to be 34.2 µM.

### *Mechanistic investigations*

#### *Contractile activity*

Functional tests should be appropriate for the characteristic cell type. For neonatal myocytes, a simple and effective functional test is the rate of spontaneous contractions.[6,60,61] Beating rates are relatively easy to measure microscopically and are reproducible provided the temperature remains constant. In contrast, cultured adult cardiac myocytes exhibit little to no spontaneous contractions.

#### *Cellular energy supply*

The main energy supply of the heart is mitochondrial β-oxidation of fatty acids. Since heart tissue utilizes ATP at high rates, toxicant-induced changes of reactants (ATP) and enzymes (e.g. succinate dehydrogenase, and glucose-6-phosphate dehydrogenase) in high-energy phosphate metabolism are important to overall cardiotoxicity. For example, 50 µM doxorubicin exposure of cardiac myocyte cultures resulted in an inhibition of glucose-6-phosphate dehydrogenase (E. Chacon, R.G. Ulrich and D. Acosta, unpublished observations) concomitant with decreased ATP levels.[19] Other assays to estimate cellular energy capacity include

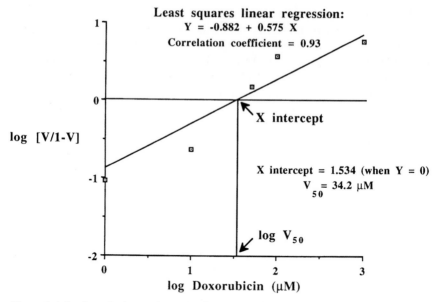

*Figure 3.4* Logit analysis to estimate $V_{50}$ for doxorubicin after 24 h in neonatal rat cardiac myocytes. The concentration of doxorubicin required to kill 50 percent ($V_{50}$) of the myocytes after 24 h was estimated at 34.2 μM by solving for the *x* intercept when $y = 0$.

measurements of mitochondrial respiratory enzymes such as succinate dehydrogenase activity (MTT assay), oxygen consumption, and mitochondrial membrane potential. Estimation of mitochondrial membrane potential and the MTT assay are discussed in the following sections as both of these assays have been suggested for cytotoxicity screening.

### SUCCINATE DEHYDROGENASE ACTIVITY (MTT ASSAY)

The MTT assay has been widely used to assess cell viability.[17,24] The MTT assay is a colorimetric reaction that measures the ability of a cell to reduce 3-(4,5-dimethylthiazole-2-yl)-2,5-diphenyltetrazolium bromide (MTT) to a blue formazan product. The assay is based on the assumption that only live cells can reduce MTT to MTT-formazan. The enzymatic reduction of MTT is catalyzed by mitochondrial succinate dehydrogenase. Hence, the MTT assay is dependent on mitochondrial respiration and indirectly serves to assess the cellular energy capacity of a cell. Moreover, formation of MTT-formazan is easily measured with multiwell plate readers,[24] making the MTT assay suitable for high-volume/high-capacity cytotoxicity screening.

### MITOCHONDRIAL MEMBRANE POTENTIAL

Rhodamine 123, a cationic fluorescent probe, distributes into negatively charged compartments in accordance with the Nernst equation: [22,62,63]

$$\Delta\psi = -60 \log(F_{in}/F_{out}) \tag{3.3}$$

where $\Delta\psi$ is membrane potential in mV and $F_{in}$ and $F_{out}$ are fluorophore concentrations inside and outside the compartment. The validity of this method for estimating electrical potential depends on ideal behavior of the fluorophore. However, many fluorescent cationic dyes, including rhodamine 123, quench when taken up into mitochondria and show non-specific binding independent of the electrical potential.[22,64] Correction factors may be applied to adjust for these effects, but each correction introduces a new degree of uncertainty to overall precision and accuracy. Other fluorophores, such as tetramethylrhodamine methyl ester, seem to lack these undesirable qualities and may be more suited to monitoring mitochondrial membrane potential.[62,65–67]

We have used laser scanning confocal microscopy to measure electrical potentials inside cultured myocytes.[66,67] Confocal microscopy creates images representing a thickness through the cell approaching 0.5 μm. In conventional fluorescence microscopy, depth of field is much greater and light from out-of-focus planes degrades image resolution. In confocal microscopy, the smaller depth of field and rejection of out-of-focus light combine to produce images that are remarkably detailed. The improved resolving power of confocal microscopy permits measurement of the Nernstian distribution of cationic fluorophores. Based on the intensity of fluorescence inside cells, electrical potentials are estimated using the Nernst equation and displayed in pseudocolor. Thus, a functional parameter such as $\Delta\psi$ can provide informative mechanistic data relating to potential functional and structural alterations that are not apparent in the sarcolemmal breakdown assay (Figure 3.1, phase I).

### HYDROGEN ION GRADIENTS

Because increasing evidence targets the mitochondria as sites of insult by xenobiotics,[3,19] it is likely that the importance of measurements of mitochondrial function for toxicologic research will only increase. The high energy state that drives ATP synthesis, ion transport, and many other energy-requiring reactions in mitochondria is the electrochemical difference of protons across the inner mitochondrial membrane ($\Delta\mu H^+$).[69,70] $\Delta\mu H^+$ comprises two components, a charge difference or membrane potential ($\Delta\psi$) and a concentration difference or pH gradient ($\Delta pH$), where:

$$\Delta\mu H^+ = \Delta\psi + 60 \, \Delta pH \tag{3.4}$$

Confocal microscopy measurements of cells loaded with tetramethylrhodamine methyl ester to measure $\Delta\psi$ and seminaphthorhodafluor (SNARF)-1 to measure $\Delta pH$ allows both components of $\Delta\mu H^+$ to be evaluated within mitochondria of living cells.[66,67] SNARF-1 is a single-excitation dual-emission fluorophore that can be calibrated against hydrogen ion concentrations by comparing its emission spectral shifts ratios. SNARF-1 is loaded into cells using its lipid-soluble acetoxymethyl ester derivative. Inside the cell, the pH-sensitive free acid is liberated by endogenous esterases. SNARF-1 is similar to other ion-sensitive fluorophores in that it does not load exclusively into the cytosol. In particular, mitochondria possess esterases and may load heavily with ion-reporting probes.[7,19,71–73] Measurements of hydrogen ion gradients serve to define mechanisms of cytotoxicity.

As fluorescence microscopy examination of xenobiotic-induced functional changes often evaluates only a single cell, these types of functional assays are often inappropriate as initial assessments of cytotoxicity. Hence, high-volume/high-capacity screening is not possible in fluorescence microscopy. However, the new technologies in fluorescence microscopy provide powerful tools to investigate mechanisms of toxicant actions.

### Calcium homeostasis

The role of calcium in the regulation of various cell functions has been an area of intense investigation.[74] Therefore, it is not surprising that a great deal of interest has been directed at studying alterations in intracellular calcium and how such effects may contribute to the cell injury process.[19,75–78] Alterations of calcium by toxicants may perturb the regulation of cellular functions beyond the normal range of physiologic control. Intracellular calcium overload has been proposed to result in the loss of high-energy phosphates.[79] Other cytotoxic effects proposed by calcium overload are blebbing of the plasma membrane,[80] activation of calcium-dependent phospholipases,[81] stimulation of calcium-dependent neutral proteases,[82] calcium-activated DNA fragmentation,[83,84] and the production of intracellular reactive oxygen species.[3] However, reports have shown that irreversible cell damage can occur without changes in cytosolic calcium.[25,77,85]

The development of selective calcium fluorophores[86] has facilitated quantitation of intracellular calcium levels using digitized fluorescence imaging.[7,12,19,25] However, interpretation of the results may be misleading as the dyes have been shown to sequester within intracellular organelles.[7,19,71–73] In particular, mitochondria sequester the dyes when loaded as their ester derivatives. Efforts to minimize subcellular sequestration must be taken if a cytosolic estimation of calcium is required. Mere changes in intracellular calcium do not serve as reliable indicators of cytotoxicity. For example, beating myocardial cells are continuously fluctuating in cytosolic calcium. In addition, hormones have been shown to increase cytosolic calcium without detectable injury.[75] Considering the complex physiologic roles of cellular calcium, one cannot say that increases in cytosolic calcium are potentially lethal. Increased levels of cytosolic calcium may be an effect of alterations in homeostatic capacity rather than the cause of cell death. Assessments of intracellular calcium may serve as adjunct tests in evaluating mechanisms of actions. Fluorescence microscopy estimates of intracellular calcium are effective in mechanistic investigations but are limited in high-volume/high-capacity cytotoxicity screening.

## Summary and conclusions

Cell culture models are promising alternatives that will minimize the use of animals and reduce the burden of cost of bringing new products to the market place. *In vitro* cell culture models may be developed to fulfill validation objectives in cytotoxicity assessment. Cytotoxicity assays should have a biologic basis that links them to the cell injury process; they should be technically reliable and easy to conduct, and must correlate with the *in vivo* biologic response being modeled. In the preceding sections, we reviewed different assays that could be used to assess potential cytotoxic responses of cells in culture. Assays based on alterations of physiologic functions for initial cytotoxicity screening are inefficient for initial cytotoxicity screening. In the heart, necrosis is the event leading to long-lasting and permanent impairment of cardiac function and reserve. Therefore, it is logical to undertake initial cytotoxicity assessments based on the occurrence of cell death. Cell death is an abrupt all-or-nothing phenomenon that occurs as the consequence of abrupt breakdown of the plasma membrane. Cell killing can be easily quantitated using multiwell readers. Differing lag times and rates of cell killing are characteristic of toxicants acting by different mechanisms. Thus, it is necessary to evaluate the kinetics of cell killing over times as long as 24 h to establish dose dependency of cell killing. Comparison with known cytotoxic agents serves as a basis for evaluating the relative toxicity of unknown test agents. Once the dose and time dependencies of toxic action are established, mechanistic studies based on functional assays can proceed to identify the molecular and cellular basis for toxicant action.

## Acknowledgments

This work was supported, in part, by grants AG07218 and DK30874 from the National Institutes of Health, grant N00014-89-J-1433 from the Office of Naval Research, Procter and Gamble, Upjohn Laboratories, and a Burroughs Wellcome Scholar in Toxicology Award to D.A. E.C. was a recipient of a National Research Service Award through grant T32ES07126 to the University of North Carolina at Chapel Hill, Curriculum in Toxicology, from the National Institute of Environmental Health Sciences.

## References

1. Ohata H, Chacon E, Tesfai SA, Harper IS, Herman B and Lemasters JJ. Mitochondrial $Ca^{2+}$ transients in caridac myocytes during the excitation–contraction cycle: effects of pacing and hormonal stimulation. *J Bioenerg Biomembr* 1998; 30: 207–222.
2. Chacon E, Acosta D and Lemasters JJ. Primary cultures of cardiac myocytes as in vitro models for pharmacological and toxicological assessments. In: Castell JV and Gomez-Lechon MJ, ed. *In Vitro Methods in Pharmaceutical Research.* New York: Academic Press, 1997; 209–223.

3. Chacon E and Acosta D. Mitochondrial regulation of superoxide by calcium: an alternate mechanism for the cardiotoxicity of doxorubicin. *Toxicol Appl Pharmacol* 1991; 107: 117.

4. Ito H, Miller SC, Billingham ME, Akimoto H, Torti SV, Wade R, Gahlmann R, Lyons G, Kedes L and Torti FM. Doxorubicin selectively inhibits muscle gene expression in cardiac cells in vivo and in vitro. *Proc Natl Acad Sci USA* 1990; 87: 4275.

5. Shirhatti MG, Chenery R and Krishna G. Structural requirements for inducing cardiotoxicity by anthracycline antibiotics: studies with neonatal rat cardiac myocytes in culture. *Toxicol Appl Pharmacol* 1986; 84: 173.

6. Acosta D, Wenzel DG and Wheatley JW. Beating duration of cultured rat heart cells as affected by drugs and other factors. *Pharmacol Res Commun* 1974; 6: 263.

7. Nieminen A-L, Gores GJ, Dawson TL, Herman B and Lemasters JJ. Toxic injury from mercuric chloride in rat hepatocytes. *J Biol Chem* 1990; 265: 2399.

8. Acosta D and Puckett M. Ischemic myocardial injury in cultured heart cells: preliminary observations in morphology and beating activity. *In Vitro* 1977; 13: 818.

9. Gores GJ, Flarsheim CE., Dawson TL. Nieminen A-L, Herman B and Lemasters JJ. Swelling, reductive stress, and cell death during chemical hypoxia in hepatocytes. *Am J Physiol* 1989; 257: C347.

10. Ramos K, Combs AB and Acosta D. Role of calcium in isoproterenol cytotoxicity to cultured myocardial cells. *Biochem Pharmacol* 1984; 33: 1989.

11. Cook JA and Mitchell JB. Viability measurements in mammalian cell systems. *Anal Biochem* 1989; 179: 1.

12. Lemasters JJ, DiGuiseppi J, Nieminen A-L and Herman B. Blebbing, free $Ca^{2+}$ and mitochondrial membrane potential preceding cell death in hepatocytes. *Nature* 1987; 325: 78.

13. Tolnai S. A method for viable cell count. *Proc Man* 1975; 1: 37.

14. Leeder JS, Dosch H-M, Harper PA, Lam P and Spielberg SP. Fluorescence-based viability assays for studies of reactive drug intermediates. *Anal Biochem* 1989; 177: 364.

15. Ramos K and Acosta D. Prevention by 1-(1) ascorbic acid of isoproterenol-induced cardiotoxicity in cultured primary cultures of rat myocytes. *Toxicology* 1983; 26: 81.

16. Mitchell DB, Santone KS and Acosta D. Evaluation of cytotoxicity in cultured cells by enzyme leakage. *J Tissue Cult Methods* 1980; 6: 113.

17. Hsieh GC and Acosta D. Dithranol-induced cytotoxicity in primary cultures of rat epidermal keratinocytes. *Toxicol Appl Pharmacol* 1991; 107: 16.

18. Goodman HS. A general method for the quantitation of immune cytolysis. *Nature* 1961; 190: 269.

19. Chacon E, Ulrich R and Acosta D. A digitized fluorescence imaging study of mitochondrial calcium increase by doxorubicin in cardiac myocytes. *Biochem J* 1992; 281: 871.

20. Bond JM, Herman B and Lemasters JJ. Recovery of cultured rat neonatal myocytes from hypercontracture after chemical hypoxia. *Res Commun Chem Pathol Pharmacol* 1991; 71: 195.

21. Wettermark G, Stymne H, Brolin SE and Petersson B. Substrate analyses in single cells. *Anal Biochem* 1975; 63: 293.

22. Emaus RK, Grunwald R and Lemasters JJ. Rhodamine 123 as a probe of transmembrane potential in isolated rat-liver mitochondria: spectral and metabolic properties. *Biochim Biophys Acta* 1986; 880: 436.

23. Bruener LH, Kain DJ, Roberts DA and Parker RD. Evaluation of seven in vitro alternatives for ocular safety testing. *Fundam Appl Toxicol* 1991; 17: 136.

24. Carmichael J, DeGraff WG, Gazdar AF, Minna JD and Mitchell JB. Evaluation of a tetrazolium-based semiautomated colorimetric assay: assessment of chemosensitivity testing. *Cancer Res* 1987; 47: 936.

25. Swann JD, Ulrich R and Acosta D. Lack of changes in cytosolic ionized calcium in primary cultures of rat kidney cortical cells exposed to cytotoxic concentrations of gentamicin: a fluorescent digital imaging method for assessing changes in cytosolic ionized calcium. *Toxicol Methods* 1991; 1: 161.

26. Gores GJ, Nieminen A-L, Wray BE, Herman B and Lemasters JJ. Intracellular pH during "chemical hypoxia" in cultured rat hepatocytes: protection by intracellular acidosis against the onset of cell death. *J Clin Invest* 1989; 83: 386.

27. Maki A, Berezesky IK, Fargnoli J, Holbrook NJ and Trump BF. Role of $[Ca^{2+}]_i$ in induction of c-fos, c-jun, and c-myc mRNA in rat PTE after oxidative stress. *FASEB J* 1992; 6: 919.

28. Edwards MJ, Dykes PJ, Donovan MRO, Merrett VR, Morgan HE and Marks R. Induction of heat shock proteins as a measure of chemical cytotoxicity. *Toxicol In Vitro* 1990; 4: 270.

29. Welder AA, Grant R, Bradlow J and Acosta D. A primary culture system of adult rat heart cells for the study of toxicologic agents. *In Vitro Cell Dev Biol* 1991; 274: 921.

30. Hayflick L. The limited in vitro lifetime of human diploid cell strains. *Exp Cell Res* 1965; 37: 614.

31. Hill RP and Stanley JA. The lung-colony assay: extension to the lewis lung tumor and the B16 melanoma-radiosensitivity of B16 melanoma. *Int J Radiat Biol* 1975; 27: 377.

32. Roper PR and Drewinko B. Comparison of in vitro methods to determine drug-induced cell lethality. *Cancer Res* 1976; 36: 2182.

33. Sanger JW and Sanger JM. Surface and shape changes during cell division. *Cell Tissue Res* 1980; 209: 177.

34. Frazier JM, Gad SC, Goldberg AM and McCulley JP. A critical evaluation of alternatives to ocular irritation testing. In: *Alternative Methods in Toxicology*, Vol. 4. New York: Liebert, 1987.

35. Herman B, Nieminen A-L, Gores GJ and Lemasters JJ. Irreversible injury in anoxic hepatocytes precipitated by abrupt increase in plasma membrane permeability. *FASEB J* 1988; 2: 146.

36. Herman B, Gores GJ, Nieminen A-L, Kawanishi T, Harman A and Lemasters JJ. Calcium and pH in anoxic and toxic injury. *Crit Rev Toxicol* 1990; 21: 127.

37. Gores GJ, Nieminen A-L, Dawson TL, Herman B and Lemasters JJ. Extracellular acidosis delays the onset of cell death in ATP-depleted hepatocytes. *Am J Physiol* 1988; 255: C315.

38. Acosta D and Li CP. Actions of extracellular acidosis on primary cultures of rat myocardial cells deprived of oxygen and glucose. *J Mol Cell Cardiol* 1980; 12: 1459.

39. Pentilla A and Trump BF. Extracellular acidosis protects Ehrlich tumor cells and rat renal cortex against anoxic injury. *Science* 1974; 185: 272.

40. McQuenn CA. *In Vitro Toxicology: Model Systems and Methods.* New Jersey: Telford Press, 1989.

41. Acosta D, Sorensen EM, Anuforo DC, Mitchell DB, Ramos K, Santone KS and Smith MA. An in vitro approach to the study of target organ toxicity of drugs and chemicals. *In Vitro Cell Dev Biol* 1985; 21: 495.

42. Wenzel DG, Wheatley JW and Byrd GD. Effects of nicotine in cultured heart cells. *Toxicol Appl Pharmacol* 1970; 17: 774.

43. Ulrich RG, Elliget KA and Rosnick DK. Purification of neonatal rat cardiac cells by centrifugal elutriation. *J Tissue Cult Methods* 1989; 11: 217.

44. Spahr R, Jacobson SL, Siegmund B, Schwartz P and Piper HM. Substrate oxidation by adult cardiomyocytes in long-term primary culture. *J Mol Cell Cardiol* 1989; 21: 175.

45. Probst I, Spahr R, Schweickhardt C, Hunneman DH and Piper HM. Carbohydrate and fatty acid metabolism of cultured adult cardiac myocytes. *Am J Physiol* 1986; 250: H853.

46. Chang TD and Cummings GR. Chronotropic responses of human heart tissue cultures. *Circ Res* 1972; 30: 628.

47. Jacobson SL. Cultures of spontaneously contracting myocardial cells from adult rats. *Cell Struct Funct* 1977; 2: 1.

48. Spieckermann PG and Piper HM. *Isolated Adult Cardiac Myocytes.* New York: Steinkopff Verlag Darmstadt, 1978.

49. Haworth RA, Hunter DR and Berkoff HA. The isolation of $Ca^{2+}$-resistant myocytes from the adult rat. *J Mol Cell Cardiol* 1980; 12: 715.

50. Haddad J, Decker ML, Hsieh L-C, Lesch M, Samarel AM and Decker RS. Attachment and maintenance of adult rabbit cardiac myocytes in primary cell culture. *Am J Physiol* 1988; 255: C19.

51. Nieminen A-L, Gores GJ, Bond JM, Imberti RI, Herman B and Lemasters JJ. A novel cytotoxicity screening assay using a multi-well fluorescence scanner. *Toxicol Appl Pharmacol* in press.

52. Pipsisewa M, Nieminen A-L, Harper RA, Herman B and Lemasters JJ. Cytotoxicity screening of surfactant-based shampoos using a multiwell fluorescence scanner: correlation with draiz eye scores. *Toxicology In Vitro* in press.

53. Nieminen A-L, Gores GJ, Dawson TL, Herman B and Lemasters JJ. Inhibitors of metalloprotease and phospholipase protect against cell death in cultured hepatocytes during chemical hypoxia. *FASEB J* 1991; 3: A626.

54. Acosta D and Ramos K. Cardiotoxicity of tricyclic antidepressants in cultured rat myocardial cells. *J Toxicol Environ Health* 1984; 14: 137.

55. Butler AW, Smith MA, Farrar RP and Acosta D. Ethanol toxicity in primary cultures of rat myocardial cells. *Toxicology* 1985; 36: 61.

56. Chacon E, Acosta D, Bond JM, Nieminen A-L and Lemasters JJ. Procedures for assessment of in vitro cardiotoxicity. In: Nadolney C, ed. *Handbook of In Vitro Toxicology*, Vol. 1. Boca Raton: CRC Press, 1995.

57. Gad SC and Weil CS. Modeling. In: Gad SC and Weil CS, eds. *Statistics and Experimental Design for Toxicologists.* New Jersey: Telford Press, 1986; Ch. 8.

58. Glantz SA and Slinker BK. Regression with a qualitative dependent variable. In: Gantz SA and Slinker BK, eds. *Primer of Applied Regression and Analysis of Variance.* New York: McGraw-Hill, 1990; Ch. 11.

59. Woolson RF. Least-squares regression methods: predicting one variable from another. In: Woolson RF, ed. *Statistical Methods for the Analysis of Biomedical Data*. New York: John Wiley & Sons, 1987; Ch. 9.

60. Butler AW, Farrar RP and Acosta D. The effects of cardioactive drugs on the beating activity of myocardial cell cultures isolated from the offspring of trained versus untrained rats. *In Vitro* 1984; 20: 629.

61. Wenzel DG and Innis JD. Arrhythmogenic and antiarrhythmic effects of lipolytic factors on cultured heart cells. *Res Commun Chem Pathol Pharmacol* 1983; 41: 383.

62. Lemasters JJ, Nieminen A-L, Chacon E, Imberti R, Reece JM and Herman B. Use of fluorescent probes to monitor mitochondrial membrane potential in isolated mitochondria, cell suspensions, and cultured cells. In: Lash LH and Jones DP, eds. *Mitochondrial Dysfunction*. San Diego: Academic Press, 1992.

63. Chen LB. Mitochondrial membrane potential in living cells. *Annu Rev Cell Biol* 1988; 4: 155.

64. Bunting JR, Phan TV, Kamali E and Dowben RM. Fluorescent cationic probes of mitochondria. *Biophys J* 1989; 56: 979.

65. Ehrenberg B, Montana V, Wei M-D, Wuskell JP and Loew LM. Membrane potentials can be determined from the nernstian distribution of cationic dyes. *Biophys J* 1988; 53: 785.

66. Lemasters JJ, Chacon E, Zahrebelski G, Reece JM and Nieminen A-L. Laser scanning confocal microscopy in living cells. In: Herman B and Lemasters JJ, eds. *Optical Microscopy: New Technologies and Applications*. San Diego: Academic Press, 1992; Ch. 11.

67. Chacon E, Reece JM, Nieminen A-L, Zahrebelski G, Herman B and Lemasters JJ. Intracellular distribution of electrical potentials, pH, free $Ca^{2+}$, and cell volume during chemical hypoxia in cultured adult rabbit cardiac myocytes: a multiparameter digitized confocal microscopic study. *Biophys J* 1994; 66: 942.

68. Nieminen A-L, Dawson TL, Gores GJ, Kawanishi T, Herman B and Lemasters JJ. Protection by acidotic pH and fructose against lethal cell injury to rat hepatocytes from mitochondrial inhibitors, ionophores, and oxidant chemicals. *Biochem Biophys Res Commun* 1990; 167: 600.

69. Lemasters JJ. ATP stoichiometries of mitochondrial oxidative phosphorylation: a reevaluation by nonequilibrium thermodynamics. *Comments Mol Cell Biophys* 1985; 3: 99.

70. Smith EL, Hill RL, Lehman IR, Lefkowitz RJ, Handler P and White A. *Biological Oxidations I*. In: Smith EL, Hill RL, Lehman IR, Lefkowitz RJ, Handler P and White A, eds. *Principles of Biochemistry*. New York: McGraw-Hill, 1983; Ch. 15.

71. Lemasters JJ, Nieminen A-L, Gores GJ, Dawson TL, Wray BE, Kawanishi T, Tanaka Y, Florine-Casteel K, Bond JM and Herman B. Multiparameter digitized video microscopy (MDVM) of hypoxic cell injury. In: Herman B and Jacobson KA, eds. *Optical Microscopy for Biology*. New York: Alan R Liss, 1990; 523–542.

72. Steinberg SF, Bilezikian JP and Al-Awqati Q. Fura-2 fluorescence is localized to mitochondria in endothelial cells. *Am J Physiol* 1987; 253: C744.

73. Gunter TE, Restroepo D and Gunter KK. Conversion of esterified fura-2 and indo-1 to $Ca^{2+}$ sensitive forms by mitochondria. *Am J Physiol*, 1988; 255: C304.

74. Carafoli R. Intracellular calcium homeostasis. *Annu Rev Biochem* 1987; 56: 395.

75. Kawanishi T, Nieminen A-L, Herman B and Lemasters JJ. Suppression of $Ca^{2+}$ oscillations in cultured rat hepatocytes by chemical hypoxia. *J Biol Chem* 1991; 266: 20062.

76. Combs A, Acosta D and Ramos K. Effects of doxorubicin and verapamil on calcium uptake in primary cultures of rat myocardial cells. *Biochem Pharmacol* 1985: 34: 1115.

77. Lemasters JJ, Nieminen A-L, Gores GJ, Wray BE and Herman B. Cytosolic free calcium and cell injury in hepatocytes. In: Fiskum G, ed. *Cell Calcium Metabolism.* New York: Plenum Press, 1989; Ch. 48.

78. Trump BF, Berezesky IK, Laiho KV, Osornio AR, Mergner WJ and Smith MW. The role of calcium in cell injury. In: Becker RP and Johari O, eds. *Scanning Electron Microscopy.* Chicago: SEM, 1980; 492.

79. Fleckenstein A, Janke J, Doring HJ and Pachinger O. Calcium overload as the determinant factor in production of catecholamine-induced myocardial lesions. In: Bajusz E and Rona G, eds. *Recent Advances in Studies on Cardiac Structure and Metabolism.* Baltimore: University Park, 1987; 455.

80. Jewell SA, Bellomo G, Thor H, Orrenius S and Smith MT. Bleb formation in hepatocytes during metabolism is caused by disturbances in thiol and calcium homeostasis. *Science* 1982; 217: 1257.

81. Chien KR, Abrams S, Pfarr RG and Farber JL. Prevention by chlorpromazine of ischemic liver cell death. *Am J Physiol* 1977; 88: 539.

82. McConley DJ, Nicotera P, Hartzell P, Bellomo G, Wyllie AH and Orrenius S. Glucocorticoids activate a suicide process in thymocytes through an elevation of cytosolic calcium concentration. *Arch Biochem Biophys* 1989; 269: 365.

83. Cantoni O, Sestili P, Catteberi F, Bellomo G, Pou S, Cohen M and Cerutti P. Calcium chelator quin 2 prevents hydrogen-peroxide-induced DNA breakage and cytotoxicity. *Eur J Biochem* 1989; 182: 209.

84. Jones DP, McConkey DJ, Nicotera P and Orrenius S. Calcium activated DNA fragmentation in rat liver nuclei. *J Biol Chem* 1989; 264: 6398.

85. Swann JD, Ulrich R and Acosta D. Lack of changes in cytosolic calcium in primary cultures of rat kidney cortical cells exposed to cytotoxic concentrations of gentamicin. *Toxicol Appl Pharmacol* 1990; 106: 3.

86. Grynkiewicz G, Poenie M and Tsien RY. A new generation of calcium indicators with greatly improved fluorescence properties. *J Biol Chem* 1985; 260: 3440.

# 4

# MONITORING OF CARDIOVASCULAR DYNAMICS IN CONSCIOUS ANIMALS

*Stephen F. Vatner, Thomas A. Patrick, Amelia B. Kudej,*
*You-Tang Shen, and Kuniya Asai*

*Cardiovascular Research Institute, University of Medicine and*
*Dentistry, New Jersey Medical School, Hackensack, NJ, USA*

The role of a variety of occupational and environmental toxins in the development and progression of cardiovascular disease is of growing public health interest.[1,2] Although the importance of tobacco smoke in the pathogenesis of atherosclerosis is well established, the cardiovascular effects of other potentially important toxins, such as ethanol, cocaine, anthracyclines, and heavy metals, are less well understood. What knowledge we do have is largely a product of observational studies in humans and is, therefore, subject to confounding influences such as self-reporting and selection biases. Apparent associations generated by these observations can be confirmed or refuted, and mechanisms defined, by the use of appropriate experimental animal models in which precise measurements of cardiovascular function can be monitored over an extended period of time.

The goal of this chapter is to describe a number of physiologic monitoring techniques that have been utilized routinely in our laboratory for the chronic and continuous assessment of cardiovascular function in conscious animals. The importance of studying the cardiovascular effects of various agents in conscious, unsedated, and unrestrained animals cannot be overstated. Conscious studies avoid the confounding influences of anesthetics, all of which alter virtually every aspect of circulatory function, including heart rate, the level of myocardial contractile state, vascular resistance in regional beds,[3,4] and, particularly, the control of these parameters by the autonomic nervous system.[5] These techniques also permit sequential studies in the same animals under normal conditions and following the induction of any of a number of cardiac disease states such as hypertrophy, ischemia, and failure.

For many years, studies using conscious, chronically instrumented animals were restricted to larger species such as dogs and pigs. Recent advances in transgenic models have raised interest in carrying out similar studies in smaller species. While the technology does not yet exist to perform studies of the level of complexity routinely carried out in larger species, we are now able to measure accurately a number of cardiovascular parameters in conscious mice. Measurements of intravascular and intracardiac pressures, dimensions, and blood flows represent the fundamental cardiovascular measurements and these are stressed in this chapter.

This chapter is divided into two sections: (1) concerning instrumentation techniques for use in large animal models and (2) those techniques that have been developed more recently for use in smaller murine models. The small animal model techniques have the advantage of lower cost than the large animal model, but the instrumentation needs are more severely constrained as to size, power consumption, and variety of measurement possible. However, they represent a growing influence, particularly with the advent of transgenic murine technology and as more refined measurement approaches are developed, and offer exciting advances in the study of toxicology.

## Large animal techniques for measurement of cardiovascular parameters

### *Arterial and ventricular pressures*

Miniature solid-state pressure transducers can be used routinely for chronic measurement of arterial pressure, as well as pressure in the left[6] (Figure 4.1) and right ventricles.[7] These transducers, which were originally developed by Van Citters and Franklin,[8] have been used in our laboratory for more than three decades[9–11] in studies in unrestrained, conscious dogs,[12] pigs,[13,14] sheep,[15] and primates.[9,11] Solid-state pressure transducers offer a number of advantages over commonly used fluid-filled catheter-strain gauge manometer systems for use in chronic implants. The most important of these are (1) wide frequency, (2) high sensitivity, which facilitates their use with radiotelemetry systems, and (3) relative freedom from signal distortion that occurs in fluid-filled systems from catheter clotting or kinking or acceleration effects upon the fluid system. A pressure transducer must have a high-frequency response in order to reproduce accurately the rapidly changing phases of a pressure signal, such as the leading edge of systole in ventricular pressure. Furthermore, the time derivative of ventricular pressure ($dP/dt$) is often used as an index of cardiac contractility, and to obtain this parameter by analog differentiation the higher-frequency components of the pressure signal must be preserved (Figure 4.1).

The pressure transducer used in our laboratory is a small (5–7 mm diameter, 1 mm thickness), hermetically sealed, cylindrical chamber with a titanium diaphragm, on the back of which are bonded four silicon strain gauge elements arranged in a Wheatstone bridge configuration (Konigsberg Instruments Models P4–P7, Pasadena, CA, USA). The transducer senses pressure changes as a deformation of the diaphragm, which in turn unbalances the bridge and generates an offset signal proportional to the applied pressure. This signal is subsequently

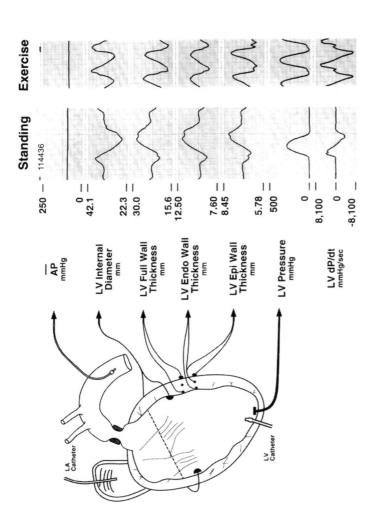

*Figure 4.1* Schematic illustration of the instrumentation used to assess global and regional left ventricular (LV) function. Catheters were implanted in the left atrium and the descending thoracic aorta for pressure measurement and to use the radioactive microsphere technique. Piezoelectric crystals were implanted on opposing subendocardial surfaces of the left ventricle to measure LV diameter. Two sets of three miniature crystals were implanted in the subendocardium, epicardium, and mid-myocardium to measure regional wall motion in the subepicardium, subendocardium, and transmurally. Typical phasic waveforms are shown before exercise (left) and then during exercise (right). Reproduced with permission from Hittinger *et al.*[43]

amplified and recorded as an analog reproduction of the pressure wave. During each experiment, the solid-state transducer undergoes an initial *in vitro* calibration before surgical implantation, and during each experiment is cross-calibrated *in vivo* against a strain gauge transducer connected to fluid-filled, chronically implanted catheters positioned in the aorta, right ventricle, and left atrium. Arterial pressure can be measured by implanting the solid-state transducer in the thoracic or abdominal aorta through a 1- to 2-cm longitudinal incision closed by interrupted sutures. The right ventricular transducer can be inserted through a stab wound in the mid-anterior free wall of the right ventricle, and the left ventricular transducer is most often inserted through a stab wound in the apex of the left ventricle. The ventricular transducers are secured by purse string sutures. As with all implants of this type, the transducer leads are exteriorized through the chest wall and routed subcutaneously to the interscapular area of the animal. The exteriorized transducer leads are protected by shrink tubing and a tear-resistant nylon vest (dogs, pigs, sheep). In intractable animals (e.g. primates), the wires are not externalized but are buried subcutaneously until the time of the experiment.

Several features of the solid-state pressure transducer make it preferable for use in experiments involving radiotelemetry of the pressure signal, although alternative systems using catheters and external strain gauges are available.[16] Fluid-filled pressure transducers are larger in size and quite fragile and, as noted above, are susceptible to distortion artifacts in the pressure signal. For these reasons, the solid-state pressure transducers are well suited to investigations in which the mobility of the animal is of primary importance.

The major disadvantages of implantable solid-state pressure transducers for use in chronic implants are drift in zero offset and sensitivity. These problems become critical because it is impossible at the time of the experiment to calibrate the implanted transducer in terms of absolute pressure. It becomes necessary therefore to cross-calibrate these transducers with a calibrated system when experiments are conducted. An electronic calibration of the overall pressure-measuring system, exclusive of the transducer, is made at the start and at the end of the experiment. The output of the implanted solid-state pressure transducer is then compared with a directly calibrated catheter-strain gauge manometer. This procedure overcomes the problem of changes that may have occurred in the solid-state transducer's transfer function since the last *in vitro* calibration. In our experience, this procedure should be repeated approximately every week for arterial implants, but daily cross-calibration is necessary for experiments in which small variations in zero pressure level are critical (e.g. measurement of intracardiac end-diastolic pressure).

Although there are many problems associated with the measurement of pressures in animals with long-term chronic implants, it is clear that the inherent advantages of the solid-state transducer make it very attractive. Reduction in size of the transducer and cable should eventually allow application to experiments using smaller animals, including mice.

### Blood flow measurements

The electromagnetic and ultrasonic techniques for measuring phasic blood flows in conscious animals are indirect, i.e. blood flow *per se* is not measured. Rather, the effects of moving blood on induced wave energy are transduced to obtain a signal that is proportional to blood flow. The signal obtained is usually small and its use depends on appropriate amplification and simultaneous rejection of extraneous signals. Each technique has both advantages and disadvantages that direct its application to particular types of flow measurements and experimental protocols. The electromagnetic flow technique will be compared with two different ultrasonic approaches, the pulsed Doppler and transit time methods.

### Electromagnetic flow technique

This technique[17,18] is an adaptation of Faraday's law of magnetic induction, using the principle that when flowing blood (a moving conductor) crosses a magnetic field induced through a blood vessel a voltage is generated that is proportional to the blood velocity, the magnetic field strength, and the length of the moving conductor. If the magnetic field strength is constant, the signal from this measurement is considered to be proportional to volume flow. Advantages of the electromagnetic flowmeter include the ability to sense direction of flow and a relative insensitivity to changes in velocity profile. The directional flow-sensing ability is important in experiments involving measurement of blood flow where a component of the flow is retrograde.[19] The insensitivity to velocity profile is important when, for example, coronary blood flow is measured in the presence of a partial coronary artery stenosis. There are several disadvantages of the electromagnetic flowmeter, including variability in the electrical zero, which makes it necessary to establish zero flow mechanically by means of temporary vessel occlusion with a hydraulic occluder. Additionally, the transducers are more massive than the ultrasonic Doppler transducers, which increases the incidence of kinking or occlusion of small vessels (e.g. coronary artery). Finally, the large excitation currents required to establish adequate electrical signals can cause significant localized heating of the vessel and must be chosen with care to minimize vessel damage. For these reasons, electromagnetic flowmeters are of primarily historical importance.

### Doppler ultrasonic flow technique

The Doppler principle for velocity measurement of blood flow, in its various implementations, is an important component in conscious animal instrumentation. The advantage of lightweight, long-lasting transducers and the accurate and stable zero that is independent of the transducer or implant conditions greatly facilitate this technique's use.

The development of the ultrasonic Doppler flowmeter has proceeded from the original, non-directional, continuous wave (CW) implementation to directional CW and, more recently, to pulsed, directional design; the last is the most commonly used device today. All use the common principle that ultrasound reflected from a target (e.g. the moving blood cells) exhibits a shift in frequency proportional to the velocity of the target. Ultrasound is directed diagonally into the bloodstream, and a part of this energy is reflected from moving blood cells. The shift in frequency caused by this process provides an average of the instantaneous velocity profile across the vessel lumen and is determined by extracting the frequency difference between transmitted and reflected sonic waves.

The fact that, at zero velocity, no Doppler shift exists results in a capability for determination of true zero flow at any time by electrical calibration, without the necessity for mechanical occlusion of the vessel. This is an important advantage over the other ultrasonic technique in use (the transit time flowmeter), as well as the electromagnetic flow measurement technique, in that accurate and stable zero determinations can be made at any time without manipulating the vessel under study. A measure of volume flow is determined by knowledge of the average velocity and internal cross-sectional area of the vessel. The relationship between velocity and volume flow has been demonstrated repeatedly and confirmed by means of timed collection of blood[20, 21] and by simultaneous comparison on a left circumflex coronary artery.[22]

The flow transducers are made of lightweight materials, most commonly hinged polystyrene half shells or cast epoxy rings with a small gap to allow the transducer to be placed on the vessel. The function of the transducer is to hold the piezoelectric crystals that generate and detect the ultrasound and to constrain the diameter of the vessel for accurate volume flow determination. Electrical connections to the crystals are made with silver-plated, stranded copper wire, with an implant lifetime of greater than 6 months. For longer chronic implants, stranded stainless-steel wire has been successfully used. The primary disadvantage of the Doppler ultrasonic flowmeter is that the Doppler effect measures velocity. Volume flow must be determined by *in vivo* calibrations or by measuring the cross-sectional area of the vessel within the lumen. While this has not been a problem for chronic implants, it does raise serious concerns for acute measurements in which turbulence or relative movement of the probe and the vessel can distort the flow waveform. Moreover, measurement of blood flow in a stenotic vessel may also lead to disruption of the normal velocity profile and inaccurate volume flow determinations.

The CW, non-directional Doppler flowmeter, as developed by Franklin *et al.*,[23] has been used in our laboratory for the measurement of coronary,[24–28] cerebral, renal, mesenteric, and iliac blood flows[29–33] using telemetry techniques for remote sensing of blood flow in conscious, unrestrained animals. These flowmeters are small (1.5 cm × 7.5 cm × 12.5 cm), lightweight, battery-powered units that use a radio frequency carrier that is frequency modulated by the Doppler signal to telemeter the flow information. The ability to telemeter the signals along with aortic pressure enables experiments with intractable animals, as well as experiments in which free-ranging exercise is to be studied.

The non-directional flowmeter is unable to sense the difference between forward and backward flow in the vessel, reporting all flow measurements in one direction. This is a disadvantage in the measurement of blood flow in arteries in which flow reversals take place, such as the iliac artery. Additionally, the quality of the received Doppler signal is more critical in low-flow velocity measurement situations as the detection of spurious noise causes a positive shift in the perceived flow. This problem has been addressed by the implementation of a quadrature, phase-shift detector technique[34] to provide the CW flowmeter with direction-sensing capability.

Both the directional and the non-directional CW flowmeters discussed above are very susceptible to pulse interference, which precludes their use with transit time dimension measurements (as described later). This problem has been circumvented by the development of the pulsed Doppler flowmeter,[35,36] which sends a repetitive burst of ultrasound diagonally into the bloodstream and senses the Doppler-shifted return energy at a moment in time that can be related to a position within the blood vessel. Additionally, it is practical to synchronize this flowmeter to other instruments, and the range-sensing capability of the design makes it practical either to measure the instantaneous average velocity across the vessel or to make simultaneous measurements of the velocity in several areas within the vessel, and thus determine the velocity profile of blood flow.[35,36] The pulsed Doppler instrument in primary use in our laboratory is a 10-MHz directional device, with large area piezocrystals to average the instantaneous velocity of flow across the vessel.[36] Commonly available flow transducers use small, 20-MHz crystals, which are used to focus the measurement at the center stream of the flow. This requires that the velocity profile be assumed and can result in underestimation of blood flow if the velocity profile changes from parabolic to blunt, as in reactive hyperemia with temporary occlusion of coronary arteries.

### *Ultrasonic transit time determination of flow velocity*

The measurement of the change in velocity of ultrasound waves propagated through a moving medium predates the development of the Doppler shift flowmeter. This technique, also developed by Franklin *et al.*,[37] uses opposed pairs of piezoelectric crystals acting alternately as transmitters and receivers. As the ultrasound moves through the blood, any movement of the blood will change the velocity of the ultrasound. By alternately transmitting upstream and then downstream, a difference in the transit time of the sound may be determined, thus measuring blood velocity. The differential transit times that are to be measured can be as small as 10 ns at maximum velocity, thus putting severe constraints on the design of the measurement electronics. This technique does not rely on a tight fit of the transducer, as does the electromagnetic sensor; consequently, zero stability and performance at low vascular pressures are better with the transit time technique.

A more recent implementation (Transonic Systems, Ithaca, NY, USA) uses transducer crystals with a reflector to increase the path length, and thus increase the transit time difference for a given velocity.[38] The transit time of the sound is spatially averaged over the cross-section of the lumen, thus enabling the instrument to be calibrated in terms of volume flow. This transducer design uses a flat metal reflector on one side of the artery, with both piezocrystals mounted at an angle in an epoxy shell, which fits on the other side of the artery. This transducer geometry uses two passes of the ultrasound at complementary angles through the lumen of the vessel, which reduces errors due to implant angle differences between the flowprobe and the vessel. Although the transducer design is larger and heavier than either the Doppler or the electromagnetic types, implantation and stable flow measurements are still routinely possible. This design does not require a tight fit function, but for optimum use the transducer should be allowed to stabilize on the artery by the growth of connective tissue before its operation.

In theory, zero velocity should result in a zero time difference, with primary stability of zero determined by the electronic design. In practice, zero flow offset and gain can be affected by non-uniform tissue density within the measurement area of the transducer, such as growth of fatty tissue, thus causing a static change in the speed of sound being measured. Additionally, if the probe axis does not align properly with the flow axis, a position-related zero flow offset can be observed. A third problem occurs with sensitivity changes if the probe is placed axially on a curved artery. Implantation on large arteries such as the aorta of dogs (18–24 mm) results in performance with minimum zero offset; however, somewhat larger zero offsets can be experienced with smaller probes because alignment is more of a problem. In use, stable flow sensitivity and little change in the zero offset are typical with chronic implants in our laboratory, after the 2–3 weeks required to allow the growth of stabilizing connective tissue.

The transit time flowmeter is a pulsed sampling device, and therefore it can be synchronized to work simultaneously with ultrasonic dimension measurements. Its pulse transmission duration (20 s), however, is incompatible with the pulsed Doppler design (pulse repetition rate of 10–16 μs), thus not allowing mixed instrumentation models with these instruments.

### *Ventricular dimensions*

The ultrasonic transit time dimension gauge, as originally described by Rushmer *et al.*[39] and developed by Patrick and co-workers,[11,40] can be used for the measurement of left ventricular internal diameter, right and left ventricular wall thickness, and right and left ventricular regional segment length[7,41–45] (Figure 4.1). This technique uses pairs of small piezoelectric transducers operating in the frequency ranges of 3–7 MHz, depending on the application. In operation, a burst of sound from one transducer propagates to the second transducer. If the speed of sound is known in the intervening medium ($1.58 \times 106$ mm s$^{-1}$ for blood), the separation of the transducers can be determined by measuring the transit time of the sound. This one-way, two-transducer technique contrasts with the ultrasonic echo technique used clinically in cardiac diagnosis that uses a single transducer to emit ultrasound, which is then reflected from the internal structures of the body. Although the two-transducer technique is invasive and is limited to a discrete straight line measurement, the capability for enhanced and more discrete reception of the ultrasonic signal can radically improve the accuracy and resolution of dimension measurements. This permits the detection of more subtle changes in regional function than the pulsed echo technique.

In operation, the dimension gauge measures the acoustic transit time of bursts of ultrasound (center frequencies ranging from 3 to 7 MHz) propagated between two piezoelectric crystals placed on opposing surfaces of the left ventricular cavity (internal diameter), or placed on opposing surfaces of the right or left ventricular free walls (wall thickness), or propagated among multiple pairs of piezoelectric crystals inserted into the free walls of the right or left ventricles approximately 1–2 cm apart (segmental length). The transit time dimension gauge can be synchronized to measure up to twelve simultaneous dimensions, thus allowing a multiple assessment of regional myocardial function (Figure 4.1). The signals can also be differentiated to obtain the rate of myocardial fiber shortening, an index of regional cardiac function (Figure 4.1). In addition, the intramyocardial electrogram from each of the transducers can be assessed, using the standard limb lead arrangements as an indifferent reference (Figure 4.1).

The theoretical resolution of the ultrasonic dimension technique is one-quarter of the wavelength, with the wavelength being determined by the thickness of the crystal. To achieve improved resolution, it is necessary to use thin, high-frequency piezoelectric crystals when possible. We are currently using 7-MHz crystals (0.3 mm thick and 2.0 mm in diameter) for myocardial segment length determination because transducer separation is typically 1 cm and the signal strength is not adversely affected by this distance. At the other extreme, transducers used for the measurement of ventricular diameter are 3-MHz crystals (0.7 mm thick and 3–4 mm in diameter) because the distance measured is in the 3- to 4-cm range and attenuation of the sound is greater, being proportional to both distance and frequency. Transducers for wall thickness determination are intermediate, with a 2-mm-diameter, 5-MHz crystal used for the endocardial surface. A similar transducer with a small Dacron patch is sutured to the epicardium to complete the implant. To measure regional subendocardial and subepicardial wall thickness, an additional crystal is implanted in the mid-wall.[43] A short (6 cm) length of small, very flexible, twisted pair of stainless-steel wires is used to connect these crystal elements to the regular transducer wire.

### Vascular dimensions

The study of the elastic properties of the aortic wall is fundamental for the understanding of the coupling between the heart and peripheral circulation, the characteristics of vascular mechanoreceptors, and the pathogenesis of important disease states, such as atherosclerosis and hypertension. Moreover, the concept of large coronary artery vasoconstriction as a possible mechanism for Prinzmetal's variant angina,[46] as well as typical angina pectoris and myocardial infarction,[47,48] underlines the importance of making direct continuous measurements of peripheral vascular dimensions.

The design of the transit time dimension gauge has recently been modified to permit the measurement of both large[40] and small[49,50] vessel dimensions. These modifications involve refinement of the electronics as well as construction of smaller transducers. The transducers (1 mm × 3 mm) are constructed from 7-MHz piezoelectric material, with stainless-steel wiring and a thin coat of epoxy. To minimize mass loading of the vessel and to facilitate alignment at surgery, these transducers have been constructed without lenses, although a small Dacron patch is attached to the back of the transducer with epoxy for stabilization purposes. The transducers are implanted on opposing sides of the vessel and secured with 5–0 suture material. Resistive loading is used to minimize the instrument ringing artifact. The inhibit pulse is shortened to be adjustable over the range of 0.5–10 μs, and the sensitivity of the post-detection amplifiers is increased to compensate for the smaller signal developed by the shorter transit time. These modifications result in an instrument that is stable enough to resolve 0.05-mm changes in the diameter of a 3-mm vessel. The measurements are repeatable and constitute a sensitive and accurate method of assessing changes in coronary artery diameter under a variety of interventions in the conscious animal.[49]

### Telemetry of pressures, flows, and dimensions

Extension of the measurement techniques described above to include radiotelemetry of the biologic signals has obvious utility in situations in which the experimental design precludes the use of cables, tethers, and the laboratory environment. Examples include activities such as free-ranging exercise, the recording of data from intractable animals such as large primates[51] (Figure 4.2), as well as studies of animals in their natural habitat.[52] Because our laboratory has been interested in this area,[9–12,28–33,52–54] the design of the instruments previously described has been planned to include the parameters of low-power requirements, battery operation, small size, and minimum parts to facilitate the telemetry of these parameters. The telemetry systems we have developed fall into two categories: flow pressure systems and pressure dimension systems. The uniqueness of both the CW ultrasonic Doppler flowmeter and the pulsed transit time dimension gauge generally preclude their simultaneous use, owing to the generation of mutual interference. However, the electromagnetic flow system can be compatible with the ultrasonic dimension system.

### Instrumentation for smaller animals

Most of the instrumentation techniques described in this chapter are too large for use in smaller animals such as the rat or mouse. Developments in smaller transducer

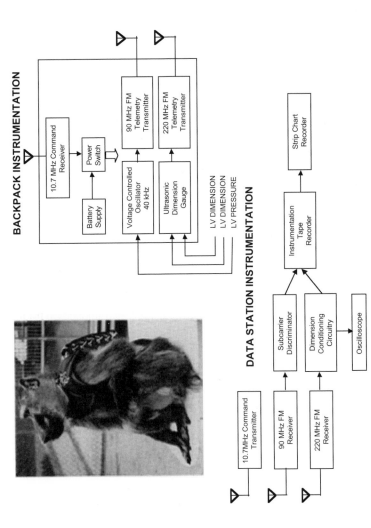

*Figure 4.2* Radiotelemetry of physiologic measurements in conscious, unrestrained baboons. The instrumentation carried by the baboon in a backpack is shown schematically. The backpack contained the dual dimension/pressure telemetry apparatus plus batteries, which were used to power the system. A radio frequency-controlled interrogator was used to activate a motor-driven pump to infuse 1000 ml of saline. The electronic instrumentation in the remote data station, used to receive and process the electronic signals, is schematically depicted at the bottom. Reproduced with permission of the American Society for Clinical Investigation from Zimpfer and Vatner.[51]

design – along with improvements in tether systems, which can couple fluid catheters to external transducers as well as accommodate the wiring from flow and dimension transducers – now make it feasible to adapt some of these measurement techniques for smaller animals. In our laboratory, as well as in others, small tether systems containing two to three fluid couplings and as many as ten electrical circuits allow chronic continuous measurements from conscious rats, instrumented with an in-dwelling catheter for infusion of fluids, a catheter in the left ventricle for the measurement of left ventricular pressure and d$P$/d$t$, and either an electromagnetic or transit time flow probe around the ascending aorta to measure cardiac output.[55]

The catheters must be maintained through the tether system, by slow infusion of a small amount of heparin, to maintain long-term potency of the catheters. The small size of tubing necessary for implant [0.96 mm, outside diameter (o.d.)] restricts the nominal use of the catheters to measurement and infusion, as withdrawal of blood is difficult and avoidance of clotting is a problem, both in the catheter and in the fluid swivel. The transit time flowmeter seems to be more stable on the aorta of these chronically instrumented animals than the electromagnetic probe, because the fit of the electromagnetic probe is extremely critical for success with such a small artery (3 mm). The relaxed constraint on fit associated with the transit time probe ensures a better chance of success in this application, although the *in vitro* calibration may require adjustment because of the curved section of artery on which the flow probe is implanted. While the use of these types of chronic instrumentation in rats is becoming commonplace, it remains a challenge in the significantly smaller murine models; however, a great deal of work has been and continues to be directed toward instrumentation for the measurement of cardiovascular parameters in conscious mice. Several of these are summarized below.

### *Arterial pressure*

#### *Invasive measurement*

The majority of reports of conscious blood pressure measurements in mice have involved surgical placement of arterial catheters, variable periods of post-operative recovery, and measurements conducted at baseline and during acute interventions. Catheters have been placed in the carotid[56–59] and femoral[60–63] arteries. Catheters can be purchased from vendors or constructed by flame stretching PE50 or PE10 tubing. Surgical placement is generally accomplished with the aid of a dissecting microscope. The mouse is anesthetized, the area over the carotid of the femoral artery is shaved, and the mouse is placed supine on a warmed surface. The artery is isolated and ligated distally and a microsurgical clip is placed proximally. One or more sutures are loosely placed proximally. An arteriotomy is performed with microsurgical scissors or a 25-gauge or smaller needle and the catheter is threaded into the vessel lumen. The sutures are tightened and the clip is carefully released, checking for adequate hemostasis. The catheter is tunneled subcutaneously and the incision is closed in layers. The catheter is flushed with a dilute heparin solution, heat sealed, and stored on the dorsum in a retaining device (small plastic cap or pouch) sutured to the animal. Intravenous catheters can be placed at the same time (usually in the internal jugular vein) for later delivery of fluid or drugs. Prophylactic antibiotics are recommended following surgery. At the time of recording, catheters are freed, flushed, and connected to modified strain gauge transducers or micromanometers. Mice are lightly restrained and allowed to accommodate to the restraining chamber.

Numerous studies have reported directly measured conscious arterial pressure in wild-type and transgenic mice.[56-64] Normal values for systolic blood pressure measured by arterial catheter in wild-type mice appear to range from 120 to135 mmHg, with mean arterial pressures ranging from 95 to 120 mmHg. This contrasts with the lower values reported in most studies of anesthetized mice. Although interstrain differences make comparison difficult, it is evident from published reports and unpublished observations that inadequate post-operative recovery time yields lower blood pressures and either lower or higher heart rates than recordings made after more prolonged periods of recovery (see below). This seems to be true even when the animal appears to have recovered fully from anesthesia as judged by a return to normal motor activity. These observations illustrate the importance of techniques for the measurement of blood pressure in fully conscious mice to the full understanding of the potentially complex cardiovascular effects of toxic exposures and specific genetic manipulations.

### *Cardiac output*

Cardiac output can be measured in mice using a number of techniques. Measurements in anesthetized mice using transthoracic echocardiographically determined aortic dimensions and Doppler-derived aortic velocities have been reported, but this technique is not feasible in the conscious state.[65] The radioisotope dilution technique was first used in anesthetized mice several decades ago.[66] Barbee *et al.*[67] more recently reported measurements of cardiac output in conscious mice using radioactive microspheres. This technique, well established in large animal studies[68,69] and previously used in rats[70] and anesthetized mice,[71,72] involves central administration of a known quantity of radiolabeled microspheres with simultaneous withdrawal of a measured quantity of peripheral arterial blood. Radioactivity is then measured using a gamma counter, and cardiac output is calculated by an established formula. Prior work had demonstrated a high rate of inadequate mixing of microspheres.[67,72] This was largely overcome in Barbee *et al.*'s study by the use of specially constructed catheters with tip diameters of < 400 μm, allowing catheter placement into the left ventricle (LV) without significant outflow tract obstruction or aortic insufficiency in the majority of cases.[67] Using this technique, the authors reported a mean cardiac output of $16 \pm 1$ ml min$^{-1}$ (cardiac index $591 \pm 49$ ml min$^{-1}$ kg$^{-1}$) in conscious mice studied 4 h after recovery from Avertin anesthesia and surgical placement of LV (via the right carotid artery) and femoral artery catheters. Stroke volume was calculated to be $26 \pm 2$ µl, and post-mortem tissue sampling and analysis were performed for the calculation of regional cardiac output distribution, which largely mirrored prior reports in rats. The authors pointed out that the technique could be repeated acutely at least once without any significant impact on peripheral resistance. Concerns remain, however, regarding hemodynamic effects of blood withdrawal (Barbee reported a 10 percent fall in mean arterial pressure during withdrawal) and potential vessel occlusion by the microspheres.[71]

Recently, Vogel[73] reported measurement of cardiac output in anesthetized and conscious mice using a measure of blood conductivity during intravenous bolus injection of 20 µl of a 5 percent glucose solution. This technique involves surgical placement of a femoral arterial platinum electrode and femoral venous catheter as well as placement of a rectal reference electrode. Blood conductivity following the bolus of glucose is converted into cardiac output using an established formula. The author included validation studies in rats where the cardiac output determinations by blood conductivity correlated well with those determined by an indicator dilution technique.

The blood conductivity technique yielded a mean cardiac index of $592 \pm 78$ ml min$^{-1}$ kg$^{-1}$ in the conscious state (1-h recovery from halothane/N$_2$O anesthesia). Vogel[73] also reported decreases in cardiac index with hemorrhage-induced hypovolemia, but no change with saline-induced hypervolemia. Although this method has the significant benefit of allowing virtually any number of determinations in a single animal during the course of an experiment, its utility for measurements in fully conscious unrestrained animals remains to be assessed.

## *Heart rate*

### *Non-invasive measures*

The non-invasive tail cuff method of determining blood pressure can also be used for measurement of heart rate. Heart rate is derived from the pulsatile waveform generated by the photosensor. This method appears to yield heart rates slightly greater than invasive methods, likely due to agitation of the mice caused by heating or cuff inflation.

### *Invasive measures*

The simplest technique for recording conscious heart rate in mice is via surgically placed subcutaneous electrodes. The animal is anesthetized, the lateral thorax and interscapular regions shaved and sterilely prepared. Three 10-cm lengths of 0.0014″ stainless-steel wire are stripped of insulation over the distal 10 mm and inserted subcutaneously via small skin incisions, one each on either side of the thorax and the third tunneled subcutaneously along the back. The thoracic leads are tunneled subcutaneously to the interscapular region, where all leads are externalized and stored in a small plastic cap sutured to the animal's back. The animal is allowed to recover for at least 48 h. At the time of study, the animal is placed in a loose restraint, and the leads are freed from the cap and connected to an EKG monitor with or without an on-line tachometer.

Conscious heart rate can also be measured from arterial pressure tracings taken from in-dwelling arterial catheters. The frequency responses of the strain gauges or micromanometers used to transduce pressure are generally adequate for heart rate determinations over the range seen in conscious mice. The inconsistency of signal quality makes this method less well suited to the analyses required for heart rate variability studies (see below).

Conscious heart rate is measured best with the use of implanted telemetry devices. Commercially available units are surgically implanted in the peritoneal cavity with paired wire electrodes placed subcutaneously over the thorax. Following recovery, conscious heart rate can be recorded on a multichannel tape recorder (Figure 4.3).[64,74]

### Respiratory rate

Conscious respiratory rate in the mouse can be measured using surgically implanted sonomicrometry crystals to record thoracic dimension changes during the respiratory cycle. The mouse is anesthetized and prepared as for implantation of subcutaneous electrodes. Piezoelectric ultrasonic dimension crystals are placed on either side of the thoracic cage and connected to an ultrasonic transit time

## Telemetered ECG

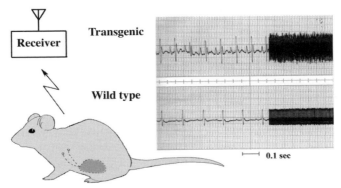

*Figure 4.3* EKG recording using telemetric system from a free-ranging transgenic mouse (top) and a wild-type control mouse (bottom). The telemetry implant is shown in the abdominal cavity of the mouse. The recorded heart rates were higher in the transgenic mice. Reproduced with permission from Uechi et al.[64]

dimension gauge. Crystal position is adjusted to optimize the signal and sutured in place. Following signal calibration, the crystal wires are tunneled subcutaneously, externalized, and stored. After recovery, the wires are reattached to the gauge and recalibrated using impulses of known duration from a crystal-controlled pulse generator. The respiratory rates of lightly restrained conscious mice have been reported to range from 160 to 270 min$^{-1}$.[64,75]

## *Ventricular function*

There are as yet no proven techniques for the measurement of LV function in fully conscious mice. Several investigators have reported ventricular function data from murine isolated working heart preparations.[76,77] Others have reported echocardiographic measures of ejection phase indices[78–81] and high-fidelity pressure transducer-derived measures of isovolumic indices of LV contractility[79,82–85] in anesthetized mice. LV d$P$/d$t$ measurements have been made in both open chest[83–85] and intact preparations.[79,82,85] Recently, relatively load-insensitive measures of LV function have been reported in intact mice.[86,87] Although these measures so far have not been reported in conscious mice, recently LV d$P$/d$t$ values in mice recovering from anesthesia[88,89] and in mice anesthetized with a-chloralose/urethane[90] were found to be nearly four- and threefold greater, respectively, than those obtained in mice fully anesthetized with more commonly used agents. This suggests that the reported values for some measures of ventricular contractility in anesthetized mice may underestimate those in conscious mice by several fold, calling into question the utility of the reported ventricular responses to inotropic stimuli in these studies. The technology of sonomicrometry has just recently started to be applied to measuring function in rats and mice. Using the bidirectional 0.2-mm crystals (Sonometrics, Canada), it is possible to measure short axis and possibly wall thickness in mice.

## *Future directions*

Significant advances have permitted the acquisition of detailed cardiovascular physiologic data in conscious mice. There remain, however, several parameters for which we lack the ability to make consistent measures in the fully conscious state. It is likely that further refinement in equipment and technique will allow for surgical placement of intraventricular catheters (either solid state or fluid filled) for the measurement of ventricular pressures in conscious mice. We have, in fact, recently instrumented a mouse with epicardial and endocardial sonomicrometry crystals and a left ventricular high-fidelity pressure gauge. It is conceivable that a recently described conductance catheter used for the simultaneous measurement of left ventricular pressure and volume in mice[90] could be used in conscious animals if it could be surgically implanted in the LV or reliably advanced via an in-dwelling arterial catheter. This device would have the important added advantage of providing relatively load-independent measures of ventricular function. These invasive techniques seem to hold more promise for measurement of LV function in the conscious state than do the non-invasive techniques which have been successfully used in anesthetized preparations. Less readily foreseeable are techniques for analyzing vascular function in conscious mice. Given recent descriptions of murine models of myocardial infarction[91] and myocardial ischemia and reperfusion,[92] it would be of great utility to develop techniques to assess coronary flow in the mouse, and one would hope eventually to perform this in the conscious state. Continued expansion of the methods available for measuring physiologic parameters in conscious mice will allow for the full realization of the insights into cardiovascular function promised by transgenic techniques.

## Summary

The chronically instrumented conscious animal model can be used to provide an important tool for the assessment of the effects of putative toxic substances on cardiovascular function.[93] This chapter updates techniques that have been used routinely in our laboratory for the measurement of arterial and cardiac pressures, blood flows to systemic and coronary circulations, and ventricular and vascular dimensions in animals ranging in size from calves to mice.[93] The application of radiotelemetry techniques to the measurement of these physiologic variables has also been described. These techniques permit the continuous high-fidelity assessment of cardiovascular dynamics in conscious, unrestrained animals without the confounding influence of anesthesia and acute surgical trauma. Thus, direct and reflex effects of toxic substances on cardiovascular function can be continuously monitored. Finally, the effect of these environmental agents can be re-evaluated in these chronically instrumented, conscious animal models following the experimental induction of a disease state, or even after changing the genetic composition of an animal.

## Acknowledgments

This work was supported by US Public Health Service grants HL59139, HL33107, HL33065, and AG14121.

## References

1. Harlan WR, Sharrett AR, Weill H, Turino GM, Borhani NO, Resnekov L. Impact of the environment on cardiovascular disease. Report of the American Heart Association Task Force on environment and the cardiovascular system. *Circulation* 1981; 63: 243A–246A.
2. Rosenman KD. Cardiovascular disease and environmental exposure. *Br J Ind Med* 1979; 36: 85–97.
3. Vatner SF, Smith NT. Effects of halothane on left ventricular function and distribution of regional blood flow in dogs and primates. *Circ Res* 1974; 34: 155–167.

4. Manders WT, Vatner SF. Effects of sodium pentobarbital anesthesia on left ventricular function and distribution of cardiac output in dogs, with particular reference to the mechanism for tachycardia. *Circ Res* 1976; 39: 512–517.

5. Vatner SF. Effects of anesthesia on cardiovascular control mechanisms. *Environ Health Perspect* 1978; 26: 193–206.

6. Vatner SF, Baig H, Dexter L. The effects of inotropic stimulation on ischemic myocardium in conscious dogs. *Trans Assoc Am Physicians* 1978; 91: 282–293.

7. Vatner SF, Braunwald E. Effects of chronic heart failure on the inotropic response of the right ventricle of the conscious dog to a cardiac glycoside and to tachycardia. *Circulation* 1974; 50: 728–734.

8. Van Citters RL, Franklin DL. Telemetry of blood pressure in free-ranging animals via an intravascular gauge. *J Appl Physiol* 1966; 21: 1633–1636.

9. Baig H, Patrick TA, Vatner SF. Implantable pressure gauges for use in chronic animals. In: Fleming DG, Ko WH, Neuman MR, eds. *Indwelling and Implantable Pressure Transducers*. Cleveland, OH: CRC Press; 1977; pp. 35–43.

10. Franklin D, Vatner SF, Higgins CB, Patrick T, Kemper WS, Van Citters RL. Measurement and radiotelemetry of cardiovascular variables in conscious animals: techniques and applications. In: Harmison IT, ed. *Research Animals in Medicine*. Washington, DC: US Government Printing Office; 1973; pp. 1119–1133.

11. Patrick TA, Vatner SF, Kemper WS, Franklin D. Telemetry of left ventricular diameter and pressure measurements from unrestrained animals. *J Appl Physiol* 1974; 37: 276–281.

12. Vatner SF, Franklin D, Higgins CB, Patrick T, Braunwald E. Left ventricular response to severe exertion in untethered dogs. *J Clin Invest* 1972; 51: 3052–3060.

13. Foreman DL, Sanders M, Bloor CM. Total and regional cerebral blood flow during moderate and severe exercise in miniature swine. *J Appl Physiol* 1976; 40: 191–195.

14. Sanders M, White FC, Bloor CM. Myocardial blood flow distribution in miniature pigs during exercise. *Basic Res Cardiol* 1977; 72: 326–331.

15. Pagani M, Mirsky I, Baig H, Manders WT, Kerkhof P, Vatner SF. Effects of age on aortic pressure-diameter and elastic stiffness–stress relationships in unanesthetized sheep. *Circ Res* 1979; 44: 420–429.

16. Barber BJ, Quillen Jr., EW, Cowley Jr., AW. An inexpensive pressure telemetry system. *Am J Physiol* 1980; 239: H570–H572.

17. Kolin A. Electromagnetic flowmeter: principle of method and its application to blood flow measurements. *Proc Soc Exp Biol Med* 1936; 35: 53–56.

18. Wetterer E. New methods of registering rate of blood circulation in unopened vessels. *Z Biol* 1937; 98: 26–36.

19. Rutherford JD, Vatner SF. Integrated carotid chemoreceptor and pulmonary inflation reflex control of peripheral vasoactivity in conscious dogs. *Circ Res* 1978; 43: 200–208.

20. Vatner SF, Franklin D, VanCitters RL. Simultaneous comparison and calibration of the Doppler and electromagnetic flowmeters. *J Appl Physiol* 1970; 29: 907–910.

21. Vatner SF, Franklin D, Higgins CB, White S, Van Citters RL. Calibration of the ultrasonic doppler flowmeter in situ. In: McCutcheon EP, ed. *Chronically Implanted Cardiovascular Instrumentation*. New York, NY: Academic Press; 1973; pp. 63–70.

22. Vatner SF, Young M, Patrick TA. Measurement of coronary blood flow in conscious animals. In: Altobelli SA, Votles WF, Greene ER, eds. *Cardiovascular Ultrasonic Flowmeter*. New York, NY: Elsevier/North-Holland; 1985; pp. 81–99.

23. Franklin DE, Watson NW, Pierson KE, Van Citters RL. Technique for radio telemetry of blood-flow velocity from unrestrained animals. *Am J Med Electron* 1966; 5: 24–28.

24. Vatner SF, Franklin D, Van Citters RL, Braunwald E. Effects of carotid sinus nerve stimulation on blood-flow distribution in conscious dogs at rest and during exercise. *Circ Res* 1970; 27: 495–503.

25. Vatner SF, McRitchie RJ. Interaction of the chemoreflex and the pulmonary inflation reflex in the regulation of coronary circulation in conscious dogs. *Circ Res* 1975; 37: 664–673.

26. Vatner SF, Higgins CB, Braunwald E. Effects of norepinephrine on coronary circulation and left ventricular dynamics in the conscious dog. *Circ Res* 1974; 34: 812–823.

27. Vatner SF, Higgins CB, Franklin D, Braunwald E. Effects of a digitalis glycoside on coronary and systemic dynamics in conscious dogs. *Circ Res* 1971; 28: 470–479.

28. Vatner SF, Franklin D, Higgins CB, Patrick T, White S, Van Citters RL. Coronary dynamics in unrestrained conscious baboons. *Am J Physiol* 1971; 221: 1396–1401.

29. Higgins CB, Vatner SF, Franklin D, Braunwald E. Effects of experimentally produced heart failure on the peripheral vascular response to severe exercise in conscious dogs. *Circ Res* 1972; 31: 186–194.

30. Millard RW, Higgins CB, Franklin D, Vatner SF. Regulation of the renal circulation during severe exercise in normal dogs and dogs with experimental heart failure. *Circ Res* 1972; 31: 881–888.

31. Vatner SF. Effects of exercise and excitement on mesenteric and renal dynamics in conscious, unrestrained baboons. *Am J Physiol* 1978; 234: H210–H214.

32. Vatner SF, Higgins CB, White S, Patrick T, Franklin D. The peripheral vascular response to severe exercise in untethered dogs before and after complete heart block. *J Clin Invest* 1971; 50: 1950–1960.

33. Franklin D, Vatner SF, Van Citters RL. Studies on peripheral vascular dynamics using animals models. In: *Animal Models for Biomedical Research*, Vol. IV. Washington, DC: National Academy of Sciences; 1971; pp. 74–84.

34. McLeod Jr., FD, Directional doppler demodulation. *ACEMB*. 1967; 27.1 (abstract).

35. Baker DW. Pulsed ultrasonic doppler flow-sensing. *IEEE Trans SU* 1970; 17: 170–185.

36. Hartley CJ, Hanley HG, Lewis RM, Cole JS. A multi-channel directional doppler flowmeter. *ACEMB* 1974; 339 (abstract).

37. Franklin D, Ellis R, Rushmer R. A pulsed ultrasonic flowmeter. *IRE Trans Med Electron* 1959; 6: 204–206.

38. Drost C. Vessel diameter-independent volume flow measurements using ultrasound. *Proceedings of the San Diego Biomedical Symposium* 1978; 17: 299–302.

39. Rushmer RF, Franklin D, Ellis RM. Left ventricular dimensions recorded by sonocardiometry. *Circ Res* 1956; 4: 684–688.

40. Pagani M, Baig H, Sherman A, Manders WT, Quinn P, Patrick T, Franklin D, Vatner SF. Measurement of multiple simultaneous small dimensions and study of arterial pressure–dimension relations in conscious animals. *Am J Physiol* 1978; 235: H610–H617.

41. Vatner SF, Higgins CB, Franklin D, Braunwald E. Extent of carotid sinus regulation of the myocardial contractile state in conscious dogs. *J Clin Invest* 1972; 51: 995–1008.

42. Heyndrickx GR, Millard RW, McRitchie RJ, Maroko PR, Vatner SF. Regional myocardial functional and electrophysiological alterations after brief coronary artery occlusion in conscious dogs. *J Clin Invest* 1975; 56: 978–985.

43. Hittinger L, Patrick T, Ihara T, Hasebe N, Shen YT, Kalthof B, Shannon RP, Vatner SF. Exercise induces cardiac dysfunction in both moderate, compensated and severe hypertrophy. *Circulation* 1994; 89: 2219–2231.

44. Theroux P, Ross Jr., J, Franklin D, Kemper WS, Sasyama S. Regional myocardial function in the conscious dog during acute coronary occlusion and responses to morphine, propranolol, nitroglycerin, and lidocaine. *Circulation* 1976; 53: 302–314.

45. Vatner SF. Correlation between acute reductions in myocardial blood flow and function in conscious dogs. *Circ Res* 1980; 47: 201–207.

46. Prinzmetal M, Kennamer R, Mertiss R, Wada T, Bor N. Angina pectoris. 1. A variance form of angina pectoris. *Am J Med* 1959; 27: 375–388.

47. Hillis LD, Braunwald E. Coronary-artery spasm. *N Engl J Med* 1978; 299: 695–702.

48. Maseri A, L'Abbate A, Baroldi G, Chierchia S, Marzilli M, Ballestra AM, Severi S, Parodi O, Biagini A, Distante A, Pesola A. Coronary vasospasm as a possible cause of myocardial infarction. A conclusion derived from the study of "preinfarction" angina. *N Engl J Med* 1978; 299: 1271–1277.

49. Vatner SF, Pagani M, Manders WT, Pasipoularides AD. Alpha adrenergic vasoconstriction and nitroglycerin vasodilation of large coronary arteries in the conscious dog. *J Clin Invest* 1980; 65: 5–14.

50. Vatner SF, Pagani M, Manders WT. Alpha adrenergic constriction of coronary arteries in conscious dogs. *Trans Assoc Am Physicians* 1979; 92: 229–238.

51. Zimpfer M, Vatner SF. Effects of acute increases in left ventricular preload on indices of myocardial function in conscious, unrestrained and intact, tranquilized baboons. *J Clin Invest* 1981; 67: 430–438.

52. Van Citters RL, Franklin DL, Vatner SF, Patrick T, Warren JV. Cerebral hemodynamics in the giraffe. *Trans Assoc Am Physicians* 1969; 82: 293–304.

53. Vatner SF, Patrick TA. Radio telemetry of blood flow and pressure measurements in untethered conscious animals. *Bibl Cardiol* 1974; 34: 1–11.

54. Franklin D, Patrick TA, Kemper S, Vatner SF. A system for radiotelemetry of blood pressure, blood flow, and ventricular dimensions from animals: a summary report. *Proceedings of the International Telemetry Conference*, Washington, DC. 1971; pp. 244–250.

55. Shen YT, Young MA, Ohanian J, Graham RM, Vatner SF. Atrial natriuretic factor-induced systemic vasoconstriction in conscious dogs, rats, and monkeys. *Circ Res* 1990; 66: 647–661.

56. Madeddu P, Varoni MV, Palomba D, Emanueli C, Demontis MP, Glorioso N, Dessi-Fulgheri P, Sarzani R, Anania V. Cardiovascular phenotype of a mouse strain with disruption of bradykinin $B_2$-receptor gene. *Circulation* 1997; 96: 3570–3578.

57. Link RE, Desai K, Hein L, Stevens ME, Chruscinski A, Bernstein D, Barsh GS, Kobilka BK. Cardiovascular regulation in mice lacking alpha$_2$-adrenergic receptor subtypes b and c. *Science* 1996; 273: 803–805.

58. Hein L, Barsh GS, Pratt RE, Dzau VJ, Kobilka BK. Behavioural and cardiovascular effects of disrupting the angiotensin II type-2 receptor in mice [published erratum appears in *Nature* 1996; 380: 366]. *Nature* 1995; 377: 744–747.

59. Tian B, Meng QC, Chen YF, Krege JH, Smithies O, Oparil S. Blood pressures and cardiovascular homeostasis in mice having reduced or absent angiotensin-converting enzyme gene function. *Hypertension* 1997; 30: 128–133.

60. Johns C, Gavras I, Handy DE, Salomao A, Gavras H. Models of experimental hypertension in mice. *Hypertension* 1996; 28: 1064–1069.

61. Merrill DC, Thompson MW, Carney CL, Granwehr BP, Schlager G, Robillard JE, Sigmund CD. Chronic hypertension and altered baroreflex responses in transgenic mice containing the human renin and human angiotensinogen genes. *J Clin Invest* 1996; 97: 1047–1055.

62. Lembo G, Rockman HA, Hunter JJ, Steinmetz H, Koch WJ, Ma L, Prinz MP, Ross Jr., J, Chien KR, Powell-Braxton L. Elevated blood pressure and enhanced myocardial contractility in mice with severe IGF-1 deficiency. *J Clin Invest* 1996; 98: 2648–2655.

63. Barbee RW, Perry BD, Re RN, Murgo JP, Field LJ. Hemodynamics in transgenic mice with overexpression of atrial natriuretic factor. *Circ Res* 1994; 74: 747–751.

64. Uechi M, Asai K, Osaka M, Smith A, Sato N, Wagner TE, Ishikawa Y, Hayakawa H, Vatner DE, Shannon RP, Homcy CJ, Vatner SF. Depressed heart rate variability and arterial baroreflex in conscious transgenic mice with overexpression of cardiac Gsalpha. *Circ Res* 1998; 82: 416–423.

65. Hartley CJ, Michael LH, Entman ML. Noninvasive measurement of ascending aortic blood velocity in mice. *Am J Physiol* 1995; 268: H499–H505.

66. Broulik PD, Kochakian CD, Dubovsky J. Influence of castration and testosterone propionate on cardiac output, renal blood flow, and blood volume in mice. *Proc Soc Exp Biol Med* 1973; 144: 671–673.

67. Barbee RW, Perry BD, Re RN, Murgo JP. Microsphere and dilution techniques for the determination of blood flows and volumes in conscious mice. *Am J Physiol* 1992; 263: R728–R733.

68. Hoffbrand BI, Forsyth RP. Validity studies of the radioactive microsphere method for the study of the distribution of cardiac output, blood flow, and resistance in the conscious rhesus monkey. *Cardiovasc Res* 1969; 3: 426–432.

69. Domenech RJ, Hoffman JI, Noble MI, Saunders KB, Henson JR, Subijanto S. Total and regional coronary blood flow measured by radioactive microspheres in conscious and anesthetized dogs. *Circ Res* 1969; 25: 581–596.

70. Ishise S, Pegram BL, Yamamoto J, Kitamura Y, Frohlich ED. Reference sample microsphere method: cardiac output and blood flows in conscious rat. *Am J Physiol* 1980; 239: H443–H449.

71. Kobayashi N, Kobayashi K, Kouno K, Horinaka S, Yagi S. Effects of intra-atrial injection of colored microspheres on systemic hemodynamics and regional blood flow in rats. *Am J Physiol* 1994; 266: H1910–H1917.

72. Sarin SK, Sabba C, Groszmann RJ. Splanchnic and systemic hemodynamics in mice using a radioactive microsphere technique. *Am J Physiol* 1990; 258: G365–369.

73. Vogel J. Measurement of cardiac output in small laboratory animals using recordings of blood conductivity. *Am J Physiol* 1997; 273: H2520–H2527.

74. Mansier P, Medigue C, Charlotte N, Vermeiren C, Coraboeuf E, Deroubai E, Ratner E, Chevalier B, Clairambault J, Carre F, Dahkli T, Bertin B, Briand P, Strosberg D, Swynghedauw B. Decreased heart rate variability in transgenic mice overexpressing atrial beta 1-adrenoceptors. *Am J Physiol* 1996; 271: H1465–H1472.

75. Onodera M, Kuwaki T, Kumada M, Masuda Y. Determination of ventilatory volume in mice by whole body plethysmography. *Jpn J Physiol* 1997; 47: 317–326.

76. Grupp IL, Subramaniam A, Hewett TE, Robbins J, Grupp G. Comparison of normal, hypodynamic, and hyperdynamic mouse hearts using isolated work-performing heart preparations. *Am J Physiol* 1993; 265: H1401–H1410.

77. Brooks WW, Apstein CS. Effect of treppe on isovolumic function in the isolated blood-perfused mouse heart. *J Mol Cell Cardiol* 1996; 28: 1817–1822.

78. Tanaka N, Dalton N, Mao L, Rockman HA, Peterson KL, Gottshall KR, Hunter JJ, Chien KR, Ross Jr., J. Transthoracic echocardiography in models of cardiac disease in the mouse. *Circulation* 1996; 94: 1109–1117.

79. Iwase M, Bishop SP, Uechi M, Vatner DE, Shannon RP, Kudej RK, Wight DC, Wagner TE, Ishikawa Y, Homcy CJ, Vatner SF. Adverse effects of chronic endogenous sympathetic drive induced by cardiac GS alpha overexpression. *Circ Res* 1996; 78: 517–524.

80. Hoit BD, Khoury SF, Kranias EG, Ball N, Walsh RA. In vivo echocardiographic detection of enhanced left ventricular function in gene-targeted mice with phospholamban deficiency. *Circ Res* 1995; 77: 632–637.

81. Gardin JM, Siri FM, Kitsis RN, Edwards JG, Leinwand LA. Echocardiographic assessment of left ventricular mass and systolic function in mice. *Circ Res* 1995; 76: 907–914.

82. Lorenz JN, Kranias EG. Regulatory effects of phospholamban on cardiac function in intact mice. *Am J Physiol* 1997; 273: H2826–H2831.

83. Milano CA, Allen LF, Rockman HA, Dolber PC, McMinn TR, Chien KR, Johnson TD, Bond RA, Lefkowitz RJ. Enhanced myocardial function in transgenic mice overexpressing the beta 2-adrenergic receptor. *Science* 1994; 264: 582–586.

84. Hunter JJ, Tanaka N, Rockman HA, Ross Jr., J, Chien KR. Ventricular expression of a MLC-2v-ras fusion gene induces cardiac hypertrophy and selective diastolic dysfunction in transgenic mice. *J Biol Chem* 1995; 270: 23173–23178.

85. Hoit BD, Ball N, Walsh RA. Invasive hemodynamics and force–frequency relationships in open- versus closed-chest mice. *Am J Physiol* 1997; 273: H2528–H2533.

86. Fentzke RC, Korcarz CE, Shroff SG, Lin H, Sandelski J, Leiden JM, Lang RM. Evaluation of ventricular and arterial hemodynamics in anesthetized closed-chest mice. *J Am Soc Echocardiogr* 1997; 10: 915–925.

87. Hoit BD, Khan ZU, Pawloski-Dahm CM, Walsh RA. In vivo determination of left ventricular wall stress-shortening relationship in normal mice. *Am J Physiol* 1997; 272: H1047–H1052.

88. Rockman HA, Choi DJ, Rahman NU, Akhter SA, Lefkowitz RJ, Koch WJ. Receptor-specific in vivo desensitization by the G protein-coupled receptor kinase-5 in transgenic mice. *Proc Natl Acad Sci USA* 1996; 93: 9954–9959.

89. Palakodeti V, Oh S, Oh BH, Mao L, Hongo M, Peterson KL, Ross Jr., J. Force–frequency effect is a powerful determinant of myocardial contractility in the mouse. *Am J Physiol* 1997; 273: H1283–H1290.

90. Georgakopoulos D, Mitzner WA, Chen CH, Byrne BJ, Millar HD, Hare JM, Kass DA. In vivo murine left ventricular pressure–volume relations by miniaturized conductance micromanometry. *Am J Physiol* 1998; 274: H1416–H1422.

91. Manning WJ, Wei JY, Katz SE, Douglas PS, Gwathmey JK. Echocardiographically detected myocardial infarction in the mouse. *Lab Anim Sci* 1993; 43: 583–585.

92. Michael LH, Entman ML, Hartley CJ, Youker KA, Zhu J, Hall SR, Hawkins HK, Berens K, Ballantyne CM. Myocardial ischemia and reperfusion: a murine model. *Am J Physiol* 1995; 269: H2147–H2154.
93. Vatner SF, Patrick TA, Murray PA. Monitoring of cardiovascular dynamics in conscious animals. In: Van Stee EW, ed. *Cardiovascular Toxicology*. New York: Raven Press; 1982; pp. 35–55.

# Part III

# PRINCIPLES OF MYOCARDIAL CELL INJURY

# 5

# CELL INJURY AND CELL DEATH

## Apoptosis, oncosis, and necrosis

*Benjamin F. Trump,*† Seung H. Chang,‡
Patricia C. Phelps,‡ and Raymond T. Jones‡*

*\*Warwick Research Institute, Baltimore, MD, USA;
†AMC Cancer Research Center, Denver, CO, USA;
and ‡Department of Pathology, University of Maryland
School of Medicine, Baltimore, MD, USA*

The purpose of this chapter is to review current knowledge concerning the cellular and molecular basis of cell injury and cell death. Knowledge in this area has progressed rapidly during the past 30 years, with most studies currently involving elucidation of the cellular and molecular mechanisms involved in both lethal and sublethal injury as well as in acute and chronic cell injury. This chapter will focus, in particular, on the morphologic, metabolic, and genetic events involved and also on the effects of altered ion homeostasis. A number of reviews are available on the pathophysiology of cell injury in general and in the heart in particular, including Trump and Ginn (1969), Trump and Arstila (1971), Trump and Mergner (1974), Bowen and Lockshin (1981), Trump et al. (1982), Combs and Acosta (1990), Mergner et al. (1990), and Trump and Berezesky (1992, 1998).

## Characteristics of cellular response following a lethal injury

### *General*

A cell injury may be defined as a stimulus or event that results in altering cellular homeostasis beyond the normal range (Trump and Ginn, 1969; Trump and Arstila, 1971; Trump and Mergner, 1974). These alterations may be transient or prolonged and can, therefore, represent acute or chronic states. The injuries may also be lethal, which are those injuries that result in cell death, or sublethal, which even if prolonged may be compatible with continued survival of the cell through an altered homeostatic condition. Examples of lethal injury in the myocardium include the effects of total inhibition of ATP synthesis, e.g. anoxia, ischemia, or inhibitors of respiration and glycolysis. Examples of chronic sublethal injury include myocardial hypertrophy, fatty metamorphosis following exposure to a variety of toxic agents, or chronic mitochondrial abnormalities.

At the present time, two principal types of prelethal responses have been defined: *oncosis* and *apoptosis* (Figure 5.1). Both have been described thoroughly in the cardiovascular system, and the characteristics of each are given below. Following cell death, the changes are termed *oncotic necrosis* and *apoptotic necrosis* respectively.

It is very important to note that the changes in the prelethal phase may or may not be reversible using present technology. This important concept has caused considerable confusion in the literature. Although it is true that reversibility does

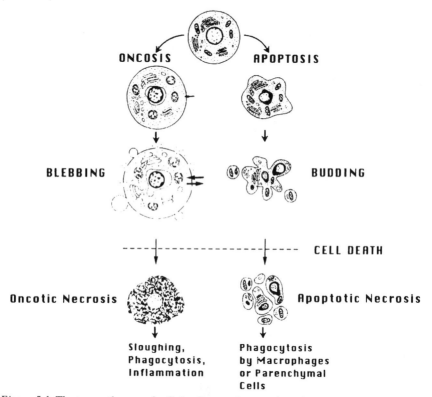

*Figure 5.1* The two pathways of cell death, namely oncosis and apoptosis, which lead a normal cell (top) to necrosis. The left side of the figure depicts schematically a cell entering and passing through oncosis, whereas the right side shows that of apoptosis. Note the differences in morphology, for example cell swelling with blebbing and increased permeability of the plasma membrane (arrows) in oncosis, whereas in apoptosis there is cell shrinkage with budding and karyorrhexis. Note also the marked nuclear chromatin clumping with near-normal cell organelles in apoptosis. Both pathways pass through the "point of no return" or cell death and onto necrosis. In oncotic necrosis, changes include sloughing, phagocytosis, and inflammation, while in apoptotic necrosis cells break up into clusters of apoptotic bodies with phagocytosis by macrophages or parenchymal cells. Modified from Majno and Joris, 1995.

confirm that the cells are alive, we have now learned enough from several experimental systems to recognize that in some cases we do not presently know how to resuscitate other cells in other conditions prior to cell death. However, numerous studies on the morphology and functional characteristics of injured cells allow us to define prelethal and post-lethal (necrotic) changes.

## Oncosis

Oncosis (from *onkos*, the Greek word for swelling) is so named because a prominent cell characteristic is swelling (Majno and Joris, 1995). This type of change occurs in widespread areas such as myocardial infarcts without reflow and/or areas targeted by toxins such as $HgCl_2$ in the proximal tubule of the kidney or $CCl_4$ toxicity in the liver. We have studied this extensively, beginning with the definition of the ultrastructural changes that characterize the reversible phase, the phase of cell death itself, and the phase of oncotic necrosis. Briefly summarized, these involve changes in the volume of cellular organelles, predominantly swelling; decreased ATP and inhibited ATP synthesis; marked changes in the concentration of intracellular ions including increased $[Na^+]_i$, $[Cl^-]_i$ and water; decreases in $[K^+]_i$; and significant increases of $[Ca^{2+}]_i$, an important signal in terms of many other responses. Such $Ca^{2+}$-mediated events include mediation of the mitochondrial permeability transition (MPT) and activation of phospholipases, proteases, endonucleases, and kinases, including those involved in induction of immediate–early genes. Key factors involved in cell death include loss of mitochondrial membrane potential ($\Delta\Psi_m$), activation of the MPT, and loss of plasmalemmal integrity.

### *Stages*

Some years ago, we investigated the reversible and irreversible changes in a variety of cell systems following lethal and sublethal injury (see for example Trump and Benditt, 1962; Goldblatt *et al.*, 1965; Trump *et al.*, 1965; Trump and Ginn, 1969; Trump and Arstila, 1971; Glaumann and Trump, 1975). These are the changes typical of oncosis. Based on these studies, we later characterized and classified these changes into stages of oncotic cell injury (Figure 5.2) to permit the correlation of structure and function and then to codify the changes so as to be able to compare differing injuries (for a review, see Trump and Berezesky, 1998). The structural and functional characteristics of each stage will be briefly discussed below.

### *Stage 1*

#### *Structure*

Stage 1 is the normal cell (Figure 5.3A). The mitochondria are in orthodox conformation and have well-defined granules. The nuclear chromatin is dispersed

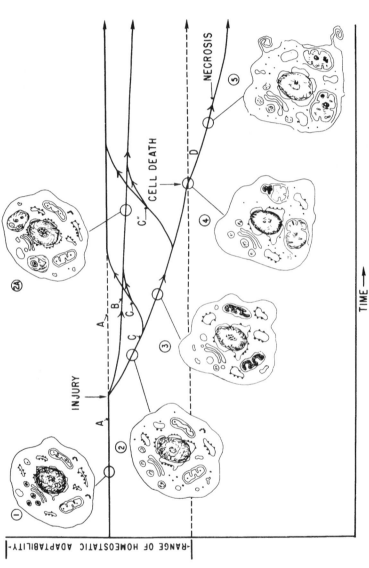

*Figure 5.2* Diagrammatic conceptualization of the stages of cell injury. As described in the text, stage 1 depicts a cell in a normal steady state (curve A). At the arrow, an injury is applied that may be acutely lethal or sublethal. In the case of a lethal injury, the cell loses homeostatic ability along curve C. Before the point of cell death, however, recovery can occur if the injurious stimulus is removed. Such recovery may then proceed along curve C' or curve C''. Note that incomplete recovery during the reversible phases after lethal injury might also result in a new steady state depicted by the right-hand limb of curves C' and C''. Reproduced with permission from Trump and Arstila (1971).

and numerous polysomes are located on the rough endoplasmic reticulum (ER) and in the cytosol.

## Stage 2

### Structure

The earliest changes are seen in this stage, often occurring within seconds after initiation of the injury. Cytoplasmic blebs form along cell surfaces; most prominently along free cell surfaces, such as lumens or capillary surfaces. These blebs have a low refractive index and are of low density, as observed by transmission electron microscopy (Figure 5.2). They usually contain free polysomes and other cytosolic components, but few organelles (Elliget *et al.*, 1991). Actin and tubulin fibers are detached from the plasma membrane and do not appear in the bleb itself; actin bundles do, however, appear at the bases of the blebs (Phelps *et al.*, 1989; Elliget *et al.*, 1991). Elsewhere in the cytosol, there is disorganization of the F-actin bundles. As the blebs grow, some constrict at the base and then detach, floating into the extracellular space. If the injury is removed prior to this point, the blebs are reabsorbed into the cytoplasm. At this phase, the ER becomes dilated and the lumen contains sparse flocculent filamentous material. This correlates with the changes in cellular volume and ion regulation. In the cytoplasm, the mitochondria often show loss of the normal matrix granules. There is clumping of the nuclear chromatin along the nuclear envelope and around the nucleolus (Trump *et al.*, 1976).

### Function

In this stage of cell injury, cellular ion shifts have begun. Depending on the type of injury, $[Ca^{2+}]_i$ may increase within a few seconds and $[Na^+]_i$, $[Cl^-]_i$, and water content also begin to increase, whereas $[K^+]_i$ decreases. In the case of anoxic injury, $[ATP]_i$ decreases rapidly, whereas $[ADP]_i$ increases (Mergner *et al.*, 1979). Coincident in time with the chromatin clumping, immediate–early genes, for example c-*fos* and c-*jun*, begin to be expressed at higher levels (Cerutti *et al.*, 1988; Cerutti and Trump, 1991; Maki *et al.*, 1992).

## Stage 3

### Structure

The principal additional change in this stage is condensation of the inner mitochondrial compartments, which become reduced in volume and become electron dense, while, at the same time, the intracristal spaces become correspondingly enlarged (Trump and Ginn, 1969). The ER continues to dilate, sometimes markedly so, creating large light microscopically visible cytoplasmic

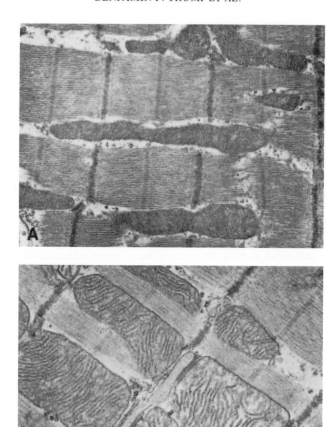

*Figure 5.3* Transmission electron micrographs (TEM) of dog myocardium. (A) Control. Bands of myofilaments comprising the A and Z bands can be seen with mitochondria arranged in rows between the myofibrils. Stage 1. ×14 000. (B) Following 15 min of *in vivo* ischemia, note marked mitochondrial swelling of inner compartments. Stage 4a. ×20 000. Reproduced with permission from Trump *et al.* (1976). (C) Following 60 min of *in vivo* ischemia, all mitochondria are markedly swollen and contain large flocculent densities, the hallmark of irreversibility. Stage 5. ×20 000. Reproduced with permission from Trump *et al.* (1976). (D) Following 120 min of *in vivo* ischemia plus 24 h of reflow, mitochondria are swollen and contain large flocculent densities and occasional calcifications (arrows). Stage 5c. ×24 000. Reproduced with permission from Trump *et al.* (1981b).

vacuoles. The former term for this was "hydropic degeneration." As the dilatation is usually shared by the nuclear envelope, which is continuous with the ER, so-called large perinuclear vacuoles often represent both dilated rough ER and dilated nuclear envelope.

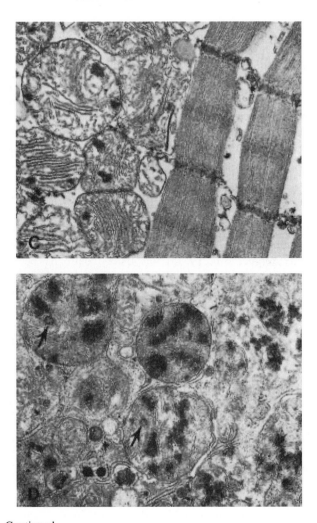

*Figure 5.3* Continued.

## Function

Condensed mitochondria typically occur under conditions in which respiration and/or oxidative phosphorylation are inhibited. Thus, in stage 3, there are markedly reduced levels of ATP (Mergner *et al.*, 1979). As long as the mitochondria remain condensed, however, they seem to be reversibly altered, and, if reoxygenated or isolated at this stage and put into a phosphorylating medium, they will synthesize ATP and generate a normal membrane potential. This condensed appearance of the mitochondria is similar to that seen in mitochondria isolated in 0.25 M sucrose (Trump and Mergner, 1974). The condensed conformation cannot apparently be maintained if significant damage to the inner membrane takes place, a change that also probably correlates with loss of the mitochondrial membrane potential.

## *Stages 4 and 4a*

### *Structure*

In these transitional stages toward irreversibility, the mitochondria show marked swelling of the inner compartment (Figure 5.3B). This can be correlated with increased inner membrane permeability, as measured in isolated mitochondria, and with a decreasing ability to maintain a proton gradient. As the inner compartment swells, mitochondrial matrical enzymes have more access to, and also probably leak into, the surrounding cytosol.

### *Function*

Functionally, the mitochondria have lost permeability control of the inner compartment, although if ATP–magnesium ($Mg^{2+}$) is added permeability control can be restored (Mergner *et al.*, 1977a). Respiratory control has been largely lost, but if cells are restored to a normal environment or mitochondria are isolated and placed in a phosphorylating medium recovery will occur. The changes in inner membrane permeability are related to modification of inner membrane phospholipids which are modified and decreased in parallel with an increase of free fatty acids. If the injurious stimulus can be removed at this point, repair of the inner membranes takes place.

## Principal mechanisms of oncosis

Direct interference with cell membrane function is a common initial injurious action from a variety of toxic and injurious agents (Figure 5.4). These include activation of the C5–9 complement sequence (Shin and Carney, 1988; Papadimitriou *et al.*, 1991), oxidant stress (Fridovich, 1978), and a variety of sulfhydryl-reactive compounds (Sahaphong and Trump, 1971), including mercurials (Gritzka and Trump, 1968). Interference with cellular energy metabolism commonly results from conditions that inhibit mitochondrial and/or glycolytic generation of ATP. Such conditions include anoxia or ischemia (Taimor *et al.*, 1999) and inhibitors of respiration, such as CN, uncouplers, such as 2,4-dinitrophenol (DNP), inhibitors of glycolysis, such as iodoacetic acid (IAA), activation of oxidants and free radicals, and inhibitors of ATPases, such as oligomycin (Gunther *et al.*, 1999).

Changes in cellular metabolism constitute the fabric of the cellular reactions to acute and chronic injury. Previous studies from our laboratory have characterized many changes and, at the present time, we are engaged in determining the precise critical mechanisms involved in cell killing, cell recovery, and cell proliferation.

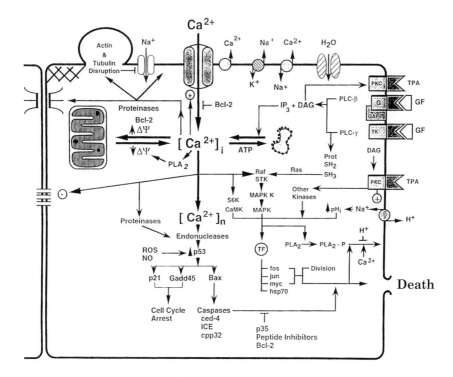

*Figure 5.4* A diagrammatic representation of a cell illustrating our current working hypothesis concerning the role of [Ca$^{2+}$]$_i$ in cell injury. Modified with permission from Trump and Berezesky (1990).

### Ion homeostasis

Ion homeostasis, and its role in the mechanism of subcellular events that follow acute and chronic cell injury, has become widely recognized and studied over the years by both our own laboratory (Trump and Berezesky, 1984, 1985a,b, 1987, 1989a,b, 1990; Trump *et al.*, 1981a) and those of others (Nicotera *et al.*, 1986; Lemasters *et al.*, 1987; Orrenius *et al.*, 1989; Van Rooijen, 1991). There is now no doubt that a variety of cellular events in cell injury are initiated by intracellular ion deregulation, particularly that of [Ca$^{2+}$]$_i$, [Na$^+$]$_i$, and [H$^+$]$_i$. Cell alterations involving changes in the metabolism and regulation of intracellular ions are extremely important as they form the basis of signaling, volume control, and energy metabolism control, and also have an increasingly evident role in division and differentiation (Trump and Berezesky, 1987; Trump *et al.*, 1989).

With the development of technologies such as energy-dispersive X-ray microanalysis, total bound elements can be measured in unfixed, freeze-dried tissues and cells (Figures 5.5–5.7). The advent of even newer methodologies such as image analysis paired with photon counting, digital imaging fluorescence microscopy, and confocal laser scanning microscopy plus the development of fluoroprobes for $Ca^{2+}$, $Na^+$, $K^+$, $Mg^{2+}$, and $\Delta\Psi_m$ is rapidly continuing the understanding of ion homeostasis and the effects on it when deregulation occurs following cell injury. These last two techniques have allowed the investigator to image living cells and not only to measure concentration levels of these various cations but also to observe the exact location of their fluctuations (see Lemasters *et al.*, 1987; Morris *et al.*, 1989; Trump *et al.*, 1989; Nieminen *et al.*, 1990; Trump and Berezesky, 1990, 1995; Bond *et al.*, 1991; Smith *et al.*, 1991, 1992; Swann *et al.*, 1991).

## *Calcium*

### *Normal regulation*

Normally, $[Ca^{2+}]_i$ (Figures 5.7–5.10) is regulated at levels of about 100 nM by a combination of transport systems at the plasma membrane, the mitochondria, the ER, and subsets thereof (Carafoli, 1987; Rasmussen, 1989). Each of these systems

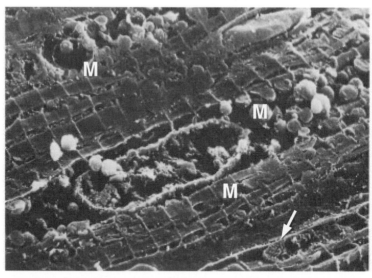

*Figure 5.5* Scanning electron micrograph (SEM) of dog myocardium following 60 min *in vivo* ischemia. A specimen was frozen following processing and then fractured to observe internal structures. Note the parallel rows of myofibrils and mitochondria (M) arranged in rows in the interfibrillar spaces and in the perinuclear region, as well as the ellipsoidal nucleus and chromatin clumping within. Also note the fractured mitochondrion (arrow) with its cristae. ×3500. Reproduced with permission from Trump *et al.* (1982).

is energy dependent and also contains specific ion channels to control membrane permeation.

## Plasma membrane

The plasmalemma constitutes a major pathway for $[Ca^{2+}]_i$ regulation (Figure 5.4). Calcium ion entry may occur through gated or ungated channels and efflux through $Ca^{2+}$-ATPase-dependent pathways. In several cell types, particularly excitable cells including the myocardium, $Na^+/Ca^{2+}$ exchange represents a major participant in $[Ca^{2+}]_i$ regulation (Pritchard and Ashley, 1986) and, therefore, toxins that interfere with the $Na^+/K^+$-ATPase or that otherwise modify $Na^+$ will have rapid secondary effects on $[Ca^{2+}]_i$. Modification of the plasmalemmal $Ca^{2+}$ regulation, therefore, constitutes a major site of toxic effects on cell injury (Figures 5.5 and 5.6). Examples include complement (Papadimitriou et al., 1991), natural killer cell-induced cytotoxicity (McConkey et al., 1990), and oxidative stress (Swann et al., 1991).

## Mitochondria

Mitochondrial calcium uptake and release systems have been well characterized and, in many cells, including the myocardium, represent large capacity systems. Uptake is energy dependent and is coupled with the generation of the proton gradient. Release occurs after cellular energy depletion or increase of nicotinamide

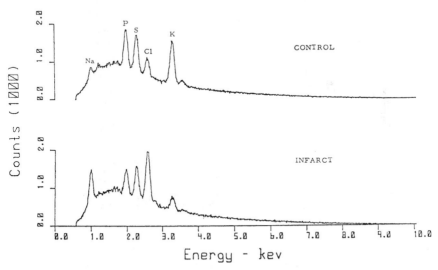

*Figure 5.6* Typical energy dispersive X-ray microanalysis spectra taken over freeze-dried 4-μm cryosections of myocardium from a patient who presented with a myocardial infarction. Note the increases in Na and Cl and the decrease in K in the infarct sample. Ca also is increased, but its small peak is obscured by the K beta peak.

adenine dinucleotide phosphate (NADPH). Cellular $[Ca^{2+}]_i$ increases after inhibition of ATP synthesis (Nicotera *et al.*, 1986; Lemasters *et al.*, 1987).

### *Endoplasmic reticulum*

The ER uptake and release pathways have also been well characterized, especially in muscle. The uptake system consists of $Ca^{2+}$-ATPase(s), which is sensitive to the compound thapsigargin and which causes immediate release of $Ca^{2+}$ from the lumen (Figure 5.4). The related species of $Ca^{2+}$-ATPases in the sarcoplasmic reticulum (SR) or endoplasmic reticulum are now referred to as the SERCA gene family, which has at least five different protein products (Lytton *et al.*, 1991). Thapsigargin inhibits all of the SERCA enzymes with equal potency. This compartment is also sensitive to metabolites of the phosphoinositide signaling pathway, especially inositol 1,4,5-trisphosphate ($IP_3$), which stimulates rapid

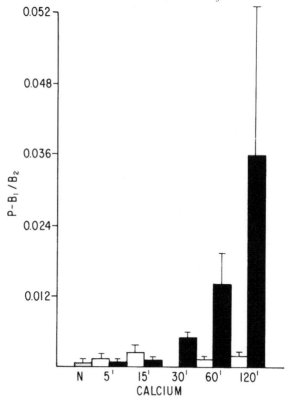

*Figure 5.7* Bar graph illustrating peak to background ratios ($P–B_1/B_2$) for calcium from energy-dispersive X-ray microanalysis measurements obtained over 4-μm freeze-dried cryosections of rat myocardium following 5, 15, 30, 60, and 120 min occlusion of the coronary artery. N, normal unoperated animals; white bars, control right ventricle; black bars, ischemic left ventricle. Reproduced with permission from Osornio-Vargas *et al.* (1981).

release of $Ca^{2+}$ and appears to represent a major link in transmembrane signaling (Berridge and Galione, 1988; Gill *et al.*, 1989). This particular $Ca^{2+}$ interaction appears to represent an important link between the effects of acute injury and toxicity and those of chronic injury, including control of growth and differentiation (Schontal *et al.*, 1991).

The release of $Ca^{2+}$ from the ER through channels occurs by two pathways, including the $IP_3$-gated channel and a calcium-gated, ryanodine-sensitive receptor (Iino *et al.*, 1988). Release of $Ca^{2+}$ from the ER following $IP_3$ stimulation is followed by a sustained $Ca^{2+}$ entry from the extracellular space. Thapsigargin has a similar effect, although it bypasses the $IP_3$ step and inhibits a $Ca^{2+}$-ATPase (Figure 5.4) (Lytton *et al.*, 1991). $Ca^{2+}$ release can also be regulated by sulfhydryl groups.

*Deregulation following injury*

Because of its central role in the mediation of a number of intracellular events,

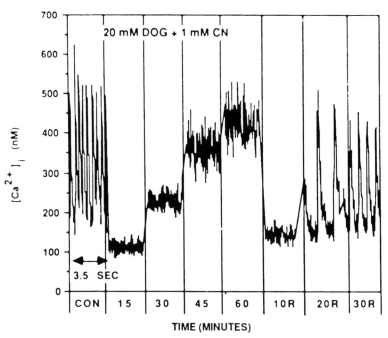

*Figure 5.8* $[Ca^{2+}]_i$ measurements, nanomolar calibration, obtained from cultured neonatal rat ventricular myocytes loaded with Fura-2 and treated with 20 mM 2-deoxy-D-glucose and 1 mM KCN for 60 min before return to control medium for 30 min. Measurements were obtained using excitation of 340/380 nm produced by a microspectrofluorometer coupled by a quartz fiber optic to a microscope epi-illuminator. Emission (510 nm) was measured by photon counting. Note cessation of $[Ca^{2+}]_i$ upon exposure to 2-deoxy-D-glucose (DOG) + CN, initial decrease in $[Ca^{2+}]_i$, and then its increase to peak systolic levels. Upon return to control medium, normal $[Ca^{2+}]_i$ transients are restored. Reproduced with permission from Morris *et al.* (1989).

acute or chronic deregulation of $[Ca^{2+}]_i$ by a cell injury would be expected to result in a variety of events. These events include activation of enzymes such as proteases, nucleases, and lipases; interaction with calmodulin; modulation of a variety of protein kinases; and alterations in cytoskeletal proteins. Some of these events may lead to terminal differentiation (Hennings *et al.*, 1989). Following injury, $[Ca^{2+}]_i$ deregulation can occur by any combination of the following: (1) influx from the extracellular space; (2) redistribution from the mitochondria; and (3) redistribution from the ER or parts thereof.

## *Sodium*

### *Normal regulation*

$Na^+$ (Figure 5.4) entry into the cell is balanced by active extrusion via the ouabain-sensitive $Na^+/K^+$-ATPase, which is sensitive to cardiac glycosides (e.g. ouabain).

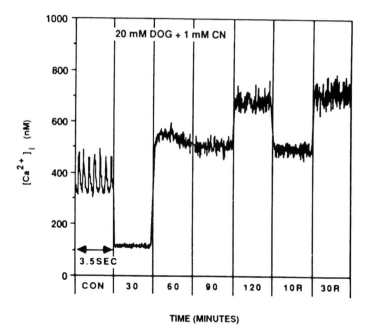

**TIME (MINUTES)**

*Figure 5.9* Same conditions as in Figure 5.8 except the treatment was for 120 min before return to the control medium. DOG–CN results in an initial decrease followed by a sustained increase in $[Ca^{2+}]_i$. Upon return to the control medium, there is a slight decrease in $[Ca^{2+}]_i$ followed by a then persistent increase. Reproduced with permission from Morris *et al.* (1989).

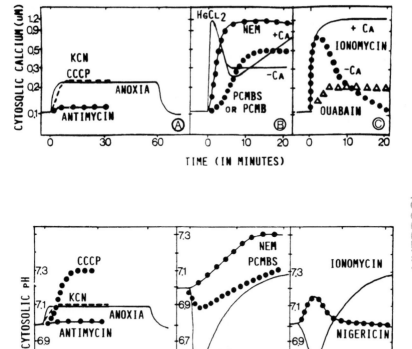

*Figure 5.10* The effect of different types of injury on cytosolic calcium of rabbit proximal tubule epithelial (PTE) cells. Cells were cultured for 8–12 days, loaded with Fura-2 (5 μM Fura-2-AM, 60 min, 25°C), and suspended by trypsinization. Spectrofluorometric measurements were made in HBSS + 10 mM Hepes, 1.37 mM $CaCl_2$, and 1 mg ml$^{-1}$ glucose at 25°C. (A) The effect of mitochondrial inhibitors on $[Ca^{2+}]_i$; anoxia, 5 mM KCN, 4 μM carbonyl-cyanide *m*-chlorophenylhydrazone (CCCP), and 5 μM antimycin. The increase in $[Ca^{2+}]_i$ seen with each is independent of $[Ca^{2+}]_e$ and is presumably due to release from mitochondria. Reoxygenation of anoxic cells leads to recovery of $[Ca^{2+}]_i$ to control levels. (B) The effect of sulfhydryl inhibition with 250 μM *N*-ethylmaleimide (NEM), 1 mM PCMBS (parachloromercuribenzenesulfonate), and 50 μM $HgCl_2$. The increased $[Ca^{2+}]_i$ seen with NEM and PCMBS is independent of $[Ca^{2+}]_e$ and is attributed mostly to release from the ER. $HgCl_2$ initially triggers release by $Ca^{2+}$ from the ER followed by activation of a plasma membrane $Ca^{2+}/H^+$ pump and then by influx of $[Ca^{2+}]_e$ when $[Ca^{2+}]_e$ is present. (C) The effect of 5 μM ionomycin with 1.37 mM $Ca^{2+}$ or less than 5 μM $Ca^{2+}$ and 500 μM ouabain. Ionomycin causes redistribution of $Ca^{2+}$ from the ER and mitochondria as well as influx of $[Ca^{2+}]_e$. In the absence of $[Ca^{2+}]_e$, $[Ca^{2+}]_i$ recovers in part by means of a plasma membrane $Ca^{2+}/H^+$-ATPase. The elevation of $[Ca^{2+}]_i$ following inhibition of $Na^+/K^+$-ATPase with ouabain is the result of increased $Na^+/Ca^{2+}$ activity in response to elevated $[Na^{2+}]_i$. Reproduced with permission from Trump *et al.* (1988).

## Deregulation

[Na$^+$]$_i$ regulation is intimately related to cell volume regulation (Figure 5.6). Cell volume regulation can be achieved in many cells if the Na$^+$/K$^+$-ATPase remains active. Following injury, however, when this is directly or indirectly inhibited, cells commonly swell and [Na$^+$]$_i$ increases, sometimes markedly. Any condition which lowers extracellular Na$^{2+}$ or raises [Na$^{2+}$]$_i$ will favor the accumulation of [Ca$^{2+}$]$_i$.

## *pH*

### *Normal regulation*

Normal intracellular pH (pH$_i$) appears to be significantly lower than plasma or tissue culture fluid, being about 7.2 (Chen and Boron, 1991). However, the actual pH of the interstitial fluid, bathing most cells, is considerably more difficult to measure and probably approximates pH$_i$. Cellular pH is regulated by three principal mechanisms: cation (Na$^+$/Ca$^{2+}$) exchange; anion (HCO$_3^-$) exchange; and H$^+$-ATPases (Chen and Boron, 1991). The Na$^+$/H$^+$ exchanger is activated by low pH$_i$ and by [Na$^+$]$_i$ increase. The activity of this exchanger can be stimulated by growth factors, probably involving phosphorylation, and, under basal conditions, works to regulate pH at about 7.0 (Figure 5.4). Following stimulation, the set point changes to 7.25 and, therefore, growth factors will result in alkalinization if the medium is below 7.2. However, this increase is minimized in the presence of normal amounts of HCO$_3^-$ which, in most proliferating cells, raises pH$_i$ by Na$^+$-dependent Cl$^-$/HCO$_3^-$ exchange.

### *Deregulation*

Considerable current interest is attached to the regulation (Figure 5.6) of pH$_i$ in relation to transmembrane signaling, effects of growth factors, and regulation of viability following toxic injury. The relation to cell division is striking following fertilization of marine eggs, where division is preceded by an influx of Ca$^{2+}$ and a rise in pH$_i$, which is apparently related to the Na$^+$/H$^+$ antiport and can be inhibited by the diuretic amiloride (Epel, 1982). Under appropriate conditions (HCO$_3^-$-free medium), amiloride or weak acids will inhibit proliferation and alkalinization of the medium will promote it. Perona and Serrano (1988) observed that chronically raising pH$_i$, by transfecting NIH-3T3 cells with yeast P-type H$^+$-ATPase, induced growth in soft agar, growth factor-independent proliferation, and tumorigenicity. Studies by Gillies *et al.* (1990) indicate that at least some human tumor cells possess enough V-type H$^+$-ATPases to raise pH$_i$ chronically.

Acidification of cells, on the other hand, appears to exert protective effects against a variety of toxic injuries. Penttila and Trump (1974), for example, found that reduction of extracellular pH (pH$_e$) from 7.4 to 6.9 could double the life span of cells subjected to complete anoxia (see also Shanley and Johnson, 1991).

Protection is also conferred against lethal injury by thermal injury as well as by chemical toxins, including $HgCl_2$. Lemasters' group reported that reducing the $pH_e$ of the perfusion medium ameliorated the reperfusion injury in ischemic myocardium (Bond *et al.*, 1991). This observation led these investigators to term this phenomenon the "pH paradox." The explanation for these effects is incomplete. Suggestions have included reduction of cell $[Na^+]_i$ and secondary $[Ca^{2+}]_i$ through the $Na^+/H^+$ and $Na^+/Ca^{2+}$ exchange mechanisms, respectively, prevention of $Ca^{2+}$ entry, and competition between $H^+$ and $Ca^{2+}$ for effects, resulting in inhibition of $Ca^{2+}$-mediated harmful events (e.g. phospholipase or protease activation).

## Potassium

### Normal regulation

$[K^+]_i$ is regulated by a process similar to that for $[Na^+]_i$ using the $Na^+/K^+$-ATPase; however, different channels exist for this cation (Figure 5.4). A variety of $K^+$ channels participate in a variety of cellular functions and participate in signaling, at least in excitable cells. Research is exploring the mechanism of this genetic diversity (Chung *et al.*, 1991). A number of genes encoding $K^+$ channel polypeptides have been cloned on the basis of their similarity to the *Drosophila* shaker locus.

### Deregulation

$[K^+]_i$ regulation is lost early and rapidly following a variety of acute injuries as a result of decreased cellular ATP and/or inhibition of the $Na^+/K^+$-ATPase at the plasmalemma (Figure 5.6).

## Magnesium

### Normal regulation

$Mg^{2+}$ is an essential element in cell function, participating in cellular energy metabolism in both photosynthesis and oxidative phosphorylation (Aikawa, 1981). In the case of oxidative phosphorylation, all ATP-requiring reactions are catalyzed by $Mg^{2+}$, which associates with ATP and other related compounds. $Mg^{2+}$ does not form highly stable chelates with organic complexes and can be dissociated from ATP.

$Mg^{2+}$ is essential for oxidative phosphorylation and changes in $[Mg^{2+}]_i$ are probably involved in its regulation. $[Mg^{2+}]_i$ participates in many other aspects of normal cell metabolism, including ribosomal structure and function and in $[Ca^{2+}]_i$ regulation where $[Mg^{2+}]_i$ is a co-factor and participates in the mediation or regulation. In the nucleus, $Mg^{2+}$ exhibits strong binding to DNA, and it appears that sections of chromosomes are maintained structurally by $Mg^{2+}$ and $Ca^{2+}$.

## *Deregulation*

Changes in $[Mg^{2+}]_i$ in relation to altered cell structure and function have not, thus far, been thoroughly characterized – principally because, until recently, methods for its measurement have not been available. More recently, however, with the development of the fluorescent probe Mag Fura-2, insights are beginning to accrue concerning its role in altered cell metabolism.

It is known that $Mg^{2+}$ is essential for mitochondrial contraction following swelling and it is often added *in vitro* as a $Mg^{2+}$–ATP complex. Similarly, the effects of $Mg^{2+}$–ATP on resuscitation of patients and animals following hemorrhagic shock have been established (Chaudry, 1990). Rats maintained on magnesium-deficient diets developed mitochondrial swelling within 10 days. Changes in total cellular $Mg^{2+}$ have not been observed in our experience until very late after cell injury, probably during the necrotic phase, in contrast to changes in total sodium, potassium, and chloride (Osornio-Vargas *et al.*, 1981). Thus, significant loss of total $[Mg^{2+}]_i$ probably represents a manifestation of rather later effects of lethal injury. On the other hand, we and others have noted rapid increases in $[Mg^{2+}]_i$ within seconds or minutes following models of anoxic or ischemic injury or treatment of cells with uncouplers of mitochondrial oxidative phosphorylation. Increases in $[Mg^{2+}]_i$, therefore, probably represent a loss from the mitochondrial compartment coupled with dissociation of $Mg^{2+}$–ATP complexes and, as such, increases in $[Mg^{2+}]_i$ probably can be used to reflect mitochondrial energy production. In addition to the effects of $[Mg^{2+}]_i$ on mitochondrial function and structure, protein synthesis, and DNA transcription, alterations of $[Mg^{2+}]_i$ may also play a role in cytoskeletal organization.

## Energy metabolism

There are many types of important cell injuries that exert a primary effect on energy metabolism, predominantly on mitochondrial ATP synthesis, although some affect primarily anaerobic glycolysis, whereas other injuries, such as ischemia, affect both eventually (Weinberg, 1991). Effects on mitochondrial ATP synthesis can be classified as follows. (1) Inhibitors of electron transport, including anoxia or ischemia, and chemical inhibitors of electron transport, including KCN, CO, antimycin, and rotenone. (2) Primary uncouplers of mitochondrial oxidative phosphorylation, including halogenated phenols such as 2,4-DNP and pentachlorophenol and hydralizines such as carbonyl cyanide *p*-(trifluoro-methoxy)-phenylhydrazone (FCCP). These compounds disperse the mitochondrial potential and proton gradient, some acting as proton ionophores. Mitochondrial uncoupling can also occur secondary to other injuries, resulting, for example, from increased $[Ca^{2+}]_i$ or primary damage to the mitochondrial inner membrane (e.g. phospholipase attack). (3) Inhibitors of oxidative phosphorylation (e.g. oligomycin) which inhibit the $H^+$-ATPase of the inner membrane. Treatment of cells or tissues *in vivo* or *in vitro* with any of these conditions results in rapid arrest of ATP synthesis within the cell and, in the case of agents which change plasma membrane permeability, acute loss of ATP from the cells. The rate of ATP decline can be extremely rapid, requiring, for example, only a few seconds or minutes in the case of the kidney cortex following clamping of the renal artery (Mergner *et al.*, 1977b). This results in transient increases in the adenosine diphosphate (ADP)/ATP ratio within cells, followed by continued conversion of ATP to ADP and of adenosine monophosphate (AMP) to xanthine, ultimately reducing total adenine nucleotides. The rate of ATP decline is related to the rate of utilization of ATP by the cell, which is dependent on ATPases. Therefore, reduction of temperature or inhibition of ATPases can retard the decline of ATP and prolong cell survival. Chaudry (1990) has reported that addition of extracellular $Mg^{2+}$-ATP can reverse some aspects of cell injury.

## Altered gene expression

### *Background*

During the past few years, it has become evident that one of the early reactions to toxic injury is the expression of a variety of immediate–early genes, stress genes, and tumor-suppressor genes such as *p53*. These are extremely important in the cellular reaction to toxic injury, and can therefore be used as early detection methods for its diagnosis. The total functions of gene expressions are incompletely understood at the present time. However, many of the proteins act as transcription factors for later genes, thus amplifying the responses of the cell. Furthermore, some of these later genes are involved in cell division and, therefore, become part of the regenerative process. Other later genes, such as *p53*, are involved in control of cell death and cell division and others, such as the stress genes, have been implicated in restricting the extent of cell injury and in protecting the cell against a repeat injury. Future understanding of these promises to be of importance in understanding the mechanisms of cell injury as well as in devising therapeutic interventions for its diagnosis, treatment, and prevention.

### *Immediate–early genes*

The oncogene c-*fos* is an example of an immediate gene that is activated by a number of acute cell injuries or stimuli, including oxidant stress (Figures 5.11 and 5.12), toxins such as heavy metals, calcium ionophores (Crawford *et al.*, 1988; Curran and Franza, 1988; Cowley *et al.*, 1989; Herbst *et al.*, 1991; Maki *et al.*, 1992), growth factors, and reflow after ischemic injury (Schiaffonati *et al.*, 1990; Rosenberg and Paller, 1991). All of the functions of c-*fos* are however still not known. It appears to relate to the early events in cell division, although it is reported also to increase in terminally differentiated cells, such as neurons, following appropriate stimulation.

How does cell injury result in activation of these genes? As the calcium

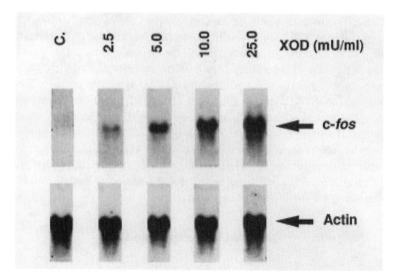

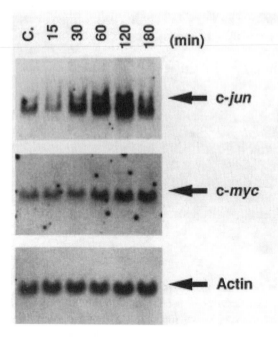

*Figure 5.11* (A) Northern blot analysis showing the dose response of c-*fos* expression by X/XOD in primary cultures of rat PTE. Cultures were treated with 500 μM xanthine (X) and 2.5–25 mU ml$^{-1}$ xanthine oxidase (XOD) for 30 min. The same membrane was rehybridized with an actin probe to ensure that the same amount of mRNA was loaded to each lane. Reproduced with permission from Maki *et al.* (1992). (B) Kinetics of the expression of c-*myc* and c-*jun* in rat PTE primary cultures following X/XOD (500 μM/ 25 mU ml$^{-1}$) treatment for 15, 30, 60, 120, and 180 min. Reproduced with permission from Maki *et al.* (1992).

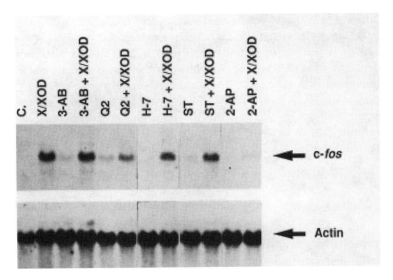

*Figure 5.12* Modification of c-*fos* expression by X/XOD in rat primary PTE cultures. X/ XOD is the sample treated with 500 μM X and 25 mU ml⁻¹ XOD for 30 min. The following samples were incubated in 3-aminobenzimide (3-AB) (10 mM), Quin 2/AM (Q2) (30 μM), H-7 (1-(5-isoquinolinesulfonyl)-2-methylpiperazine hydrochloride; 25 nM), staurosporine (ST) (50 nM), and 2-aminopurine (2-AP) (10 mM) alone or with X/XOD. C, control from an untreated culture. Reproduced with permission from Maki *et al.* (1992).

ionophore A23187 and thapsigargin (Schontal *et al.*, 1991) readily activate c-*fos*, a role for $[Ca^{2+}]_i$ seems likely. Furthermore, the cell injuries studied thus far, for example oxidant stress, also induce early increases in $[Ca^{2+}]_i$ (Swann *et al.*, 1991) which precede the stimulation of c-*fos* (Maki *et al.*, 1992). Such increases in $[Ca^{2+}]_i$ may also be associated with calcium endonuclease-induced breaks in DNA which, in turn, induce poly-ADP ribosylation. Cerutti *et al.* (1988) have proposed a role for poly-ADP ribosylation of proteins in c-*fos* induction. Pretreatment of cells with Quin 2 to buffer $[Ca^{2+}]_i$ increases has been found to be preventive against DNA strand breaks (Cantoni *et al.*, 1989).

### Stress genes

Much of the original work on stress genes has involved the so-called "heat shock proteins" (hsp), originally described in *Drosophila*. These proteins, which have now been extensively subdivided into families (see reviews by Lindquist, 1988; Welch, 1990), are evoked in virtually all prokaryotic and eukaryotic forms, and various classes are induced by a variety of stressors including heat, ATP depletion, heavy metal intoxication, ischemia (Cairo *et al.*, 1985), and oxidant stress (Blake *et al.*, 1990).

Typically, the shock response is characterized by specific and transient induction of heat shock gene expression, blockade of normal translation with preferential translation of heat shock proteins, and induction of thermotolerance or, in some cases, protection against other forms of cell injury (Ghosh *et al.*, 1991; Yamamoto *et al.*, 1993). Hsp70 and hsp90 have been investigated the most extensively. Hsp90 represents the non DNA-binding component of the steroid receptor and appears to be involved in complexes with several oncogenic tyrosine-specific kinases including v-*src*. Hsp70 is associated with a variety of cell phenomena involving binding to unfolded proteins in an ATP-dependent manner. Such unfolding may occur during normal turnover or during exposure to denaturing conditions, as often occurs after lethal cell injury (Majno and Joris, 1996).

## p53

### Background

Overexpression of wild-type *p53* occurs following a number of apoptosis-producing injuries in the kidney and elsewhere (Harris *et al.*, 1996). In the kidney, overexpression of *p53* has been observed in a number of models and situations, including microinjection of p53, ischemia/reflow, chemical models of ischemia, nitric oxide exposure, oxidant injury, mercuric chloride, and cisplatin. In each case, overexpression appears to be linked to apoptosis.

Thus far, possible mechanisms can be classified as transcription dependent and transcription independent. Most is known about the transcription-dependent pathway. Phosphorylated p53 is a potent transcription factor for several genes associated with apoptosis and cell cycle arrest. These include *Bax*, *Gadd45*, *p21* (*Waf*), *mdm-2* and others. Vogelstein's group (Polyak *et al.*, 1997) has observed fourteen genes that were markedly expressed in *p53*-expressing cells. Most of these encoded proteins that could generate or respond to oxidative stress. This led them to propose that *p53* results in apoptosis through a three-step process: (1) transcriptional induction of redox-related genes; (2) the formation of reactive oxygen species; and (3) the oxidative degradation of mitochondrial components, culminating in cell death. Our group has indeed found evidence that overexpression of *p53* does induce oxygen stress in cultured cells. This leads to the fascinating idea that not only does oxidant stress induce *p53* overexpression but that *p53* overexpression leads to oxidant stress – thus developing a vicious cycle.

## Hypothesis of [Ca$^{2+}$] and oncosis

Through the years, based on our experiments and those in the literature, we have continued to develop a working hypothesis of the response of cells to acute, lethal, and sublethal injury as ideas are proposed and data are confirmed (Figure 5.13). This hypothesis has focused, and continues to focus, on the role of ion deregulation, especially that of [Ca$^{2+}$]$_i$ (Trump *et al.*, 1981a,b; 1989; 1990; Trump and Berezesky, 1987, 1989a,b, 1990).

## *Regulation of [Ca²⁺]ᵢ*

Regulation of $[Ca^{2+}]_i$ at normal levels approximates 100 nM. In Figure 5.13, note the ATP-dependent regulation by the plasma membrane, the mitochondria, and the ER. Several of the $Ca^{2+}$-activated systems are shown, including $Ca^{2+}$-activated proteases, phospholipases, and nucleases; integrity of gap junctions, and affects on calmodulin and calmodulin-dependent processes, including modulation of the cytoskeleton.

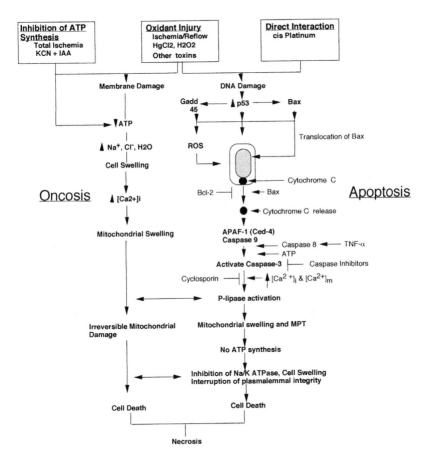

*Figure 5.13* Diagram showing the contrast and similarity between events leading to apoptosis and oncosis. Note that the pathways converge after cell death.

## *Relationship to signaling*

For relationship to signaling, see the right-hand side of Figure 5.14. Note that signaling, involving ion deregulation, can either be initiated by growth factors or by other extracellular stimuli binding to receptors and activating pathways involving cyclic GMP or cyclic AMP at the cell membrane. In the case of G protein signaling, calcium-dependent phospholipase *c* appears to be involved in the liberation of membrane phosphoinositide metabolites, such as $IP_3$ and diacylglycerol (DAG) (Berridge and Irvine, 1984). $IP_3$ results in rapid loss of $Ca^{2+}$ from the ER, thus increasing $[Ca^{2+}]_i$, which may, in turn, induce further signal transmission. Furthermore, increases of $[Ca^{2+}]_i$ in many cells open calcium channels at the cell membrane, causing an influx of $Ca^{2+}$. DAG is capable of activating protein kinase C (PKC), which is also directly activated by phorbol esters such as TPA (Nishizuka, 1984). Actually, it is a growing family of PKC whose total function is not currently understood. Several of these are calcium dependent and increases of $[Ca^{2+}]_i$ may act synergistically with direct stimulation, e.g. by 12-*O*-tetradecanoylphorbol-13-acetate (TPA). Other protein kinases are activated by cyclic AMP kinases, some of which stimulate phosphorylation of calcium-reactive sites on the SR, such as phospholamban, and on the troponin–tropomyosin complex.

Regulation of the membrane G proteins in the active versus the inactive state is accomplished through regulator proteins, including GTPase-activating protein (GAP), which interacts with the protein to down-regulate it to the inactive state, thus stopping a signal. It has been observed that mutations in G proteins, such as those induced by mutations of the oncogene *ras*, interfere with this regulation and that the modified protein can remain in the active state, thus perpetuating the signaling process (Freissmuth *et al.*, 1989). Other activities of PKC include activation of the $Na^+/H^+$ antiport which is involved in regulation of $[pH]_i$ and, under appropriate conditions, can result in alkalinization of the cytoplasm.

The action of the signaling pathway on the ER through $IP_3$ can be simulated by compounds, such as thapsigargin, which induce release of $Ca^{2+}$ from the ER by inhibition of uptake (Ghosh *et al.*, 1991). This can result in activation of many of the processes, including gene expression, that are triggered by growth factor or hormone stimulation. This area thus provides an important link between xenobiotic treatment of cells or other types of cell injury and normal stimulation. The normal control mechanisms can return calcium homeostasis to normal through the normal calcium translocation systems described above; however, if these are modified, for example with *ras* mutations or with continued increase in $[Ca^{2+}]_i$ by changes of membrane permeability, continued and inappropriate signaling will occur.

## *Cytoskeleton*

Alterations of the cytoskeleton appear to play an active and possibly fundamental role in many sublethal and lethal reactions to injury. These can involve actin and associated proteins, tubulin, and intermediate filaments, including keratin. Regulation of $[Ca^{2+}]_i$ can be involved in the modification of all components of the cytoskeleton. Some of these interactions involve phosphorylation, for example phosphorylation of tubulin may be a controlling factor in mitosis, and formation of the spindle and interactions with troponin C permits actin and myosin interactions.

Some of the early changes following sublethal injury include bleb formation (Figure 5.14), which clearly results from increased $[Ca^{2+}]_i$ (Nicotera et al., 1986; Lemasters et al., 1987; Phelps et al., 1989; Nieminen et al., 1990) and modification of actin and tubulin (Figures 5.15 and 5.16) (Elliget et al., 1991). The detachment of actin from the membrane in the region of the bleb and possibly contraction by forming a band of actin at the base of the bleb seem to be common to many types of bleb formation. In ruffles, phospholipase $A_2$ has been localized in blebs (Bar-Sagi et al., 1988). At least some of this appears to involve calcium-activated proteases because inhibitors such as leupeptin and antipain can markedly modify bleb formation. Kolber et al. (1990) have observed that modification with actin and cytochalasin results in DNA strand breaks.

In terminal differentiation in the skin, epithelium, and bronchial epithelium, increased $[Ca^{2+}]_i$ seems to modify expression of keratin intermediate filaments and formation of cross-linked bundles of keratin (Yuspa et al., 1988; Miyashita et al., 1989).

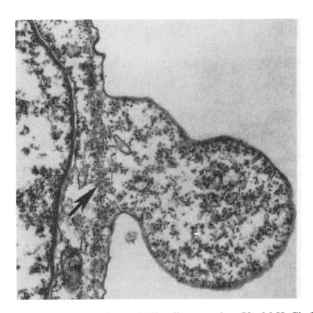

*Figure 5.14* TEM of a portion of a rat PTE cell exposed to 50 μM $HgCl_2$ for 4 min at 37°C with low $[Ca^{2+}]_e$. Note the bands of fine filaments, probably representing actin, at the base of the blebs (arrow). ×25 000. Reproduced with permission from Phelps et al. (1989).

## *Gene activation*

As shown in Figure 5.14, modification of cell ions can modify gene expression. Increases in $[Ca^{2+}]_i$ result in activation of several immediate–early and stress genes, including c-*fos*, c-*jun*, c-*myc* (Morgan and Curran, 1988; Kolber *et al.*, 1990), and hsp70 (Welch *et al.*, 1990). Some of this activation appears to result from phosphorylation of regulatory proteins. In some cases, poly-ADP ribosylation seems to represent a control mechanism. Poly-ADP ribosylation is stimulated by DNA strand breaks, which, in turn, can result from calcium activation of endonucleases (e.g. following oxidant injury). The role of altered $[pH]_i$ in this process is currently being investigated; however, regulation in the physiologic range is essential for DNA replication and transcription to occur.

## *Changes in cell junctions*

Increases in $[Ca^{2+}]_i$ result in decreased cell–cell communications or changes in GAP junction proteins. It has been proposed that decreased cell–cell communication is an early change in tumor promotion and can, in fact, be used as a screening test for putative tumor promoters. Decreased concentrations of $[Ca^{2+}]_e$ also affect cell–cell communication and, if prolonged, can result in detachment of desmosomes, intermediate junctions, and tight junctions.

A

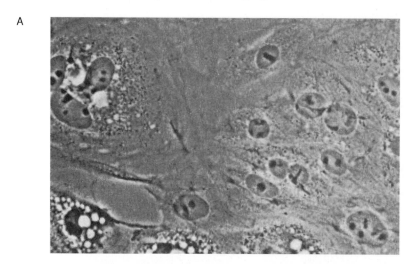

*Figure 5.15* Photomicrographs of untreated, 4-day, control cultures of rat PTE. The phase-contrast photomicrograph (A) shows the spread-out, flat appearance typical of these cultured cells. Fluorescein phalloidin staining (B, the same field as A) shows abundant stress fibers as long, fluorescent cables spanning the long axis of control cells. In (B), heavy staining is identified with the nuclear area in (A). ×260. Reproduced with permission from Elliget *et al.* (1991). Photomicrographs of PTE stained with fluorescein phalloidin after exposure to 100 μM $HgCl_2$ for 2 min (C) and 10 min (D). ×260. Reproduced with permission from Elliget *et al.* (1991).

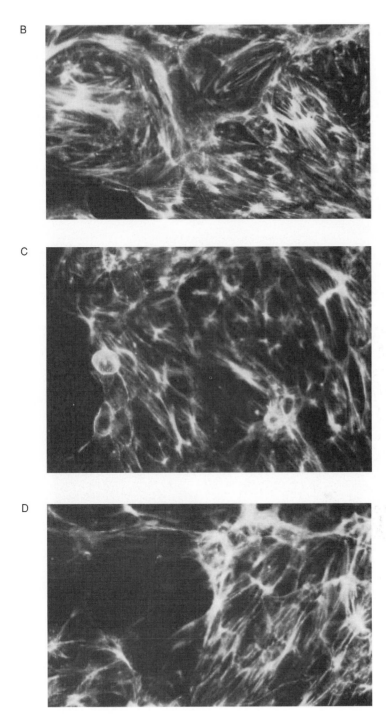

*Figure 5.15* Continued.

A

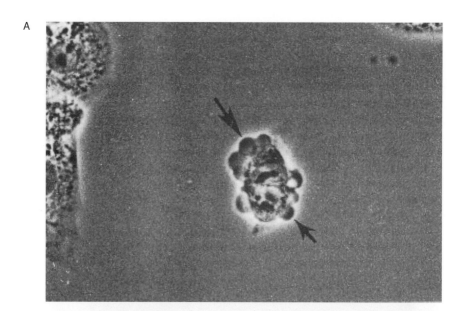

B

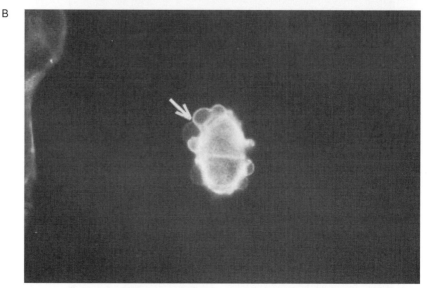

*Figure 5.16* Phase-contrast (A) and fluorescent (B) photomicrographs of PTE after 6-min exposure to 100 μM HgCl₂. Actin filaments are absent in the cytoplasm and interior of blebs (arrows), but there is a clear band of fluorescent staining around each cell and four of the blebs (B). ×260. Reproduced with permission from Elliget *et al.* (1991).

## Changes in cell membranes

During the progression from sublethal to lethal injury, marked alterations in membrane integrity occur that involve all membranes within the cell. In mitochondria, for example, change from the condensed to the swollen conformation is a result of mitochondrial swelling and modification of inner membrane phospholipids. The entire cell undergoes swelling due largely to the Donnan effect in the absence of ion regulation, especially $[Na^+]_i$. The cytoplasmic blebs become more numerous and, ultimately, marked increases of plasmalemmal permeability occur, permitting escape of cytosolic enzymes and ultimately leading to cell death. These membrane effects appear to be the direct result of activation of calcium-dependent phospholipases and proteases. Although initially these are apparently repairable (e.g. mitochondrial swelling even of the high-amplitude variety can reverse), they ultimately become irreversible, an event which appears to correlate with the point of cell death.

# Apoptosis

The term "apoptosis" is derived from two Greek words *apo*, meaning away from, and *ptosis*, to fall. Apoptosis (Figures 5.17–5.27) is, therefore, literally a falling away. This term thus refers to the blebbing and fragmentation of the cells undergoing this phenomenon. It was first described by Kerr (1971) and given the name apoptosis by Kerr *et al.* (1972). In a sense, the phenomenon is similar to apocrine secretion, which is a type of secretion in which part of the cytoplasm is budded away and enters the extracellular space (Bowen and Lockshin, 1981; Wyllie, 1981; Bowen and Bowen, 1990).

The phenomenon of apoptosis occurs in a variety of physiologic and pathologic conditions, including normal development, hormone withdrawal as in the prostate gland following castration, turnover of lymphocytes, development of the nervous system including the eye, and many other examples which have been well reviewed by Wyllie (1981).

The typical changes of apoptosis are well known and need not be repeated here. However, it is important to note that the mechanisms of apoptosis leading from injury to cell death are considerably less well understood than those in oncosis. Part of this is, of course, because it has not been recognized as an important entity until recently. Pathologists had previously referred to this change as "single cell necrosis" or "shrinkage necrosis." However, because of the rapid turnover of apoptotic cells, evaluation of the magnitude of apoptosis becomes virtually impossible to estimate from observations of single sections at any one point in time. In addition, the apoptotic fragments are typically phagocytosed by adjacent parenchymal or mesenchymal cells, leading to further deterioration of apoptotic cells within the phagolysosomal system of these cells.

Apoptosis occurs in the kidney following a variety of types of cell injury (see Figure 5.13 and review by Davis and Ryan, 1998). These include a variety of

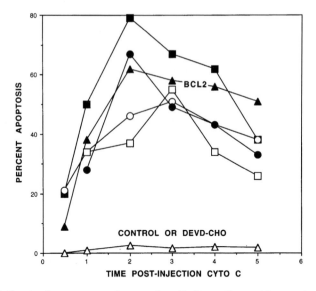

*Figure 5.17* Graph of percentage of apoptotic cells (in medium with serum) seen over a 6-h time period in four experiments after microinjection with cytochrome *c* and in one experiment where cells were microinjected with Bcl-2 plasmid (pD5-neo-Bcl-2) 24 h before cytochrome *c* microinjection. Also shown is a curve representing cells that were incubated with 50 mmol $l^{-1}$ Ac-DEVD-CHO for 1.5 h before, during, and after microinjection with cytochrome *c* which shows minimal apoptosis similar to that of control cells. Reproduced with permission from Chang *et al.* (2000).

congenital and acquired diseases of the kidney, including polycystic kidney; ischemia/reflow (Raafat *et al.*, 1997) and chemical models thereof; renal allograft rejection (Wever *et al.*, 1998); Fas binding (Schelling *et al.*, 1998); toxic injury including $HgCl_2$ (Nath *et al.*, 1996), cadmium, okadaic acid (Davis *et al.*, 1994; Nguyuza *et al.*, 1997), gentamicin, lipopolysaccharide, nitric oxide (Muhl *et al.*, 1996, Traylor and Mayeux, 1997; Paller *et al.*, 1998) and *cis*-platinum; urinary tract obstruction; growth factors including TGF-β; and a variety of types of oxidative injury *in vivo* and *in vitro*. Significantly, several immediate–early genes including c-*fos*, c-*jun* (Ishikawa *et al.*, 1997), and c-*myc* also can trigger apoptosis. We have observed that all of these can be induced by oxidant stress in the kidney (Maki *et al.*, 1992; Yamamoto *et al.*, 1993). Oxidative injury is common to many of these and, therefore, because of its widespread involvement appears to be one of the best models for studying the mechanisms involved. In addition, oxidant injury can clearly induce either oncosis or apoptosis, depending on unknown factors which we will investigate. Another important characteristic of oxidant injury to the kidney is that it can be reversible (Nowak *et al.*, 1998). We have utilized microinjection of cytochrome *c* to study this (Figures 5.17 and 5.18).

The phenomenon of apoptosis begins with striking changes in both the cytoplasm and the nucleus. The cytoplasm undergoes marked blebbing at the cell

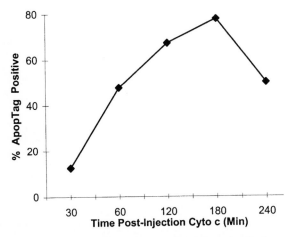

*Figure 5.18* Graph of percentage of cytochrome *c* microinjected cells that were positive for ApopTag staining over a period of 4 h, indicating DNA strand breaks characteristic of apoptosis. Reproduced with permission from Chang *et al.* (2000).

periphery, undoubtedly due to mediated changes in cytoskeletal membrane interactions. Such interactions result in constriction of the blebs, pinching off and ultimately phagocytosis of the budded portions of cytoplasm by adjacent parenchymal or connective tissue cells. These buds then enter the phagolysosomal system of the phagocytosing cell and initially form large eosinophilic cytoplasmic inclusions, of which the Councilman body in the liver is a classic example. Also, very early in the process, there is clumping of nuclear chromatin along the nuclear envelope and the beginning of fragmentation of the nucleus. This morphologic change in chromatin is accompanied by double-stranded DNA breaks which typically occur at internucleosomal regions, giving a characteristic "ladder" pattern on gels. This pattern is maintained and is particularly prominent in certain cells, such as lymphocytes.

As the process continues, the cytoplasm condenses and the nuclei become pyknotic, leading to the formation of so-called "apoptotic" bodies, readily visible in hematoxylin- and eosin-stained sections. These bodies are typical of hormone withdrawal in hormone-dependent organs and also occur prominently during development in several systems. Ultimately, the death of the fragments occurs and they undergo necrotic changes either in the extracellular space or within the phagolysosomes of the phagocytosing cell.

### Kinetics and stages of apoptosis

It is clear from our studies that the progress of apoptosis can be subdivided into at least four phases. This conclusion is based on our own work using time-lapse video microscopy correlated with a number of other techniques, but it also has

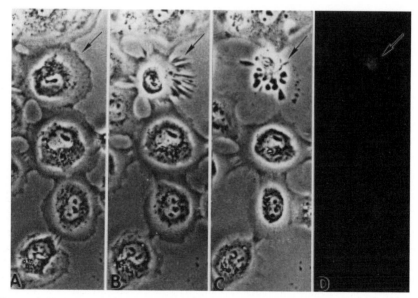

*Figure 5.19* Series of phase-contrast images of the same group of live cells after microinjection of cytochrome *c* (original magnification, ×785). (A) Just after microinjection. (B) Thirty minutes after microinjection, showing a cell beginning to shrink (arrow). (C) Thirty-two minutes after microinjection, showing the start of active phase apoptosis (arrow). (D) A fluorescent image (UV filter) of the cells stained with Hoechst 33342 at 35 min, demonstrating early chromatin condensation in the apoptotic cell (arrow). Reproduced with permission from Chang *et al.* (2000).

drawn on the classic and excellent studies by Bessis (1964) on cell death using time-lapse cinematography.

In our studies, we utilized the microinjection of cytochrome *c*, a common intermediate mediator for apoptosis in many cell systems and following a variety of injuries. Cytochrome *c* microinjection begins to induce apoptosis within 25 min and peaks at 2–3 h in NRK-52E cells (Chang *et al.*, 2000).

### Initiation phase

In this phase, the cells show an initial slight swelling followed by retraction and cell rounding, leaving long retraction processes on the substrate. The extent of the perimeter of these processes roughly outlines the periphery of the original cell margins.

### Active phase

In this phase, pseudopods begin to appear around the entire periphery of the cells (Figures 5.20–5.24). In time-lapse recordings (accelerated 60×), this process is very dramatic and pseudopods are readily observed to extend rapidly and contract

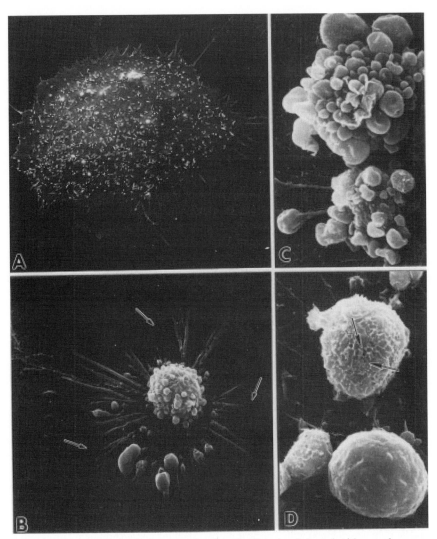

*Figure 5.20* Scanning EM of a control cell and cells microinjected with cytochrome *c*. (A) A typical untreated epithelial cell with many short microvilli and thin peripheral processes (original magnification, ×2400). (B) A contracted cell in the early (1 h) active phase of apoptosis, showing multiple pseudopods on the cell body and on remnant cytoplasmic strands (arrows) (original magnification, ×2800). (C) Cells in late active phase (2 h) that have formed aggregates and show large pseudopods. The upper group includes three or four active phase cells (original magnification, ×3100). (D) Two spherical phase cells (4 h), identified by shape and lack of pseudopods. Occasional pitted areas are seen at the cell surface (arrows) (original magnification, ×3500). These areas are presumed to correspond to vacuoles, as seen in Figure 5.21D. Reproduced with permission from Chang *et al.* (2000).

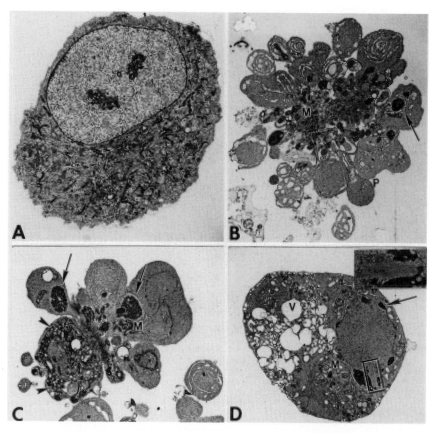

*Figure 5.21* (A) Transmission EM of a normal untreated cell, showing a nucleus and elongated mitochondria (original magnification, ×3750). (B and C) Active phase cells after microinjection, showing multiple pseudopods, often containing annular patterns of rough endoplasmic reticulum (RER) profiles, dense free ribosomes, and nuclear fragments or processes (arrows). Cellular organelles are concentrated in one area, mitochondria (M) are mostly condensed or slightly swollen, and the RER is dilated (original magnification, ×4500). In B at lower left, note a process of a necrotic cell (arrowhead). Also note at middle right a pseudopod with a nuclear process showing dense chromatin (arrow). In C at lower left, there is a narrow band region of chromatin with nuclear pores (arrowheads), also note two pseudopods with a nuclear process (arrows). (D) A spherical phase cell with an eccentric nucleus having peripheral patches of dense chromatin, nuclear budding (arrow), highly dilated RER, swollen mitochondria (M), and large apical vacuoles (V) (original magnification, ×3000). An outlined area of nuclear filaments is enlarged (inset) (original magnification, ×8250). Reproduced with permission from Chang *et al.* (2000).

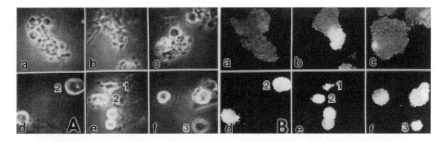

*Figure 5.22* Phase-contrast images of Fura 2-loaded cells after microinjection with cytochrome *c*. (A) a, b, and c: Active phase cells at 2 h, 2 h, and 3 h respectively. (A) d, e, and f: Spherical phase cells at 5 h, 5.25 h, and 6 h respectively. (B) Ratioed and normalized images of the identical cells in A. Cells were analyzed for $[Ca^{2+}]_i$ by digital imaging fluorescence microscopy. Images are displayed in gray tone, ranging from ~200 nmol $l^{-1}$ (darkest) to 900 nmol $l^{-1}$ calcium (lightest). The calcium range for the active phase cells was from 150 to 200 nmol $l^{-1}$ (B, b and c), and for the spherical cells the maximum range was 900 nmol $l^{-1}$ (B, d, cell 2), 500 nmol $l^{-1}$ (B, e, cells 1 and 2), and 500 nmol $l^{-1}$ (B, f, cell 3). Reproduced with permission from Chang *et al.* (2000).

multiple times (Chang *et al.*, 2000). It is also common to observe secondary pseudopods arising from the longer primary pseudopods; occasionally, we have observed the detachment of portions of a pseudopod which then drifts into the medium. This process is, therefore, very active and presumably energy requiring. At this time, the actin filaments become disorganized, although the status of actin-associated proteins, such as gelsolin, is not yet known. It has, however, been reported that caspase-3 cleaves gelsolin, some fragments of which appear to cut actin. Detailed observations of individual cells show that this active phase may continue for several hours.

Electron microscopy of this phase shows an extremely electron-dense cytosol, clustering of organelles around the nucleus, marked nuclear irregularity with clumping of chromatin, and numerous pseudopods which contain only a dense cytosol and free polyribosomes (Chang *et al.*, 2000). The mitochondria are either normal or have slight condensation of the matrix. The $\Delta\Psi_m$ remains intact, as seen by rhodamine 123 fluorescence.

### *Quiescent spherical phase*

When the cells enter this phase, the active pseudopod formation ceases and the cells become spherical and quiescent. The plasma membrane is relatively smooth except for some invaginations. The mitochondria begin to show swelling by phase-contrast and electron microscopy. $[Ca^{2+}]_i$ also begins to increase, but the $\Delta\Psi_m$ is still intact (Figures 5.20, 5.21, 5.24, 5.26).

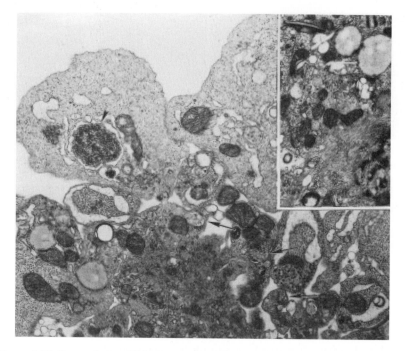

*Figure 5.23* Transmission EM of an active phase cell showing portions of several pseudopods and part of the central organelle area. Mitochondria appear to be slightly swollen and rounded, and the RER is dilated. Pseudopods contain a few mitochondria, free ribosomes, RER, and an occasional nuclear process with condensed chromatin (left pseudopod, arrowhead). Within the organelle region are phagolysosomes (arrows) and areas of filaments measuring ~200 nm (original magnification, ×16 500). The inset shows a prominent area of filaments from another active phase cell (original magnification, ×16 500). Reproduced with permission from Chang *et al.* (2000).

### Apoptotic necrosis

In this phase, the cells become more swollen, and the mitochondria and ER are markedly swollen. The mitochondria exhibit typical flocculent densities characteristic of necrotic cells. The cells detach from the coverslips or dishes at this phase.

## Principal proposed mechanisms of apoptosis

### Cell volume and ion regulation

A striking morphologic characteristic of apoptotic cells is the marked shrinkage that occurs. The loss of water renders the cytosol dense by both phase-contrast and electron microscopy. Current evidence indicates that the shrinkage is secondary to loss of $K^+$ and $Cl^-$ from the cytosol, although the precise mechanism of this loss has not been characterized. The relationship of cell shrinkage and $K^+$ loss to other

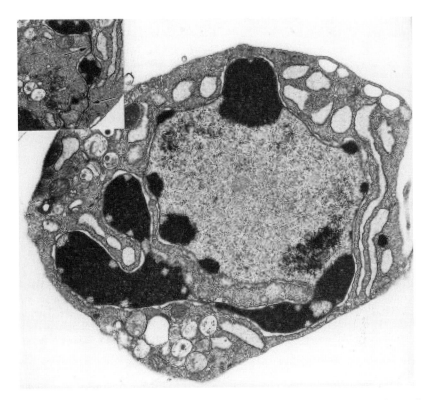

*Figure 5.24* Transmission EM of a spherical phase cell showing areas of intense chromatin clumping and a large, dramatic nuclear chromatin bud with a bilobular configuration (original magnification, ×15 600). The inset shows a smaller nuclear chromatin process, which can be identified by the presence of a nuclear envelope and small strands that connect the process with the main body of the nucleus (arrows) (original magnification, ×13 000). Reproduced with permission from Chang *et al.* (2000).

steps in apoptosis has been questioned by Cidlowski and co-workers (Bortner *et al.*, 1997; Hughes *et al.*, 1997). They found that $K^+$ at normal concentrations inhibits DNA fragmentation and caspase-3 activity, suggesting an important early role for the $K^+$ loss. They suggested a role for the shrinkage and found that hypotonically treated cells with the same $K^+$ loss exhibited no apoptosis.

## *Regulation of $[Ca^{2+}]_i$*

There is considerable evidence that deregulation of $[Ca^{2+}]_i$ plays an important role in apoptosis, as it does in oncosis (Figure 5.22). We have reviewed this subject in detail (Trump and Berezesky, 1998). Although entry of $Ca^{2+}$ from the extracellular fluid can clearly induce apoptosis in several cell types, increased $[Ca^{2+}]_i$ can also result from $Ca^{2+}$ redistribution, e.g. from the ER. Treatment of thymocytes with thapsigargin clearly induces rapid apoptosis. With other types of

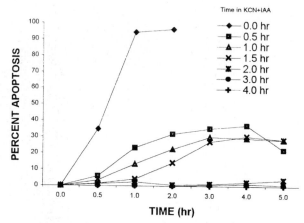

*Figure 5.25* Graph of percentage of apoptotic cells in medium without serum over a 5-h period after different pretreatment times with 0.25 mmol l⁻¹ KCN + 0.25 mmol l⁻¹ IAA followed by microinjection of cytochrome *c*. Zero time represents the time of microinjection. Control cells (no chemical treatment) had almost 100 percent apoptosis by 1–2 h. Cells pretreated for up to 1.5 h before microinjection showed a reduction to about 30 percent apoptosis by 4 h, and cells pretreated for 2 h or longer before microinjection had no apoptotic cells. Reproduced with permission from Chang *et al.* (2000).

apoptosis induction in the kidney, such as that following treatment with okadaic acid, overexpression of p53 or microinjection of cytochrome *c*, we observed that the increase in $[Ca^{2+}]_i$ occurred later – during the inactive spherical phase described above but prior to cell death. One hypothesis is that this later $Ca^{2+}$ entry induces the MPT. Furthermore, we reported an important role for $Ca^{2+}$ regulation in the protective effects exerted by overexpression of Bcl-2 (Ichimiya *et al.*, 1998).

### Induction of p53

The mechanisms involved in the induction of *p53* overexpression are incompletely understood, but do not seem to involve transcription; instead, the half-life of p53 is extended through decreased protein turnover (Harris, 1996a,b). Most of the overexpressed protein is in the nucleus where it can readily be demonstrated by immunohistochemistry. Damage to DNA induced by ionizing or ultraviolet irradiation, chemotherapeutic agents or oxidant injury from a variety of toxins and drugs is one important inducing factor. The precise mechanism(s) whereby induction of p53 leads to apoptosis in any cell type has not yet been determined.

### Cytochrome c

Cytochrome *c* release from mitochondria into the cytosol appears to be a major mechanistic step following many different inducers of apoptosis, including oxidant

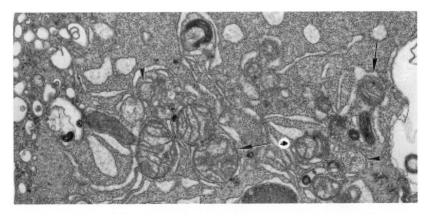

*Figure 5.26* Transmission EM of the perinuclear area of a spherical phase cell. A dense chromatin area in the nucleus is just visible at the bottom of the micrograph. Mitochondria are rounded (arrows) and show high-amplitude swelling of the inner compartment, the cytoplasm is densely packed with free ribosomes, the RER is dilated, and phagolysosomes are present (arrowheads) (original magnification, ×15 600). Reproduced with permission from Chang *et al.* (2000).

stress and p53 overexpression. It, therefore, is an important mechanism to investigate as it is part of the pathway with diverse agents. Normally found in the outer compartment of mitochondria, cytochrome *c* can be released following appropriate stimulation. It can then be detected in the cytosol using immunohistochemistry and/or Western blotting. The mechanism of release to the cytosol is unknown, but two principal mechanisms have been proposed: (1) rupture of the outer mitochondrial membrane secondary to mitochondrial swelling, and (2) release through some type of pore in the membrane. It becomes important to distinguish between these possibilities as the first is a relatively late event, occurring after the MPT, while the second may occur relatively early and may be related to the antiapoptotic properties of Bcl-2 and the proapoptotic protein Bax.

Following such release, it has been suggested that cytochrome *c* can induce apoptosis through pathways of which some at least apparently involve activation of caspase-3 (Figure 5.17). Previously, we confirmed that microinjection of cytochrome *c*, indeed, induces rapid apoptosis in NRK-52E cells. We also observed that caspase-3 inhibition totally protected against all stages of apoptosis, as mentioned above.

### *The* Bcl-2 *gene family*

This important gene family (at least fifteen family members thus far defined) includes both anti-death genes (such as *Bcl-2*) and pro-death genes (such as *Bax*) which are highly conserved in animal species. These proteins seem to be important regulators of apoptosis and are apparently involved in normal cell and tissue homeostasis, embryonic development, and response to pathogens or other cellular

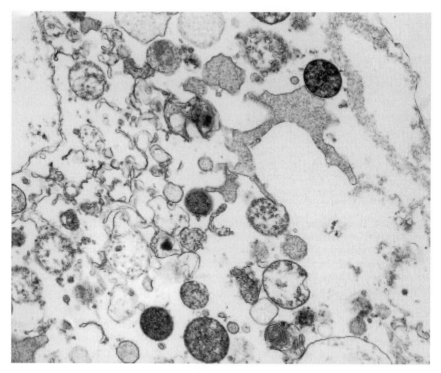

*Figure 5.27* Necrotic cell following injection of *p53* genes. Note the swollen cytosol, nuclear karyolysis, flocculent densities in the swollen mitochondria, and extreme dilatation of ER with fragmentation of cell membranes. Notice the similarity to oncotic necrosis in Figure 5.3C.

injuries. Inappropriate expression of members of this family may, by preventing cell death, exert deleterious effects in the prognosis of cancer.

We, and others, have observed that Bcl-2 also protects against oncosis and necrosis following other types of injury such as ischemia, chemical models of ischemia, and oxidant injury (Ichimiya *et al.*, 1998). This broad spectrum of protection conferred by Bcl-2 and related family members deserves considerable attention as it may provide important clues to diverse types of cell injury response as well as to novel therapeutic or preventive approaches.

The mode of action of these proteins is thus receiving considerable attention (Adams and Cory, 1998). Bcl-2 is located on the cytoplasmic face of the mitochondrial outer membrane, in the ER, and in the nuclear envelope. Studies using MRI and related techniques have revealed that these proteins can insert into membranes, forming channels which may permit transfer of ions and/or proteins. The Bcl-XL three-dimensional structure resembles that of diphtheria toxin and bacterial colicins. Interestingly, while Bcl-2, Bax, and Bcl-XL can all form channels in synthetic membranes, they have opposing effects on cell life and death. There is good evidence that the Bcl-2/Bax ratio can regulate an antioxidant pathway that leads to cell death (Korsmeyer *et al.*, 1993). Furthermore, there is good evidence that Bax can be targeted to the mitochondria.

Several possible mechanisms for cell death protection have been suggested by recent studies, including (1) modification or buffering of increased $[Ca^{2+}]_i$ resulting from cell injury (Murphy *et al.*, 1996; Ichimiya *et al.*, 1998); (2) prevention of cytochrome *c* release from the outer mitochondrial compartment to the cytosol; (3) inhibition of caspases; (4) shifting the cellular redox potential to a more reduced state, thus preventing oxidative stress (Ellerby *et al.*, 1996)

### Immediate–early genes and kinase pathways

During the past several years, it has become apparent that induction of immediate–early genes such as c-*fos*, c-*jun*, and c-*myc* is an early reaction of many cells to acute injury. We, for example, have shown that this occurs in the rat kidney following injuries such as oxidant stress, $HgCl_2$ and other toxins including sulfonyl ureas, and ischemia/reflow. The possible functions of these early genes is incompletely understood, as often the induction occurs within 15 min in cells that are destined to die in 1–2 h. It is possible, therefore, that such proteins might be part of some pathway(s) that ultimately result in cell death. Both c-*jun* and c-*myc* have, under some conditions, been related to the initiation of apoptosis. As we have observed that induction of c-*fos*, c-*jun*, and c-*myc* following oxidant injury is dependent on increased $[Ca^{2+}]_i$, this provides another link between increased $[Ca^{2+}]_i$ and cell death.

### The caspases

Activation of various members of the caspase family has been identified following various types of apoptosis-inducing agents (Thornberry and Lazebnik, 1998). The role of these enzymes, if any, in oncosis has not been studied. It also appears that different caspases may be activated in different apoptosis initiation programs. For example, caspase-8 may be part of the Fas pathway and may not be in the p53 pathway. Other caspases such as caspase-3 may be common to several pathways. Elucidation of such details could be of importance in development of therapeutic strategies for different types of injury.

### Alterations of mitochondrial function

Changes in mitochondrial structure and function occur during the later phases of apoptosis. These changes consist of high-amplitude swelling of the matrix, rupture of the outer mitochondrial membrane, loss of $\Delta\Psi_m$, and activation of MPT (Lemasters *et al.*, 1998). Our time-lapse video microscopy findings clearly show that these occur during the transition from the active phase of pseudopod formation to the more quiescent spherical phase. Later, in the necrotic phase these mitochondria will show intramatrical flocculent densities.

## *Phospholipases*

While major attention has been directed toward activation of cytosolic phospholipases such as cPLA2 during oncosis and oncotic necrosis, little attention has been given to them in apoptosis. However, Wissing *et al.* (1997) have demonstrated that cPLA2 can be activated by cleavage with caspase-3 and that specific inhibition of cPLA2 partially inhibited tumor necrosis factor-induced apoptosis without inhibition of caspase activity.

## *The cytoskeleton*

Major activity in the structure and function of the cytoskeletal elements must occur during the active pseudopod formation. Several efforts to delineate the nature of these changes indicate a role for actin, vinculin, gelsolin, and fodrin. Fodrin and gelsolin can be substrates for caspase-3 (Kothakota *et al.*, 1997) and overexpression of gelsolin can inhibit Fas-induced apoptosis (Ohtsu *et al.*, 1997). Furthermore, caspase-cleaved gelsolin fragments cleave actin in a $Ca^{2+}$-dependent manner. Expression of the gelsolin cleavage product in several cell types resulted in cellular rounding up, detachment, and nuclear fragmentation (Kothakota *et al.*, 1997).

## *Necrosis*

We and others have extensively characterized the structural, biochemical and functional aspects of the necrosis that follows oncosis. Thus far, our results indicate that the necrosis following apoptosis is very similar (Figure 5.27). *In vivo*, of course, the apoptotic cells are usually phagocytosed rapidly by adjacent cells while they are still viable. Necrotic changes, therefore, only occur in the phagolysosomal system of the phagocytosing cell. *In vitro*, however, the changes can be carefully compared.

Majno and Joris (1995) suggest that, in some cases at least, the cells with apoptotic necrosis have a more dense cytosol – a remnant of the originally shrunken cytosol during the prelethal active phase. In our observations, however, this does not occur *in vitro* after apoptosis induced by okadaic acid, overexpression of p53, or injection of cytochrome *c*. In these examples, the cytosol is swollen, as are the mitochondria, the ER and the Golgi components. The nucleus ultimately displays total lysis of the chromatin (karyolysis), as in any other type of necrosis.

# What determines whether an injury leads to apoptosis or oncosis

As more has been learned about both apoptosis and oncosis, it has become important to determine the fundamental reasons why some injuries in some situations induce the one whereas under different conditions the other is induced. There are many examples of etiologic agents that can induce either oncosis or apoptosis, even in the same cell type, depending on other conditions in the cellular micro- or macroenvironments. An excellent example of this is oxidant injury, which can induce either pathway in various cell types including the kidney. Elucidation of these differences and the mechanism of the signaling "switches" involved could have a major impact in the development of intervention strategies for either prevention or treatment (Figure 5.13).

One major difference between apoptotic and oncotic cells is, of course, cell volume regulation. The shrinkage that is typical of apoptosis seems to occur despite a decreased $[K^+]_i$. The mechanism of this appears to involve $K^+$ channels and may be related to $Ca^{2+}$ stimulation. It also implies a maintenance of cellular energy stores, because, in the absence of available ATP, cell volume control is lost, $Na^+$, $Cl^-$, and water increase and the cell swells. Cidlowski's group (Bortner et al., 1997; Hughes et al., 1997) even have data that the cell shrinkage in apoptosis may relate to subsequent changes such as chromatin degradation. Although the signaling involved in this is totally unclear, the possible role of the cytoskeleton in this signaling cannot be dismissed.

Loss of ATP synthesis rapidly results in loss of cell volume control primarily because the $N^+/K^+$ transport system at the plasmalemma is inactive. It has been proposed that ATP concentration is at least one factor that determines whether a given injury will lead to oncosis or apoptosis. Indeed, in our current experiments inducing apoptosis with microinjection of cytochrome $c$, pretreatment with KCN + IAA to inhibit ATP synthesis totally seems to inhibit the apoptotic response totally and leads to an explosive reaction of the cells which is rapidly followed by death (Figure 5.25).

Also fascinating in this regard is the action of cell death protection proteins such as the Bcl-2 family members. We observed that overexpression of Bcl-2 in NRK-52E cells is equally protective against either apoptosis or oncosis following oxidant stress. Other investigators have noted this in other cells with other types of injury. One clear protective function of Bcl-2 is increased mitochondrial buffering of increased $[Ca^{2+}]_i$, as shown by Ichimiya et al. (1998) in kidney proximal tubule epithelial cells and by Murphy et al. (1996) in neural cells. Possibly related is the work of Ellerby et al. (1996), who showed that it also shifted the cellular oxidation–reduction potential in neural cells.

Also in the area of ion regulation is the possible role of pH as a signaling point. It is quite clear from work in our laboratory that reduction of extracellular pH is inhibitory to oncosis from diverse causes including hypoxia, $HgCl_2$, and heat (Pentilla et al., 1976). Although little, if anything, is known concerning the role of pH in renal apoptosis, some studies in neurons suggest that acidosis reduces apoptosis (Xu et al., 1998), whereas other studies suggest the opposite.

Proteases may also play differential roles in apoptosis and oncosis. Beginning with the work on nematodes, caspases have mainly attracted attention in apoptosis (Cryns and Yuan, 1998). At the same time, there are recent data that they may also be involved in oncosis and necrosis (Dong et al., 1997, 1998). Finally, while calpains clearly have a role in oncosis and oncotic necrosis (Elliget et al., 1994), the nature and distinction between these pathways is unclear. Among the possibilities is the evidence of Wood *et al.* (1998) that Bax cleavage is mediated by calpains.

Studies of human intimal hyperplasia associated with arteriosclerosis in arteriovenous fistulas in dialysis have shown that there is remodeling of smooth muscle cells (SMCs). This appears to be mediated by proliferation of SMCs and apoptosis but not by oncosis (Hayakawa *et al.*, 1999). The apoptosis is associated with overexpression of Bax and an increase of the Bax/Bcl-2 ratio. On the other hand, activation of poly-(ADP ribose) polymerase (PARP) occurs early in oxidant-induced cell death in endothelial cells by depleting $NAD^+$. The subsequent cell death was associated with oncosis, not apoptosis; but when PARP was inhibited by 2-aminobenzamide or 1,5-dihydroxyquinoline, the pattern shifted to apoptosis with activation of caspase-3 (Walisser and Thies, 1999).

When acute ischemia of the myocardium for 30 min was followed by 0, 30 min, 2 h or 4 h of reperfusion, only oncosis and no apoptosis occurred in the 2- and 4-h groups, in spite of the fact that DNA ladders and terminal deoxynucleotidyl-mediated biotin–dUTP nick-end labeling (TUNEL) staining were observed. This suggests strongly that ATP levels were critical as myocardial ATP is already very low by 30 min (Ohno *et al.*, 1998).

## Cell death

Although cell death (the point of no return) is often said to be defined as the point at which cells can no longer reproduce by division, such a definition has obvious limitations in the case of cells arrested in $G_1$ or in the case of most neurons which, using current *in vivo* conditions, cannot divide. If injured cells can still divide, after the cells are restored to a normal environment, the changes observed must be prelethal. On the other hand, for cells such as neurons or cells for which tests of division are not appropriate or are impossible to conduct, other definitions are needed. This has led to the development of other tests which can be applied to cells fixed by chemical agents or by freezing; cells killed by homogenization that are used for chemical or functional studies of organelles; and DNA, RNA, and proteins or metabolic pathways. Such pathways include cytosolic enzymes which are released with interruption of plasmalemmal permeability and trypan blue or propidium iodide staining, which only occurs after cell death. Another reliable marker, seen by electron microscopy in both oncotic and apoptotic cell death, is matrical density within the mitochondria. Trypan blue has the marked advantage that it does not kill cells and can thus be utilized in experiments where multiple time points prior to cell death need to be studied, including mitosis; staining can be observed by *in vivo* microscopy, biochemical or molecular methods, or after fixation or rapid freezing by electron microscopy.

# Necrosis

The term "necrosis" is used to refer to the phase of degradation of cell components following irreversible injury *in vivo* (Trump *et al.*, 1965; Trump and Ginn, 1969) following either oncosis or apoptosis.

## *Stages*

Necrosis is characterized by breakdown of cell macromolecules, including membranes, nucleic acids, and proteins, and, over a period of time, converts the cell to debris which eventually reaches equilibrium with the environment. At the light microscopic level, the characteristic changes of necrosis include increasing eosinophilia of the cytoplasm, presumed to be due to denaturation of cytoplasmic proteins; nuclear chromatin clumping and shrinkage; and finally karyolysis, in which the chromosomes are totally digested and the nucleus is only visible as a faint shadow. Gradually, the cellular debris is liquefied and/or removed by mononuclear phagocytes. *In vivo*, a zone of acute intense inflammation often surrounds the necrotic cells which activates complement and other pathways, leading to the inflammatory response. In many cases, it is believed that the inflammatory response also contributes to further damage of cells at the margin of necrotic zones through release of injurious mediators, such as active oxygen species.

### *Stages of oncotic necrosis*

#### *Stage 5*

##### STRUCTURE

This stage represents the irreversibly altered cell (Figure 5.3C) (Trump and Ginn, 1969; Trump and Arstila, 1971). The markedly swollen mitochondria have enlarged and now contain dense intramatrical inclusions known as "flocculent densities" and which represent precipitates of mitochondrial matrix protein (Collan *et al.*, 1981). In addition, following certain types of injury, mitochondria exhibit calcium phosphate precipitates (Figure 5.3D). These begin as small amorphous deposits, often near the cristae, which sometimes form annular aggregates; one mitochondrial profile often can have several such aggregates. If this process continues, the precipitates grow and become confluent. Also, the precipitates may become crystalline, forming aggregates of hydroxyapatite in the mitochondria (Gritzka and Trump, 1968; Osornio-Vargas *et al.*, 1981).

Mitochondrial calcification in stage 5 occurs only after certain types of injury. It has been observed that such calcification, even in dead cells, is an active process requiring electron transport. Accordingly, cells following injuries such as total ischemia (Figure 5.5) or anoxia or injury from metabolic inhibitors such as CN or 2,4-DNP do not exhibit this calcification. Occasionally, intramitochondrial calcifications can be observed within myocardial infarcts *in vivo* or at the edges of ischemic areas. These calcifications are within cells near collaterals or at the border zone of the infarct where oxygen and substrates are available even to dying cells. As can be noted from the above morphologic descriptions, mitochondrial changes are important in stage classification; these changes are illustrated diagrammatically in Figure 5.28.

FUNCTION

In this stage, cells are beginning to reach equilibrium. $[Na^+]_i$, $[Cl^-]_i$, $[Ca^{2+}]_i$, and water content are high; $[K^+]_i$ and $[Mg^{2+}]_i$ are low. Most enzyme activities are reduced; an exception is the lysosomal acid hydrolases which typically maintain full activity in this stage. Mitochondrial phosphorylating ability is irreversibly lost and mitochondrial matrix enzymes are in equilibrium with the cytosol. As the integrity of the cell membrane is violated, soluble enzymes, for example lactic dehydrogenase, escape from the cytosol into the extracellular space. Plasmalemmal membrane functions are lost, including $Na^+/K^+$-ATPase.

*Stages 6 and 7*

STRUCTURE

These stages occur during the necrotic phase, with cell morphology now significantly altered by chromatin breakdown, marked membrane shape changes, myelin figure formation, etc.

FUNCTION

Lysosomal hydrolases, although active long after cell death, have, at these stages, escaped from their compartments and catalyzed macromolecules in the cytoplasm, the organelles, and the nucleus. As time progresses, these cells find large amounts of $Ca^{2+}$ and calcifications occur. The other cations reach equilibrium in the extracellular space. Finally, the cells also return to total equilibrium, although, *in vivo*, necrotic debris is phagocytosed by adjacent cells and digested within the phagolysosomal system of epithelium and macrophages.

### Stages of apoptotic necrosis

Although the changes here are basically similar to those of oncotic necrosis, there are some very important differences. These differences mainly apply in tissue cells *in vitro* in that the cells are usually shrunken and very dense in the cytosol, probably mainly through loss of $K^+$ as mentioned above, especially in the earlier phases. This difference is, however, usually not seen because in these stages the cells or their processes are normally phagocytosed except in excretory ducts such

150

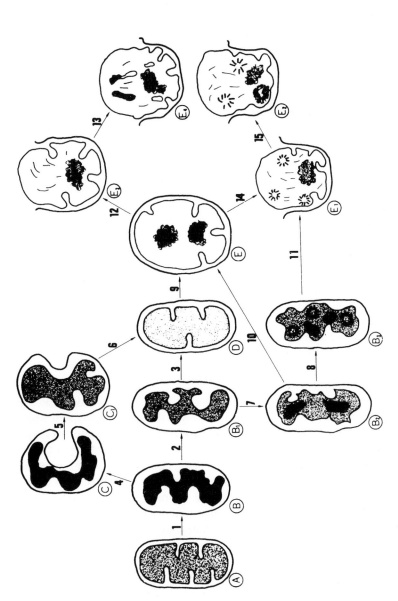

*Figure 5.28* A diagrammatic representation of mitochondrial profiles following cell injury. (A) Orthodox mitochondria (stage 1). (B) Condensed (stage 3); $B_1$, transitional form of condensed; $B_2$ and $B_3$, condensed mitochondria with flocculent densities or calcifications (stage 3c). (C and $C_1$) Ring-formed condensed mitochondria. (D) Slightly swollen (stage 4a). (E, $E_1$, $E_2$, $E_3$, and $E_4$) Various forms of highly swollen mitochondria with flocculent densities (stage 5) or calcifications (stage 5c). Reproduced with permission from Trump and Mergner (1974).

as the kidney tubule, where they are passed to the extracellular space – in this case, the urine.

*In vitro*, however, the apoptotic cells and their processes are usually phagocytosed when still alive and eventually enter the lysosome system, where they die and contribute to the formation of "residual bodies" and lipofuscin or aging pigment. This point has been largely overlooked in the literature and explains why for a long time the importance of apoptosis was underestimated until another group of pathologists recognized and named it (Kerr *et al.*, 1972).

Isolated cells, however, when they undergo apoptosis have the same characteristics of shrinkage during the prelethal phase but show swelling and all of the changes described above for stage 5 after they die. It is thus very difficult to recognize apoptotic death *in vitro* in hematoxylin- and eosin-stained tissue sections.

## Other terms and concepts used in reference to cell death

### *Instantaneous cell death*

Instantaneous cell death is usually within less than a second, occasioned by such treatments as ultra-rapid freezing or immersion in or perfusion with fixatives, such as glutaraldehyde or osmium tetroxide. This type of death is rare in living animals, but is important because it distinguishes between the concepts of cell death and necrosis. With these types of instantaneous cell death, necrosis never occurs as the enzymes and factors responsible for degradation of cellular macromolecules are also rapidly inactivated.

### *Autophagocytosis*

Autophagocytosis is a process whereby organelles such as mitochondria, ER, and peroxisomes are turned over by sequestration into the lysosomal system where extensive digestion and conversion to debris and residual bodies develops (Marzella and Glaumann, 1987; Lee and Marzella, 1994). Autophagy is seen in virtually all cells and, in most cases, consists of budding of portions of cytoplasm-containing organelles into the lumens of the cisternae of the ER. The subsequent double-membrane limited bodies, thus formed, ultimately fuse with primary and/or secondary lysosomes, resulting in the digestion of the sequestered organelles and the formation of a secondary lysosome. Autophagy is a common phenomenon under sublethal states of stress, including starvation, hormonal stimulation, and hypoxia, and represents a normal mechanism for organelle turnover. The residual bodies formed by autophagocytosis accumulate in the cytoplasm and become auto-oxidized, forming lipofuscin pigment. Such accumulations are commonly observed in myocardial cells, where they increase as a function of age. By light microscopy, they can be observed as yellowish-brown autofluorescence cytoplasmic inclusions.

Autophagy, thus, represents a type of cell death and necrosis of organelles occurring within the lysosomal system where they mix with other debris taken into the cell by endo- or phagocytosis. During the process of apoptosis, discussed below, cell fragments are commonly detached from apoptotic cells, undergo phagocytosis by adjacent parenchymal or mesenchymal cells, and then add heterophagic granules to the portfolio of the secondary lysosome. As these fragments may also contain organelles, including mitochondria, ER, and microbodies, it can be confusing to distinguish apoptosis from the process of autophagocytosis.

Extensive autophagocytosis has been described in cells to the point where the cytoplasm becomes virtually filled with engorged secondary lysosomes. It is still difficult to be certain whether or not this event is capable of leading the cell in question to death, although unquestionably the organelles within the autophagic vacuole are themselves dying and undergo necrosis.

### Programmed cell death

The term "programmed cell death" is now used to refer to cells that die in a more or less predictable manner, following some type of scheduled agent, such as hormonal changes, alterations in growth factors, and alterations in nutrition, among others (Bowen and Bowen, 1990). Usually, the precise stimulus is not known. Since, however, this occurs in otherwise disease-free animals and plants, the term has thus been used to distinguish between a natural or so-called "programmed" cell death, which permits normal turnover of cells (as in maturation of the epidermal cells in the skin), as contrasted with "accidental" cell death, which refers to cell death occurring from environmental or other factors including trauma, ischemia, anoxia, or xenobiotic chemicals. On the other hand, there is no doubt that overlap between these categories does occur and that, although certain types of biologic cell responses typify programmed cell death, such as terminal differentiation and apoptosis, necrosis is typical of accidentally and environmentally induced cell death. However, it is also apparent that the two types may overlap in a particular case as more is learned.

### Terminal differentiation

The phrase "terminal differentiation" has been commonly used to apply to a type of cell death often induced by growth factors, hormones, or other environmental changes by which cells in the mitotic cycle leave the cycle, usually from $G_1$, and, instead of remaining available for recruitment back into the cycle, as in the case of renal tubular epithelium or hepatic parenchymal cells, undergo an irreversible program of commitment to a new phenotype. This new phenotype contains a variety of new expressed genes, which lead the cell to one that cannot divide and, therefore, which undergoes atrophy and death. A classic example is the keratin layer of the epidermis. During maturation from the basal layer, the epidermal cells undergo a terminal differentiation program and develop new cytoskeletal keratin proteins and active RNA and DNA synthesis; the cells then atrophy and

153

form a keratinized cornified layer. A similar type of differentiation also occurs following injury in the bronchial epithelium, forming areas of so-called "squamous metaplasia" (McDowell and Trump, 1983). A variety of stimuli, including phorbol esters and growth factors such as TGF-$\beta_1$ (Pfeifer *et al.*, 1989) and serum (Lechner *et al.*, 1984), induce this in bronchial epithelium. Ionized cytosolic calcium ($[Ca^{2+}]_i$) seems to be involved in one type of signaling leading to this terminal differentiation program (Miyashita, 1989) and, in the case of keratinocytes, varying the extracellular ionized calcium ($[Ca^{2+}]_e$) is sufficient to induce such differentiation (Yuspa *et al.*, 1988). It is of interest that many compounds and inflammatory agents that may be tumor promoters differentially induce this phenomenon in normal compared with initiated cells, thus giving the initiated cells a growth advantage; this is one current hypothesis of tumor promotion (Hennings *et al.*, 1989).

## Conclusions

For many years, the study of ischemic and toxic cell injury has been one in which the understanding of the relationship between basic cellular structure and function and the disease process has been of paramount importance. As these studies have evolved, relating molecular mechanisms to aid in our understanding of these phenomena has also become important. Cell injury and cell death play important roles, not only in disease but also in the normal process of cell development and embryonic maturation. From the above discussion, it can be seen that we now know that a variety of cellular events in both acute and chronic cell injury, including neoplasia, are closely related, if not initiated by intracellular ion deregulation. This conclusion has been made possible through the recent development of new methodologies, such as digital imaging fluorescence microscopy. It is through the use of this technique that investigators can now image living cells and, using appropriate fluorescent probes such as Fura-2 for $[Ca^{2+}]_i$, locate and measure concentration levels. Although $[Ca^{2+}]_i$ appears to be of particular importance, other ions are important as well, especially $[Na^+]_i$ and $[H^+]_i$. Examples include the fact that $Ca^{2+}$-activated endonucleases may well play a role in DNA damage following an acute non-mutagenic toxic injury, such as that induced by oxidative stress, and that $[Ca^{2+}]_i$ deregulation and alkalinization of the cytoplasm may ultimately lead to prolonged states of disordered cell division and cell differentiation. Although much more needs to be clarified before any conclusions can be made, it is quite clear that toxic cell injury is a fundamental biologic process and that further understanding of the cellular and molecular mechanisms involved could well lead to modification of the cell to toxic insults. It is our hypothesis, based upon many years of experimentation, that a wide variety of phenomena which occur following cell injury are due to ion deregulation.

## Acknowledgments

This work was supported by NIH grant DK 15440, a grant from the Warwick Research Institute and Navy grant N00014-88-K-0427. This is contribution no. 4038 from the Cellular Pathobiology Laboratory.

## References

Adams, J.M. and Cory, S. 1998. The Bcl-2 protein family: Arbiters of cell survival. *Science* 281: 1322–1326.

Aikawa, J.K. 1981. *Magnesium: Its biological significance*. Boca Raton: CRC Press.

Bar-Sagi, D., Suhan, J.P., McCormick, F., and Feramisco, J.R. 1988. Localization of phospholipase A2 in normal and ras-transformed cells. *J Cell Biol* 106: 1649–1658.

Berridge, M.J. and Galaione, A. 1988. Cytosolic calcium oscillations. *FASEB J* 230: 3074–3082.

Berridge, M.J. and Irvine, R.F. 1984. Inositol triphosphate, a novel second messenger in cellular signal transduction. *Nature* 312: 315–321.

Bessis, M. 1964. Studies on cell agony and death: An attempt at classification. In: *Cellular Injury*. deReuck, A.V.S., and Knight, J. (eds), pp. 287–328. London: J & A Churchill.

Blake, M.J., Gershon, D., Fargnoli, J., and Holbrook, N.J. 1990. Discordant expression of heat shock protein mRNAs in tissues of heat-stressed rats. *J Biol Chem* 265: 15275–15279.

Bond, J.M., Herman, B., and Lemasters, J.J. 1991. Protection by acidotic pH against anoxia/reoxygenation injury to rat neonatal cardiac myocytes. *Biochem Biophys Res Commun* 179: 798–803.

Bortner, C.D., Hughes, Jr., F.M., and Cidlowski, J.A. 1997. A primary role for $K^+$ and $Na^+$ efflux in the activation of apoptosis. *J Biol Chem* 272: 32436–32442.

Bowen, I.D. and Bowen, S.M. 1990. *Programmed Cell Death in Tumours and Tissues*. London: Chapman & Hall.

Bowen, I.D. and Lockshin, R.A. 1981. *Cell Death in Biology and Pathology*. London: Chapman and Hall.

Cairo, G., Bardella, L., Schiaffonati, L., and Bernelli-Zazzera, A. 1985. Synthesis of heat shock proteins in rat liver after ischemia and hyperthermia. *Hepatology* 5: 357–361.

Cantoni, O., Sestili, P., Cattabeni, F., Bellomo, G., Pou, S., Cohen, M., and Cerutti, P. 1989. Calcium chelator quin 2 prevents hydrogen-peroxide-induced DNA breakage and cytotoxicity. *Eur J Biochem* 182: 209–212.

Carafoli, E. 1987. Intracellular calcium homeostasis. *Annu Rev Biochem* 56: 395–433.

Cerutti, P.A. and Trump, B.F. 1991. Inflammation and oxidative stress in carcinogenesis. *Cancer Cells* 3: 1–7.

Cerutti, P., Larsson, R., Krupitza, G., Muehlematter, D., Crawford, D., and Amstad, P. 1988. Pathophysiological mechanisms of oxidants. In: *Oxy-radicals in Molecular Biology and Pathology*. Cerutti, P.A., Fridovich, I., and McCord, J.M. (eds), pp. 493–507. New York: Alan R. Liss, Inc.

Chang, S.H., Phelps, P.C., Ebersberger, M.L., Berezesky, I.K., and Trump, B.F. 2000. Studies on the mechanisms and kinetics of apoptosis induced by microinjection of cytochrome C in rat kidney tubule epithelial cells (NRK-52). *Am J Pathol* 156: 637–649.

Chaudry, I.H. Use of ATP following shock and ischemia. *Ann NY Acad Sci* 1990; 603: 130–141.

Chen, L.K. and Boron, W.F. 1991. Intracellular pH regulation in epithelial cells. *Kidney Int Suppl* 40: S11–S17.

Chung, S., Reinhart, P.H., Martin, B.L., Brautigan, D., and Levitan, I.B. 1991. Protein kinase activity closely associated with a reconstituted calcium-activated potassium channel. *Science* 253: 560–562.

Collan, Y., McDowell, E.M., Trump, B.F. 1981. Studies on the pathogenesis of ischemic cell injury. VI. Mitochondrial flocculent densities in autolysis. *Virchows Arch [B]* 35: 189–199.

Combs, A.B. and Acosta D. 1990. Toxic mechanisms of the heart: A review. *Toxicol Pathol* 18: 583–596.

Cowley, Jr., B.D., Chadwick, L.J., Grantham, J.J., and Calvet, J.P. 1989. Sequential protooncogene expression in regenerating kidney following acute renal injury. *J Biol Chem* 264: 8389–8393.

Crawford, D., Zbinden, I., Amstrad, P., and Cerutti, P. 1988. Oxidant stress induces the proto-oncogenes c-fos and c-myc in mouse epidermal cells. *Oncogene* 3: 27–32.

Cryns, V.L. and Yuan, J. 1998. The cutting edge: Caspases in apoptosis and disease. In: *When Cells Die: A Comprehensive Evaluation of Apoptosis and Programmed Cell Death.* Lockshin, R.A., Zakeri, Z., and Tilly, J.L. (eds), pp. 177–210. New York: Wiley-Liss.

Curran, T. and Franza, B.R. 1988. Fos and jun: the AP-1 connection. *Cell* 55: 395–397.

Davis, M.A. and Ryan, D.H. 1998. Apoptosis in the kidney. *Toxicol Pathol* 26: 810–825.

Davis, M.A., Smith, M.W., Chang, S.H., and Trump, B.F. 1994. Characterization of a renal epithelial cell model of apoptosis using okadaic acid and the NRK-52E cell line. *Toxicol Pathol* 22: 595–605.

Dong, Z., Saikumar, P., Weinberg, J.M., and Venkatachalam, M.A. 1997. Internucleosomal DNA cleavage triggered by plasma membrane damage during necrotic cell death. Involvement of serine but not cysteine proteases. *Am J Pathol* 151: 1205–1213.

Dong, Z., Saikumar, P., Griess, G.A., Weinberg, J.M., and Venkatachalam, M.A. 1998. Intracellular $Ca^{2+}$ thresholds that determine survival or death of energy-deprived cells. *Am J Pathol* 152: 231–240.

Ellerby, L.M., Ellerby, H.M., Park, S.M., Holleran, A.L., Murphy, A.N., Fiskum, G., Kane, D.J., Testa, M.P., Kayalar, C., and Bredesen, D.E. 1996. Shift of the cellular oxidation–reduction potential in neural cells expressing Bcl-2. *J Neurochem* 67: 1259–1267.

Elliget, K.A., Phelps, P.C., and Trump, B.F. 1991. $HgCl_2$-induced alteration of actin filaments in cultured primary rat proximal tubule epithelial cells labelled with fluorescein phalloidin. *Cell Biol Toxicol* 7: 263–280.

Elliget, K.A., Phelps, P.C., and Trump, B.F. 1994. Cytosolic $Ca^{2+}$ elevation and calpain inhibitors in $HgCl_2$ injury to rat kidney proximal tubule epithelial cells. *Pathobiology* 62: 298–310.

Epel, D. 1982. The cascade of events initiated by rises in cytosolic $Ca^{2+}$ and pH following fertilization in sea urchin eggs. In: *Ions, Cell Proliferation and Cancer.* Boynton, A.L., McKeehan, W.L., and Whitfield, J.F. (eds), pp. 327–340. New York: Academic Press.

Fridovich, I. 1978. The biology of oxygen radicals. *Science* 210: 878–880.

Freissmuth, M., Casey, P.J., and Gilman, A.G. 1989. G proteins control diverse pathways of transmembrane signaling. *FASEB J* 3: 2125–2131.

Ghosh, T.K., Bian, J.H., Rybak, S.L., and Gill, D.L. 1991. Persistent intracellular calcium pool depletion by thapsigargin and its influence on cell growth. *J Biol Chem* 266: 24690–24697.

Gill, D., Ghosh, T., and Mullaney, J. 1989. Calcium signaling mechanisms in endoplasmic reticulum activated by inositol 1,4,5-triphosphate and GTP. *Cell Calcium* 10: 363–374.

Gillies, R.J., Martinez-Zaguilan, R., Martinez, G.M., Serrano, R., and Perona, R. 1990. Tumorigenic 3T3 cells maintain an alkaline intracellular pH under physiological conditions. *Proc Natl Acad Sci USA* 87: 7414–7418.

Glaumann, B. and Trump, B.F. 1975. Studies on the pathogenesis of ischemic cell injury. III. Morphological changes of the proximal pars recta tubules (P3) of the rat kidney made ischemic in vivo. *Virchows Arch [B]* 19: 303–323.

Goldblatt, P.J., Trump, B.F., and Stowell, R.E. 1965. Studies on necrosis of mouse liver in vitro. Alterations in some histochemistry demonstrable hepatocellular enzymes. *Am J Pathol* 47: 183–208.

Gritzka, T.L. and Trump, B.F. 1968. Renal tubular lesions caused by mercuric chloride. Electron microscopic observations: Degeneration of the pars recta. *Am J Pathol* 52: 1225–1277.

Gunther, M.R., Sampath, V., and Caughey, W.S. 1999. Potential roles of myoglobin in myocardial ischemia-reperfusion injury. *Free Radical Biol Med* 26: 1388–1395.

Harris, C.C. 1996a. p53 tumor suppressor gene: from the basic research laboratory to the clinic – an abridged historical perspective. *Carcinogenesis* 17: 1187–1198.

Harris, C.C. 1996b. Structure and function of the p53 tumor suppressor gene: Clues for rational cancer therapeutic strategies. (Review). *J Natl Cancer Inst* 88: 1442–1455.

Hayakawa, Y., Takemura, G., Misao, J., Kanoh, M., Ohno, M., Ohashi, H., Takatsu, H., Ito, H., Fkuda, K, Fujjiwara, T., Minatoguchi, S., and Fumiwara, H. 1999. Apoptosis and overexpression of bax protein and bax mRNA in smooth muscle cells within intimal hyperplasia of human radial arteries: analysis with arteriovenous fistulas used for hemodialysis. *Arteriosclerosis Thromb Vasc Biol* 19: 2066–2077.

Hennings, H., Kruszewske, F.H., Yuspa, S.H., and Tucker, R.W. 1989. Intracellular calcium alterations in response to increased external calcium in normal and neoplastic keratinocytes. *Carcinogenesis* 10: 777–780.

Herbst, H., Milani, S., Schuppan, D., and Stein, H. 1991. Temporal and spatial patterns of proto-oncogene expression at early stages of toxic liver injury in the rat. *Lab Invest* 65: 324–333.

Hughes, Jr., F.M., Bortner, C.D., Purdy, G.D., and Cidlowski, J.A. 1997. Intracellular $K^+$ suppresses the activation of apoptosis in lymphocytes. *J Biol Chem* 272: 30567–30576.

Ichimiya, M., Chang, S.H., Liu, H., Berezesky, I.K., Trump, B.F., and Amstad, P.A. 1998. Effect of bcl-2 on oxidant-induced cell death and intracellular $Ca^{2+}$ mobilization. *Am J Physiol* 275: C832–C839.

Iino, M., Kkobayashi, T., and Endo, M. 1988. Use of ryanodine for functional removal of the calcium store in smooth muscle cells of the guinea-pig. *Biochem Biophys Res Commun* 152: 417–422.

Ishikawa, Y., Yokoo, T., and Kitamura, M. 1997. c-Jun/AP-1, but not NF-kappa B, is a mediator for oxidant-initiated apoptosis in glomerular mesangial cells. *Biochem Biophys Res Commun* 240: 496–501.

Kerr, J.F.R. 1971. Shrinkage necrosis: a distinct mode of cellular death. *J Pathol* 105: 13–29.

Kerr, J.F.R., Wyllie, A.H., and Currie, A.R. 1972. Apoptosis: a basic biological phenomenon with wide-ranging implications in tissue kinetics. *Br J Cancer* 26: 239–257.

Kolber, M.A., Broschat, K.O., and Landa-Gonzalez, B. 1990. Cytochalasin B induces cellular DNA fragmentation. *FASEB J* 4: 3021–3027.

Korsmeyer, S.J., Shutter, J.R., Veis, D.J., Merry, D.E., and Oltvai, Z.N. 1993. Bcl-2/Bax: a rheostat that regulates an anti-oxidant pathway and cell death. *Sem Cancer Biol* 4: 327-332.

Kothakota, S., Azuma, T., Reinhard, C., Klippel, A., Tang, J., Chu, K., McGarry, T.J., Kirschner, M.W., Koths, K., Kwiatkowski, D.J., and Williams, L.T. 1997. Caspase-3-generated fragment of gelsolin: effector of morphological change in apoptosis. *Science* 278: 294–298.

Lechner, J.F., Haugen, A., McClendon, I.A., and Shamsuddin, A.K.M. 1984. Induction of squamous differentiation of normal human bronchial epithelial cells by small amounts of serum. *Differentiation* 25: 229–237.

Lee, H.K. and Marzella, L. 1994. Regulation of intracellular protein degradation with special reference to lysosomes: role in cell physiology and pathology. *Int Rev Exp Pathol* 135: 39–147.

Lemasters, J.J., DiGuiseppi, J., Nieminen, A., and Herman, B. 1987. Blebbing, free $Ca^{2+}$ and mitochondrial membrane potential preceding cell death in hepatocytes. *Nature* 325: 78–81.

Lemasters, J.J., Nieminen, A.L., Qian, T., Trost, L.C., Elmore, S.P., Nishimura, Y., Crowe, R.A., Cascio, W.E., Bradham, C.A., Brenner, D.A., and Herman, B. 1998. The mitochondrial permeability transition in cell death: a common mechanism in necrosis, apoptosis and autophagy. *Biochim Biophys Acta* 1366: 177–196.

Lindquist, S. 1988. The heat shock protein. *Annu Rev Genet* 22: 631–77.

Lytton, J., Westlin, M., and Hanley, M.R. 1991. Thapsigargin inhibits the sarcoplasmic or endoplasmic reticulum Ca-ATPase family of calcium pumps. *J Biol Chem* 266: 17067–17071.

McConkey, D.J., Chow, S.C., Orrenius, S., and Jondal, M. 1990. NK cell-induced cytotoxicity is dependent on a $Ca^{2+}$ increase in the target. *FASEB J* 4: 2661–2664.

McDowell E.M. and Trump, B.F. 1983. Histogenesis of preneoplastic and neoplastic lesions in tracheobronchial epithelium. *Surv Synth Pathol Res* 2: 235–279.

Majno, G. and Joris, I. 1995. Apoptosis, oncosis, and necrosis. An overview of cell death. *Am J Pathol* 146: 3–15.

Majno, G. and Joris, I. 1996. *Cells, Tissues, and Disease: Principles of General Pathology.* Cambridge, MA: Blackwell Science.

Maki, A., Berezesky, I.K., Fargnoli, J., Holbrook, N.J., and Trump, B.F. 1992. Role of $[Ca^{2+}]_i$ in induction of c-fos, c-jun, and c-myc RNA in rat PTE after oxidative stress. *FASEB J* 6: 919–924.

Marzella, L. and Glaumann, H. 1987. Autophagy, microautophagy and crinophagy as mechanisms for protein degradation. In: *Lysosomes: Their Role in Protein Breakdown.* Glaumann, H. and Ballard, J. (eds), pp. 319–367. London: Academic Press.

Mergner, W.J., Smith, M.A., and Trump, B.F. 1977a. Studies on the pathogenesis of ischemic cell injury. IV. Alteration of ionic permeability of mitochondria from ischemic rat kidney. *Exp Mol Pathol* 26: 1–12.

Mergner, W.J., Marzella, L.L., Mergner, G., Kahng, M.W., Smith, M.W., and Trump, B.F. 1977b. Studies on the pathogenesis of ischemic cell injury. VII. Proton gradient and respiration of renal tissue cubes, renal mitochondria and submitochondrial particles following ischemic injury. *Beitr Pathol* 161: 260–271.

Mergner, W.J., Chang, S.H., Marzella, L., Kahng, M.W., and Trump, B.F. 1979. Studies on the pathogenesis of ischemic cell injury. VII. ATPase of rat kidney mitochondria. *Lab Invest* 40: 686–694.

Mergner, W.J., Jones, R.T., and Trump, B.F. 1990. *Cell Death. Mechanisms of Acute and Lethal Injury*, Vol. 1. New York: Field and Wood Medical Publishers.

Miyashita, M., Smith, M.W., Willey, J.C., Lechner, J.F., Trump, B.F., and Harris, C.C. 1989. Effects of serum, transforming growth factor type, or 12-O-tetradecanol-phorbol-13-acetate on ionized cytosolic calcium concentration in normal and transformed human bronchial epithelial cells. *Cancer Res* 49: 63–67.

Morgan, J.I. and Curran, T. 1989. Regulation of c-fos expression by voltage-dependent calcium channels. In: *Cell Calcium Metabolism. Physiology, Biochemistry, Pharmacology, and Clinical Implications*. Fiskum, G. (ed.), pp. 305–312. New York: Plenum Press.

Morris, A.C., Hagler, H.K., Willerson, J.T., and Buja, L.M. 1989. Relationship between calcium loading and impaired energy metabolism during $Na^+$, $K^+$, pump inhibition and metabolic inhibition in cultured neonatal cardiac myocytes. *J Clin Invest* 83: 1876–1887.

Muhl, H., Sandau, K., Brune, B., Briner, V.A., and Pfeilschifter, J. 1996. Nitric oxide donors induce apoptosis in glomerular mesangial cells, epithelial cells and endothelial cells. *Eur J Pharmacol* 317: 137–49.

Murphy, A.N., Bredesen, D.E., Cortopassi, G., Wang, E., and Fiskum, G. 1996. Bcl-2 potentiates the maximal calcium uptake capacity of neural cell mitochondria. *Proc Natl Acad Sci USA* 93: 9893–9898.

Nath, K.A., Croatt, A.J., Likely, S., Behrens, T.W., and Warden, D. 1996. Renal oxidant injury and oxidant response induced by mercury. *Kidney Int* 50: 1032–43.

Nguyuza, N., Ichimiya, M., Amstad, P.A., Trump, B.F., and Davis, M.A. 1997. The roles of ERK-2 and Bcl-2 in okadaic acid-induced apoptosis of NRK-52E renal epithelial cells. *The Toxicologist* 36: 250.

Nicotera, P., Hartzell, P., Davis, G., and Orrenius, S. 1986. The formation of plasma membrane blebs in hepatocytes exposed to agents that increase cytosolic $Ca^{2+}$ is mediated by activation of a non-lysosomal proteolytic system. *FEBS Lett* 209: 139–144.

Nieminen, A., Gores, G., Dawson, T., Herman, B., and Lemasters, J. 1990. Toxic injury from mercuric chloride in rat hepatocytes. *J Biol Chem* 265: 2399–2408.

Nishizuka, Y. 1984. The role of protein kinase C in cell surface signal transduction and tumour promotion. *Nature* 308: 693–698.

Nowak, G., Aleo, M.D., Morgan, J.A., and Schnellmann, R.G. 1998. Recovery of cellular functions following oxidant injury. *Am J Physiol* 274: F509–F515.

Ohno, M., Takemua, G., Ohno, A., Misao, J., Hayahawa, Y., Mintoguchi, S., Fujiwara, T., and Fujiwara, H. 1998. "Apoptotic" myocytes in infarct area in rabbit hearts may be oncotic myocytes with DNA fragmentation: analysis by immunogold electron microscopy combined with in situ nick end-labeling. *Circulation* 98: 1422–1430.

Ohtsu, M., Sakai, N., Fujita, H., Kashiwagi, M., Gasa, S., Shimizu, S., Eguchi, Y., Tsujimoto, Y., Sakiyama, Y., Kobvayashi, K., and Kauzumaki, N. 1997. Inhibition of apoptosis by the actin-regulatory protein gelsolin. *EMBO J* 16: 4650–4656.

Orrenius, S., McConkey, D.J., Bellomo, G., Nicortera, P. 1989. Role of $Ca^{2+}$ in toxic cell killing. *Trends Pharmacol Sci* 10: 281–285.

Osornio-Vargas, A.R., Berezesky, I.K., and Trump, B.F. 1981. Progression of ion movements during acute myocardial infarction in the rat. An x-ray microanalysis study. *Scan Electron Microsc* 2: 463–472.

Paller, M.S., Weber, K., and Patten, M. 1998. Nitric oxide-mediated renal epithelial cell injury during hypoxia and reoxygenation. *Renal Failure* 20: 459–469.

Papadimitriou, J.C., Ramm, L.E., Drachenberg, C.B., Trump, B.F., and Shin, M.L. 1991. Quantitative analysis of adenine nucleotides during the prelytic phase of cell death mediated by C5b-9. *J Immunol* 147: 212–217.

Pentilla, A., Glaumann, H., and Trump, B.F. 1976. Studies on the modification of extracellular acidosis against anoxia, thermal, etc. *Life Sci* 18: 1419–1430.

Penttila, A. and Trump, B.F. 1974. Extracellular acidosis protects Ehrlich ascites tumor cells and rat renal cortex against anoxic injury. *Science* 185: 277–278.

Perona, R. and Serrano, R. 1988. Increased pH and tumorigenicity of fibroblasts expressing a yeast proton pump. *Nature* 334: 438–440.

Pfeifer, A.M., Lechner, J.F., Masui, T., Reddel, R.R., Mark, G.E., and Harris, C.C. 1989. Control of growth and squamous differentiation in normal human bronchial epithelial cells by chemical and biological modifiers and transferred genes. *Environ Health Perspect* 80: 209–220.

Phelps, P.C., Smith, M.W., and Trump, B.F. 1989. Cytosolic ionized calcium and bleb formation after acute cell injury of cultured rabbit renal tubule cells. *Lab Invest* 60: 630–642.

Polyak, K., Xia, Y., Zweier, J.L., Kinzler, K.W., and Vogelstein, B. 1997. A model for p53-induced apoptosis. *Nature* 389: 300–305.

Pritchard, K. and Ashley, C.C. 1986. $Na^+/Ca^{2+}$ exchange in isolated smooth muscle cells demonstrated by the fluorescent calcium indicator fura-2. *FEBS Lett* 195: 23–27.

Raafat, A.M., Murray, M.T., McGuire, T., DeFrain, M., Franko, A.P., Zafar, R.S., Palmer, K., Diebel, L., and Dulchavsky, S.A. 1997. Calcium blockade reduces renal apoptosis during ischemia reperfusion. *Shock* 8: 186–192.

Rasmussen, H. 1989. The cycling of calcium as an intracellular messenger. *Sci Am* 108: 66–73.

Rosenberg, M.E. and Paller, M.S. 1991. Differential gene expression in the recovery from ischemic renal injury. *Kidney Int* 39: 156–1161.

Sahaphong, S. and Trump, B.F. 1971. Studies of cellular injury in isolated kidney tubules of the flounder. V. Effects of inhibiting sulfhydryl groups of plasma membrane with the organic mercurials PCMB (parachloromercuribenzoate) and PCMBS (parachloromercuribenzenesulfonate). *Am J Pathol* 63: 277–297.

Schelling, J.R., Nkemere, N., Kopp, J.B., and Cleveland, R.P. 1998. Fas-dependent fratricidal apoptosis is a mechanism of tubular epithelial cell deletion in chronic renal failure. *Lab Invest* 78: 813–24.

Schiaffonati, L., Rappocciolo, E., Tacchini, L., Cairo, G., and Bernelli-Zazzera, A. 1990. Reprogramming of gene expression in postischemic rat liver: Induction of proto-oncogenes and hsp 70 gene family. *J Cell Physiol* 143: 79–87.

Schontal, A., Sugarman, J., Brown, J.H., Hanley, M.R., Feramisco, J.R. 1991. Regulation of c-fos and c-jun protooncogene expression by the $Ca^{2+}$-ATPase inhibitor thapsigargin. *Proc Natl Acad Sci USA* 88: 7096–7100.

Shanley, P.F. and Johnson, G.C. 1991. Calcium and acidosis in renal hypoxia. *Lab Invest* 65: 298–305.

Shin, M.L. and Carney, D.F. 1988. Cytotoxic action and other metabolic consequences of terminal complement proteins. *Prog Allergy* 40: 44–81.

Smith, M.W., Phelps, P.C., and Trump, B.F. 1991. Cytosolic $Ca^{2+}$ deregulation and blebbing after $HgCl_2$ injury to cultured rabbit proximal tubule cells as determined by digital imaging microscopy. *Proc Natl Acad Sci USA* 88: 4926–4930.

Smith, M.W., Phelps, P.C., and Trump, B.F. 1992. Injury-induced changes in cytosolic $Ca^{2+}$ in individual rabbit proximal tubule cells. *Am J Physiol* 262: F647–F655.

Swann, J.D., Smith, M.W., Phelps, P.C., Maki, A., Berezesky, I.K., and Trump, B.F. 1991. Oxidative injury induces influx-dependent changes in intracellular calcium homeostasis. *Toxicol Pathol* 19: 128–137.

Taimor, G., Lorenz, H., Hofstaetter, B., Schluter, K.D., and Piper, H.M. 1999. Induction of necrosis but not apoptosis after anoxia and reoxygenation in isolated adult cardiomyocytes of rat. *Cardiovasc Res* 41: 147–156.

Thornberry, N.A. and Lazebnik, Y. 1998. Caspases: enemies within. *Science* 281: 1312–1316.

Traylor, L.A. and Mayeux, P.R. 1997. Superoxide generation by renal proximal tubule nitric oxide synthase. *Nitric Oxide* 1: 432–438.

Trump, B.F. and Arstila, A.U. 1971. Cell injury and cell death. In: *Principles of Pathobiology*. LaVia, M.F., and Hill, Jr., R.B. (eds), pp. 9–95. New York: Oxford University Press.

Trump, B.F. and Benditt, E.P. 1962. Electron microscopic studies of human renal disease. Observations of normal visceral glomerular epithelium and its modification in disease. *Am J Pathol* 11: 753–781.

Trump, B.F. and Berezesky, I.K. 1984. The role of sodium and calcium regulation in toxic cell injury. In: *Drug Metabolism and Drug Toxicity*. Mitchell, J.R., and Horning, M.G. (eds), pp. 261–300. New York: Raven Press.

Trump, B.F. and Berezesky, I.K. 1985a. The role of calcium in cell injury and repair. A hypothesis. *Surv Synth Pathol Res* 4: 248–256.

Trump, B.F. and Berezesky, I.K. 1985b. Cellular ion regulation and disease: A hypothesis. In: *Current Topics in Membranes and Transport*. Vol. 25. *Regulation of Calcium Transport Across Muscle Membranes*. Shamoo, A.E. (ed.), pp. 279–319. New York: Academic Press.

Trump, B.F. and Berezesky, I.K. 1987. Mechanisms of cell injury in the kidney: The role of calcium. In: *Mechanisms of Cell Injury: Implications for Human Health*. Fowler, B.A. (ed.), pp. 135–151. Chichester: John Wiley and Sons.

Trump, B.F. and Berezesky, I.K. 1989a. Cell injury and cell death. The role of ion deregulation. *Comments Toxicology* 3: 47–67.

Trump, B.F. and Berezesky, I.K. 1989b. Ion deregulation in injured proximal tubule epithelial cells. In: *Nephrotoxicity. In Vitro to In Vivo Animals to Man*. Bach, P.H. and Lock, E.A. (eds), pp. 731–741. New York: Plenum Press.

Trump, B.F. and Berezesky, I.K. 1990. The importance of calcium regulation in toxic cell injury. Studies utilizing the technology of digital imaging fluorescence microscopy. *Clin Lab Methods* 10: 531–547.

Trump, B.F. and Berezesky, I.K. 1992. Cellular and molecular basis of toxic cell injury. In: *Cardiovascular Toxicity*, Vol. 2. Acosta, D. (ed.), pp. 77–113. New York: Raven Press.

Trump, B.F. and Berezesky, I.K. 1995. Calcium-mediated cell injury and cell death. *FASEB J* 9: 219–228.

Trump, B.F. and Berezesky, I.K. 1998. The reactions of cells to lethal injury: oncosis and necrosis – the role of calcium. In: *When Cells Die: A Comprehensive Evaluation of Apoptosis and Cell Death*. Lockshin, R.A., Tilly, J.L., and Zakeri, Z. (eds), pp. 57–96. New York: Wiley-Liss.

Trump, B.F. and Ginn, F.L. 1969. The pathogenesis of subcellular reaction to lethal injury. In: *Methods and Achievements in Experimental Pathology*, Vol. IV. Bajusz, E. and Jasmin, G. (eds), pp. 1–29. Basle: Karger.

Trump, B.F. and Mergner, W.J. 1974. Cell injury. In: *The Inflammatory Process*, Vol. 1. Zweifach, B.W., Grant, L., and McClusky R.T. (eds), pp. 115–257. New York: Academic Press.

Trump, B.F., Goldblatt, P.J., and Stowell, R.E. 1965. Studies of mouse liver necrosis in vitro. Ultrastructural and cytochemical alterations in hepatic parenchymal cell nuclei. *Lab Invest* 14: 1969–1999.

Trump, B.F., Mergner, W.J., Kahng, M.W., and Saladino, A.J. 1976. Studies on the subcellular pathophysiology of ischemia. *Circulation* (Suppl. I) 53: 17–26.

Trump, B.F., Berezesky, I.K., and Phelp, P.C. 1981a. Sodium and calcium regulation and the role of the cytoskeleton in the pathogenesis of disease: a review and hypothesis. *Scan Electron Microsc* 2: 434–454.

Trump, B.F., Berezesky, I.K., and Osornio-Vargas, A. 1981b. Cell death and the disease process. The role of cell calcium. In: *Cell Death in Biology and Pathology*. Bowen, I.D. and Lockshin, R.A. (eds), pp. 209–242. London: Chapman and Hall.

Trump, B.F., Berezesky, I.K., and Cowley, RA. 1982. The cellular and subcellular characteristics of acute and chronic injury with emphasis on the role of calcium. In: *Pathophysiology of Shock, Anoxia, and Ischemia*. Cowley, R.A. and Trump, B.F. (eds), pp. 6–46. Baltimore: Williams and Wilkins.

Trump, B.F., Smith, M.W., Phelps, P.C., Regec, A.L., and Berezesky, I.K. 1988. The role of ionized calcium in acute and chronic cell injury. In: *Integration of Mitochondrial Function*. Lemasters, J.J., Hackenbrook, C.R., Thurman, R.G., and Westerhoff, H.V. (eds), pp. 437–444. New York: Plenum Press.

Trump, B.F., Berezesky, I.K., Smith, M.W., Phelps, P.C., and Elliget, K.A. 1989. The role of ion deregulation in cell injury and carcinogenesis. *Methodological Surveys in Biochemistry and Analysis: Biochemical Approaches to Cellular Calcium* 19: 439–452.

Trump, B.F., Jones, T.W., Elliget, K.A., Smith, M.W., Phelps, P.C., Maki, A., and Berezesky, I.K. 1990. Relation between toxicity and carcinogenesis in the kidney: an heuristic hypothesis. *Renal Failure* 12: 183–191.

Van Rooijen, N. 1991. High and low cytosolic $Ca^{2+}$ induced macrophage death? Hypothesis. *Cell Calcium* 12: 381–384.

Walisser, J.A. and Thies, R.L. 1999. Poly(ADP-ribose) polymerase inhibition in oxidant-stressed endothelial cells prevents oncosis and permits caspase activation and apoptosis. *J Exp Cell Res* 251: 401–413.

Weinberg, J.M. 1991. The cell biology of ischemic renal injury. *Kidney Int* 39: 476–500.

Welch, W.J. 1990. The mammalian stress response: Cell physiology and biochemistry of stress proteins. In: *Stress Proteins in Biology and Medicine*. Morimoto Tissieres, R. and Georgopoulos, C. (eds), pp. 223–278. Cold Spring Harbor, NY: Cold Spring Harbor Laboratory Press.

Wever, P.C., Aten, J., Rentenaar, R.J., Hack, C.E., Koopman, G., Weening, J.J., and ten Berge, I.J. 1998. Apoptotic tubular cell death during acute renal autograph rejection. *Clin Nephrol* 49: 28–34.

Wissing, D., Mouritzen, H., Egeblad, M., Porier, G.G., and Jaattela, M. 1997. Involvement of caspase-dependent activation of cytosolic phospholipase A2 in tumor necrosis factor-induced apoptosis. *Proc Natl Acad Sci USA* 94: 5073–5077.

Wood, D.E., Thomas, A., Devi, L.A., Berman, Y., Beavis, R.C., Reed, J.C., and Newcomb, E.W. 1998. Bax cleavage is mediated by calpain during drug-induced apoptosis. *Oncogene* 17: 1069–1078.

Wyllie, A.H. 1981. Cell death: a new classification separating apoptosis from necrosis. In: *Cell Death in Biology and Pathology*. Bowen, I.D. and Lockshin, R.A. (eds), pp. 9–34. London: Chapman and Hall.

Xu, L., Glassford, A.J., Giaccia, A.J., and Giffard, R.G. 1998. Acidosis reduces neuronal apoptosis. *Neuroreport* 9: 875–879.

Yamamoto, N., Maki, A., Swann, J.D., Berezesky, I.K., and Trump, B.F. 1993. Induction of immediate early and stress genes in rat proximal tubule epithelium following injury: the significance of cytosolic ionized calcium. *Renal Failure* 15: 63–171.

Yuspa, S., Hennings, H., Tucker, R., Jaken, S., Kilkenny, A., and Roop, D. 1988. Signal transduction for proliferation and differentiation in keratinocytes. *Ann NY Acad Sci* 548: 191–196.

# 6

# PATHOBIOLOGY OF MYOCARDIAL ISCHEMIC INJURY

*L. Maximilian Buja*

*Department of Pathology and Laboratory Medicine,*
*The University of Texas-Houston Medical School, USA*

## Introduction

Myocardial ischemia is a state of myocardial impairment, which results from inadequate coronary perfusion of oxygenated blood relative to the metabolic demands of the myocardium.[1-3] Thus, ischemic heart disease involves an imbalance in the normal integrated function of the coronary vasculature and the myocardium. The major consequences of myocardial ischemia are depressed myocardial contractile function, arrhythmias, and myocardial necrosis (infarction).

## Role of coronary alterations in myocardial ischemia

### *Observations in humans*

Atherosclerosis leads to progressive narrowing of the coronary arteries and predisposes to the development of ischemic heart disease.[4-7] However, the pathogenesis of acute ischemic heart disease involves the occurrence of an acute pathophysiologic alteration in the presence of coronary atherosclerosis of variable severity.[7-16] The acute pathophysiologic event may involve a stress-induced increase in myocardial oxygen demand or an impairment in the oxygen-carrying capacity of the blood. However, many cases of acute ischemic heart disease result from a primary alteration in the coronary vasculature leading to decreased delivery of blood to the myocardium. These alterations involve platelet aggregation, vasoconstriction (coronary spasm), and thrombosis superimposed on atherosclerotic lesions (Figure 6.1).

An acute alteration of an atherosclerotic plaque often initiates acute narrowing or occlusion of the coronary artery. Acute changes in plaques consist of fissures, ulceration, and rupture, with injury to the endothelium and surface cap of the plaque as the initiating event.[7,12] Precipitation of these changes likely requires chronic or recurrent injury that involves toxic effects of products produced by degeneration of the plaque constituents, inflammation, and hemodynamic

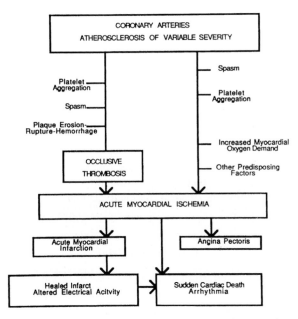

*Figure 6.1* Pathogenetic mechanisms of acute ischemic heart disease and potential clinical outcomes. Adapted with permission from Buja *et al.*[8]

trauma.[17–19] Occlusive coronary thrombi overlying fissured, ulcerated, or ruptured plaques are found in over 90 percent of cases of acute transmural myocardial infarction.[12,13] This finding is the basis for the successful application of thrombolytic therapy for the treatment of acute myocardial infarction by coronary reperfusion.[20,21] In syndromes of ischemic heart disease other than acute myocardial infarction, including unstable angina pectoris and sudden cardiac death, acute alterations of the coronary arteries also are frequently observed. These include endothelial disruption, plaque fissuring, platelet aggregation, and non-occlusive or occlusive thrombi.[7–16,22]

### Observations in experimental models

Insights into the role of coronary factors in the pathogenesis of acute myocardial ischemia have been provided by a canine model in which coronary stenosis with endothelial injury has been produced by placement of a plastic constrictor on a roughened area of the left anterior descending coronary artery.[14,16] Coronary injury in the model results in the development of cyclic blood flow alterations which are characterized by periods of progressive reduction to a nadir of blood flow, followed by abrupt restoration of blood flow. These cyclic blood flow alterations are due to recurrent platelet aggregation at the site of coronary stenosis. There is evidence that the process is driven by several platelet-derived mediators, including thromboxane $A_2$ ($TxA_2$) and serotonin.[10,11,14,15] The cyclic blood flow alterations

165

are mediated both by anatomic obstruction of the coronary artery by aggregated platelets as well as by excessive vasoconstriction produced by TxA$_2$, serotonin, and possibly other products released from the platelets (Figure 6.2). Endothelial damage, leading to loss of prostacyclin and endothelium-derived relaxing factor (nitric oxide), also contributes to the process. The cyclic blood flow alterations can be inhibited by treatment with TxA$_2$ synthesis inhibitors, TxA$_2$ receptor antagonists, and serotonin receptor antagonists.[10,11] In a chronic model with cyclic blood flow alterations for several days, the animals develop intimal proliferation at the site of coronary stenosis with further narrowing of the lumen.[16] This process is likely mediated by multiple growth factors, including platelet-derived growth factor (PDGF) released from platelets. The intimal proliferation can be attenuated by treatment with inhibitors of leukocyte and platelet receptors and chemical mediators.[16,23]

### *Clinical correlates*

The observations derived from the canine cyclic blood flow model have implications for the pathogenesis of acute ischemic heart disease.[7–16,22] Endothelial injury developing at a site of coronary stenosis can initiate changes leading to impaired coronary perfusion and myocardial ischemia. Endothelial injury predisposes to recurrent platelet aggregation, which produces anatomic obstruction compounded by vasoconstriction. TxA$_2$ and serotonin are important mediators of

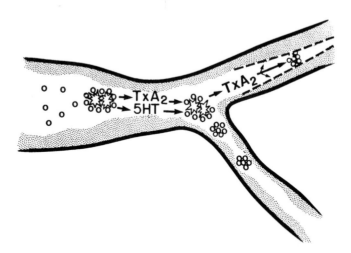

*Figure 6.2* A schematic diagram indicating the role of platelet-mediated mechanisms of induction of acute myocardial ischemia. Platelet aggregation develops in atherosclerotic coronary arteries at sites of endothelial injury. Aggregating platelets release mediators, including thromboxane A$_2$ (TxA$_2$) and serotonin (5HT), which cause further platelet aggregation downstream and vasoconstriction. Reproduced with permission of Elsevier Science and Lippincott Williams & Wilkins from Hirsh *et al.*,[10] as modified by Willerson *et al.*[15]

the process. Recurrent episodes of platelet aggregation may lead to further coronary stenosis as a result of intimal proliferation.[16-23] A clinical counterpart of the last phenomenon may be the intimal proliferation that frequently occurs following percutaneous transluminal coronary angioplasty (PTCA) in man. The process of recurrent platelet aggregation may result at any stage in the development of occlusive coronary thrombosis, although spontaneous resolution is also possible. Studies in man have also provided evidence of platelet aggregation as well as release of $TxA_2$ and serotonin in patients with unstable angina pectoris.[7,10,11] Anti-platelet therapies, including glycoprotein IIA/IIIB receptor antagonists, are clinically effective in patients with acute coronary syndromes.[22,24] Thus, there is strong evidence that endothelial injury and platelet aggregation are key factors in the mediation of acute ischemic heart disease.

## Mechanisms of myocardial ischemic injury

### *Metabolic alterations*

The major metabolic alterations induced by myocardial ischemia involve impaired energy and substrate metabolism.[1-3] Oxygen deprivation results in a rapid inhibition of mitochondrial oxidative phosphorylation, the major source of cellular ATP synthesis. Initially, there is compensatory stimulation of anaerobic glycolysis for ATP production from glucose. However, glycolysis leads to the accumulation of hydrogen ions and lactate with resultant intracellular acidosis and inhibition of glycolysis.[1-3,25] Fatty acid metabolism as well as glucose metabolism is impaired.[3,26] Free fatty acids in the ischemic myocardium are derived from endogenous as well as exogenous sources, the magnitude of the latter depending upon the degree of collateral perfusion. Inhibition of mitochondrial β-oxidation leads to the accumulation of long-chain acylcarnitine, long-chain acyl coenzyme A (CoA), and free fatty acids. Initially, the free fatty acids are esterified into triglycerides, giving rise to fatty change in the myocardium. However, as esterification becomes blunted, free fatty acids increase (Figure 6.3).

Myocardial ischemia is initially manifested by impaired excitation contraction coupling with resultant reduction in contractile activity of the ischemic myocardium.[1-3] The sudden regional loss of intravascular pressure appears to be the primary cause of the immediate decline in contractile function following coronary occlusion.[27] Subsequent progression of contractile failure is related to the associated early metabolic changes, including a declining ATP level, leakage of potassium from myocytes, intracellular acidosis, and accumulation of inorganic phosphate.[1-3] The loss of contractile activity probably has a beneficial secondary effect by prolonging myocardial viability as a result of a major reduction in the demand for ATP.

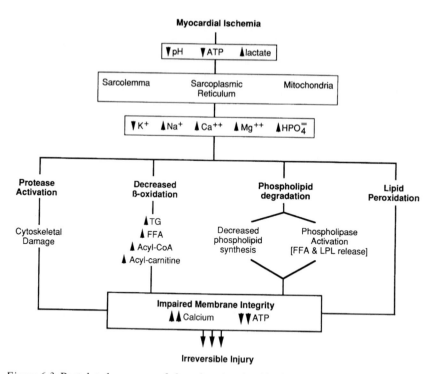

*Figure 6.3* Postulated sequence of alterations involved in the pathogenesis of irreversible myocardial ischemic injury. Oxygen deficiency induces metabolic changes, including decreased ATP, decreased pH, and lactate accumulation, in ischemic myocytes. The altered metabolic milieu leads to impaired membrane transport with resultant derangements in intracellular electrolytes. An increase in cytosolic $Ca^{2+}$ may trigger the activation of proteases and phospholipases with resultant cytoskeletal damage and impaired membrane phospholipid balance. Lipid alterations include increased phospholipid degradation with release of free fatty acids and lysophospholipids (LPLs) and decreased phospholipid synthesis. Lipid peroxidation occurs as a result of attack by free radicals produced at least in part by the generation of excess electrons in oxygen-deprived mitochondria. Free radicals also may be derived from metabolism of arachidonic acid and catecholamines, metabolism of adenine nucleotides by xanthine oxidase in endothelium (species dependent), and activation of neutrophils and macrophages. The irreversible phase of injury appears to be mediated by severe membrane damage produced by phospholipid loss, lipid peroxidation, and cytoskeletal damage. Reproduced with permission from Buja.[26]

## *Altered ionic homeostasis*

The metabolic derangements discussed above lead to dysfunction of membrane pumps and channels with resultant derangements in intracellular electrolyte homeostasis. The earliest manifestation of membrane dysfunction is a net loss of potassium due to accelerated efflux of the ion from ischemic myocardial cells.[1–3,28–30] Although the potassium efflux occurs before a severe reduction in ATP, more rapid depletion of a localized component or compartment of ATP may lead to activation of ATP-dependent $K^+$ efflux channels.[29] Once ATP reduction is of sufficient magnitude, impaired function of the sodium/potassium-ATPase occurs. This is accompanied by an accumulation of sodium, chloride, and water in the cells; further loss of potassium; loss of cell volume regulation; and cell swelling.[31] Another early change involves an initial increase in free intracellular magnesium levels followed by progressive loss of magnesium.[30] This is related in part to release of magnesium–ATP complexes as ATP depletion occurs. Finally, progressive changes in intracellular calcium homeostasis occur that may be of particular importance in the development of lethal cell injury.

### Role of calcium

The intracellular calcium level regulates normal cardiac function, and deranged calcium balance contributes significantly to the pathogenesis of myocardial cell injury.[32–34] The intracellular calcium level is regulated by several processes.[32] At the level of the sarcolemma, the voltage-dependent calcium channel is responsible for the slow inward current of the normal action potential, the sodium–calcium exchanger modulates intracellular calcium levels, and the calcium-ATPase mediates a calcium efflux pathway. At the level of the sarcoplasmic reticulum, the calcium magnesium-ATPase and phospholamban mediate calcium uptake and release on a beat-to-beat basis. Intracellular calcium levels also are modulated by uptake and storage of calcium in the mitochondria and binding of calcium to calcium-binding proteins.

The total intracellular calcium concentration is in the order of 1–2 mM, with most of this calcium bound to cellular proteins.[32–34] The free cytosolic ionized calcium ($Ca^{2+}$) concentration is approximately 100–300 nM during diastole and approximately 1 μM during systole. Beat-to-beat regulation of the cell calcium level involves voltage-dependent calcium influx across the sarcolemma followed by calcium-induced calcium release from the sarcoplasmic reticulum, with the latter providing the major source of the calcium that binds to the myofilaments and activates cardiac contraction. Diastole is mediated by a reuptake of calcium into the sarcoplasmic reticulum, thereby lowering the cytosolic free calcium level.

Recent studies have confirmed that, at an early stage of myocardial hypoxic and ischemic injury, normal calcium transients are lost and the cytosolic free calcium concentration increases into the micromolar range.[35–38] Multiple mechanisms may be involved, including a net influx of calcium across the sarcolemma as well as loss of calcium from intracellular storage sites in the sarcoplasmic reticulum and mitochondria.[32–38] These changes reflect membrane dysfunction, which is induced by ATP depletion and intracellular acidosis. The postulated consequences of an increase in cytosolic calcium include activation of phospholipases, proteinases, and calcium-dependent ATPases. Contractile depression persists in spite of the increase in cytosolic calcium as a result of damage to the myofibrillar proteins, thereby decreasing their sensitivity to calcium.[3]

## *Progressive membrane damage*

The conversion from reversible to irreversible myocardial injury is mediated by progressive membrane damage (Figure 6.3). A number of factors may contribute to the more advanced stages of membrane injury. Cellular and organellar membranes consist of a phospholipid bilayer containing cholesterol and glycoproteins. The phospholipid bilayer is maintained by a balance between phospholipid degradation and synthesis. In myocardial ischemia, progressive phospholipid degradation occurs, probably as a result of the activation of one or more phospholipases secondary to an increase in cytosolic calcium or possibly other metabolic derangements.[3] Phospholipase A- and phospholipase C-mediated pathways may be involved. Phospholipid degradation results in a transient increase in lysophospholipids, which are subsequently degraded by other lipases, as well as the release of free fatty acids. Thus, phospholipid degradation contributes to the accumulation of various lipid species in ischemic myocardium. These lipids include free fatty acids, lysophospholipids, long-chain acyl CoA, and long-chain acylcarnitines.[1,3,39,40] These molecules are amphiphiles (molecules with hydrophilic and hydrophobic portions). As a result of their amphipathic property, these molecules accumulate in the phospholipid bilayer, thereby altering the fluidity and permeability of the membranes.[41]

Initially, phospholipid degradation appears to be balanced by energy-dependent phospholipid synthesis. However, degradation eventually becomes predominant, with the result that net phospholipid depletion in the order of approximately 10 percent of total phospholipid content occurs after 3 h of coronary occlusion. Although this net change in total phospholipid content is relatively small, it is associated with the development of significant permeability and structural defects which are inhibited by agents that inhibit phospholipid degradation.[42]

Myocardial ischemia also induces the generation of free radicals and toxic oxygen species derived from several sources.[43–46] As a result of impaired oxidative metabolism, ischemic mitochondria generate an excess number of reducing equivalents that may initiate the generation of free radicals. Free radicals also can be produced by the enzymatic and non-enzymatic metabolism of arachidonic acid derived from phospholipid degradation and of catecholamines released from nerve terminals (see below). Endothelium of several species contains xanthine dehydrogenase, which may be converted to xanthine oxidase during ischemia. The xanthine oxidase can then metabolize adenine nucleotides derived from the metabolism of ATP. Neutrophils and macrophages invading ischemic tissue represent another source of free radicals. One major free radical cascade involves a generation of superoxide anions followed by the production of toxic oxygen species, including the hydroxyl radical. Another major free radical cascade involves the production of excessive amounts of nitric oxide (NO).[47,48] A major target of free radicals is cell membranes, where the free radicals act on unsaturated fatty acids in membrane phospholipids leading to their peroxidation. Thus, free radicals can be generated during myocardial ischemia and this process can be accelerated by reoxygenation.

An additional factor in membrane injury involves disruption of the cytoskeleton, thereby affecting the anchoring of the sarcolemma to the interior of the myocyte.[49–51] Vinculin has been identified as a cytoskeletal protein involved in this process. It is postulated that ischemia leads to disruption of cytoskeletal filaments connecting the sarcolemma to the myofibrils as a result of activation of proteases by increased cytosolic calcium or other mechanisms. After such disruption, the ischemic myocyte becomes more susceptible to the effects of cell swelling following accumulation of sodium and water. This process leads to the formation of subsarcolemmal blebs followed by rupture of the membrane.

Such injury culminating with cell swelling (oncosis) and rupture is accelerated by the effects of reperfusion, which allows for increased sodium, chloride, water, and calcium accumulation in the injured cells. Marked reactivation of contraction occurs as a result of marked calcium influx coupled with transient regeneration of ATP by mitochondria resupplied with oxygen. The resultant hypercontracture will accelerate membrane rupture following cytoskeletal disruption. The processes just described are important mechanisms of reperfusion injury.[52,53]

Thus, the transition from reversible to irreversible myocardial damage appears to be mediated by membrane injury secondary to progressive phospholipid degradation, free radical effects, and damage to the cytoskeletal anchoring of the sarcolemma. The consequences of this vicious cycle are loss of membrane integrity and further calcium accumulation with secondary ATP depletion (Figure 6.3).

### Oncosis, apoptosis, and necrosis

The above description presents the well-documented pathophysiology of cell injury and cell death in cardiac myocytes subjected to a major ischemic or hypoxic insult. However, it is now known that other pathophysiologic mechanisms may contribute to myocardial cell injury and death. Following the recognition of apoptosis as a major and distinctive mode of cell death, multiple reports have implicated apoptosis in myocardial infarction, reperfusion injury, and other forms of cardiovascular pathology.[3,54,55] Apoptosis is characterized by a series of molecular and biochemical events, including (1) gene activation (programmed cell death); (2) perturbations of mitochondria, including membrane permeability transition and cytochrome $c$ release; (3) activation of a cascade of cytosolic aspartate-specific cysteine proteases (caspases); (4) endonuclease activation leading to double-stranded DNA fragmentation; and (5) altered phospholipid distribution of cell membranes and other surface properties with preservation of selective membrane permeability. Apoptosis is also characterized by distinctive morphologic alterations featuring cell and nuclear shrinkage and fragmentation. In contrast, numerous studies have reported ischemic myocardial damage to be characterized by cell swelling and altered cellular ionic composition as a result of altered membrane permeability. This pattern of cell injury and death with cell swelling has been termed oncosis. Although some reports have proposed a major role for apoptosis in myocardial ischemic injury and infarction, such a role for apoptosis may be overstated because of overinterpretation of evidence of DNA fragmentation, which is not specific for apoptosis.[3,54,55] Although certain assays have been proposed to be more reliable for detection of patterns of DNA fragmentation characteristic of apoptosis, the overall sensitivity and specificity of these assays need confirmation.[3,55] Nevertheless, work using caspase inhibitors does suggest that apoptosis as well as oncosis may contribute to the overall magnitude of ischemic necrosis.[3,55] The rate and magnitude of ATP reduction may be a critical determinant of whether an injured myocyte progresses to death by apoptosis or oncosis, because an ATP analogue, deoxyadenosine 5′-triphosphate (d-ATP), is a key component of a molecular complex that mediates cytochrome $c$ release with activation of the caspase cascade and apoptotic death.[3,55] It is likely then that severely ischemic myocytes progress rapidly to cell death with swelling (oncosis), whereas less severely ischemic myocytes may progress to cell death by apoptosis.

### *Autonomic alterations and arrhythmogenesis*

Myocardial ischemia is accompanied by significant alterations in the autonomic nervous system. A major acute ischemic episode generates a stress reaction that leads to elevation of circulating catecholamines. Within the ischemic myocardium, norepinephrine is released from injured nerve terminals, resulting, initially, in a redistribution of catecholamines followed by their eventual depletion.[56] Alterations in adrenergic receptors develop, including increases in the numbers of β- and α-adrenergic receptors expressed on the sarcolemmal membrane.[57,58] Initially, excess catecholamine stimulation is coupled to increased intracellular metabolism mediated in part through the adenylate cyclase system. However, eventually, uncoupling occurs between intracellular metabolism and receptor stimulation. However, this coupling can be restored and heightened upon reperfusion. Excess catecholamine stimulation can have a number of untoward consequences, including enhanced intracellular calcium influx as well as arrhythmogenesis.

Arrhythmias and conduction disturbances occur commonly in association with myocardial ischemia and may range from mild alterations to ventricular fibrillation. Arrhythmias are particularly common during the early phase of an ischemic episode as well as at the onset of reperfusion.[2,59] It is likely that different mechanisms operate in different phases of ischemic arrhythmias. The arrhythmias may be mediated by metabolic alterations, including a high concentration of potassium in the extracellular space adjacent to cardiac myocytes and nerve terminals;[2] accumulation of lysophospholipids, long-chain acyl compounds, and free fatty acids in myocardial membranes;[26,40] the alterations in the adrenergic system described above;[56-58] and intracellular electrolyte alterations, including accumulation of intracellular calcium.[60]

# Evolution of myocardial infarction

## *Progression of myocardial ischemic injury*

In humans, the left ventricular subendocardium is the region most susceptible to myocardial ischemic injury. This is also true for the dog, which is the most common species used for experimental studies of myocardial ischemia. The susceptibility of the subendocardium relates to a more tenuous oxygen supply–demand balance in this region versus the subepicardium. This in turn is related to the pattern of distribution of the collateral circulation as well as local metabolic differences in subendocardial versus subepicardial myocytes.

Following coronary occlusion, the myocardium can withstand up to about 20 min of severe ischemia without developing irreversible injury. However, after about 20–30 min of severe ischemia, irreversible myocardial injury develops. The subsequent degradative changes give rise to recognizable myocardial necrosis. In the human and dog, myocardial necrosis first appears in the ischemic subendocardium because this area generally has a more severe reduction in perfusion than the subepicardium. Over the ensuing 3–6 h, irreversible myocardial injury progresses in a wavefront pattern from the subendocardium into the subepicardium.[2,61] In the experimental animal, and probably in humans as well, most myocardial infarcts are completed within approximately 6–8 h after the onset of coronary occlusion. However, a slower pattern of evolution of myocardial infarction can occur when the coronary collateral circulation is particularly prominent and/or when the stimulus for myocardial ischemia is intermittent, e.g. in the case of episodes of intermittent platelet aggregation before occlusive thrombosis.

## *Histologic and ultrastructural changes*

Established myocardial infarcts have distinct central and peripheral regions (Figure 6.4).[2,34,61,62] In the central zone of severe ischemia, the necrotic myocytes exhibit clumped nuclear chromatin; stretched myofibrils with widened I bands; mitochondria containing amorphous matrix (flocculent) densities composed of denatured lipid and protein and linear densities representing fused cristae; and defects (holes) in the sarcolemma. In the peripheral region of an infarct, which has some degree of collateral perfusion, many necrotic myocytes exhibit disruption of the myofibrils with the formation of dense transverse (contraction) bands; mitochondria containing calcium phosphate deposits as well as the amorphous matrix densities; variable amounts of lipid droplets; and clumped nuclear chromatin. A third population of cells at the outermost periphery of infarcts contain excess numbers of lipid droplets but do not exhibit the features of irreversible injury just described. The pattern of injury seen in the infarcted periphery is also characteristic of myocardial injury produced by temporary coronary occlusion followed by reperfusion. In general, the most reliable ultrastructural features of

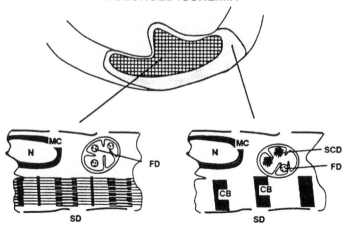

## A PROLONGED ISCHEMIA

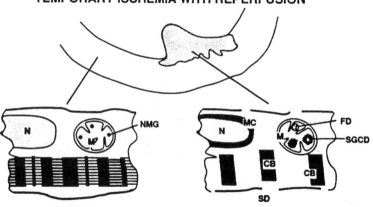

## B TEMPORARY ISCHEMIA WITH REPERFUSION

*Figure 6.4* Schematic diagram of morphologic features of myocardial cell injury present in different regions of transmural infarcts produced by permanent coronary occlusion (A) and subepicardial infarcts produced by temporary ischemia followed by reperfusion (B). With prolonged coronary occlusion, myocardial necrosis is established in the subendocardium within 40–60 min, progresses in a wavefront pattern into the subendocardium of the region at risk (risk zone), and is completed by 3–6 h. With prolonged coronary occlusion, the myofibrils of myocytes in the central infarct region are hyper-relaxed compared with those in the normal tissue depicted in (A), and the mitochondria contain flocculent densities composed of denatured lipid and protein. The myofibrils of myocytes in the peripheral infarct region are formed into contraction bands and the mitochondria show calcium deposits as well as flocculent densities. With temporary ischemia and reperfusion, injury is limited to the subendocardium and is characterized by myofibrillar contraction bands and early mitochondrial calcification. N, nucleus; MC, marginated chromatin; M, mitochondria; SD, sarcolemmal defect; FD, flocculent (amorphous) density; NMG, normal matrix granule; CB, contraction band; SCD, spicular calcium deposit; SGCD, small (granular) calcium deposit. Reproduced with permission of Kluwer Academic publishers from Hagler and Buja.[34]

irreversible injury are the amorphous matrix densities in the mitochondria and the sarcolemmal defects.

## *Determinants of myocardial infarct size*

The myocardial bed-at-risk, or risk zone, refers to the mass of myocardium that receives its blood supply from a major coronary artery that develops occlusion.[61] Following occlusion, the severity of the ischemia is determined by the amount of pre-existing collateral circulation into the myocardial bed-at-risk. The collateral blood flow is derived from collateral channels connecting the occluded and non-occluded coronary systems. With time, there is progressive increase in coronary collateral blood flow. However, much of this increase in flow may be too late to salvage significant amounts of myocardium.[2,61–63]

The size of the infarct is determined by the mass of necrotic myocardium within the bed-at-risk.[2,61–63] The bed-at-risk will also contain viable but injured myocardium. The border zone refers to the non-necrotic but dysfunctional myocardium within the ischemic bed-at-risk. The size of the border zone varies inversely with the relative amount of necrotic myocardium, which increases with time as the wavefront of necrosis progresses. The border zone exists primarily in the subepicardial half of the bed-at-risk and has very little lateral dimension owing to a sharp demarcation between vascular beds supplied by the occluded and patent major coronary arteries.

Thus, the major determinants of ultimate infarct size are the duration and severity of ischemia, the size of the myocardial bed-at-risk, and the amount of collateral blood flow available shortly after coronary occlusion.[2,61–63] Infarct size can also be influenced by the major determinants of myocardial metabolic demand, which are heart rate, wall tension (determined by blood pressure), and myocardial contractility.

## *Measurement of myocardial infarct size*

Pathologic analysis of infarct size has provided a "goal standard" in accessing the accuracy of various non-invasive diagnostic tests for myocardial infarction. Although extensive investigation in this area has been conducted, non-invasive determination of infarct size remains a challenge.[63] Techniques that have been utilized have included various electrocardiographic methods, quantitation of serum enzyme release, and various scintigraphic approaches. Our group has extensively evaluated the use of technetium stannous pyrophosphate scintigraphy for detection and sizing of myocardial infarcts, while other groups have evaluated the other approaches. Further work is need to perfect methods for non-invasive detection and quantification of the myocardial bed-at-risk. This then will allow an analysis of absolute infarct size as well as infarct size as a percentage of the bed-at-risk.

# Modulation of myocardial ischemic injury

## *Modulating influences of preconditioning, stunning, and reperfusion*

A number of factors can significantly modulate the myocardial response and subsequent outcome following an ischemic episode.[3] The progression of myocardial ischemia can be profoundly influenced by reperfusion. However, the effects of reperfusion are complex.[52,53,64] Reperfusion clearly can limit the extent of myocardial necrosis if instituted early enough after the onset of coronary occlusion. However, reperfusion also changes the pattern of myocardial injury by causing hemorrhage within the severely damaged myocardium and by producing a pattern of myocardial injury characterized by contraction bands and calcification. Reperfusion also accelerates the release of intracellular enzymes from damaged myocardium. This may lead to a marked elevation of serum levels of these enzymes without necessarily implying further myocardial necrosis. The timing of reperfusion is critical to the outcome, with the potential for myocardial salvage being greater with earlier intervention. Although reperfusion can clearly salvage myocardium, it may also induce additional injury. The concept of reperfusion injury implies the development of further damage, as a result of the reperfusion, to myocytes that were injured but that remained viable during a previous ischemic episode. Such injury may involve functional impairment, arrhythmia, and/or progression to cell death.[52,53,64]

The rate of progression of myocardial necrosis can be influenced by prior short intervals of coronary occlusion and reperfusion. Specifically, experimental evidence indicates that the extent of myocardial necrosis after 60–90 min of coronary occlusion is significantly less in animals that had been pretreated with one or more 5-min intervals of coronary occlusion before the induction of permanent occlusion.[61,65,66] However, after 120 min of coronary occlusion, the effect on infarct size is lost. This phenomenon is known as preconditioning.[3,65,66] Recent evidence has indicated that a reduced rate of ATP depletion correlates with the beneficial effects of preconditioning.[65,66] Further studies have suggested that activation of adenosine receptors and ATP-dependent potassium channels may mediate the process of preconditioning.[67,68] After a refractory period, a second late phase of myocardial protection during a subsequent ischemic event develops.[69] This phenomenon, known as the second window of protection, is related to ischemia-induced gene activation with production of various gene products, including stress (heat shock) proteins and nitric oxide synthase.[3,69]

Prolonged functional depression, requiring up to 24 h or longer for recovery, develops on reperfusion even after relatively brief periods of coronary occlusion, in the order of 15 min, which are insufficient to cause myocardial necrosis. This phenomenon has been referred to as myocardial stunning.[3] A related condition, termed hibernation, refers to chronic depression of myocardial function owing to a chronic moderate reduction of perfusion.[3] Preconditioning and stunning are independent phenomena as the preconditioning effect is short term, is transient, and is not mediated through stunning. Free radical effects and calcium loading have been implicated in the pathogenesis of stunning, as well as other components of reperfusion injury.[70,71] After longer intervals of coronary occlusion, in the order of 2–4 h, necrosis of the subendocardium develops and even more severe and persistent functional depression occurs.[72] In experimental studies, after 2 h of coronary occlusion, left ventricular (LV) regional sites of moderate dysfunction during ischemia recovered normal or near-normal regional contractile function after 1–4 weeks of reperfusion, whereas after 4 h of coronary occlusion contractile dysfunction persisted after 4 weeks of reperfusion.[72]

Therefore, depending on the interval of coronary occlusion before reperfusion, various degrees of contractile dysfunction, necrosis, or both are seen with reperfusion. These observations emphasize the need for early intervention to salvage myocardium.[3,61] On balance, early reperfusion results in a major net positive effect, thus making early reperfusion an important goal in the treatment of acute ischemic heart disease.[20,21]

### Therapeutic interventions

Continuing efforts have been made to develop therapeutic approaches to limiting infarct size because the extent of myocardial necrosis is a major determinant of prognosis following myocardial infarction. Experimental studies have shown that evaluation of a therapeutic agent should take into account both the influence of the size of the myocardial bed-at-risk and the amount of collateral perfusion over a given time interval of coronary occlusion.[63,73] If an intervention produces a smaller infarct as a percentage of the bed-at-risk at any given level of residual perfusion, then it can be concluded that the intervention has an independent effect on myocardial ischemic cell injury. Various pharmacologic approaches have been aimed at improving myocardial metabolism, increasing myocardial blood flow, reducing cellular calcium overload, and preventing free radical-mediated effects.[63,73] The most important advance in recent years has been the advent of thrombolytic therapy to provide reperfusion of the ischemic myocardium. This approach has initiated a new era of treatment of acute myocardial infarction.[20,21] Ongoing investigations are aimed at developing pharmacologic interventions which can be coupled with thrombolytic therapy to provide optimal protection and salvage of the ischemic myocardium.

### Pathology of interventionally treated coronary artery disease

Percutaneous transluminal coronary angioplasty (PTCA) can produce a variety of acute effects, including dilatation of the vessel caused by stretching of the intima and media, damage to the endothelial surface, multiple fissures in the plaque, and dissection of the media.[74,75] The acute injury initiates a reparative response which leads to intimal proliferation.[16,74,75] Similar effects occur after atherectomy and laser angioplasty.[76,77] The resultant fibrocellular tissue is composed of modified smooth muscle cells (myofibroblasts) and connective tissue matrix without lipid deposits. A similar lesion is seen in animal models of arterial injury.[16] Experimental evidence supports a role for platelet activation in the pathogenesis of the lesion.[16] This process of intimal proliferation leads to restenosis of lesions in 30–40 percent of cases within 6 months. The use of vascular stents in conjunction with angioplasty has significantly improved the long-term patency rates, although the stents do invoke some intimal reaction.[78,79]

Saphenous vein coronary artery bypass grafts (SVCABG) develop diffuse fibrocellular intimal thickening, medial degeneration and atrophy, and vascular dilatation within several months after implantation.[80–82] Subsequently, the grafts are prone to development of eccentric intimal plaques with lipid deposition (atherosclerosis). Plaque fissuring and thrombosis may also develop. Therefore, all of the changes seen in naturally occurring atherosclerosis may also develop in the saphenous veins, thereby creating a finite limit to the beneficial effects of these grafts. With improvements in surgical technique, the use of internal mammary arteries for coronary bypass has taken on more widespread application. The internal mammary arteries are more resistant to the intimal injury and intimal proliferation observed in saphenous veins and, therefore, the arterial bypass grafts have prolonged potency.[83,84]

## New approaches to myocardial modulation

A new era in the treatment of ischemic heart disease is developing based on the therapeutic application of new insights regarding the pathogenesis of myocardial ischemic disease. Ongoing work is being conducted to successfully achieve genetic manipulation (gene therapy) of the processes accountable for the response of the arterial wall to injury, with the goals of retarding or preventing intimal proliferation and thrombosis at sites of coronary injury.[85–87] New pharmacologic interventions are being tested based on the possible contribution of apoptosis as well as oncosis to myocardial infarction.[3] The debate regarding whether or not cardiac myocytes are terminally differentiated has been revived.[88,89] Molecular mechanisms responsible for the mitotic block of mature myocytes is under investigation, with the potential for genetic manipulation of myocyte proliferation.[88,89] Other approaches are being explored, including microinjection of genetically engineered myocytes for repopulation of damaged myocardium.[90,91] Alternative approaches are also being explored for the treatment of intractable angina pectoris.[92,93] One surgical approach is the use of transmyocardial laser treatment to create new myocardial microvasculature.[93–96] An alternate approach is the intravascular delivery of genetically engineered growth factors, including vascular endothelial growth factor (VEGF) and fibroblast growth factor (FGF).[97–100] These approaches have considerable promise for the treatment of ischemic myocardial disease.

# References

1. Hillis LD, Braunwald E. 1977. Myocardial ischemia. *N Engl J Med* 296: 971–978, 1034–1041, 1093–1096.
2. Reimer KA, Ideker RE. 1987. Myocardial ischemia and infarction: anatomic and biochemical substrates for ischemic cell death and ventricular arrhythmias. *Human Pathol* 18: 462–475.
3. Buja LM. 1998. Modulation of the myocardial response to ischemia. *Lab Invest* 78: 1345–1373.
4. Ross R. 1993. The pathogenesis of atherosclerosis: a perspective for the 1990s. *Nature* 362: 801–809.
5. Munro JM, Cotran RS. 1988. The pathogenesis of atherosclerosis: atherogenesis and inflammation. *Lab Invest* 58: 249–261.
6. Buja LM, Clubb Jr., FJ, Bilheimer DW, Willerson JT. 1990. Pathobiology of human familial hypercholesterolemia and a related animal model, the Watanabe heritable hyperlipidemic rabbit. *Eur Heart J* 11 (Suppl. E): 41–52.
7. Fuster V, Badimon L, Badimon JJ, Chesebro JH. 1992. The pathogenesis of coronary artery disease and the acute coronary syndromes. *N Engl J Med* 326: 242–250, 310–318.
8. Buja LM, Hillis, LD, Petty CS, Willerson JT. 1981. The role of coronary arterial spasm in ischemic heart disease. *Arch Pathol Lab Med* 105: 221–226.
9. Davies MJ, Thomas AC, Knapman PA, Hangartner JR. 1986. Intramyocardial platelet aggregation in patients with unstable angina pectoris suffering sudden ischemic cardiac death. *Circulation* 73: 418–427.
10. Hirsh PD, Campbell WB, Willerson JT, Hillis LD. 1981. Prostaglandins and ischemic heart disease. *Am J Med* 71: 1009–1026.
11. Fitzgerald DJ, Roy L, Catella F, Fitzgerald GA. 1986. Platelet activation in unstable coronary disease. *N Engl J Med* 315: 983–989.
12. Buja LM, Willerson JT. 1987. The role of coronary artery lesions in ischemic heart disease: insights from recent clinicopathologic, coronary arteriographic, and experimental studies. *Human Pathol* 18: 451–461.
13. Buja LM, Willerson JT. 1991. Relationship of ischemic heart disease to sudden cardiac death. *J Forensic Sci* 36: 25–33.
14. Willerson JT, Hillis LD, Winniford M, Buja LM. 1986. Speculation regarding mechanisms responsible for acute ischemic heart disease syndromes. *J Am Coll Cardiol* 8: 245–250.
15. Willerson JT, Golino P, Eidt J, Campbell WB, Buja LM. 1989. Specific platelet mediators and unstable coronary artery lesions: experimental evidence and potential clinical implications. *Circulation* 80: 198–205.
16. Willerson JT, Yao S-K, McNatt J, Benedict CR, Anderson HV, Golino P, Murphree SS, Buja LM. 1991. Frequency and severity of cyclic flow alternations and platelet aggregation predict the severity of neointimal proliferation following experimental coronary stenosis and endothelial injury. *Proc Natl Acad Sci USA* 88: 10624–10628.
17. Casscells W, Hathorn B, David M, Krabach T, Vaughn WK, McAllister HA, Bearman G, Willerson JT. 1996. Thermal detection of cellular infiltrates in living atherosclerotic plaques: possible implications for plaque rupture and thrombosis. *Lancet* 347: 1447–1451.

18. Burke AP, Farb A, Malcom GT, Liang Y-H, Smialek JE, Virmani R. 1999. Plaque rupture and sudden death related to exertion in men with coronary artery disease. *J Am Med Assoc* 281: 921–926.

19. Burke AP, Farb A, Malcom GT, Liang Y, Smialek J, Virmani R. 1998. Effect of risk factors on the mechanism of acute thrombosis and sudden coronary death in women. *Circulation* 97: 2110–2116.

20. Gunnar RM, Passamani ER, Bourdillon PD, Pitt B, Dixon DW, Rapaport E, Fuster V, Reeves TJ, Karp RB, Russell Jr., RO, *et al.* 1990. Guidelines for the early management of patients with acute myocardial infarction. *J Am Coll Cardiol* 16: 249–292.

21. Ryan TJ, Anderson JL, Antman EM, Braniff BA, Brooks NH, Califf RM, Hillis LD, Hiratzka LF, Rapaport E, Riegel BJ, Russell RO, Smith, III, EE, Weaver WD. 1996. ACC/AHA guidelines for the management of patients with acute myocardial infarction. *J Am Coll Cardiol* 28: 1328–1428.

22. Théroux P, Fuster V. 1998. Acute coronary syndrome: unstable angina and non-Q wave myocardial infarction. *Circulation* 97: 1195–1206.

23. Golino P, Ambrosio G, Ragni M, Cirillo P, Esposito N, *et al.* 1997. Inhibition of leucocyte and platelet adhesion reduces neointimal hyperplasia after arterial injury. *Thromb Haemost* 77: 783–788.

24. Schulman SP, Goldschmidt-Clermont PJ, Topol EJ, Califf RM, Navetta FI, *et al.* 1996. Effects of integrelin, a platelet glycoprotein IIb/IIIa receptor antagonist, in unstable angina. A randomized multicenter trial. *Circulation* 94: 2083–2089.

25. Neely JR, Grotoyohann LW. 1984. Role of glycolytic products in damage to ischemic myocardium: dissociation of adenosine triphosphate levels and recovery of function of reperfusion ischemic hearts. *Circ Res* 55: 816–824.

26. Buja LM. 1991. Lipid abnormalities in myocardial cell injury. *Trends Cardiovasc Med* 1: 40–45.

27. Koretsune Y, Corretti MC, Kusuoka H, Marban E. 1991. Mechanism of early ischemic contractile failure: Inexcitability, metabolite accumulation or vascular collapse? *Circ Res* 68: 255–262.

28. Carmeliet E. 1984. Myocardial ischemia: reversible and irreversible changes. *Circulation* 70: 149–151.

29. Venkatesh N, Lamp ST, Weiss JN. 1991. Sulfonylureas, ATP-sensitive $K^+$ channels, and cellular $K^+$ loss during hypoxia, ischemia, and metabolic inhibition in mammalian ventricle. *Circ Res* 69: 623–637.

30. Thandroyen FT, Bellotto D, Katayama A, Hagler HK, Miller J, Willerson JT, Buja LM. 1992. Subcellular electrolyte alterations during hypoxia and following reoxygenation in isolated rat ventricular myocytes. *Circ Res* 71: 106–119.

31. Buja LM, Willerson JT. 1981. Abnormalities of volume regulation and membrane integrity in myocardial tissue slices after early ischemic injury in the dog: effects of mannitol, polyethylene glycol, and propranolol. *Am J Pathol* 103: 79–95.

32. Braunwald E. 1982. Mechanism of action of calcium-channel-blocking agents. *N Engl J Med* 307: 1618–1627.

33. Buja LM, Hagler HK, Willerson JT. 1988. Altered calcium homeostasis in the pathogenesis of myocardial ischemic and hypoxic injury. *Cell Calcium* 9: 205–217.

34. Hagler HK, Buja LM. 1990. Subcellular calcium shifts in ischemia and reperfusion. In: *Pathophysiology of Severe Ischemic Myocardial Injury*, Piper HM (ed.). Kluwer Academic Publishers, Dordrecht, pp. 283–296.

35. Morris ACI Hagler HK, Willerson JT, Buja LM. 1989. Relationship between calcium loading and impaired energy metabolism during Na⁺, K⁺ pump inhibition and metabolic inhibition in cultured neonatal rat cardiac myocytes. *J Clin Invest* 83: 1876–1887.

36. Lee HC, Smith N, Mohabir R, Clusin WT. 1987. Cytosolic calcium transients from the beating mammalian heart. *Proc Natl Acad Sci USA* 84: 7793–7797.

37. Marban E, Kitakaze M, Kusuoka H, Porterfield JK, Yue DT, Chacko VP. 1987. Intracellular free calcium concentrations measured with 19F NMR spectroscopy in intact ferret hearts. *Proc Natl Acad Sci USA* 84: 6005–6009.

38. Steenbergen C, Murphy E, Levy L, London RE. 1987. Elevation in cytosolic free calcium concentration early in myocardial ischemia in perfused rat heart. *Circ Res* 60: 700–707.

39. Katz AM, Messineo FC. 1981. Lipid–membrane interactions and the pathogenesis of ischemic damage in the myocardium. *Circ Res* 481: 1–16.

40. Corr PB, Gross RW, Sobel BE. 1984. Amphipathic metabolites and membrane dysfunction in ischemic myocardium. *Circ Res* 55: 135–154.

41. Buja LM, Miller JC, Krueger GRF. 1991. Altered membrane fluidity occurs during metabolic impairment of cardiac myocytes. *In Vivo* 5: 239–243.

42. Jones RL, Miller JC, Hagler HK, Chien KR, Willerson JT, Buja LM. 1989. Association between inhibition of arachidonic acid release and prevention of calcium loading during ATP depletion in cultured neonatal rat cardiac myocytes. *Am J Pathol* 135: 541–556.

43. Burton KP. 1985. Superoxide dismutase enhances recovery following myocardial ischemia. *Am J Physiol* 248: H637–H643.

44. Burton KP. 1988. Evidence of direct toxic effects of free radicals on the myocardium. *Free Radical Biol Med* 4: 15–24.

45. McCord JM. 1985. Oxygen-derived free radicals in postischemic tissue injury. *N Engl J Med* 312: 159–163.

46. Burton KP, Morris AC, Massey KD, Buja LM, Hagler HK. 1990. Free radicals alter ionic calcium levels and membrane phospholipids in cultured rat ventricular myocytes. *J Mol Cell Cardiol* 22: 1035–1047.

47. Ferdinandy P, Appelbaum Y, Csonka C, Blasig IE, Das DK, Tosaki A. 1998. The role of nitric oxide and TPEN, a potent metal chelator, in ischemic and reperfused rat hearts. *Clin Exp Pharmacol Physiol* 25: 496–502.

48. Zhang X, Xie YW, Nasjletti A, Xu X, Wolin MS, Hinze TH. 1997. ACE inhibitors promote nitric oxide accumulation to modulate myocardial oxygen consumption. *Circulation* 95: 176–182.

49. Steenbergen C, Hill ML, Jennings RB. 1985. Volume regulation and plasma membrane injury in aerobic, anaerobic, and ischemic myocardium in vitro: effects of osmotic cell swelling on plasma membrane integrity. *Circ Res* 57: 864–875.

50. Steenbergen C, Hill ML, Jennings RB. 1987. Cytoskeletal damage during myocardial ischemia: changes in vinculin immunofluorescence staining during total in vitro ischemia in canine heart. *Circ Res* 60: 478–486.

51. Ganote CE, VanderHeide RS. 1987. Cytoskeletal lesions in anoxic myocardial injury: a conventional and high-voltage electron microscopic and immunofluorescence study. *Am J Pathol* 129: 327–334.

52. Weisfeldt ML. 1987. Reperfusion and reperfusion injury. *Clin Res* 35: 13–20.

53. Hearse, DJ, Bolli R. 1991. Reperfusion-induced injury: manifestations, mechanisms and clinical relevance. *Trends Cardiovasc Med* 1: 233–240.

54. Takashi E, Ashraf M. 2000. Pathologic assessment of myocardial cell necrosis and apoptosis after ischemia and reperfusion with molecular and morphological markers. *J Mol Cell Cardiol* 32: 209–224.

55. Buja LM, Entman ML. 1998. Modes of myocardial cell injury and cell death in ischemic heart disease (editorial). *Circulation* 98: 1355–1357.

56. Muntz KH, Hagler HK, Boulas JH, Willerson JT, Buja LM. 1984. Redistribution of catecholamines in the ischemic zone of dog heart. *Am J Pathol* 114: 64–78.

57. Sharma AD, Saffitz JE, Lee BI, Sobel RE, Corr PB. 1983. Alpha adrenergic-mediated accumulation of calcium in reperfused myocardium. *J Clin Invest* 72: 802–818.

58. Thandroyen FT, Muntz KH, Buja LM, Willerson JT. 1990. Alterations in beta-adrenergic receptors, adenylate cyclase, and cyclic AMP concentrations during acute myocardial ischemia and reperfusion. *Circulation* 82 (Suppl. II): II30–HH37.

59. Zipes DP, Wellens HJJ. 1998. Sudden cardiac death. *Circulation* 98: 2334–2351.

60. Thandroyen FT, Morris AC, Hagler HK, Ziman B, Pai L, Willerson JT, Buja LM. 1991. Intracellular calcium transients and arrhythmia in isolated heart cells. *Circ Res* 69: 810–819.

61. Reimer KA, Jennings RB. 1979. The "wavefront phenomenon" of myocardial ischemic cell death. II. Transmural progression of necrosis within the framework of ischemic bed size (myocardium at risk) and collateral flow. *Lab Invest* 40: 633–644.

62. Buja LM, Tofe AJ, Kulkarni PV, Mukherjee A, Parkey RW, Francis MD, Bonte FJ, Willerson JT. 1977. Sites and mechanisms of localization of technetium-99m phosphorus radiopharmaceuticals in acute myocardial infarcts and other tissues. *J Clin Invest* 60: 724–740.

63. Buja LM, Willerson JT. 1987. Infarct size – can it be measured or modified in humans? *Prog Cardiovasc Dis* 29: 271–289.

64. Virmani R, Kolodgie FD, Forman MB, Farb A, Jones RM. 1992. Reperfusion injury in the ischemic myocardium. *Cardiovasc Pathol* 1: 117–130.

65. Murry CE, Jennings RB, Reimer KA. 1986. Preconditioning with ischemia: a delay of lethal cell injury in ischemic myocardium. *Circulation* 74: 1124–1136.

66. Murry CE, Richard VJ, Reimer KA, Jennings RB. 1990. Ischemic preconditioning slows energy metabolism and delays ultrastructural damage during a sustained ischemic episode. *Circ Res* 66: 913–931.

67. Liu GS, Thornton J, Van Winkle DM, Stanley AW, Olsson RA, Downey J. 1991. Protection against infarction afforded by preconditioning is mediated by $A_1$ adenosine receptors in rabbit heart. *Circulation* 84: 350–356.

68. Cleveland Jr., JC, Meldrum DR, Rowland RT, Banerjee A, Harken AH. 1997. Adenosine preconditioning of human myocardium is dependent upon the ATP-sensitive $K^+$ channel. *J Mol Cell Cardiol* 29: 175–182.

69. Kuzuya T, Hoshida S, Yamashita N, Fuji H, Oe H, Hori M, Kamada T, Tada M. 1993. Delayed effects of sublethal ischemia on the acquisition of tolerance to ischemia. *Circ Res* 72: 1293–1299.

70. Bolli R, Patel BS, Jeroudi MO, Lai EK, McCay PB. 1988. Demonstration of free radical generation in "stunned" myocardium of intact dogs with the use of the spin trap alpha-phenyl N-tert-butyl nitrone. *J Clin Invest* 82: 476–485.

71. Kusuoka H, Porterfield JK, Weisman HF, Weisfeldt ML, Marban E. 1987. Pathophysiology and pathogenesis of stunned myocardium: depressed $Ca^{2+}$ activation of contraction as a consequence of reperfusion-induced cellular calcium overload in ferret hearts. *J Clin Invest* 79: 950–961.

72. Bush LR, Buja LM, Tilton G, Wathen M, Apprill P, Ashton J, Willerson JT. 1985. Effects of propranolol and diltiazem alone and in combination on the recovery of left ventricular segmental function after temporary coronary occlusion and long term reperfusion in conscious dogs. *Circulation* 72: 413–430.

73. Reimer KA, Jennings RB, Cobb FR, Murdock RH, Greenfield Jr., JC, *et al.* 1985. Animal models for protecting ischemic myocardium (AMPIM): Results of the NHLBI Cooperative Study. Comparison of unconscious and conscious dog models. *Circ Res* 56: 651–665.

74. Buja LM, Willerson JT, Murphree SS. 1991. Pathobiology of arterial wall injury, atherosclerosis, and coronary angioplasty. In: *Complications of Coronary Angioplasty*, Black AJR, Anderson HV, Ellis SG (eds). Marcel Dekker, New York, pp. 11–33.

75. Waller BF. 1989. "Crackers, breakers, stretchers, drillers, scrapers, shavers, burners, welders and melters" the future treatment of atherosclerotic coronary artery disease? A clinical-morphologic assessment. *J Am Coll Cardiol* 13: 969–987.

76. Farb A, Roberts DK, Pichard AD, Kent KM, Virmani R. 1995. Coronary artery morphologic features after coronary rotational atherectomy: insights into mechanisms of lumen enlargement and embolization. *Am Heart J* 129: 1058–1067.

77. Topaz O, McIvor M, Stone GW, Krucoff MW, Perin EC, Eoschi AE, Sutton J, Nair R, de Marchena E. 1998. Acute results, complications, and effect of lesion characteristics on outcome with the solid-state, pulsed-wave, mid-infrared laser angioplasty system: final multicenter registry report. *Lasers Surg Med* 22: 228–239.

78. Farb A, Lindsay Jr., J, Virmani R. 1999. Pathology of bailout coronary stenting in human beings. *Am Heart J* 137: 621–631.

79. Farb A, Sangiorgi G, Carter AJ, Walley VM, Edwards WD, Schwartz RS, Virmani R. 1999. Pathology of acute and chronic coronary stenting in humans. *Circulation* 99: 44–52.

80. Lie JT, Laurie GM, Morris Jr., GC. 1977. Aortocoronary bypass saphenous vein graft atherosclerosis: anatomic study of 99 vein grafts from normal and hyperlipoproteinemic patients up to 75 months postoperatively. *Am J Cardiol* 40: 906–913.

81. Bulkley BH, Hutchins GM. 1978. Pathology of coronary artery bypass graft surgery. *Arch Pathol Lab Med* 102: 273–280.

82. Grondin CM, Campeau L, Lesperance J, *et al.* 1979. Atherosclerotic changes in coronary vein grafts six years after operation: angiographic aspects in 100 patients. *J Thorac Cardiovasc Surg* 77: 24–31.

83. Loop FD, Lytle BW, Cosgrove DM, Stewart RW, Goormastic M, Williams GW, Golding LA, Gill CC, Taylor PC, Sheldon WC, *et al.* 1986. Influence of the internal-mammary-artery graft on 10-year survival and other cardiac events. *N Engl J Med* 314: 1–6.

84. Shelton ME, Forman MB, Virmani R, Bajaj A, Stoney WS, Atkinson JB. 1988. A comparison of morphologic and angiographic findings in long-term internal mammary artery and saphenous vein bypass grafts. *J Am Coll Cardiol* 11: 297–307.

85. Nabel EG. 1995. Gene therapy for cardiovascular diseases. *Circulation* 91: 541–548.

86. Simari RD, Sam H, Rekhter M, Ohno T, Gordon D, Nabel GJ, Nabel EG. 1996. Regulation of cellular proliferation and intimal formation following balloon injury in atherosclerotic rabbit arteries. *J Clin Invest* 98: 225–235.

87. Zoldhelyi P, McNatt J, Xu XM, Loose-Mitchell D, Meidell RS, Clubb Jr., FJ, Buja LM, Willerson JT, Wu KK. 1996. Prevention of arterial thrombosis by adenovirus-mediated transfer of cyclooxygenase gene. *Circulation* 93: 10–17.

88. Anversa P, Kajstura J. 1998. Ventricular myocytes are not terminally differentiated in the adult mammalian heart. *Circ Res* 83: 1–14.

89. Soonpoa MH, Field LJ. 1998. Survey of studies examining mammalian cardiomyocyte DNA synthesis. *Circ Res* 83: 15–26.

90. Mar JH, McNatt JM, Wang Y, Clubb FJ, Zoldhelyi P, Willerson JT. 1996. Fetal canine cardiomyocytes to enhance adult canine myocardium cell numbers. *Circulation* 94 (Suppl.): I-171.

91. Mar JH, McNatt JM, Barasch E, Clubb FJ, Wang Y, Zoldhelyi P, Willerson JT. 1997. Improving function of infarcted canine myocardium by transplanting canine fetal cardiac myocytes. *Circulation* 96 (Suppl.): I-566.

92. Mulcahy D, Knight C, Stables R, Fox K. 1994. Lasers, burns, cuts, tingles and pumps: a consideration of alternative treatments for intractable angina. *Br Heart J* 71: 406–407.

93. Schoebel FC, Frazier OH, Jessurun GAJ, DeJongste MJL, Kadipasaoglu KA, Jax TW, Heintzen MP, Cooley DA, Strauer BE, Leschke M. 1997. Refractory angina pectoris in end-stage coronary artery disease: evolving therapeutic concepts. *Am Heart J* 134: 587–602.

94. Sundt, III, TM, Rogers JG. 1997. Transmyocardial laser revascularization for inoperable coronary artery disease. *Curr Opin Cardiol* 12: 441–446.

95. Kwong KF, Kanellopoulos GK, Nickols JC, Pogwizd SM, Saffitz JE, Schuessler RB, Sundt, III, TM. 1997. Transmyocardial laser treatment denervates canine myocardium. *J Thoracic Cardiovasc Surg* 114: 883–889.

96. Schumacher B, Pecker P, von Specht BU, Stegmann T. 1998. Induction of neoangiogenesis in ischemic myocardium by human growth factors: first clinical results of a new treatment of coronary heart disease. *Circulation* 97: 645–650.

97. Losordo DW, Vale PR, Symes JF, Dunnington CH, Esakof DD, Maysky M, Ashare AB, Lathi K, Isner JM. 1998. Gene therapy for myocardial angiogenesis: initial clinical results with direct myocardial injection of phVEGF165 as sole therapy for myocardial ischemia. *Circulation* 98: 2800–2804.

98. Folkman J. 1998. Angiogenic therapy of the human heart. *Circulation* 97: 628–629.

99. Folkman J, D'Amore PA. 1996. Blood vessel formation: what is its molecular basis? *Cell* 87: 1153–1155.

100. Nabel EG. 1999. Delivering genes to the heart – right where it counts! *Nature Med* 5: 141–142.

# Part IV

# CARDIOTOXICITY

# 7

# CARDIOVASCULAR TOXICITY OF ANTIBACTERIAL ANTIBIOTICS

*J. Kevin Kerzee,\* Kenneth S. Ramos,\* Janet L. Parker,†
and H. Richard Adams\**

*\*Department of Physiology and Pharmacology, College of
Veterinary Medicine, and †Department of Medical Physiology,
College of Medicine, Texas A & M University,
College Station, TX, USA*

## Introduction

The toxicity of clinically important antibacterial antibiotics can often be explained either by hypersensitivity (allergic reactions) or by cytotoxic lesions in susceptible tissues after repeated treatment. Occasionally, however, untoward patient responses to antibiotics are encountered that can be explained neither by immunologic mechanisms nor by overt cytotoxicity damage. Rather, the chemical structures of some antibiotic molecules allow them to pose as native ligands and therefore to be recognized by specific binding domains on excitable membranes of eukaryotic cells. The resulting interaction between the antibiotic ligand and the receptive membrane binding site modulates or even prevents the normal membrane functions associated with these sites, thereby leading to dysfunction of homeostatic regulatory activities of the affected host cell.

Indeed, there is considerable evidence that the pharmacodynamic profiles of certain antibiotic agents encompass direct actions on peripheral cardiorespiratory control mechanisms that can be explained best by antibiotic interaction with membrane binding sites of host cells. Antibiotics chemically related to neomycin and streptomycin (i.e. the aminoglycosides) are exemplary in this respect (Adams *et al.*, 1973, 1974, 1976a,b, 1979a,b; Adams and Goodman, 1974; Adams, 1975a–d, 1976; Adams and Durrett, 1978, 1981; Parker and Adams, 1982). These drugs retard somatic neuromuscular function via an inhibitory action at the prejunctional terminal of motor axons (Pittinger and Adamson, 1972); they also disrupt excitation–contraction coupling across the sarcolemmal membrane of vascular smooth muscle and myocardium (Adams, 1975d, 1976; Adams and Durrett, 1981; Parker and Adams, 1982). These actions share a common basic mechanism in that aminoglycoside antibiotics reversibly interact with $Ca^{2+}$ binding domains on excitable membranes of neurons, vascular smooth muscle, and cardiac myocyte (Pittinger and Adamson, 1972; Adams *et al.*, 1976b; Adams and Durrett, 1978).

Much less is known about the mechanisms whereby other types of antibiotics disrupt cardiovascular functions.

The clinical significance of the direct cardiovascular depressant actions of antibiotics remains conjectural, but several case reports can be interpreted as support for this contention. Cardiac asystole (Ream, 1963; Daubeck *et al.*, 1974), circulatory collapse (Pittinger *et al.*, 1970), cardiopulmonary arrest (Waisbren, 1968), cardiac dysrhythmias (Nattel *et al.*, 1990), cardiac decompensation in congestive heart failure (Daynes, 1974), and hypotensive episodes (Cohen *et al.*, 1970; Pittinger *et al.*, 1970; Hall *et al.*, 1972) have been linked to antibiotic administration. However, little definitive information is available about either the clinical importance of antibiotic-related cardiovascular problems or the precise mechanisms responsible for such activities. This chapter gives an overview of this problem area with primary emphasis on the direct cardiovascular actions of the aminoglycoside antibiotics. The authors reviewed this field more than a decade ago (Adams and Durrett, 1981; Parker and Adams, 1982); the present chapter comprises a condensation of this earlier information along with an update on more recent publications focusing on cardiovascular toxicity and related membrane actions of antibiotics, as well as a brief discussion of the cardiovascular effects of bacterial infection. Neither an exhaustive examination of all antibiotics nor a review of all related publications was attempted. Rather, our goal was to consider selected key reports that best typify the types of cardiovascular toxicities that can be associated with direct membrane actions of antibacterial antibiotics. Circulatory disturbances associated with anaphylactic reactions to antibiotics or cytotoxicity of antineoplastic antibiotics were not considered in this discussion.

## Clinical reports

Direct cardiovascular toxicity of antibiotics is encountered infrequently during the therapy of bacterial infections, thus leading to the general understanding that antibacterial antibiotics are innocuous to the heart and vasculature. Certainly, this assumption is valid relative to the management of uncomplicated infections in otherwise uncompromised patients. However, appropriate antimicrobial therapy and its unquestionable beneficial results have led to the frequent use of these drugs without consideration by the clinician of potential cardiovascular toxicities. Although antibiotics are rarely considered when untoward hemodynamic responses are examined for etiologic or iatrogenic factors, episodes of circulatory dysfunction related to antibiotics occasionally have been detected in individuals with primary circulatory disease or serious systemic illness.

In an early report, Swain *et al.* (1956) referred to "peripheral circulatory disturbances" and anginal syndrome in tubercular patients treated with large doses of streptomycin; circulatory collapse was seen with chloramphenicol. In a case study involving a 9-month-old infant, post-operative circulatory collapse was attributed to impaired left ventricular function induced as a result of chloramphenicol treatment (Suarez and Ow, 1992). However, complete recovery was seen when chloramphenicol was removed from the child's system. More recently, a 5-month-old infant and a 12-month-old infant suffered cardiac arrest following a bolus infusion of vancomycin (Trentesaux *et al.*, 1998). Both infants were promptly resuscitated and recovered fully. The mechanism of cardiac dysfunction was attributed to anaphylactic shock and direct cardiac toxicity (Trentesaux *et al.*, 1998). Hypotensive episodes occurred during therapy with gentamicin (Warner and Sanders, 1971; Hall *et al.*, 1972; Hagiwara and Byerly, 1981), streptomycin (Cohen *et al.*, 1970; Pittinger *et al.*, 1970; Wakabayashi and Yamada, 1972), neomycin (Pittinger *et al.*, 1970), lincomycin (Daubeck *et al.*, 1974), and kanamycin (Ream, 1963). Such hemodynamic responses usually were not attributed to direct cardiovascular depressant effects of the involved antibiotics but were unexplained or assumed to be secondary to bacteremia or respiratory depression. For instance, cardiorespiratory arrest occurred shortly after intravenous administration of a kanamycin overdose in a patient seriously ill with an abdominal abscess, and Ream (1963) assumed that this episode of cardiac standstill was secondary to apnea and hypoxemia. However, the immediate onset of cardiac asystole suggests that direct myocardial depression was involved.

More than 250 case reports of acute adverse patient responses to antibiotic therapy were reviewed by Pittinger *et al.* (1970). The majority of these problems were associated with the concurrent administration of anesthetics, muscle relaxants, or other antibiotics. Most attention was directed toward the respiratory depressant effects of the antibiotics as responsible mechanisms. Several cases of circulatory collapse, some terminating in death, were reported (Pittinger *et al.*, 1970).

Hypotension was detected by Cohen *et al.* (1970) in a patient treated with streptomycin during the post-operative period after heart surgery. These investigators believed that a myocardial depressant action of streptomycin was responsible because of an accumulation of the antibiotic in the serum secondary to renal dysfunction (Cohen *et al.*, 1970); they did not consider the related possibility that myocardial depression associated with surgery could have predisposed the heart to the deleterious action of streptomycin.

In 1990, Nattel *et al.* (1990) reported on several clinical episodes of a bizarre type of cardiac dysrhythmia produced by erythromycin. This antibiotic can induce a long QT syndrome with accompanying ventricular tachycardia characterized as a form of "torsades de pointes." Clarithromycin, a newly developed macrolide antibiotic which differs from erythromycin only in the methylation of the hydroxyl group at position 6, has been reported to have similar effects (Kundu *et al.*, 1997; Lee *et al.*, 1998). Nattel *et al.* (1990) cautioned that electrocardiogram (ECG) monitoring may be wise when intravenous erythromycin is used in patients with predisposing factors for long QT syndrome, such as hypokalemia and hypomagnesemia or pretreatment with antiarrhythmic drugs. The mechanism of long QT syndrome and "torsades de pointes" has been attributed to the inhibition of the rapidly activating component of the delayed rectifier potassium current (IKr) (Antzelevitch *et al.*, 1996), which can be inhibited by mexiletin, an inhibitor of the tetrodotoxin-sensitive $Na^+$ current (Fazekas *et al.*, 1998). A recent report has suggested that women are more prone to erythromycin-induced arrythmias than men by 67 percent compared with 33 percent respectively (Drici *et al.*, 1998).

Although controlled studies in humans are not available, the nature of antibiotic-induced cardiovascular effects is no doubt dependent on the rate and route of administration as well as on the total amount of the drug. With lincomycin, for example, Novak *et al.* (1971) found that intravenous infusion of up to 1.5 g over 60 min produced no significant cardiovascular changes. However, Waisbren (1968) reported on four cases of cardiopulmonary arrest after rapid intravenous administration of large doses of this antibiotic. Daubeck *et al.* (1974) successfully resuscitated a lincomycin-treated patient after 90 min of cardiac arrest; arrest was attributed to massive intravenous overdose of the antibiotic.

Daynes (1974) associated streptomycin administration with an exacerbation of heart failure in patients with advanced pulmonary tuberculosis. A considerable number of the tuberculous patients with chronic congestive heart failure died soon after beginning therapy with streptomycin, isoniazid, and ethionamide. Daynes (1974) suggested that the myocardial depressant action of streptomycin was involved, and he reported a decreased mortality rate when kanamycin was substituted for streptomycin. However, as kanamycin can also depress cardiac function (Ramos *et al.*, 1961; Cohen *et al.*, 1970; Adams *et al.*, 1979a), the causal relationship between streptomycin and heart failure in these cases is tenuous.

Indeed, it should be emphasized that a direct causal relationship between antibiotics and cardiovascular depression was rarely established in the above-mentioned reports. Evaluation of adverse patient responses was retrospective and evidence for antibiotic participation usually was circumstantial at best. However, because of the serious outcome of some of the clinical episodes, investigators have attempted to identify and characterize cardiovascular depressant actions of antibiotics using laboratory animals as test subjects. Based on such studies, the circulatory effects of certain antibiotics reflect a net response dependent on changes in several different physiologic systems. Some antibiotics, for instance, can (1) directly depress the heart and vasculature, (2) indirectly affect these tissues secondarily to respiratory insufficiency, and (3) even disrupt autonomic control of the circulation.

In contrast to the role of antibacterial antibiotics in cardiovascular disease, azithromycin treatment after exposure to *Chlamydia pneumoniae*, a common respiratory pathogen, can prevent intimal thickening induced by this bacterial infection (Muhlestein *et al.*, 1998). The role of antibiotics in cardiovascular toxicology is complex, as evidenced by reports which suggest a causal role for infectious agents in cardiovascular disease (reviewed in Noll, 1998). This topic was previously suggested at the turn of the twentieth century, but was ignored for almost 100 years without adequate investigation. In recent years, this topic has been revisited and is the subject of much of the current clinical investigation of cardiovascular disease, particularly atherosclerotic disease.

Various viral and bacterial pathogens have been implicated in atherosclerosis, including herpes, cytomegalovirus, and *Helicobacter pylori*. A pathogen that has received much attention is *C. pneumoniae*. Seroepidemiologic evidence has demonstrated the presence of *C. pneumoniae* in atherosclerotic lesions of coronary arteries (Kuo *et al.*, 1995), of the aorta (Grayston *et al.*, 1995), as well as of other peripheral diseased vessels, while there have been no reports of detection in non-diseased arteries. Maass *et al.* (1998) identified chlamydial DNA in 21 percent of atherosclerotic samples, while non-atherosclerotic samples were all negative. Chlamydial DNA was detected in vascular tissue from coronary revascularization procedures and carotid artery stenosis, as well as aortic and iliac artery samples (Maass *et al.*, 1998).

Various strains of *C. pneumoniae* involved in cardiovascular dysfunction have been identified, including AR-39 (Godzik *et al.*, 1995) and TWAR (Grayston *et al.*, 1995). TWAR is the name formed by the combination of TW-183 and AR-39 (Grayston *et al.*, 1989), two bacterial strains. These strains share homology with *Chlamydia*, and the name has become synonymous with *Chlamidia pneumoniae* (TWAR). AR-39 has been localized to endothelial cells, smooth muscle cells, and macrophages derived from peripheral blood monocytes (Grayston *et al.*, 1995), while infection was primarily localized to smooth muscle cells (Yamashita *et al.*, 1998). Interestingly, all of these cells are capable of supporting *C. pneumoniae* growth *in vitro* (Godzik *et al.*, 1995). Melnick *et al.* (1993) found that 73 percent of patients with asymptomatic atherosclerosis were positive for TWAR antibodies compared with 63 percent of controls, and this association was stronger for individuals aged 45–54 years than for those aged 55–64 years. Kuo *et al.* (1995) demonstrated the presence of *C. pneumoniae* in coronary lesions in young adults age 15–34 years with atherosclerosis.

The interaction between bacterial and antibacterial antibiotics in cardiovascular disease has gone almost completely without investigation. An overdose of Micotil 300, a new macrolide antibiotic for the treatment of bovine respiratory disease complex, can result in positive chronotropic and negative inotropic cardiovascular effects (Jordon *et al.*, 1993; Main *et al.*, 1996). This is of particular importance when investigating the clinical aspects of bacterial and antibiotic toxicity because it demonstrates the complexity that may arise if antibiotic treatment of bacterial infections may itself lead to cardiovascular dysfunctions.

## Respiratory depressant actions: link to cardiovascular function

Clinical recognition of respiratory depressant actions of antibiotics can be traced to Pridgen (1956). He reported that two infants developed apnea and later died subsequent to intraperitoneal lavage with neomycin. Pridgen (1956) suggested that the antibiotic exerted a neuromuscular blocking effect that led to respiratory paralysis. Numerous clinical and research studies have validated that neomycin and other aminoglycosides do indeed possess neuromuscular blocking properties (Pittinger *et al.*, 1970; Dretchen *et al.*, 1972; Pittinger and Adamson, 1972; Prado *et al.*, 1978; Molgo *et al.*, 1979; Bruckner *et al.*, 1980; Matsukawa *et al.*, 1997; Gilbert *et al.*, 1998). Considerably less information is available about the neuromuscular effects of other antibiotics that also exert this action, such as the tetracyclines, lincomycin, and polymyxins (Dretchen *et al.*, 1972; Pittinger and Adamson, 1972; Rubbo *et al.*, 1977; Durant and Lambert, 1981).

The actions of antibiotics at the somatic neuromuscular junction are important to the present discussion for two major reasons. First, and obviously, if the respiratory depressant effects are sufficient to impede pulmonary exchange of oxygen and carbon dioxide, then the cardiovascular system will be affected by hypoxemia, acidemia, and autonomic reflex adjustments. Second, the mechanism of the inhibitory action of the aminoglycosides at the motor end plate has provided important information about the basic interaction of these agents with excitable membranes.

The neuromuscular blocking effect of aminoglycoside antibiotics involves two separate mechanisms. First, they exert a prejunctional effect by decreasing the release of the neurotransmitter acetylcholine from the motor neuron (Vital Brazil and Prado-Franceschi, 1969a,b). Second, they also exert a "curare-like" post-junctional blocking effect either by altering the sensitivity of the nicotinic receptor of the skeletal myofiber to acetylcholine or by modulating receptor-coupled ion channel conductance. The prejunctional inhibitory action is generally viewed as the dominant mechanism, but species and even muscle differences may exist (Pittinger *et al.*, 1970; Dretchen *et al.*, 1973; Adams *et al.*, 1976a).

To delineate prejunctional from post-junctional actions of gentamicin, Torda (1980) measured the quantal content of end-plate potential (EPP) along with miniature end-plate potentials (MEPPs) and miniature end-plate currents (MEPCs) in a toad sartorius nerve–muscle preparation. Torda (1980) observed a marked reduction in the quantal content of the EPP, confirming that gentamicin inhibited neuromuscular transmission by preventing transmitter release from the cholinergic axon terminal. The effects of gentamicin on post-junctional events were not evident until the concentration of gentamicin was increased to an order of magnitude above that necessary for neuromuscular blockade (Torda, 1980). The presynaptic effects of neomycin, streptomycin, and gentamicin were found to occur as a consequence of a reduction in $Ca^{2+}$ currents and acetylcholine release in the motor nerve terminal (Redman and Silinsky, 1994). The reduction observed in $Ca^{2+}$ currents was most potent with neomycin, streptomycin, and gentamicin respectively.

Caputy and co-workers (1981) studied the effects of fourteen antibiotics on neuromuscular transmission in a rat nerve–muscle preparation; conclusions from this study were that neomycin has both pre- and post-junctional effects, whereas tobramycin acts predominantly prejunctionally and netilmicin acts post-junctionally. Fiekers (1983a) concurred with previous workers and concluded that the major mechanism of neuromuscular blockade by aminoglycosides is a competitive antagonism with $Ca^{2+}$ at a prejunctional site. Fiekers (1983b) also reported that neomycin and streptomycin have different post-junctional mechanisms. Neomycin interacts with the open configuration of the ionic channels associated with the acetylcholine receptor, whereas streptomycin seemingly blocks the receptor (Fiekers, 1983b).

To describe more clearly the mechanism of antibiotic action at the prejunctional site, Talbot (1987) studied the effects of pH on transmitter release and $Ca^{2+}$ antagonism by aminoglycosides in a frog nerve–muscle preparation. Talbot (1987) found that a decrease in pH caused potentiation of the inhibitory aminoglycoside actions, possibly as a result of a pH-dependent regulation of the voltage-dependent $Ca^{2+}$-mediated release of acetylcholine. Atchison and colleagues (1988) examined the effects of antibiotics on calcium uptake into isolated nerve terminals; they studied aminoglycosides, lincosamides, tetracyclines, and polymyxins. The results of their experiments confirmed other studies, indicating that the prejunctional mechanism by which aminoglycoside antibiotics induce neuromuscular blockade is by antagonism of $Ca^{2+}$ entry through voltage-gated calcium channels across the axon terminal membrane. In another study of isolated neurons, Nation and Roth (1988) proposed that neomycin's prejunctional inhibitory activity is dependent on binding of the antibiotic to axonal membrane phospholipids.

In summary, numerous types of antibiotics can disrupt somatic neuromuscular function, but the responsible mechanisms are varied and often poorly delineated. The neuromuscular actions of the aminoglycoside antibiotics have been relatively well defined. Although aminoglycosides disrupt post-junctional receptor events, their dominant neuromuscular blocking action depends on a decrease in the release of acetylcholine from cholinergic neurons; these agents interfere with the participation of $Ca^{2+}$ in the excitation–secretion coupling process of the axon terminal membrane (Vital Brazil and Prado-Franceschi, 1969a,b; Pittinger and Adamson, 1972). This action is reversed by $Ca^{2+}$ in a competitive-like manner (Prado et al., 1978); in certain details, it simulates the inhibitory effects of magnesium; and it depends on a binding of the antibiotic to plasma membrane phospholipids where $Ca^{2+}$ is normally distributed. Studies with other tissues have shown clearly that the $Ca^{2+}$ antagonistic activity of the aminoglycosides is not restricted to somatic nerve terminals. Indeed, it is manifested in excitable membranes of different tissues in which $Ca^{2+}$ serves as a coupling agent between membrane depolarization and cellular events such as muscle contraction and exocytotic release of neurotransmitters.

## Autonomic effects

In view of basic similarities at all peripheral cholinergic neuroeffector junctions, it is not surprising that antibiotics that inhibit motor end-plate function also interfere with neurotransmission in autonomic ganglia (Corrado, 1958; Corrado and Ramos, 1958; Singh et al., 1978). The ganglionic blocking effect of the aminoglycosides seems to be due principally to a $Ca^{2+}$-related decrease in the discharge of acetylcholine from the presynaptic neuron (Wright and Collier, 1976). Wright and Collier (1976) reported that aminoglycosides similarly decrease the release of the sympathetic neurotransmitter norepinephrine from adrenergic axons. Thus, the bradycardia and hypotensive responses to the aminoglycosides in intact animals (Adams, 1975a,b; Adams, et al., 1979b) could be partly due to blockade of sympathetic ganglia and adrenergic neuroeffector junctions of the heart and blood vessels.

Indeed, the fact that bradycardia rather than tachycardia occurs in conjunction with the hypotensive response suggests that these agents directly suppress the sinoatrial node, inhibit sympathetic reflex drive to the heart, or both. On the other hand, aminoglycosides depress both cardiac and arterial muscles even when these tissues are isolated *in vitro* from autonomic and humoral control factors (Adams *et al.*, 1976b; Adams *et al.*, 1979a; Adams and Durrett, 1981). The relative importance of autonomic effects in the intact subject remains questionable. The direct influence of these agents on the circulatory system is likely to be more important than effects secondary to autonomic changes, but, admittedly, more comparative information is needed in this area.

## Cardiovascular effects

### *Background*

Relatively few systematic investigations of cardiovascular actions of therapeutically useful antibiotics have been reported. In an early study, Swain *et al.* (1956) found that the canine heart–lung preparation was depressed by several chemically unrelated antibiotics such as chloramphenicol, streptomycin, and tetracycline. Mechanisms were not identified, but potential interactions with digitalis-sensitive functions were suggested. Leaders *et al.* (1960) reported that tetracycline, chloramphenicol, oleandomycin, streptomycin, and dihydro-streptomycin decreased contractile strength of perfused rabbit hearts. Mechanisms were not identified, but streptomycin also decreased coronary flow (Leaders *et al.*, 1960). As streptomycin decreased myocardial contractile force and thereby reduced myocardial oxygen demand, Leaders *et al.* (1960) did not determine whether the decrease in coronary flow produced by this antibiotic was caused by a direct vasoconstrictor action or was secondary to an autoregulated increase in coronary vascular resistance because of the fall in myocardial oxygen demand.

In an interesting study of the canine microcirculation, Stallworth *et al.* (1972) concluded that vascular reactivity and blood pressure could be influenced by commonly used anti-infectious drugs such as penicillin-G-potassium, tetracycline hydrochloride, chloramphenicol sodium succinate, nitrofurantoin sodium, and sodium cephalothin. These investigators reported that three of nine dogs treated with large doses of penicillin-G-potassium developed acute circulatory shock and died. Stallworth *et al.* (1972) attributed these responses to allergic reactions to the penicillin. However, such a high incidence of penicillin sensitivity in a random population of mongrel dogs is exceedingly unlikely, if not impossible. Stallworth *et al.* (1972) did not consider the more obvious explanation of direct cardiac toxicity owing to the large amounts of potassium these dogs received. Bolus injections of potassium salts can evoke cardiac arrest due to depolarization of excitable membranes and thus electromechanical quiescence of the heart. Penicillin-G-sodium was found to have no discernible cardiovascular effects either in control dogs or in dogs subjected to an experimental form of circulatory shock (Adams *et al.*, 1979b). Ingredients of commercial preparations of antibiotics should be considered by investigators when responsibilities for adverse responses are assigned.

For another example, Gross *et al.* (1979) reported that intravenous injection of a preparation of oxytetracycline in propylene glycol provoked transient sinoatrial arrest and circulatory collapse in unanesthetized calves. This adverse response could be reproduced by injection of propylene glycol vehicle but not by aqueous preparations of oxytetracycline (Gross *et al.*, 1979).

Oxytetracycline in ascorbic acid vehicle was reported by McCullough and Wallace (1975) to inhibit vasoconstrictor responses to norepinephrine and histamine in rabbit ear arteries, but mechanisms were not identified. The vascular and sympathetic nervous system activity of oxytetracycline was studied in more detail by Kalsner (1976) using rabbit aortic strips and perfused rabbit ear arteries. Kalsner (1976) found no evidence for an *in vitro* effect of 0.1 mM oxytetracycline on sympathetic nerve stimulation or contractile responses to norepinephrine. However, a limitation of that study is that only one concentration of oxytetracycline, 0.1 mM, was tested; larger concentrations may well have influenced sympathetic neuroeffector function or vascular reactivity.

Intravenous administration of the macrolide antibiotics erythromycin, oleandomycin, spiramycin, and leucomycin reduced blood pressure in pentobarbital-anesthetized dogs (Wakabayashi and Yamada, 1972). The response to erythromycin was not abolished by bilateral cervical sympathectomy, bilateral cervical vagotomy, spinal cord transections, or atropine. The hypotensive action of these antibiotics was not a direct effect, however, but was apparently secondary to histamine release (Wakabayashi and Yamada, 1972).

Cohen *et al.* (1970) reported on a rather detailed hemodynamic study of several antibiotics in dogs. Intravenous infusions of streptomycin, tetracycline, kanamycin, vancomycin, erythromycin, and colymycin reduced cardiovascular function in a dose-dependent manner. Streptomycin decreased left ventricular pressure and its rate of development ($+dP/dt_{max}$) in Langendorff cat heart preparations, as did tetracycline, kanamycin, vancomycin, and chloramphenicol. Cohen *et al.* (1970) proposed that electrolyte disturbances were probably involved in the cardiac depressant effect of streptomycin; however, they neither suggested nor studied $Ca^{2+}$, as claimed later by De Morais *et al.* (1978) and Sohn and Katz (1978).

### *Aminoglycoside antibiotics*

Taken in concert, the preceding series of experimental studies with various antibiotics provided little information about responsible cellular mechanisms, but yielded convincing evidence that several clinically useful antibiotics could directly affect vascular smooth muscle and cardiac function. Subsequently, studies in different laboratories were directed toward identification of hemodynamic mechanisms of different antibiotics, with much emphasis on the aminoglycosides.

## In vivo *studies*

Cardiovascular manifestations of acute toxicity of several antibiotics were studied in non-human primates and dogs anesthetized with pentobarbital (Adams, 1975a,b; Adams *et al.*, 1979b). These animals were maintained on artificial respiration, thereby avoiding circulatory effects secondary to neuromuscular blockade and respiratory insufficiency. Intravenous administration of penicillin G and cephalothin in doses from 10 to 40 mg kg$^{-1}$ body weight produced no discernible circulatory effects (Adams and Parker, 1979). In contrast, bolus intravenous injections of large amounts of neomycin, tobramycin, or gentamicin consistently depressed cardiovascular function expressed as dose-dependent reductions of systemic blood pressure, cardiac output, left ventricular contractile force (LVCF), the first derivative of LVCF ($+dP/dt_{max}$), peak systolic left ventricular pressure (LVP) $+dP/dt_{max}$, and heart rate (Adams, 1975a,b; Adams *et al.*, 1979b).

As outlined earlier, Vital Brazil and Prado-Franceschi (1969a,b) suggested that aminoglycosides compete with $Ca^{2+}$ for membrane receptive areas on the somatic nerve terminal, thereby preventing the participation of $Ca^{2+}$ in the excitation–secretion coupling process (for a review, see Pittinger and Adamson, 1972). Indirect evidence for $Ca^{2+}$-aminoglycoside antagonism in other tissues can be interpreted from early hemodynamic experiments. For example, Swain *et al.* (1956) observed that $Ca^{2+}$ exerted some antagonistic activity toward the *in vitro* cardiodepressant effects of streptomycin and dihydrostreptomycin. Similarly, Corrado (1958), Pandey *et al.* (1964), and Wolf and Wigton (1971) reported that circulatory responses to streptomycin were "reversed" or "restored" by $Ca^{2+}$. The site or specificity of such interactions was not known. Wolf and Wigton (1971) speculated that vascular tissue was affected directly, whereas Corrado (1958) and Pandey *et al.* (1964) assumed autonomic ganglia were involved.

The specificity of $Ca^{2+}$-aminoglycoside interaction was tested *in vivo* in a comparative study of the circulatory effects of $Ca^{2+}$ and two other cardiovascular stimulants, isoproterenol and norepinephrine, in primates treated with neomycin (Adams, 1975a). The catecholamines rapidly antagonized the hemodynamic depressant effects of the antibiotic, but the positive actions of the amines were only transient. Conversely, cardiovascular functions depressed by neomycin were rapidly restored to, and maintained at, control levels by a single injection of an amount of calcium chloride "equipotent" to the catecholamines. The differing responsiveness to $Ca^{2+}$ and the catecholamines in antibiotic-treated monkeys was interpreted as evidence for a reversible inhibitory action of aminoglycosides on $Ca^{2+}$-dependent functions in the heart, the vasculature, or both (Adams, 1975a).

## In vivo *studies in compromised subjects*

Although direct *in situ* cardiovascular actions of antibiotics are unlikely to be clinically relevant under usual conditions, we were concerned that such actions could be manifested in those individuals already experiencing circulatory instability. We tested this hypothesis by administering different antibiotics to control dogs and to dogs subjected to an experimental form of Gram-negative endotoxemia (Adams *et al.*, 1979b). During the circulatory shock model induced by *Escherichia coli* endotoxemia, the cardiovascular depressant actions of aminoglycoside antibiotics were indeed relatively enhanced compared with effects in control dogs, as illustrated with gentamicin in Figure 7.1. We advised that rapid intravenous injection of such antibiotics should be approached cautiously in patients with pre-existing hemodynamic dysfunctions, and we suggested that the myocardium and the vasculature could be involved in adverse cardiovascular responses of aminoglycoside antibiotics in endotoxemic subjects (Adams *et al.*, 1979b).

## *Vascular smooth muscle*

Streptomycin was reported to produce vasodilation in the perfused hindlimb preparation of the dog (Cohen *et al.*, 1970). Wolf and Wigton (1971) later confirmed the vasodilator properties of streptomycin using perfused kidneys of dogs. Importantly, $Ca^{2+}$ antagonized the vasodilator activity of streptomycin in this study (Wolf and Wigton, 1971). It was not clear, however, whether perfusion pressure changes in the hindlimb and kidney represented direct effects of the antibiotics on contractile function of vascular smooth muscle or whether vascular resistance changes were indirect and reflected autoregulatory adjustments to metabolic changes in the skeletal muscle or renal parenchymal tissues.

Direct evidence for a $Ca^{2+}$-antagonistic action of aminoglycosides was obtained initially from experiments with $^{45}Ca$ and rabbit aorta (Adams *et al.*, 1973). Arterial tissue was selected for use in this study for two reasons. First, the direct vascular effects of the aminoglycosides were believed to be important to the net hemodynamic response of mammals to these drugs. Second, vascular smooth muscle represented an excellent model system for elucidating effects of aminoglycosides that perhaps could be extrapolated to excitable membranes of other tissues. In brief, streptomycin, neomycin, gentamicin, and kanamycin characteristically decreased $^{45}Ca$ uptake and increased $^{45}Ca$ efflux in a sustained manner in vascular smooth muscle (Adams *et al.*, 1973, 1974; Adams and Goodman, 1974; Goodman *et al.*, 1974, 1975). Reciprocally, $Ca^{2+}$ inhibited the uptake and increased the efflux of [$^{14}C$]-gentamicin (Goodman, 1978a). Thus, there seemed to be some type of competition between aminoglycosides and $Ca^{2+}$ for membrane binding sites in the vascular smooth muscle cells.

Effects of aminoglycosides on $Ca^{2+}$ movement were demonstrated not only in rabbit aorta but also in different vascular beds of dogs and non-human primates. Vessels studied included the aorta and the renal, superior mesenteric, femoral,

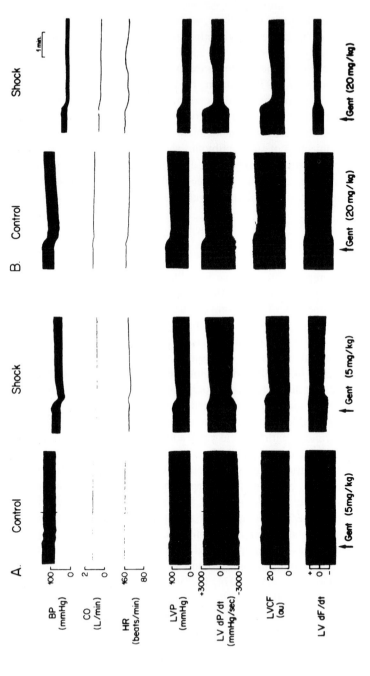

*Figure 7.1* Representative tracings illustrating the relatively greater cardiovascular depressant response to gentamicin (Gent) during *E. coli* endotoxin shock than during the control state. Studies were in dogs anesthetized with pentobarbital; intravenous bolus infections of Gent at 5 mg kg⁻¹ (A) or 20 mg kg⁻¹ (B). BP, blood pressure; CO, cardiac output; HR, heart rate; LVP, left ventricular pressure; d*P*/d*t*, first derivative of LVP; LVCF, left ventricular contractile force; d*F*/d*t*, first derivative of LVCF. Reproduced with permission from Adams *et al.* (1979b).

coronary, carotid, and terminal mesenteric arteries (Adams and Goodman, 1974; Goodman *et al.*, 1975; Goodman and Adams, 1976a). The disruptive effect of aminoglycosides on $Ca^{2+}$ homeostasis was manifested at cellular membrane sites important to contractile reactivity of the vessels. Specifically, these antibiotics inhibited arterial contractions induced by norepinephrine, angiotensin II, serotonin, histamine, $Ca^{2+}$, and depolarizing concentrations of $K^+$ (Adams and Goodman, 1974; Adams *et al.*, 1974; Goodman *et al.*, 1974, 1975).

Based on differing inhibitory effects of the antibiotics on contractile responses and $^{45}Ca$ movement, it was proposed that these drugs exert their $Ca^{2+}$ antagonistic activity by inhibiting the uptake, reuptake, and/or binding of $Ca^{2+}$ at superficial membrane sites (Adams *et al.*, 1973; Weiss, 1977; Goodman, 1978b; Adams and Durrett, 1981). We suggested that anionic binding sites of membrane phospholipids interacted with, or were in some way affected by, the polycationic aminoglycosides. The membrane phospholipid perturbation resulting from such aminoglycoside–membrane interaction would decrease the capacity of the cell membrane to bind and store $Ca^{2+}$. Such action(s) would in turn decrease the availability of membrane-bound $Ca^{2+}$ for intracellular movement to the contractile proteins of the vascular smooth muscle cell, thereby inhibiting contractile responses to vasostimulatory interventions that act through mobilization of $Ca^{2+}$ from superficial membrane stores (Adams *et al.*, 1973; Goodman *et al.*, 1975).

The $Ca^{2+}$-inhibiting activity of the aminoglycosides was more pronounced in small resistance arteries than in large conduit vessels (e.g. effects on coronary arteries and terminal mesenteric arteries > carotid arteries > aorta) (Adams and Goodman, 1974; Goodman *et al.*, 1975). It was concluded that small, highly reactive vessels such as terminal mesenteric arteries and also coronary arteries depend more on a superficial membrane source of $Ca^{2+}$ than do large conduit vessels (Adams and Goodman, 1974; Goodman *et al.*, 1975). The dependence of coronary arteries on a superficial source of $Ca^{2+}$ for norepinephrine responses was reported later by van Breeman *et al.* (1978). Thus, it seemed that the aminoglycosides might be useful as model drugs for probing $Ca^{2+}$-dependent events in excitable tissues that rely on mobilization of superficial $Ca^{2+}$ for intracellular functions.

In addition, it was postulated that the disruptive effect of aminoglycosides on $Ca^{2+}$ homeostasis at superficial membrane sites could explain the inhibitory activity of these agents in excitable tissues other than vascular smooth muscle alone (Adams *et al.*, 1973). Direct evidence for $Ca^{2+}$-aminoglycoside antagonism has been obtained in several different tissues, including sarcoplasmic reticulum of skeletal muscle (Calviello and Chiesi, 1989), inner ear tissues (Orsulakova *et al.*, 1975), intestinal smooth muscle (De Morais *et al.*, 1978), and cholinergic neurons (Wright and Collier, 1976). Based on studies with renal and inner ear isolates, Orsulakova *et al.* (1975) and Schibeci and Shacht (1977) suggested that neomycin inhibits the turnover of membrane polyphosphoinositides and their ability to bind $Ca^{2+}$. It now seems clear that the renal and ototoxicity of the aminoglycosides is associated with the interaction of these agents with membrane phospholipids that are directly or indirectly involved in $Ca^{2+}$ movements.

## Myocardium

In view of the participation of superficially localized $Ca^{2+}$ in activation of myocardial contractions, and in view of previous studies pointing toward cardiodepressant actions of aminoglycosides (Swain *et al.*, 1956; Cohen *et al.*, 1970; Adams, 1975a), it seemed likely that these antibiotics affected $Ca^{2+}$ metabolism in the heart. Gentamicin, a representative aminoglycoside, depressed isometric contractions of atrial myocardium from rats and guinea pigs in a concentration-dependent manner (Adams, 1975c, Adams and Durrett, 1978; Adams *et al.*, 1979a). Similar negative inotropic effects were seen with kanamycin, amikacin, and sisomicin in guinea pig atria (Adams *et al.*, 1979a). Using rat ventricular muscle, Sohn and Katz (1977, 1978) subsequently verified the direct myocardial depressant effects of kanamycin and streptomycin.

The negative inotropic action of large concentrations of gentamicin was antagonized by excess $Ca^{2+}$ in a competitive manner (Adams, 1975c; Adams *et al.*, 1979a). In contrast, effects of the antibiotic were only partially antagonized by norepinephrine, isoproterenol, digoxin, or increased frequency of beating (Adams, 1975c; Adams *et al.*, 1979a). These data showed that the negative inotropic action of an aminoglycoside could be completely antagonized by an increase in the concentration of interstitial $Ca^{2+}$, but not by interventions that mobilized available membrane-bound pools of $Ca^{2+}$.

The $Ca^{2+}$-related myocardial depressant action of aminoglycosides was supported by data presented in abstract form, which showed that gentamicin decreased $^{45}Ca$ tissue spaces in beating, but not in quiescent, atrial muscle of the guinea pig (Goodman and Adams, 1976b). This inhibitory action was demonstrable if the $Ca^{2+}$ concentration of the bathing medium was low (1.0 mM) rather than high (2.5 or 10.0 mM). These data were later published in a comprehensive review of aminoglycoside effects in vascular tissue (Goodman, 1978b). Lullman and Schwarz (1985) subsequently reported similar inhibition of $Ca^{2+}$ binding to atrial myocardium by gentamicin and also by sisomicin and dibekacin.

Further study showed that the cardiac depressant action of gentamicin (Adams and Durrett, 1978) and other aminoglycosides was augmented considerably when myocardial contractions were dependent on an increased influx of $Ca^{2+}$ through slow cation channels of the sarcolemma. These channels are responsible for the influx of $Ca^{2+}$ during the plateau phase of the cardiac action potential; $Ca^{2+}$ influx through slow channels couples membrane excitation to activation of the contractile proteins (Pappano, 1970; Thyrum, 1974). The inhibitory effect of gentamicin on slow $Ca^{2+}$ contractile responses provided evidence that aminoglycosides in some way affect either the transport system responsible for $Ca^{2+}$ influx through the slow channels of the cell membrane or the availability of $Ca^{2+}$ for translocation to these sites, or both. Myographic tracings illustrating the enhanced negative inotropic action of gentamicin in heart muscle contracting under $Ca^{2+}$ channel-activated conditions are presented in Figure 7.2. We proposed that aminoglycosides decrease the systolic influx of $Ca^{2+}$ in contracting myocardial cells by inhibiting the uptake or binding of $Ca^{2+}$ at superficial binding sites of the sarcolemma, thereby reducing the quantity of membrane-bound $Ca^{2+}$ available for movement into the myoplasm during depolarization of the cell membrane (Adams, 1975c; Adams and Durrett, 1978).

The inhibitory influence of gentamicin on slow inward $Ca^{2+}$ channels in heart muscle (Adams and Durrett, 1978) was later confirmed by different investigators. Hino *et al.* (1982) reported that gentamicin remarkably diminished the slow inward current measured in guinea pig papillary muscle by a single sucrose gap voltage clamp technique. Hino *et al.* (1982) also demonstrated depression of the slow inward $Ca^{2+}$ current at low concentrations of gentamicin and depression of the time-dependent outward current only at high concentrations of gentamicin. The inhibitory action of gentamicin was expressed rather selectively on the peak amplitude of the slow inward current as the antibiotic did not affect the time-course, voltage dependency of steady-state inactivation or activation, or reversal potential of the current. Addition of exogenous $Ca^{2+}$ reversed the inhibitory effects of gentamicin on the slow inward current. Concurring with previous reports (Adams and Durrett, 1978), Hino *et al.* (1982) proposed that the depressant action of gentamicin on slow inward current in myocardial cells was due to a blockade of slow channels, with the antibiotic dislocating $Ca^{2+}$ from slow channel binding sites on the external surface of the sarcolemma. In agreement with this theory, numerous studies have shown aminoglycoside inhibition of $Ca^{2+}$ binding using isolated membrane preparations (Lohdi *et al.*, 1980; Gotanda *et al.*, 1988). Lullmann and Schwarz (1985) demonstrated $Ca^{2+}$ binding abnormalities induced by gentamicin in intact cardiac muscle. They too concluded that the functional depression caused by gentamicin is not due to a decrease in extracellular $Ca^{2+}$, but rather a decrease in the amount of $Ca^{2+}$ bound to the sarcolemmal membrane of the cardiac tissue.

De la Chapelle-Groz and Athias (1988) studied the effect of gentamicin on cultured cardiac myocytes; they obtained results consistent with the above studies in that gentamicin antagonized the inotropic actions of $Ca^{2+}$. One of the main objectives in their study was to compare the actions of gentamicin with other known $Ca^{2+}$ antagonists to ascertain the binding site on the cardiac myocyte where gentamicin acts as a ligand. The actions of lanthanum ($La^{3+}$) and ethylene-diaminetetraacetate (EDTA) most closely resembled the actions of gentamicin on cardiac myocytes. This indicates that as gentamicin has been shown not to chelate $Ca^{2+}$ ions the action of gentamicin is more like that of $La^{3+}$, as also suggested by earlier studies (Durrett and Adams, 1980). Therefore, it was concluded that gentamicin binds to an extracellular site of the cardiac membrane, which normally binds $Ca^{2+}$. Hashimoto and colleagues (1989) demonstrated the close resemblance of gentamicin–$Ca^{2+}$ antagonism with cobalt ($Co^{2+}$)–$Ca^{2+}$ antagonism. Their data suggested that gentamicin may be binding to the same site as $Co^{2+}$ and $Ca^{2+}$; however, they provided no direct evidence for this proposal. $Co^{2+}$ has been shown

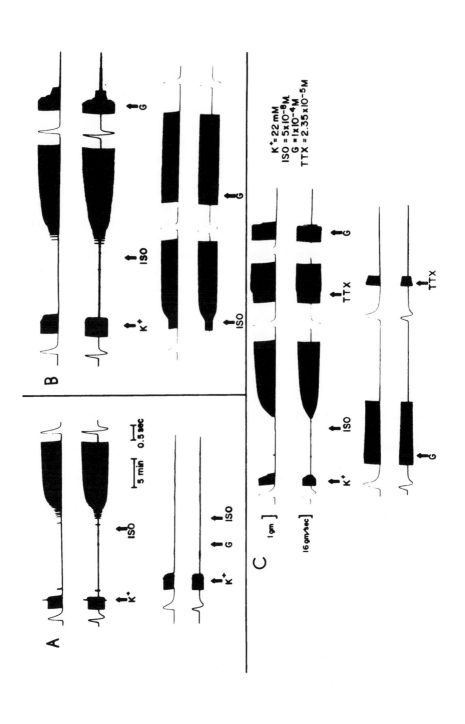

K⁺ = 22 mM
ISO = 5x10⁻⁶M
G = 1x10⁻⁴M
TTX = 2.35x10⁻⁵M

to compete with $Ca^{2+}$ for binding sites in the membrane at the site of $Ca^{2+}$ channels (Hagiwara and Byerly, 1981). These investigators also demonstrated that prolongation of the open state of the $Ca^{2+}$ channel by the $Ca^{2+}$ channel agonist BayK 8644 had little effect on the action of gentamicin or $Co^{2+}$. This is consistent with the theory that gentamicin dislocates $Ca^{2+}$ from the cardiac sarcolemmal membrane (Adams and Durrett, 1978) and that with less membrane-bound $Ca^{2+}$ there is less $Ca^{2+}$ available for entry through the opened channel irrespective of how long the channel may be open.

Calcium flow through the slow cation channels of the cardiac cell membrane is inhibited by several chemical agents referred to commonly as "$Ca^{2+}$ antagonists" or "slow channel blockers." Included in this group are the organic compounds such as verapamil and D600 and the cationic or inorganic $Ca^{2+}$ antagonists such as $La^{3+}$ and manganese ($Mn^{2+}$) (Adams and Durrett, 1978; Durrett and Adams, 1980). Based on the selective inhibitory action of small amounts of gentamicin on slow $Ca^{2+}$ contractile responses, we proposed the aminoglycosides as members of the list of slow $Ca^{2+}$ channel blockers in heart muscle (Adams and Durrett, 1978). Furthermore, combinatorial responses have been seen with clarithromycin and verapamil (Kaeser et al., 1998).

Comparative cardiac studies were carried out with $La^{3+}$, D600, and gentamicin using the inotropic response to changes in heart rate as a test inotropic intervention (Durrett and Adams, 1980). The positive inotropic response of heart muscle to increased frequency of stimulation is thought to involve increased $Ca^{2+}$ influx and/or increased releasability of membrane $Ca^{2+}$ (Durrett and Adams, 1980). The negative inotropic effect of D600 was more pronounced at high rates of stimulation ($> 1.4$ Hz) than at low rates ($< 0.8$ Hz). On the other hand, $La^{3+}$ and gentamicin decreased the positive inotropic response to increased beating rates throughout the frequency range that was examined (0.1–2.2 Hz). Further study showed that the pharmacodynamics of the myocardial effects of gentamicin were less complex than those exhibited by either $La^{3+}$ or D600 (Durrett and Adams, 1980).

For example, contractile strength of gentamicin-depressed heart muscle consistently recovered to near control values within 10 min after the muscle was placed in a drug-free control medium. Muscle treated with an equipotent

*Figure 7.2* Effects of gentamicin (G) in guinea pig left atria contracting under normal (5.4 mM $K^+$) or "slow channel activated" (22 mM $K^+$-isoproterenol) conditions. (A) Contractions (CT) ceased after 22 mM $K^+$ but were restored by isoproterenol (ISO) (upper tracings). Pretreatment with G (0.1 mM) prevented restoration of contractions by ISO (lower tracings). (B) G abolished contractions of muscle beating under high $K^+$-ISO conditions (upper tracings); however, G had no effect in the ISO-treated atria beating under normal $K^+$ (5.4 mM) conditions (lower tracings). (C) Tetrodotoxin (TTX) did not stop contractions of atria beating under high $K^+$-ISO conditions, whereas G blocked contractions (upper tracings). Conversely, under control conditions (5.4 mM $K^+$; no ISO), G had little effect, whereas TTX stopped contractions (lower tracings). The time markers in (A) and the calibration markers and drug concentrations in (C) apply to all tracings. Stimulation frequency is 0.2 Hz. Reproduced with permission from Adams and Durrett (1978).

203

concentration of La$^{3+}$ or D600 failed to regain 50 percent of basal inotropy even after recovery in normal bathing medium for 1 h. Furthermore, D600-treated muscle still displayed an inversion of the amplitude–frequency curve after the recovery period. In La$^{3+}$-treated muscle, contractile responses to high rates of stimulation were attenuated, and responses to low frequencies were actually enhanced after the recovery period. In contrast, the inhibitory activity of a similar concentration of gentamicin seemed completely reversible as inotropic responses to changes in heart rate were quite normal after recovery from this antibiotic (Durrett and Adams, 1980) compared with La$^{3+}$ and D600 (Figure 7.3).

Rapid recovery of mechanical function strongly suggested the recovery of an active physiologic process rather than cytotoxic damage inflicted on the myocytes by the antibiotic. Thus, although gentamicin inhibits slow Ca$^{2+}$ responses (Adams and Durrett, 1978), the inotropic effects of this agent could be differentiated from the poorly reversible and more complex actions of the well-known Ca$^{2+}$ antagonists D600 and La$^{3+}$ (Durrett and Adams, 1980) (Figure 7.3). We suggested that these characteristics enhance the utility of gentamicin as a model Ca$^{2+}$ channel-blocking drug for those types of studies requiring recovery of contractile function, and warrant further study for potential application in cardiologic investigations (Durrett and Adams, 1980). The negative inotropic potency of the aminoglycosides is less than that of the organic Ca$^{2+}$ antagonists D600 and verapamil, but is of a similar order of magnitude as the cationic Ca$^{2+}$ antagonists such as La$^{3+}$ and Mn$^{2+}$ (Durrett and Adams, 1980).

Cation channel blockade by aminoglycosides has now been reported not only in vascular muscle (Adams *et al.*, 1973, 1974; Adams and Goodman, 1974) and myocardium (Adams and Durrett, 1978) but also in other tissues, e.g. neomycin block of slowly inactivating Ca$^{2+}$ channels in clonal GH3 pituitary cells (Suarez-Kurtz and Reuben, 1987), aminoglycoside block of N-type Ca$^{2+}$ channel of rat brain synaptosomes (Wagner *et al.*, 1987), neomycin block of inward Ca$^{2+}$ current in paramecium (Gustin and Hennessey, 1988), gentamicin block of voltage-gated Ca$^{2+}$ channels in cochlear outer hair cells (Dulon *et al.*, 1989), and aminoglycoside block of Ca$^{2+}$-activated K$^+$ channels from rat brain synaptosomal membranes incorporated into planer lipid bilayers (Nomura *et al.*, 1990). These types of studies have substantiated clearly that toxicities of aminoglycoside antibiotics in different types of host cells depend on a common type of molecular mechanism involving disruption of Ca$^{2+}$-dependent signaling across excitable membranes.

### Other antibiotic agents

In addition to the aminoglycosides, several other antimicrobial as well as non-antimicrobial antibiotics have been reported to affect myocardial activity. In most cases, however, little is known about the mechanism(s) of their cardiac depressant actions, and interactions with cellular functions have not been intensely investigated.

Cardiac depressant effects have been described for several of the macrolide

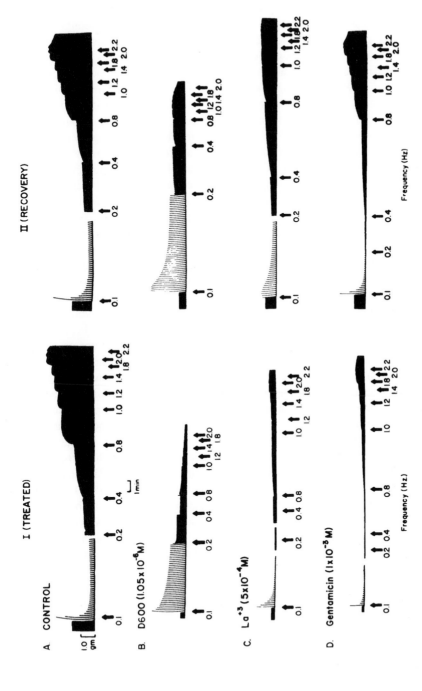

*Figure 7.3* Myographic tracings illustrating the effects of gentamicin, D600, and La³⁺ on frequency–force relationships of isolated heart muscle while the drug was present in the bathing medium (I, treated) and again 1.5–2 h after recovery in control bathing medium (II, recovery). Tension and time scales in I (A) apply to all tracings. Reproduced with permission from Durrett and Adams (1980).

antibiotics, including erythromycin and oleandomycin (Tomargo *et al.*, 1982). Leaders *et al.* (1960) reported hypotension and slowed heart rate in anesthetized rabbits treated with oleandomycin, as well as a decrease in the beating rate and contractile amplitude of isolated rabbit hearts. Intravenous injection of erythromycin was shown to produce dose-dependent decreases in both blood pressure and myocardial contractile force in anesthetized dogs (Cohen *et al.*, 1970). Regan *et al.* (1969) reported that erythromycin may cause arrhythmias and ventricular tachycardia in the ischemic ventricle or in the digitalis-treated animal, possibly by enhancing intracellular potassium loss. Clinically, erythromycin has been associated with cardiac dysrhythmias characterized by the long QT syndrome and accompanying ventricular tachycardia waveform known as "torsades de pointes" (Nattel *et al.*, 1990). Cardiac transmembrane potential experiments showed that erythromycin prolonged action potential duration and reduced phase zero depolarization rate, effects consistent with the fast $Na^+$ channel-blocking properties of quinidine and other class IA antiarrhythmic drugs (Nattel *et al.*, 1990). Alteration of ion fluxes by erythromycin is a likely factor responsible for the cardiac effects of this type of antibiotic.

Lincomycin has been shown to produce adverse effects on myocardial electrical impulse transmission. Daubeck *et al.* (1974) observed cardiac arrest and ventricular fibrillation in a patient following an inadvertent overdose of lincomycin. Spurred by the clinical incident, these investigators examined lincomycin-induced hypotension, arrhythmias, cardiac slowing, and ventricular fibrillation in subsequent canine studies. These abnormalities were dependent on rate of administration of lincomycin as well as on the amount of drug given. The arrhythmias appeared to result from decreased excitability and conduction velocity; arrhythmias caused by lincomycin may be potentiated by digitalis (Daubeck *et al.*, 1974). Chloramphenicol, in addition to its well-known toxic effects on bone marrow, has also been shown to produce negative inotropic and chronotropic effects in a number of cardiac preparations (Swain *et al.*, 1956; Leaders *et al.*, 1960; Cohen *et al.*, 1970). The myocardial depressant effects of chloramphenicol were incompletely antagonized by $Ca^{2+}$ or ouabain (Swain *et al.*, 1956) and seemed additive to the depression produced by halothane (Sohn and Katz, 1977). Isometric contractions of isolated rat heart muscle were depressed by chloramphenicol, but the degree of depression was considerably less than that obtained with kanamycin or streptomycin (Sohn and Katz, 1977, 1978). Propranolol or atropine had no effect on the response to chloramphenicol in the isolated toad heart, suggesting that the negative inotropic and chronotropic effects of this agent resulted from a myocardial cell interaction rather than an alteration in the release or response to endogenous autonomic mediators (Banerjee and Mitra, 1976). Inhibition of protein synthesis has been implicated in the altered heart beat response to chloramphenicol in explanted chick embryos (Glanzer and Peaslee, 1970).

Vancomycin reduced pressure development and $+dP/dt_{max}$ in both the left and right ventricles of anesthetized dogs (Cohen *et al.*, 1970). The cardiac depressant action of vancomycin was confirmed in isolated cat hearts (Cohen *et al.*, 1970).

Several of the polyene group of antifungal agents have been shown to depress myocardial contractility and induce electrical disturbances in isolated cardiac preparations. Arora (1965) and Arora and Arora (1970) demonstrated that eurocidine, pentamycin, fungichromin, and amphotericin B diminished the amplitude of contraction in perfused Langendorff preparations of several species. The accompanying disturbances in electrical activity in response to candicidin and amphotericin B appeared to result from changes in myocardial ion transport similar to those induced by toxic concentrations of ouabain (Arora et al., 1967). Ruiz-Ceretti et al. (1976) examined the effects of amphotericin B on electrical activity in isolated rabbit hearts and found a decrease in both amplitude and rate of depolarization of the cardiac action potential within 15 min after exposure to the drug. The authors concluded that the subsequent disappearance of the plateau phase of the action potential was due to inhibition of slow inward current by the antibiotic. This proposal is further supported by the observation that one of the first changes observed in the electrocardiogram following administration of amphotericin B is prolongation of the P–R interval (Ruiz-Ceretti et al., 1976). Since the slow current is thought to contribute as much as 30 percent to the depolarizing current in the nodal cells, inhibition of the slow current by amphotericin B could be the mechanism underlying the decrease in atrioventricular conduction seen with this drug. Using voltage clamp techniques, Schanne et al. (1977) showed that this antibiotic blocked the ionic channels involved in activation of the slow inward current and suggested this mechanism for explaining the depression of contractility observed in rabbit hearts (Schanne et al., 1977). It should be emphasized, however, that amphotericin B is not typical of a "$Ca^{2+}$ antagonist, slow channel blocker" because it affects action potential parameters other than the plateau alone. Indeed, it may also exert a blocking effect on sodium channels responsible for rapid depolarization of the transmembrane potential (Schanne et al., 1977).

To complicate further the amphotericin B story, a previous study indicated that this drug provokes in vivo renal arterial vasoconstriction (Tolins and Raij, 1988). This response was inhibited by the $Ca^{2+}$ channel-blocking agent verapamil, but not by angiotensin II receptor blockade or renal sympathectomy (Tolins and Raij, 1988). Verapamil is a vasodilator agent, and its inhibition of amphotericin B-induced renal vasoconstriction may reflect simple physiologic antagonism between a vasodilator and a vasoconstrictor. On the other hand, as amphotericin B can act as a $Ca^{2+}$ ionophore in liposomes (Ramos et al., 1989), perhaps it may also enhance $Ca^{2+}$ influx in some intact cells such as renal vascular smooth muscle.

Considering the well-known $Ca^{2+}$-chelating properties of the tetracyclines, it is not surprising that this group of antibiotics can produce toxic effects on the cardiovascular system. Cardiovascular depressant effects have been observed in intact animals and in isolated cardiac preparations from different laboratory animal species (Swain et al., 1956; Leaders et al., 1960; Cohen et al., 1970). Swain et al. (1956) used an isolated dog heart–lung preparation and reported a complete reversal of tetracycline-induced myocardial depression by $Ca^{2+}$. The possibility that this interaction was due to $Ca^{2+}$-chelating activity of tetracycline was tested by comparing tetracycline, $Ca^{2+}$, and $Na_2EDTA$. Calcium similarly reversed the effects of increasing doses of both EDTA and tetracycline. The comparison was limited, however, because of precipitate formation of the tetracycline–$Ca^{2+}$ complex. These results indicate an important difference in the mechanism by which tetracyclines exert their cardiotoxic effects in comparison with those of other antibiotics. Whereas the aminoglycosides, polyenes, and macrolides are thought to have a direct action on some myocardial cellular process, it appears that the tetracyclines may act simply by lowering $Ca^{2+}$ levels in plasma or in the extracellular space. Further studies are needed, however, to discount completely a direct cardiac action of tetracyclines independent of $Ca^{2+}$ chelation.

Considerable information about the myocardial toxicity of valinomycin, a macrocyclic antibiotic, has been obtained by Sperelakis and co-workers (Schneider and Sperelakis, 1974; Vogel and Sperelakis, 1978). Valinomycin was found to block the $Ca^{2+}$-dependent, slowly rising electrical response (slow response) induced by isoproterenol in hearts whose fast $Na^+$ channels were voltage inactivated by partial depolarization with elevated $K^+$ solution. This agent also markedly shortened the ventricular action potential plateau and lowered the ATP level. Other metabolic inhibitors, such as cyanide or dinitrophenol, also produced action potential shortening and slow response blockade concomitant with a lowering of the ATP level (Vogel and Sperelakis, 1978). Glucose elevation to 27 or 55 mM or treatment with insulin was found to reverse the effects of valinomycin and restore the $Ca^{2+}$-dependent slow responses of guinea pigs and chick embryo hearts. Vogel and Sperelakis (1978) thus concluded that, as elevated glucose uptake should lead to an increased availability of ATP, the electrophysiologic effects of valinomycin are due largely to metabolic poisoning rather than to a direct effect of the cardiac sarcolemma.

## Summary

### *Mechanisms*

The spectrum of cardiovascular effects of antibiotics, as with other types of drugs, depends on the pharmacodynamic profiles of the individual agents. Circulatory dysfunction induced by certain antibiotics can be secondary to neuromuscular paralysis and respiratory insufficiency, primary to direct depressant actions on the heart and blood vessels, or caused by a combination of direct and indirect effects.

The inhibitory influence of the aminoglycosides on $Ca^{2+}$ homeostasis in peripheral neurons, vascular smooth muscle, and the myocardium no doubt explains the capability of this particular group of antibiotics to disrupt hemodynamic control mechanisms. This characteristic of the aminoglycosides does not seem to be attributable to overt cytotoxic damage of cardiovascular tissues but is related to a reversible interaction of these agents with $Ca^{2+}$-binding sites of excitable membranes. Many of the biologic actions of aminoglycosides in mammals, including cellular damage to the kidney and inner ear tissues, also are associated in some way with perturbation of membrane phospholipids where $Ca^{2+}$ is normally distributed.

Indeed, no doubt prompted by early work from Schacht's group (Orsulakova *et al.*, 1975; Schibeci and Schacht, 1977), recent studies have shown convincingly that aminoglycosides alter interactions between $Ca^{2+}$ and polyphosphatidylinositol elements in membranes of various types of eukaryotic cells (Marche *et al.*, 1987; Cockcroft and Stutchfield, 1988; Tysnes *et al.*, 1988; Vassbotn *et al.*, 1990). The phosphoinositides are believed to represent the membrane receptors that misconstrue aminoglycosides as native ligands. Resulting interactions between the phosphoinositide and the aminoglycoside ligand displace $Ca^{2+}$ from its normal binding domain, and thereby disrupt cell membrane homeostasis and signal transduction mechanisms that depend on phosphoinositide–$Ca^{2+}$ interactions (Orsulakova *et al.*, 1975; Schibeci and Schacht, 1977; Marche *et al.*, 1987; Cockcroft and Stutchfield, 1988; Tysnes *et al.*, 1988; Vassbotn *et al.*, 1990). This paradigm is believed to account for many actions of aminoglycosides, e.g. nephro- and ototoxicity (Orsulakova *et al.*, 1975; Schibeci and Schacht, 1977; Lohdi *et al.*, 1980; Marche *et al.*, 1987), inhibition of platelet function (Tysnes *et al.*, 1988), inhibition of platelet-derived growth factor actions (Vassbotn *et al.*, 1990), and perhaps even modulation of pertussis sensitivity of G protein-regulated polyphosphoinositide phosphodiesterase activity in the promyelocytic HL60 cell (Cockcroft and Stutchfield, 1988). Future studies involving aminoglycoside antibiotics and phosphoinositides in membranes from myocardial and vascular tissues will add new critical information concerning the molecular mechanisms responsible for cardiovascular actions of this important group of antibiotics.

Relatively less is known about mechanisms of cardiovascular toxicities of other antibiotics that also can affect hemodynamics. Lincomycin can induce neuromuscular paralysis but also seems to exert direct effects on cardiac impulse conduction. Tetracyclines can influence respiratory and myocardial functions; these activities appear to be related, at least in part, to chelation of $Ca^{2+}$ or other cations. Chloramphenicol spares the somatic neuromuscular junction but, under some conditions, may affect inotropic and chronotropic responsiveness of cardiac tissue. The circulatory depressant actions of erythromycin and related antibiotics seem to depend on histamine release, but a disruption of potassium distribution in the heart may also be involved. More information is needed in this neglected field of antibiotic pharmacology/toxicology.

### Clinical aspects

Although experimental studies have established the potential for untoward cardiovascular effects of several clinically important antibiotics (Tables 7.1 and 7.2), most of the data cannot be extrapolated directly to clinical medicine. Greater-than-therapeutic doses of antibiotics administered by intravenous bolus injections were commonly studied in animals subjected to circulatory stress associated with

Table 7.1 Cardiovascular depressant effects of aminoglycoside antibiotics

| Antibiotic | Species | Preparation | Effect | Comments | References |
|---|---|---|---|---|---|
| Streptomycin | Dog | In vivo | Cardiovascular depression | During anesthesia | Cohen et al. (1970) |
| | Dog | Perfused kidney | Vasodilation | During anesthesia | Wolf and Wigton (1971) |
| | Cat, rabbit | In vitro (Langendorff) | Contractile depression | | Cohen et al. (1970) Leaders et al. (1960) |
| | Human | | Suspected cardiac depression | Tuberculous patients with congestive heart failure | Daynes (1974) |
| | Dog | In vitro (heart–lung) | Cardiac depression | | Swain et al. (1956) |
| | Dog, cat, rhesus monkey | In vivo | Hypotension | During anesthesia | Adams (1975b) Pandey et al. (1964) |
| | Rat | In vitro (ventricular muscle) | Contractile depression | Additive with halothane | Sohn and Katz (1977, 1978) |
| | Human | | Persistent hypotension | After cardiac surgery | Cohen et al. (1970) |
| | Rabbit | In vivo | Hypotension | During anesthesia; $ED_{50} = 40$ mg kg$^{-1}$ | Leaders et al. (1960) |
| Dihydrostreptomycin | Rabbit | In vitro (Langendorff) | Contractile depression | | Leaders et al. (1960) |
| | Rabbit | In vivo | Hyptension | During anesthesia; $ED_{50} = 40$ mg kg$^{-1}$ | Leaders et al. (1960) |
| | Dog | Heart–lung | Contractile depression | | Swain et al. (1956) |
| Kanamycin | Human | | Cardiac arrest | IV overdose | Ream (1963) |
| | Rabbit | In vitro (Langendorff) | Contractile depression | | Ramos et al. (1961) |
| | Dog | In vivo | Cardiovascular depression | During anesthesia | Cohen et al. (1970) |
| | Dog | In vivo | No effects | Unanesthetized, slow IV drip | Tysnes et al. (1988) |
| | Guinea pig | In vitro (atrial muscle) | Contractile depression | 30 percent depression with 3.8 mM | Adams et al. (1979a) |
| | Rat | In vitro (ventricular muscle) | Contractile depression | Additive with halothane | Sohn and Katz (1977, 1978) |

| Drug | Species | Preparation | Effect | Notes | Reference |
|---|---|---|---|---|---|
| Neomycin | Human | | Cardiovascular depression | Review of case reports | Pittinger et al. (1970) |
| | Rhesus monkey, baboons | In vivo | Cardiovascular depression | During anesthesia | Adams (1975a,b) |
| Gentamicin | Rat | In vitro (atrial muscle) | Contractile depression | Antagonized by $Ca^{2+}$ | Adams (1975c) |
| | Rhesus monkey | In vivo | Cardiovascular depression | During anesthesia antagonized by $Ca^{2+}$ | Adams (1975a) |
| | Dog | In vivo | Cardiovascular depression | Potentiated in shock | Adams et al. (1979b) |
| | Guinea pig | In vitro (ventricular muscle) | Reduced slow inward $Ca^{2+}$ current | Voltage clamp | Hino et al. (1982) |
| | Guinea pig | In vitro (atrial muscle) | Inhibited $^{45}Ca$ binding | Other aminoglycosides | Lullman and Schwarz (1985) |
| | Rat | Cultured ventricular myocytes | Negative inotrope and chronotrope | Antagonized by $Ca^{2+}$ | De la Chapella-Groz and Athias (1988) |
| | Guinea pig | In vitro (atrial muscle) | Contractile depression | Blocked slow $Ca^{2+}$-dependent contractions | Adams and Durrett (1978) |
| | Dog | Papillary muscle | Reduced contractile force | During anesthesia | Hino et al. (1982) |
| | Dog | SA node | Slowed SA rate | During anesthesia | Hino et al. (1982) |
| | Dog | AV node | AV block (large doses) | During anesthesia | Hino et al. (1982) |
| | Dog | In vitro (ventricular muscle) | Negative inotrope | Compared with $Co^{2+}$ and Bay k 8644 | Hashimoto et al. (1989) |
| | Guinea pig | In vitro (atrial muscle) | Contractile depression | Comparison with $La^{3+}$ and D600 | Durrett and Adams (1980) |
| Amikacin | Guinea pig | In vitro (atrial muscle) | Contractile depression | 34 percent depression with 4 mM | Adams et al. (1979a) |
| | Dog | In vivo | No effects | Unanesthetized; slow IV drip | Vogel and Sperelakis (1978) |
| Sisomicin | Guinea pig | In vitro (atrial muscle) | Contractile depression | 45 percent depression with 2 mM | Adams et al. (1979a) |

Table 7.2 Cardiovascular depressant effects of several antibiotics

| Antibiotic | Species | Preparation | Effect | Comments | References |
|---|---|---|---|---|---|
| Tetracyclines | Dog | *In vitro* (heart–lung) | Contractile depression | $Ca^{2+}$ chelation | Swain *et al.* (1956) |
| | Dog | *In vivo* | Cardiovascular depression | During anesthesia | Cohen *et al.* (1970) |
| | Cat, rabbit | *In vitro* (Langendorff) | Contractile depression | | Cohen *et al.* (1970) |
| | | | | | Leaders *et al.* (1960) |
| | Rabbit | *In vivo* | Hypotension | During anesthesia; $ED_{50} = 120$ mg $kg^{-1}$ | Leaders *et al.* (1960) |
| Chloramphenicol | Rabbit, cat | *In vitro* (Langendorff) | Contractile depression | | Cohen *et al.* (1970) |
| | | | | | Leaders *et al.* (1960) |
| | Rabbit | *In vivo* | Hypotension | During anesthesia; $ED_{50} = 120$ mg $kg^{-1}$ | Leaders *et al.* (1960) |
| | Dog | *In vitro* (heart–lung) | Contractile depression | | Swain *et al.* (1956) |
| | Toad | *In vitro* | Contractile depression | | Banerjee and Mitra (1976) |
| | Chick | *In vitro* | Decreased pulsatile rate | Embryonic chick heart | Glanzer and Peaslee (1970) |
| | Rat | *In vitro* (ventricular muscle) | Contractile depression | Additive with halothane | Sohn and Katz (1977, 1978) |
| Erythromycin | Cat | *In vitro* (Langerdorff) | Contractile depression | During anesthesia; histamine release | Cohen *et al.* (1970) |
| | Dog | *In vivo* | Cardiovascular depression | | Cohen *et al.* (1970) |
| | | | | | Wakabayashi and Yamada (1972) |
| | | | | | Regan *et al.* (1969) |
| | Human | Purkinje fiber | Cardiac dysrrhythmia | Torsades de pointes | Nattel *et al.* (1990) |
| | Dog | | Prolonged action potential | Inhibit $Na^+$ channel | Nattel *et al.* (1990) |
| | Rat | *In vitro* (atrial muscle) | Negative inotrope | Other macrolides | Tomargo *et al.* (1982) |
| Lincomycin | Dog | *In vivo* | Ventricular arrhythmias | After digitalis or ischemia | Regan *et al.* (1969) |
| | Human | | Cardiac arrest | Overdose IV | Daubeck *et al.* (1974) |

| | | | | | |
|---|---|---|---|---|---|
| Oleandomycin | Rabbit | In vitro (Langendorff) | Contractile depression | | Leaders et al. (1960) |
| | Rabbit | In vivo | Hypotension | During anesthesia; $ED_{50} = 80$ mg kg$^{-1}$ | Leaders et al. (1960) |
| | Dog | In vivo | Hypotension | During anesthesia | Wakabayashi and Yamada (1972) |
| Colymycin | Dog | In vivo | Cardiovascular depression | During anesthesia | Cohen et al. (1970) |
| Vancomycin | Dog | In vivo | Cardiovascular depression | During anesthesia | Cohen et al. (1970) |
| | Cat | In vitro (Langendorff) | Contractile depression | | Cohen et al. (1970) |
| Amphotericin B | Rabbit | In vitro (Langendorff) | Electromechanical depression | Decreased action potential plateau | Ruiz-Ceretti et al. (1976) |
| | Guinea pig | In vitro (Langendorff) | Contractile depression; decreased coronary flow; decreased heart rate | | Arora and Arora (1970) |
| | | | | | Arora et al. (1967) |
| Candicidin | Guinea pig | In vitro (Langendorff) | Contractile depression; systolic arrest; decreased heart rate; decreased coronary flow | | Arora et al. (1967) |
| | Rat | In vitro (Langendorff) | Contractile depression; altered electrolyte balance | | Arora (1965) |
| Valinomycin | Guinea pig | In vitro | Contractile depression | Blocks slow Ca$^{2+}$ responses by metabolic poisoning | Ramos et al. (1961) Schneider and Sperelakis (1974) |

surgical instrumentation and general anesthesia. Concentrations of antibiotics many times greater than those that occur in plasma of patients generally are needed *in vitro* to depress myocardial or arterial contractility directly. Buyiniske and Bierwagen (1975) demonstrated that even large amounts of the aminoglycosides kanamycin and amikacin exert little or no detectable hemodynamic effects when administered by slow intravenous drip to unanesthetized dogs.

On the one hand, therefore, we must conclude that cardiovascular depressant effects of antibiotics are unlikely to be clinically relevant in the routine therapy of uncomplicated infections in otherwise normal patients. The beneficial results of appropriate antibiotic therapy are unquestionable, and the present discussion should not be considered reason to withhold antibiotic treatment when sensitivity tests and clinical experience dictate otherwise.

On the other hand, however, the serious and even disastrous outcome of some of the clinical incidents should not be disregarded. Inadvertent overdose of antibiotics undoubtedly was involved in several cases, and pre-existing circulatory dysfunction or systemic illness seemed contributory. Neuromuscular effects may dominate if myoneural or pulmonary disease has decreased the margin of safety of impulse transmission in respiratory muscles. On the other hand, direct cardiovascular effects may become more important if congestive heart failure, circulatory shock, myocardial infarction, or other circulatory ailments have diminished cardiac reserve. Thus, as a few investigative groups forewarned (Cohen *et al.*, 1970; Pittinger *et al.*, 1970; Adams, 1976; Sohn and Katz, 1978; Adams *et al.*, 1979b; Parker and Adams, 1982), the circulatory effects of certain antibiotics may well become a relevant issue if the patient's cardiovascular system is compromised by disease, general anesthesia, drugs, or any other intervention that directly or indirectly depresses physiologic reactivity of the heart and the vasculature.

## Acknowledgments

Research in the Ramos laboratory is supported by NIH grants ES 04849 and ES 09106. Dr. Parker's laboratory is supported by the American Heart Association and NIH grant P01-HL52490. Dr. Adams's laboratory is supported by NIH grant HL50082.

## References

Adams H.R. 1975a. Cardiovascular depressant effects of neomycin and gentamicin in rhesus monkeys. *British Journal of Pharmacology* 54: 453–462.

Adams H.R. 1975b. Cardiovascular depressant effects of the neomycin–streptomycin group of antibiotics. *American Journal of Veterinary Research* 36: 103–108.

Adams H.R. 1975c. Direct myocardial depressant effects of gentamicin. *European Journal of Pharmacology* 30: 272–279.

Adams H.R. 1975d. Acute adverse effects of antibiotics. *Journal of the American Veterinary Medical Association* 166: 983–987.

Adams H.R. 1976. Antibiotic-induced alterations of cardiovascular reactivity. *Federation Proceedings* 35: 1148–1150.

Adams H.R. and Durrett L.R. 1978. Gentamicin blockade of slow $Ca^{2+}$ channels in atrial myocardium of guinea pigs. *Journal of Clinical Investigation* 62: 241–247.

Adams H.R. and Durrett L.R. 1981. Myocardial toxicity of antibiotics. In *Cardiac Toxicology*, Vol. 2. Balaz, T. (ed.), pp. 145–164. Boca Raton, FL: CRC Press.

Adams H.R. and Goodman F.R. 1974. Differential inhibitory effects of neomycin on contractile responses of various canine arteries. *Journal of Pharmacology and Experimental Therapeutics* 193: 393–402.

Adams H.R., Goodman F.R., Lupean V.A. and Weiss G.B. 1973. Effects of neomycin on tension and $^{45}Ca$ movements in rabbit aortic smooth muscle. *Life Sciences* 12: 279–287.

Adams H.R., Goodman F.R. and Weiss G.B. 1974. Alteration of contractile function and calcium ion movements in vascular smooth muscle by gentamicin and other aminoglycoside antibiotics. *Antimicrobial Agents and Chemotherapy* 5: 640–646.

Adams H.R., Mathew B.P., Teske R.H. and Mercer H.D. 1976a. Neuromuscular blocking effects of aminoglycoside antibiotics on fast- and slow-contracting muscles of the cat. *Anesthesia and Analgesia* 55: 500–507.

Adams H.R., Teske R.H. and Mercer H.D. 1976b. Anesthetic–antibiotic interrelationships. *Journal of the American Veterinary Medical Association* 168: 409–412.

Adams H.R., Parker J.L. and Durrett L.R. 1979a. Cardiac toxicities of antibiotics. *Environmental Health Perspectives* 26: 217–223.

Adams H.R., Parker J.L. and Mathew B.P. 1979b. Cardiovascular manifestations of acute antibiotic toxicity during *E. coli* endotoxin shock in anesthetized dogs. *Circulatory Shock* 6: 391–404.

Antzelevitch C., Sun Z.Q., Zhang Z.Q. and Yan G.X. 1996. Cellular and ionic mechanisms underlying erythromycin-induced long QT intervals and torsades de pointes. *Journal of the American College of Cardiology* 28: 1836–1848.

Arora H.R.K. 1965. Effects of polyene antifungal antibiotics on the heart: a study with amphotericin B and endomycin. *Indian Journal of Medical Research* 53: 877–881.

Arora H.R.K. and Arora V. 1970. A study on the cardiac actions of some polyene antibiotics. *Archives Internationales de Pharmacodynamie et de Therapie* 185: 234–245.

Arora V., Shah G.F. and Arora H.R.K. 1967. Effects of polyene-antifungal antibiotics on the perfused guinea pig heart. A study with F-17 c, candicidin, and amphotericin B. *Medicina et Pharmacologia Experimentalis* 17: 391–396.

Atchison W.D., Adgate I. and Beaman C.M. 1988. Effects of antibiotics on uptake of calcium into isolated nerve terminals. *Journal of Pharmacology and Experimental Therapeutics* 245: 394–401.

Banerjee S. and Mitra C. 1976. Muscle relaxant properties of chloramphenicol. *Journal of Pharmaceutical Science* 65: 704–708.

van Breeman C., Siegel B. and Hwang O. 1978. Differences in adrenergic activation of coronary and peripheral arteries. *Federation Proceedings* 37: 416 (Abstract).

Bruckner J., Thomas Jr., K.C., Bikhazi G.B. and Foldes F.F. 1980. Neuromuscular drug interactions of clinical importance. *Anesthesia and Analgesia* 59: 678–682.

Buyiniske J.P. and Bierwagen M.E. 1975. Comparative effects of kanamycin and amikacin on aortic blood pressure, cardiac rate, and surface electrocardiogram in the conscious dog. *Research Communications in Chemical Pathology and Pharmacology* 11: 327–330.

Calviello G. and Chiesi M. 1989. Rapid kinetic analysis of the calcium-release reticulum: the effect of inhibitors. *Biochemistry* 28: 1301–1306.

Caputy A.J., Kim Y.I. and Sanders D.B. 1981. The neuromuscular blocking effects of therapeutic concentrations of various antibiotics on normal rat skeletal muscle: a quantitative comparison. *Journal of Pharmacology and Experimental Therapeutics* 217: 369–378.

Cockcroft S. and Stutchfield J. 1988. Effect of pertussis toxin and neomycin on G-protein-regulated polyphosphoinositide phosphodiesterase. *Biochemical Journal* 256: 343–350.

Cohen L.S., Wechsler A.S., Mitchell J.H. and Click G. 1970. Depression of cardiac function by streptomycin and other antimicrobial agents. *American Journal of Cardiology* 26: 505–511.

Corrado A.P. 1958. Ganglioplegic action of streptomycin. *Archives Internationales de Pharmacodynamie et de Therapie* 114: 166–178.

Corrado A.P. and Ramos A.O. 1958. Neomycin – its curariform and ganglioplegic actions. *Revista Brasileria de Biologia* 18: 81–85.

Daubeck J.L., Daughety M.J. and Petty C. 1974. Lincomycin-induced cardiac arrest: a case report and experimental investigation. *Anesthesia and Analgesia* 53: 563–567.

Daynes G. 1974. Drug-induced heart failure in advanced tuberculosis. *South African Medical Journal* 48: 2352–2353.

De la Chapelle-Groz A. and Athias P. 1988. Gentamicin causes the fast depression of action potential and contraction in cultured cardiocytes. *European Journal of Pharmacology* 152: 111–120.

De Morais I.P., Corrado A.P. and Suarez-Kurtz G. 1978. Competitive antagonism between calcium and aminoglycoside antibiotics on guinea pig intestinal smooth muscle. *Archives Internationales de Pharmacodynamie et de Therapie* 231: 317–327.

Dretchen K.L., Gergis S.D., Sokoll M.D. and Long J.P. 1972. Effect of various antibiotics on neuromuscular transmission. *European Journal of Pharmacology* 18: 201–203.

Dretchen K.L., Sokoll M.D., Gergis S.D. and Long J.P. 1973. Relative effects of streptomycin on motor nerve terminal and end-plate. *European Journal of Pharmacology* 22: 10–16.

Drici M.D., Knollmann B.C., Wang W.X. and Woosley R.L. 1998. Cardiac actions of erythromycin: influence of female sex. *Journal of the American Medical Association* 280: 1774–1776.

Dulon D., Zajic G., Aran J.M. and Schacht J. 1989. Aminoglycoside antibiotics impair calcium entry but not viability and motility in isolated cochlear hair cells. *Journal of Neuroscience Research* 24: 338–346.

Durant N.N. and Lambert J.J. 1981. The action of polymyxin B at the frog neuromuscular junction. *British Journal of Pharmacology* 72: 41–47.

Durrett L.R. and Adams H.R. 1980. A comparison of the influence of $La^{3+}$, D600, and gentamicin on frequency–force relationships in isolated myocardium. *European Journal of Pharmacology* 66: 315–325.

Fazekas T., Krassoi I., Lengyel C., Varro A. and Papp J.G. 1998. Suppression of erythromycin-induced early afterdepolarization and torsades de pointes ventricular tachycardia by mexiletine. *Pacing and Clinical Electrophysiology* 21: 147–150.

Fiekers J.F. 1983a. Effects of the aminoglycoside antibiotics, streptomycin and neomycin on neuromuscular transmission. II. Postsynaptic considerations. *Journal of Pharmacology and Experimental Therapeutics* 225: 496–502.

Fiekers J.F. 1983b. Effects of the aminoglycoside antibiotics, streptomycin and neomycin, on neuromuscular transmission. I. Presynaptic considerations. *Journal of Pharmacology and Experimental Therapeutics* 225: 487–495.

Gilbert T.B., Jacobs S.C. and Quaddoura A.A. 1998. Deafness and prolonged neuromuscular blockade following single-dose peritoneal neomycin irrigation. *Canadian Journal of Anaesthesia* 45: 568–570.

Glanzer M.L. and Peaslee M.H. 1970 Inhibition of heart beat development by chloramphenicol in intact and cardia bifida explanted chick embryos. *Experientia* 26: 370–371.

Godzik K.L., O'Brien E.R., Wang S.K. and Kuo C.C. 1995. In vitro susceptibility of human vascular wall cells to infection with Chlamydia pneumoniae. *Journal of Clinical Microbiology* 33: 2411–2414.

Goodman F.R. 1978a. Distribution of 4C-gentamicin in vascular smooth muscle. *Pharmacology* 16: 17–25.

Goodman F.R. 1978b. Calcium related basis of action of vascular agents: cellular approaches. In *Calcium in Drug Action*. Weiss G.B. (ed.), p. 331. New York: Plenum Press.

Goodman F.R. and Adams H.R. 1976a. Contractile function and 45Ca movements in vascular smooth muscle of nonhuman primates: effects of aminoglycoside antibiotics. *General Pharmacology* 7: 227–232.

Goodman F.R. and Adams H.R. 1976b. Negative inotropic effects of gentamicin in guinea pig left atria. *Federation Proceedings* 35: 613 (Abstract).

Goodman F.R., Weiss G.B. and Adams H.R. 1974. Alterations by neomycin of 45Ca movements and contractile responses in vascular smooth muscle. *Journal of Pharmacology and Experimental Therapeutics* 188: 472–480.

Goodman F.R., Adams H.R. and Weiss G.B. 1975. Effects of neomycin on 45Ca binding and distribution in canine arteries. *Blood Vessels* 12: 248–260.

Gotanda K., Yanagisawa T., Satoh K. and Taira N. 1988. Are the cardiovascular effects of gentamicin similar to those of calcium antagonists? *Japanese Journal of Pharmacology* 47: 217–227.

Grayston J.T., Kuo C.-C., Coulson A.S., Campbell L.A. and Wang S.P. (1989) Chlamydia pneumoniae sp. nov. for Chlamydia sp. strain TWAR. *International Journal for Systemic Bacteriology* 39: 88–90.

Grayston J.T., Kuo C.-C., Coulson A.S., Campbell L.A., Lawrence R.D., Lee M.J., Strandness E.D. and Wang S.P. 1995. Chlamydia pneumoniae (TWAR) in atherosclerosis of the carotid artery. *Circulation* 92: 3397–4000.

Gross D.R., Kitzman J.V. and Adams H.R. 1979. Cardiovascular effects of intravenous administration of propylene glycol and of oxytetracycline in propylene glycol in calves. *American Journal of Veterinary Research* 40: 783–791.

Gustin M. and Hennessey T.M. 1988. Neomycin inhibits the calcium current of paramecium. *Biochimica et Biophysica Acta* 940: 99–104.

Hagiwara S. and Byerly L. 1981. Calcium channel. *Annual Reviews of Neuroscience* 4: 69–125.

Hall D.A., McGibbon D.H., Evans C.C. and Meadows G.A. 1972. Gentamicin, tubocurarine, lignocaine, and neuromuscular blockade: a case report. *British Journal of Anaesthesia* 44: 1329.

217

Hashimoto H., Yanagisawa T. and Taira N. 1989. Differential antagonism of the negative inotropic effect of gentamicin by calcium ions, Bay k 8644 and isoprenaline in canine ventricular muscle: comparison with cobalt ions. *British Journal of Pharmacology* 96: 906–912.

Hino N., Ochi R. and Yanagisawa T. 1982. Inhibition of the slow inward current and the time-dependent outward current of mammalian ventricular muscle by gentamicin. *Pflügers Archives, European Journal of Physiology* 394: 243–249.

Jordan W.H., Byrd R.A., Cochrane R.L., Hanasono G.K., Hoyt J.A., Main B.W., Meyerhoff R.D. and Sarazan R.D. 1993. A review of the toxicology of the antibiotic MICOTIL 300. *Veterinary and Human Toxicology* 35: 151–158.

Kaeser Y.A., Brunner F., Drewe J. and Haefeli W.E. 1998. Severe hypotension and bradycardia associated with verapamil and clarithromycin. *American Journal of Health-System Pharmacy* 55: 2417–2418.

Kalsner S. 1976. The lack of effect of oxytetracycline on response to sympathetic nerve stimulation and catecholamines in vascular tissue. *British Journal of Pharmacology* 58: 261–266.

Kundu S., Williams S.R., Nordt S.P. and Clark R.F. 1997. Clarithromycin-induced ventricular tachycardia. *Annals of Emergency Medicine* 30: 542–544.

Kuo C.C., Grayston J.T., Campbell L.A., Goo Y.A., Wissler R.W. and Benditt E.P. 1995. Chlamydia pneumoniae (TWAR) in coronary arteries of young adults (15–34 years old). *Proceedings of the National Academy of Science of the United States of America* 92: 6911–6914.

Leaders F., Pittinger C.B. and Long J.P. 1960. Some pharmacological properties of selected antibiotics. *Antibiotics and Chemotherapy* 10: 503–507.

Lee K.L., Jim M.H., Tang S.C. and Tai Y.T. 1998. QT prolongation and Torsades de Pointes associated with clarythromycin. *American Journal of Medicine* 104: 395–396.

Lohdi S., Weiner N.D., Mechigian J. and Schacht J. 1980. Ototoxicity of aminoglycosides correlated with their action on monomolecular films of polyphosphoinositides. *Biochemical Pharmacology* 29: 597–601.

Lullmann H. and Schwarz B. 1985. Effects of aminoglycoside antibiotics on bound calcium and contraction in guinea-pig atria. *British Journal of Pharmacology* 86: 799–803.

Maass M., Bartels C., Kruger S., Krause E., Engel P.M. and Dalhoff K. 1998. Endovascular presence of Chlamydia pneumoniae DNA is a generalized phenomenon in atherosclerotic vascular disease. *Atherosclerosis* 140 (Suppl. 1): S25–S30.

McCullough D.A. and Wallace W.F.M. 1975. Inhibition of constrictor responses of the rabbit ear artery by a mixture of oxytetracycline and ascorbic acid. *British Journal of Pharmacology* 54: 261.

Main B.W., Means J.F., Rinkema L.E., Smith W.C. and Sarazan R.D. 1996. Cardiovascular effects of the macrolide antibiotic tilmicosin, administered alone or in combination with propanolol or dobutamine, in conscious unrestrained dogs. *Journal of Veterinary Pharmacology and Therapeutics* 19: 225–232.

Marche P., Olier B., Girard A., Fillastre J.P. and Morin J.P. 1987. Aminoglycoside-induced alterations of phosphoinositide metabolism. *Kidney International* 31: 59–64.

Matsukawa S., Suh J.H., Hashimoto Y., Kato M., Satoh D., Saito S., Endo K. and Saishu T. 1997. Neuromuscular blocking actions of the aminoglycoside antibiotics sisomicin and micronomicin in the rabbit. *Tohoku Journal of Experimental Medicine* 181: 471–473.

Melnick S.L., Shahar E., Folsom A.R., Grayston J.T., Sorlie P.D., Wang S.P. and Szklo M. 1993. Past infection by Chlamydia pneumoniae strain TWAR and asymptomatic carotid atherosclerosis. Atherosclerosis Risk in Communities (ARIC) Study Investigators. *American Journal of Medicine* 95: 499–504.

Molgo J., Lemeignan M., Uchiyama T. and Lechat P. 1979. Inhibitory effect of kanamycin on evoked transmitter release. Reversal by 3,4-diaminopyridine. *European Journal of Pharmacology* 57: 93–97.

Muhlestein J.B., Anderson J.L., Hammond E.H., Zhao L., Trehan S., Schwobe E.P. and Carlquist J.F. 1998. Infection with Chlamydia pneumoniae accelerates the development of atherosclerosis and treatment with azithromycin prevents it in a rabbit model. *Circulation* 97: 633–636.

Nation P.N. and Roth S.H. 1988. The effects of neomycin on membrane properties and discharge activity of an isolated sensory neuron. *Canadian Journal of Physiology and Pharmacology* 66: 27–31.

Nattel S., Ranger S., Talajic M., Lemery R. and Roy D. 1990. Erythromycin-induced long QT syndrome: concordance with quinidine and underlying cellular electrophysiologic mechanism. *American Journal of Medicine* 89: 235–238.

Noll G. 1998. Pathogenesis of atherosclerosis: a possible relation to infection. *Atherosclerosis* 140 (Suppl. 1): S3–S9.

Nomura K., Naruse K., Watanabe K. and Sokabe M. 1990. Aminoglycoside blockade of $Ca^{2+}$-activated $K^+$ channel from rat brain synaptosomal membranes incorporated into planar bilayers. *Journal of Membrane Biology*. 115: 241–251.

Novak E., Vitti T.G. and Panzer J.D. 1971. Antibiotic tolerance and serum levels after intravenous administration of multiple large doses of lincomycin. *Clinical Pharmacology and Therapeutics* 12: 793–797.

Orsulakova A., Stockhurst E. and Schacht J. 1975. Effect of neomycin on phosphoinositide labeling and calcium binding in guinea pig inner ear tissues *in vivo* and *in vitro*. *Journal of Neurochemistry* 26: 285–290.

Pandey K., Kumar S. and Badola R.P. 1964. Neuromuscular blocking and hypotensive actions of streptomycin and their reversal. *British Journal of Anaesthesiology* 36: 19–25.

Pappano A.J. 1970. Calcium-dependent action potentials produced by catecholamines in guinea pig atrial muscle fiber depolarized by potassium. *Circulation Research* 27: 379–389.

Parker J.L. and Adams H.R. 1982. Cardiovascular depressant effects of antibiotics. In *Cardiovascular Toxicology*. Van Stee E.W. (ed.), pp. 327–351. New York: Raven Press.

Pittinger C. and Adamson R. 1972. Antibiotic blockade of neuromuscular function. *Annual Reviews of Pharmacology* 12: 169–184.

Pittinger C.B., Eryasa Y. and Adamson R. 1970. Antibiotic-induced paralysis. *Anesthesia and Analgesia* 49: 487–501.

Prado W.A., Corrado A.P. and Marseillan R.F. 1978. Competitive antagonism between calcium and antibiotics at the neuromuscular junction. *Archives Internationales de Pharmacodynamie et de Therapie* 231: 297–307.

Pridgen J.E. 1956. Respiratory arrest thought to be due to intraperitoneal neomycin. *Surgery* 40: 571–574.

Ramos A.O., Ramos L. and de Luca A.M. 1961. Acoes da Kanamicina nas musculatures lisa e cardiaca. *Folia Clinica Biologica* 21: 156–162.

Ramos H., de Murciano A.A., Cohen B.E. and Bolard J. 1989. The polyene antibiotic amphotericin B acts as a $Ca^{2+}$ ionophore in sterol-containing liposomes. *Biochimica et Biophysica Acta* 982: 303–306.

Redman R.S. and Silinsky E.M. 1994. Decrease in calcium currents induced by aminoglycoside antibiotics in frog motor nerve endings. *British Journal of Pharmacology* 13: 375–378.

Ream C.R. 1963. Respiratory and cardiac arrest after intravenous administration of kanamycin with reversal of toxic effects by neostigmine. *Annals of Internal Medicine* 59: 384–387.

Regan T.J., Khan M.I., Oldewurtel H.A. and Passannante A.J. 1969. Antibiotic effect on myocardial $K^+$ transport and the production of ventricular tachycardia. *Journal of Clinical Investigation* 48: 68A.

Rubbo J.T., Gergis S.D. and Sokoll M.D. 1977. Comparative neuromuscular effects of lincomycin and clindamycin. *Anesthesia and Analgesia* 56: 329–332.

Ruiz-Ceretti E., Schanne O.F. and Bonnardeaux J.L. 1976. Effects of amphotericin B on isolated rabbit hearts. *Molecular and Cellular Cardiology* 8: 77–88.

Schanne O.F., Ruiz-Ceretti E., Deslauriers Y., Payet D., Soulier P. and Demers J.M. 1977. The effects of amphotericin B on the ionic currents of frog atrial trabeculae. *Journal of Molecular and Cellular Cardiology* 9: 909–920.

Schibeci A. and Schacht J. 1977. Action of neomycin on the metabolism of polyphosphoinositides in the guinea pig kidney. *Biochemical Pharmacology* 26: 1769–1774.

Schneider J.A. and Sperelakis N. 1974. Valinomycin blockade of slow channels in guinea pig heart perfused with elevated $K^+$ and isoproterenol. *European Journal of Pharmacology* 27: 349–354.

Singh Y.N., Marshall I.G. and Harvey A.L. 1978. Some effects of the aminoglycoside antibiotic amikacin on neuromuscular and autonomic transmission. *British Journal of Anaesthesiology* 50: 109–117.

Sohn Y.Z. and Katz R.L. 1977. Interaction of halothane and antibiotics on isometric contractions of rat heart muscle. *Anesthesia and Analgesia* 56: 515–521.

Sohn Y.Z. and Katz R.L. 1978. Effects of certain antibiotics on isometric contractions of isolated heart muscle. *Canadian Anaesthesiology Society Journal* 25: 291–296.

Stallworth J.M., Rodriguez O. and Barrington B.A. 1972. Microcirculatory responses to commonly used therapeutic drugs. *Annals of Surgery* 38: 145–153.

Suarez C.R. and Ow E.P. 1992. Chloramphenicol toxicity associated with severe cardiac dysfunction. *Pediatric Research* 13: 48–51.

Suarez-Kurtz G. and Reuben J.P. 1987. Effects of neomycin on calcium channel currents in clonal GH3 pituitary cells. *Pflügers Archives, European Journal of Physiology* 410: 517–523.

Swain H.H., Kiplinger G.F. and Brody T.M. 1956. Actions of certain antibiotics on the isolated dog heart. *Journal of Pharmacology and Experimental Therapeutics* 117: 151–159.

Talbot P.A. 1987. Potentiation of aminoglycoside-induced neuromuscular blockade by protons in vitro and in *vivo*. *Journal of Pharmacology and Experimental Therapeutics* 241: 686–694.

Thyrum P.T. 1974. Inotropic stimuli and systolic transmembrane calcium flow in depolarized guinea pig atria. *Journal of Pharmacology and Experimental Therapeutics* 188: 166–179.

Tolins J.P. and Raij L. 1988. Adverse effect of amphotericin B administration on renal hemodynamics in the rat: neurohumoral mechanisms and influence of calcium channel blockade. *Journal of Pharmacology and Experimental Therapeutics* 245: 594–599.

Tomargo J., De Miguel B. and Tejerina M.T. 1982. A comparison of josamycin with macrolides and related antibiotics on isolated rat atria. *European Journal of Pharmacology* 80: 285–293.

Torda T. 1980. The nature of gentamicin-induced neuromuscular block. *British Journal of Anaesthesiology* 52: 325–329.

Trentesaux A.S., Bednarek N. and Morville P. 1998. Vancomycin and cardiac arrest in the infant. *Archives de Pediatrie* 5: 521–524.

Tysnes O.B., Steen V.M. and Holmsen H. 1988. Neomycin inhibits platelet functions and inositol phospholipid metabolism upon stimulation with thrombin, but not with ionomycin or 12-O-tetradecanoyl-phorbol 13-acetate. *European Journal of Biochemistry* 177: 219–223.

Vassbotn F.S., Langeland N. and Holmsen H. 1990. Neomycin inhibits PDGF-induced IP3 formation and DNA synthesis but not PDGF-stimulated uptake of inorganic phosphate in C3H/IOTI/2 fibroblasts. *Biochimica et Biophysica Acta* 1054: 207–212.

Vital Brazil O. and Prado-Franceschi J. 1969a. The nature of the neuromuscular block produced by neomycin and gentamicin. *Archives Internationales de Pharmacodynamie et de Therapie* 179: 78–110.

Vital Brazil O. and Prado-Franceschi J. 1969b. The neuromuscular blocking action of gentamicin. *Archives Internationales de Pharmacodynamie et de Therapie* 179: 65–77.

Vogel S. and Sperelakis N. 1978. Valinomycin blockade of myocardial slow channels is reversed by high glucose. *American Journal of Physiology* 235: H46–H51.

Wagner J.A., Snowman A.M., Olivera B.M. and Snyder S.H. 1987. Aminoglycoside effects on voltage-sensitive calcium channels and neurotoxicity. *New England Journal of Medicine* 317: 1669.

Waisbren B.A. 1968. Lincomycin in larger doses (Letter). *Journal of the American Medical Association* 206: 2118.

Wakabayashi K. and Yamada S. 1972. Effects of several macrolide antibiotics on blood pressure of dogs. *Japanese Journal of Pharmacology* 22: 799–807.

Warner W.A. and Sanders E. 1971. Neuromuscular blockade associated with gentamicin therapy. *Journal of the American Medical Association* 215: 1153.

Weiss G.B. 1977. Calcium and contractility in vascular smooth muscle. In *Advances in General and Cellular Pharmacology 11*. Narahashi T. and Bianchi C.P. (eds), pp. 71–154. New York: Plenum Press.

Wolf G.L. and Wigton R.S. 1971. Vasodilation induced by streptomycin in the perfused canine kidney. *Archives Internationales de Pharmacodynamie et de Therapie* 194: 285–289.

Wright J.M. and Collier B. 1976. The effects of neomycin upon transmitter release and action. *Journal of Pharmacology and Experimental Therapeutics* 200: 576–587.

Yamashita K., Ouchi K., Shirai M., Gondo T., Nakazawa T. and Ito H. 1998. Distribution of Chlamydia pneumoniae infection in the atherosclerotic carotid artery. *Stroke* 29: 773–778.

# 8

# BACTERIAL LIPOPOLYSACCHARIDE (ENDOTOXIN) AND MYOCARDIAL DYSFUNCTION

*Leona J. Rubin,\* Janet L. Parker,†
and H. Richard Adams‡*

*\*Department of Veterinary Biomedical Sciences,
College of Veterinary Medicine, University of Missouri –
Columbia, MO, USA; †Department of Medical Physiology,
College of Medicine and ‡Department of Veterinary
Physiology and Pharmacology, College of Veterinary Medicine,
Texas A & M University, College Station, TX, USA*

## Introduction

Circulatory shock resulting from bacterial sepsis remains the most common cause of death in medical and surgical intensive care units in the USA (Cunnion and Parrillo, 1989a; Parrillo, 1990a,b; Snell and Parrillo, 1991). Mortality rates ascribed to septicemic shock remain as high as 30–60 percent despite aggressive clinical management with antibiotics, intravascular volume expansion, cardiovascular support drugs, and other interventions (Parrillo, 1990b). The pathogenesis of shock is incompletely understood, but it unquestionably involves a highly complex and dynamic progression of hemodynamic and metabolic derangements eventually affecting virtually all organ systems. Profound cardiovascular dysfunction is believed to dominate as the ultimate cause of death in septicemic patients.

The lipopolysaccharide (LPS) constituent of the outer cell membrane of Gram-negative bacteria, commonly referred to as endotoxin, is considered to be the primary bacterial product toxin responsible for the development of host cell reactions to Gram-negative sepsis and its subsequent cardiovascular manifestations (Ravin *et al.*, 1960; Wolff and Bennett, 1974; Van Deventer *et al.*, 1988; Natanson *et al.*, 1989; Suffredini *et al.*, 1989; Danner *et al.*, 1991; Fink, 1991; Raetz *et al.*, 1991). Upon entry into the host organism's circulation, LPS interacts with different types of cells including macrophages, polymorphonuclear leukocytes, platelets, and vascular endothelial cells. Cells activated by LPS are induced to release an impressive repertoire of endogenous compounds that normally serve immunomodulatory or inflammatory functions. These factors include immunopermissive cytokines, such as tumor necrosis factor-α and interleukins, and fatty acid breakdown products, such as the eicosanoids and platelet-activating factor. In the septicemic patient, these factors become pathophysiologic progenitors and mediators of LPS toxicity instead of physiologically containing the bacterial invaders. This complex cascade culminates in the severe cardiovascular dysfunction and multiorgan failure constituting septicemic shock.

Septic shock is characterized typically by low systemic vascular resistance, generalized maldistribution of tissue blood flows, and cardiac output inadequate relative to metabolic demands. The predominate historical viewpoint emphasized the role of peripheral vascular collapse, rather than myocardial failure, in the pathogenesis of circulatory shock. However, shock-related functional depression of the heart has now been documented in numerous clinical and experimental investigations utilizing a wide variety of techniques and approaches (for reviews, see Hess *et al.*, 1981a; Parker and Adams, 1981a, 1985a; Archer, 1985; Goldfarb, 1985; Parker and Jones, 1988; Abel, 1989, 1990; Cunnion and Parrillo, 1989a,b; Parrillo, 1989, 1990a,b; Adams *et al.*, 1990; Snell and Parrillo, 1991). Current research efforts not only include validation of the presence of shock-induced myocardial depression in patients and intact animal models but they also address (1) cellular, subcellular, biochemical and molecular mechanisms of disrupted excitation–contraction coupling of the heart in shock; (2) putative endogenous toxic mediators that may be involved in producing myocardial dysfunction in shock; and (3) potential chemotherapeutic interventions that may directly or indirectly improve myocardial contractile function in shock.

This chapter provides an overview of this area, with emphasis on (1) the large body of clinical and experimental evidence indicating that impaired myocardial performance accompanies endotoxin and septic shock states; (2) cellular and biochemical mechanisms of disrupted excitation–contraction coupling processes of the cardiac myocyte in shock; and (3) potential *in vivo* mechanisms and mediators involved in the myocardial toxicity of endotoxicosis.

## Cardiac dysfunction in clinical LPS and sepsis syndromes

Generally accepted concepts relative to the function of the heart in clinical shock states have undergone major transition and considerable controversy over the past several decades. Much of the discrepancies during this period relate to changes in (1) clinical recognition and characterization of the shock state itself; (2) criteria for identification of myocardial depression; and (3) major alterations in therapeutic management of shock, particularly relating to the more recent use of aggressive fluid resuscitation. The dynamic and precarious nature of shock and limited diagnostic capabilities have further increased the difficulty of studying intrinsic cardiodynamic function in shock patients. Despite these drawbacks, a large number of clinical studies have now provided convincing evidence for significant myocardial dysfunction in endotoxemic and septicemic patients.

Historically, septic shock was characterized by a hemodynamic pattern mainly of hypotension and low cardiac output (Wiggers, 1950; Udhoji and Weil, 1965; Cunnion and Parrillo, 1989b). Aggressive administration of resuscitative fluids was not standard clinical practice during this period (prior to 1960), primarily because a convenient and accurate measure of LV end-diastolic filling volume or preload was unavailable (for reviews, see Cunnion and Parrillo, 1989a,b; Parrillo, 1989). The subsequent use of the pulmonary artery catheter to monitor pulmonary capillary wedge pressures provided information suggesting that the reduced cardiac output reported in previous studies resulted from reduced venous return and inadequate LV preload (Cunnion and Parrillo, 1989b). Septic shock patients in more contemporary investigations generally receive large volumes of resuscitative fluids to achieve optimal preload. Under these conditions, most septic patients initially exhibit a "hyperdynamic" pattern of hemodynamic and cardiac function characterized by normal to high cardiac output and low systemic vascular resistance. Increased cardiac output in the majority of septic shock patients seemed inconsistent with the presence of heart failure and it renewed doubts and controversy about the involvement of myocardial dysfunction in the early hyperdynamic stages of shock.

Subsequent findings of Siegel *et al.* (1967, 1972) indicated that septic shock patients may shift from a high cardiac output (hyperdynamic) to a low cardiac output (hypodynamic) state as circulatory shock progresses. Shoemaker (1976) similarly reported a general pattern of normal to increased cardiac output early in patients in septic shock, followed by a precipitous fall in cardiac output and cardiac work in patients who subsequently died; indeed, cardiac output at the onset of therapeutic management has been closely proportional to survival following bacterial shock (Weil and Nishijima, 1978; Vincent *et al.*, 1981). Decreased LV stroke work in relation to right-sided filling pressure was observed by Siegel *et al.* (1967) in thirty patients with bacterial shock of various causes. Those patients with hypodynamic (low output) septic shock states had poorer ventricular function relationships and tended to be the least responsive to therapy (Siegel *et al.*, 1971). Weisel *et al.* (1977) measured the transient effects of fluid challenge on LV stroke work and pulmonary artery occlusive pressure and found evidence of impaired LV function in fatal cases of sepsis. The LV stroke work index in patients with low output septic shock was only 25 percent of normal values in the presence of a 200 percent increase in central venous pressure (CVP).

The premise that a hyperdynamic state of increased cardiac output is an indicator of a better prognosis during sepsis has not been accepted by all investigators. Several studies showed that most non-survivors maintained a normal or high cardiac index (CI), even within a few hours of death (Groeneveld *et al.*, 1986; Parker *et al.*, 1987; D'Orio *et al.*, 1990; Jardin *et al.*, 1990). In 1990, D'Orio *et al.* (1990) reported an analysis of clinical, hemodynamic, and metabolic data from twenty-six consecutive septic shock patients before and during volume infusion. Mean CI was initially greater in survivors than in non-survivors (4.5 compared with 3.0 L min$^{-1}$ m$^{-2}$), but none of the initial cardiovascular variables served as a reliable predictor for survival. During fluid loading, however, only survivors exhibited a normal cardiac response, as evidenced by the change in LV stroke work index (LVSWI) for a given increase in the pulmonary capillary wedge pressure as the index of LV preload. These investigators suggested that the LVSWI response to volume loading may be a better predictor of prognosis than total CI (D'Orio *et al.*, 1990). In the same year, Jardin *et al.* (1990) evaluated serial hemodynamic measurements and two-dimensional echocardiographic studies in twenty-one patients with sepsis-related circulatory failure. Initial hemodynamic evaluation revealed severe ventricular systolic dysfunction in one-third of the patients, as evidenced by low CI and markedly reduced LV ejection fraction. The remaining patients exhibited an increased CI associated with tachycardia. As LVEF remained normal despite low peripheral vascular resistance, they concluded the presence of moderate LV systolic dysfunction, even during the apparently hyperdynamic state of septic shock. Reinhart *et al.* (1990) reported that therapeutically induced increases in oxygen delivery (via inotropic support drugs) produced measurable but small increases in oxygen consumption ($Vo_2$) in septic shock patients; $Vo_2$ increases, however, were similar in survivors and non-survivors, suggesting that factors other than tissue oxygen deficit determined patient outcome. The use of pulmonary capillary wedge pressure as an index of LV end-diastolic pressure may be inaccurate in some conditions (Lefcoe *et al.*, 1979; Hardaway, 1982; Mammana *et al.*, 1982; Snyder, 1984). Lefcoe and colleagues (1979) reported wedge pressure to be 30 mm higher than LV end-diastolic pressure in five septic patients. Snyder (1984) suggested that ventricular filling pressure may be consistently dissociated from wedge pressure in septic patients. If so, greater reliance may need to be placed on volume challenge, measurements of end-diastolic volume, or direct measures of left atrial or ventricular end-diastolic pressure to assure adequate ventricular filling.

Much insight has recently been provided by the work of Parrillo and co-workers (Cunnion and Parrillo, 1989a,b; Parrillo, 1989, 1990a,b; Snell and Parrillo, 1991), using simultaneous assessment of cardiac hemodynamics and measurements of radionuclide scan-determined LV end-systolic and end-diastolic volume indices in endotoxemic and septic shock patients. These investigators used three different methods of quantitating serial ventricular performance in their subjects: ejection fractions; shifts in the Starling ventricular function curve based on LV end-diastolic volume index versus stroke work index; and the ventricular function curve response to intravascular volume expansion. In brief, their findings indicated that septic shock produced a profound decrease in systolic LV performance that was expressed as a substantial decrease in ejection fraction. Left ventricular dysfunction was most evident during the early course (1–3 days) of sepsis and was reversible by days 7–10 after the onset of sepsis. Intravascular volume expansion partially overcame the decrease in systolic performance early in shock, but was less effective after progression of shock to the more severe stages (Cunnion and Parrillo, 1989a,b; Parrillo, 1989, 1990a,b; Snell and Parrillo, 1991). The impairment in LV systolic function was associated temporally with a dilatative increase in LV end-diastolic volume index. Dilation of the heart with increased end-diastolic volume tended to maintain the stroke volume index constant, although ejection fraction remained low. However, the diastolic enlargement was dependent on the intravascular volume expansion. The end-diastolic volume index did not increase without volume expansion; instead, it seemingly decreased (Cunnion and Parrillo, 1989b; Parrillo, 1989).

Vincent *et al.* (1981) reported the presence of biventricular cardiac failure in the fatal progression of septic shock as a result of peritonitis. In contrast to the acute survivors, the fatal cases failed to respond to fluid repletion; instead, they demonstrated disproportionate increases in both right- and left-side filling pressures, increases in pulmonary vascular resistance, and decreased right and LV work capability. Right ventricular (RV) dysfunction in septic shock patients was manifested as reduced RV ejection fraction with higher RV end-systolic volumes. Similar responses were observed by Bell and Thal (1970) in another group of septic shock patients without pre-existing heart disease. These patients responded to volume loading with a rapid rise in CVP without a concomitant increase in cardiac output. Early heart failure was suggested in some patients, although most showed evidence of cardiac failure after shock periods of longer than 24 h. Right ventricular failure in shock has also been suggested by Clowes (1974) and Krausz *et al.* (1974) to be related to increased pulmonary vascular resistance and attendant elevation of impedance to RV ejection. Indeed, Schneider *et al.* (1988) suggested that volume loading in some patients with septic shock does not result in increased forward flow because of RV failure associated with pulmonary hypertension (increased RV outflow pressure) and also coronary hypotension. Disparate changes in both preload and afterload may thus disorder biventricular working conditions and, ultimately, adversely affect output performance of both left and right ventricles in shock (Bell and Thal, 1970; Gunnar *et al.*, 1973; Clowes, 1974; Clowes *et al.*, 1974; Krausz *et al.*, 1974; Kimichi *et al.*, 1984; Dhainaut *et al.*, 1988; Schneider *et al.*, 1988; Vincent *et al.*, 1989).

In summary, numerous clinical studies have now provided considerable evidence confirming the contention that septicemic circulatory shock is associated with reduced ventricular performance. Because of major changes in cardiac filling volumes and outflow resistance seen by both the RV and LV chambers, it has been difficult to distinguish intrinsic myocardial dysfunction from an otherwise normal heart that is forced to work/pump under abnormal preload and afterload conditions (Adams *et al.*, 1990). The difficulty inherent to highly invasive monitoring in ill patients has prompted study of experimental shock models in laboratory animals.

## Cardiac dysfunction in experimental LPS and sepsis models: *in vivo* studies

The complex issues involved in the experimental evaluation of cardiodynamic adjustments during shock have been addressed previously by numerous groups

(Hess *et al.*, 1981a; Parker and Adams, 1981a; Archer, 1985; Goldfarb, 1985; Parker and Jones, 1988; Abel, 1989, 1990; Cunnion and Parrillo, 1989a,b; Parrillo, 1989, 1990a; Adams *et al.*, 1990; Snell and Parrillo, 1991). Much of the earlier investigations using experimental shock models followed a similar line of reasoning as that described in clinical reports. For instance, Weil *et al.* (1956) demonstrated that the heart appears to perform adequately in the early phase of endotoxin shock in the dog, but that the pooling of large volumes of blood in the liver and intestines elicits marked decreases in venous return and the heart is thus unable to maintain its output (Weil *et al.*, 1956). Goodyer (1967) reported no evidence of primary myocardial failure in early hemorrhagic or endotoxin shock in dogs and therefore concluded that peripheral mechanisms, rather than heart failure *per se*, were dominant in determining irreversibility in shock. Lefer (1979) reported that LV performance (calculated as stroke output corrected for filling pressure) actually increased 2 h after 0.75 mg kg$^{-1}$ endotoxin administration in dogs; significant cardiodepression was not observed until 6–7 h after endotoxin. Further evidence supportive of a lack of myocardial depression in the early phase of shock has been presented by other investigators on the basis of unaltered LV function curves (Rothe and Selkurt, 1964; Abel and Kessler, 1973; Coleman *et al.*, 1975), maximum velocity of contraction ($V_{max}$) (Guntheroth *et al.*, 1978), function of pumping heart preparations (Hinshaw *et al.*, 1971a,b, 1972a; Hinshaw, 1974), and other *in vivo* indices of cardiac contractility (Maclean and Weil, 1956; Brockman *et al.*, 1967; Wangensteen *et al.*, 1971). Indeed, Hess *et al.* (1981a) suggested that the early phase of experimental endotoxin or bacteremic shock may be analogous to the high-output/low-resistance stage of clinical septic shock in which cardiac output is relatively maintained without evidence of myocardial failure. Even in cases where decreases in LV pressure, LV maximal rate of pressure development (+d$P$/d$t_{max}$), or cardiac output were reported (Priano *et al.*, 1971; Miller *et al.*, 1977), investigators generally attributed these alterations to deficient venous return and LV preload, and did not consider myocardial depression to be a major contributing factor.

On the other hand, Solis and Downing (1966) reported initial evidence for reduced LV function curves in early endotoxemia in the cat. The initial resistance of the canine pumping heart preparation to the effects of endotoxin shock was initially shown (Archer *et al.*, 1975; Hinshaw *et al.*, 1972b, 1974a,b; David and Rogel, 1976) to deteriorate after several hours. Notable cardiac dysfunction or failure was reported to occur as early as 4–7 h following an LD$_{70}$ endotoxin administration, and was demonstrated by increased LV end-diastolic pressure, decreased cardiac power and myocardial efficiency, and depressed negative and positive d$P$/d$t_{max}$ values. These authors suggested that abnormal ventricular diastolic filling and inadequate coronary perfusion result in progressively diminishing cardiac performance, often terminating in overt failure (Hinshaw *et al.*, 1974b). Indeed, maintenance of coronary perfusion pressure and coronary blood flow has been shown to delay cardiac functional deterioration in both hemorrhagic (David and Rogel, 1976) and endotoxin (Elkins *et al.*, 1973; Hinshaw *et al.*, 1974b) shock.

As emphasized in previous reviews (Goldfarb, 1982, 1985; Adams *et al.*, 1990; Parker and Jones, 1988), the preponderance of early studies of shock cardiodynamics utilized indexes of myocardial inotropy that were sensitive to changes in preload and afterload. Such methods are limited because they cannot adequately sample intrinsic myocardial compartments independently of concurrent changes in peripheral vascular preconditions (Parker and Adams, 1981a, 1985a; Parker and Jones, 1988; Adams *et al.*, 1990). More recent studies with improved technologies have reopened the issue of early cardiac participation in LPS-related shock syndromes.

The LV end-systolic pressure–volume relationship is believed to describe the inotropic state of the heart independently of changes in preload and afterload (Sagawa, 1978; Goldfarb, 1982, 1985). Guntheroth *et al.* (1978, 1982) utilized the LV end-systolic pressure–volume ratio technique in mongrel dogs and found that evidence for depressed myocardial contractility appeared early after endotoxin injection (2–6 h) and persisted until death. This ratio technique was also utilized to obtain consistently similar evidence for an early and maintained reduction in myocardial contractility after endotoxin injection in both dogs (Mammana *et al.*, 1982; Goldfarb *et al.*, 1983, 1990; Goldfarb, 1985) and pigs (Goldfarb *et al.*, 1986; Lee *et al.*, 1988a,b). Lee *et al.* (1988b) utilized an endotoxin-loaded osmotic pump to produce a state of "hyperdynamic" sepsis in pigs characterized by elevated cardiac output, heart rate, and LV systolic pressure. Hearts of surviving pigs (ten out of fifteen) exhibited significantly depressed slope of the end-systolic pressure–diameter relationships (ESPDR) and percent shortening of short axis diameter, despite concomitant elevated rates of pressure development.

Other investigators have used basically similar end-systolic pressure–dimension relationships as an index of myocardial contractility in whole animal studies of shock but, in contrast, recorded no negative inotropism. In some studies, *in vivo* endotoxemia was even associated with enhanced myocardial contractility (Kober *et al.*, 1985; Raymond *et al.*, 1989). This controversy was resolved when Law *et al.* (1988) reported that β-adrenergic blockade with propranolol prevented the increase in end-systolic pressure–dimension ratio that they normally observed in endotoxemic animals (Kober *et al.*, 1985; Raymond *et al.*, 1989). Indeed, these investigators reported that after propranolol they now observed evidence of decreased myocardial contractility in their animal model of sepsis (Law *et al.*, 1988), consistent with studies by other investigators (Goldfarb *et al.*, 1983, 1986, 1990; Lee *et al.*, 1988a,b).

The preceding findings from different laboratories (Guntheroth *et al.*, 1978, 1982; Goldfarb *et al.*, 1983, 1986, 1990; Kober *et al.*, 1985; Law *et al.*, 1988; Lee *et al.*, 1988a,b; Raymond *et al.*, 1989) emphasize two important caveats about *in situ* hemodynamic studies in shock research (Adams *et al.*, 1990). First, compensatory release of epinephrine and norepinephrine acting on cardiac β-receptors can mask underlying myocardial depression, an often overlooked but fundamental characteristic of shock recognized years ago (Adams *et al.*, 1985a). Second, although the end-systolic pressure–volume relationship may describe myocardial inotropic state independently of cardiac loading conditions, alterations in this relationship do not differentiate underlying abnormalities in intrinsic muscle mechanics from inotropic effects evoked by extrinsic factors such as catecholamines or other neurogenic or circulating cardioactive agents.

Papadakis and Abel (1988) evaluated LV performance in canine endotoxin shock using an intact open-chest experimental model wherein cardiac function curves were constructed at constant mean arterial pressure and heart rate (Abel *et al.*, 1972). The $+dP/dt_{max}$ index of contractility was used along with LV end-diastolic pressure to assess directional changes in contractility under these controlled conditions. Interestingly, $+dP/dt_{max}$ was depressed early (60 min) during the 2-h period after intravenous endotoxin, although coronary sinus flow was significantly elevated at 2 h. These findings supported the view of an early and sustained depression of myocardial contractility in endotoxin shock unrelated to coronary hypoperfusion and its resulting detrimental effects on the myocardium. Abel and Beck (1988) reported that, with constant heart rate and preload, ventricular performance indicators tended to follow the afterload curve. The largest changes were observed in $-dP/dt_{max}$, perhaps suggesting an early disturbance in LV relaxation. These authors also appropriately expressed caution regarding the difficulty of interpreting any *in vivo* parameter of cardiac performance under conditions of changing preload, heart rate, or afterload. Recently, Abel *et al.* (2000) evaluated myocardial function in awake sheep receiving a low-dose infusion of endotoxin (20 $\mu$g kg$^{-1}$ min$^{-1}$ for 10 h). They reported decreases in LV $dP/dt_{max}$, end-systolic elastance and $P_{max}$ at constant LV preload, afterload, heart rate, cardiac output, cardiac work, and arterial pressure. Thus, this group reported the presence of early LV depression which might easily escape detection in the presence of these normal cardiac variables.

Findings from several studies utilizing non-human primates also suggest strongly that the myocardium is adversely affected during shock, based primarily on abnormal relationships between ventricular filling pressure, cardiac output, and mean arterial pressure (Cavanagh *et al.*, 1970; Geocaris *et al.*, 1973; Greenfield *et al.*, 1974; Hinshaw, 1974; Coalson *et al.*, 1975). Greenfield *et al.* (1974) found that, during fluid loading (colloid infusion) in monkeys, cardiac work in endotoxin-shocked animals was one-half that of control animals at equal end-diastolic ventricular pressures. Autopsy evaluation of these animals revealed evidence of myocardial edema and swelling of capillary endothelium in the endotoxin-treated group. Geocaris *et al.* (1973) similarly demonstrated altered LV responses to fluid loading in an intact awake shock model in baboons. Snow *et al.* (1990) reported the effects of endotoxemia on basic cardiovascular function using *in situ* hearts of rhesus monkeys. These investigators reported an impairment of the heart's ability to maintain sufficient oxygen delivery, as measured by the reduction–oxidation state of cytochrome $aa_3$ during periods of increased work and oxygen delivery.

Evidence is emerging that in addition to the LV systolic contractile dysfunction in shock the LV diastolic volume index and volume–pressure relationships are also altered. Parrillo's group (Natanson *et al.*, 1986, 1988) conducted studies relevant to their clinical work (discussed above) using a canine model that simulates human septic shock. They documented that, without intravascular volume loading, LV end-diastolic volume index fell whereas pulmonary capillary wedge pressure tended to increase (Natanson *et al.*, 1986, 1988); this set of findings suggested that septic shock *decreased* LV diastolic compliance and therefore increased its reciprocal, LV diastolic stiffness (Glantz and Parmley, 1978; Lewis and Gotsman, 1980; Momomura *et al.*, 1988). This decrease in LV compliance was especially evident in non-survivors, where it was associated with greater decrements in stroke volume and stroke work indexes (Natanson *et al.*, 1988). In contrast, intravascular volume loading resulted in an increase in LV end-diastolic volume index without a matching increase in pulmonary wedge pressure (Natanson *et al.*, 1986); this set of findings suggested that intravascular volume therapy *increased* LV diastolic compliance during sepsis (Glantz and Parmley, 1978; Lewis and Gotsman, 1980; Momomura *et al.*, 1988). This increase in LV compliance was associated with improved LV cardiodynamic indexes and survival in both dogs (Natanson *et al.*, 1986, 1988) and humans (Ognibene *et al.*, 1988; Parrillo, 1990a).

The mechanism(s) responsible for the opposing interactive effects of septicemia and intravascular volume expansion on LV diastolic pressure–volume relationships is unknown. Nevertheless, as emphasized by Adams *et al.* (1990), this series of studies by Parrillo and co-workers (Natanson *et al.*, 1986, 1988; Ognibene *et al.*, 1988; Cunnion and Parrillo, 1989a,b; Parrillo, 1989, 1990a,b; Snell and Parrillo, 1991) yielded three key findings. First, based on ejection fractions measured in conjunction with measurements of cardiac hemodynamics, the radionuclide scan technique provided substantial support for a reversible diminution of intrinsic LV contractile reserves in clinical and experimental sepsis. Second, septicemia also markedly altered LV diastolic function, first reducing end-diastolic compliance and then in some way setting the stage for ventricular dilation and an increase in LV compliance in response to intravascular volume expansion. Third, intravascular volume expansion substantially altered manifestation of the systolic and diastolic LV sequelae of septicemic shock. This third element clearly emphasized the difficulty of ascertaining changes in basal intrinsic myocardial function in patients or intact animals wherein the heart is influenced by the shock state and by numerous endogenously released factors as well as by therapeutic intervention.

Evidence for diastolic dysfunction in sepsis and endotoxin shock models has emerged from other laboratories as well. Stahl *et al.* (1990) evaluated cardiac responses to continuous high-volume fluid resuscitation in a chronic canine model of hyperdynamic sepsis. Septic animals demonstrated a significant reduction in systolic contractility, as evidenced by the use of a rate- and load-independent index of LV performance ($E_{max}$ of the end-systolic pressure–volume relationship), confirming previous work (Goldfarb *et al.*, 1983, 1986, 1990; Lee *et al.*, 1988a,b). Abnormal diastolic function was indicated by significant progressive increases in unstressed and end-diastolic ventricular volumes, but significant decreases in myocardial compliance as quantified by transmural pressure versus normalized volume–strain analysis. Thus, intravascular volume expansion increased LV chamber compliance during sepsis by inducing LV chamber dilatation. However, stiffness of the myocardium itself actually increased (Stahl *et al.*, 1990). Evidence for increased LV stiffness was also observed early (2–4 h) after endotoxemia in guinea pigs (Parker *et al.*, 1990) and sepsis in rats (Field *et al.*, 1989). Thus, fluid-induced increases in diastolic volume help to maintain global cardiac performance during endotoxemia or sepsis. However, the intrinsic diastolic response of LV myocardium itself apparently entails an early increase in stiffness and a decrease in its reciprocal compliance (Field *et al.*, 1989; Adams *et al.*, 1990; Parker *et al.*, 1990; Stahl *et al.*, 1990), whereas the LV chamber size actually may be increasing owing to fluid-induced dilatation (Stahl *et al.*, 1990). Interestingly, Walley and Cooper (1991) concluded that impaired LV function during hypovolemic shock in a pig model is due entirely to increased diastolic stiffness.

## Cardiac dysfunction in experimental LPS and sepsis models

### *Isolated tissue studies*

Different investigative groups have evaluated different types of cardiac tissue preparations isolated from experimentally shocked animals (e.g. Hess *et al.*, 1981a; Parker and Adams, 1981a; Archer, 1985; Abel, 1989; Field *et al.*, 1989; Adams *et al.*, 1990). The approach of using isolated cardiac preparations was initiated in an attempt to circumvent the confounding influence of multiple extracardiac constraints operative in all previous studies with intact subjects. The shock models studied include acute endotoxemia, chronic endotoxemia, intraperitoneal sepsis, and bacteremia. Cardiac tissues include atrial muscle, ventricular muscle, sinoatrial tissue, isovolumetric LV preparations, externally working LV preparations, and isolated cells. The underlying rationale for these studies was to compare cardiodynamic responsiveness of hearts from animals in shock with appropriate sham-shock (control) hearts under equal conditions of preload, heart rate, temperature, and coronary perfusate composition. Recently, this work also has been extended to include functional analysis of perfused hearts isolated from selected knock-out mouse models to evaluate roles of underlying mediators and molecular mechanisms (McMichael *et al.*, 2000; White *et al.*, 2000).

### *Systolic properties of the heart after LPS and sepsis*

Cardiodynamic studies with hearts isolated from shocked animals yielded basically similar results; cardiac muscle removed from the complexity of the *in situ* LPS or septic shock environment consistently displayed a decrease in systolic contractile function irrespective of shock model or animal species. This loss in contractile function was expressed as diminished length–tension curves in isolated atrial and ventricular muscles, diminished LV systolic pressure versus LV end-diastolic pressure curves in isovolumetric LV preparations, and diminished LV stroke volume versus left atrial filling pressure curves in externally working hearts. In a series of early reports (Archer *et al.*, 1975; Archer, 1985; Hinshaw *et al.*, 1971a,b, 1972a,b, 1974a,b; Lee *et al.*, 1988a), LV preparations isolated from dogs receiving LPS utilized blood-perfused pumping to document myocardial failure and decreased responsiveness to catecholamines. Similar effects on myocardial performance were obtained using a live *Escherichia coli* bacteremia model (Archer *et al.*, 1982; Archer, 1985). The concomitant presence of coronary hypotension was found to increase the incidence of endotoxin-induced myocardial failure in these preparations. These investigators suggested that myocardial edema and/or coronary hypoperfusion may contribute significantly to the endotoxin-induced reductions in myocardial function and responsiveness (Archer *et al.*, 1975).

Examination of an isovolumetric LV model after 16–18 h of *E. coli* endotoxemia in guinea pigs indicated that endotoxemia produced reductions in peak LV systolic pressure and also lowered the maximal rates for LV pressure increase ($+dP/dt_{max}$) and decrease ($-dP/dt_{max}$) (Adams *et al.*, 1985b). The contractile dysfunctions associated with this condition were not coupled to changes in heart rate, active state duration, or tissue water content; neither were they surmounted by pyruvate nor by maximally effective increments in coronary flow, end-diastolic stretch, or interstitial $Ca^{2+}$ concentration (Adams *et al.*, 1985b). These findings led to the interpretation that the pathogenesis of endotoxemia and septicemia in some way entailed a decrease in intrinsic inotropic reserves of the left ventricle that was expressed as impaired isovolumic contraction and relaxation (Adams *et al.*, 1985b). The data from crystalloid-perfused hearts provided direct corroboration of cardiac contraction–relaxation disorders observed previously in more complex preparations of endotoxemia with blood-perfused dog hearts (Hinshaw *et al.*, 1974a,b). Results obtained from crystalloid-perfused hearts also supported analogous findings obtained previously by Adams and colleagues in isolated atrial and LV papillary muscle preparations harvested from guinea pig and rat endotoxin shock models (Parker and Adams, 1979, 1981a,b, 1985a,b; Parker *et al.*, 1980, 1984; Parker and Jamison, 1981; Parker, 1983; Adams *et al.*, 1984, 1985a; Miller and Parker, 1989).

The time-course of intrinsic cardiac changes associated with shock were examined in the guinea pig endotoxemic model; based on isometric contractions of electrically paced atrial muscle, inotropic depression developed within 1–2 h after intraperitoneal injection of *E. coli* endotoxin (Parker and Adams, 1985b). Maximal loss of contractile function occurred between 6 and 16 h after endotoxemia was initiated; the endotoxin-mediated inotropic changes were reversible, with normal contractile function restored by 2 days after endotoxin injection (Parker and Adams, 1985b). Similar temporal findings after LPS injection were obtained in preliminary studies with the isovolumetric LV preparation in guinea pig hearts (Parker *et al.*, 1984). Thus, it seems that intrinsic cardiac contractile dysfunction associated with endotoxemia is not simply terminal or agonal in onset, but is present early (< 4 h) in the developmental phase of endotoxicosis. This early development of intrinsic cardiac dysfunction supports previous findings in intact dogs indicating that evidence of myocardial dysfunction in endotoxemia occurred within 2–4 h after systemic exposure to endotoxin (Guntheroth *et al.*, 1978, 1982; Goldfarb *et al.*, 1983, 1990). Thus, owing to this timely appearance, it would seem that systolic myocardial dysfunction could contribute to the development of the hemodynamic instability characteristic of endotoxin and septic shock syndromes.

McDonough and co-workers (McDonough and Lang, 1984; McDonough *et al.*, 1985a,b, 1990) examined *in vitro* cardiac function of pumping hearts isolated from rat models of hyperdynamic sepsis. These studies confirmed a relatively early onset of myocardial dysfunction in these models. Hearts removed from septic rats during the hyperdynamic stage exhibited a downward and rightward shift in work–function curves, indicative of severe depression. These *in vitro* alterations were evident despite *in vivo* demonstration of significantly elevated cardiac output, tachycardia, elevated coronary blood flow, and unaltered blood pressure (McDonough and Lang, 1984; McDonough *et al.*, 1985a,b, 1990). No significant alterations in high-energy phosphate production or substrate utilization were observed, indicating that altered myocardial metabolism is not likely to be a significant contributor to the dysfunction (McDonough *et al.*, 1985b). Furthermore, in these studies of early sepsis, the heart retained the ability to respond to β-adrenergic stimulation by catecholamines with increased inotropy and chronotropy (Smith *et al.*, 1986; Smith and McDonough, 1988; McDonough *et al.*, 1990). Smith and McDonough (1988) reported that, with maximal isoproterenol stimulation, isovolumically contracting hearts from septic animals were able to generate the same $+dP/dt_{max}$ as hearts from control animals exposed to lower levels of isoproterenol; there were no differences in inotropic indices between the two groups when expressed as a percent of the maximal $+dP/dt_{max}$ achieved. In addition, chronotropic supersensitivity of cardiac β-adrenoceptors was reported by this group to occur in this rat model of early sepsis (Smith and McDonough, 1988; Barker *et al.*, 1989). The chronotropic actions of isoproterenol and fenoterol appeared to be mediated by $\beta_2$-receptors in septic hearts and by $\beta_1$-receptors in control hearts (Barker *et al.*, 1989). These studies collectively suggest that in early sepsis the ability of the heart to modulate its inotropic state in response to β-adrenergic stimulation is operative despite intrinsic myocardial contractile dysfunction (McDonough and Lang, 1984; McDonough *et al.*, 1985a,b, 1990; Smith *et al.*, 1986; Smith and McDonough, 1988; Barker *et al.*, 1989).

Chronic administration of endotoxin in rats by subcutaneous osmotic pump was shown (Fish *et al.*, 1985) to result in reduced *in vitro* cardiac work performance in the absence of *in vivo* evidence of cardiac dysfunction. These studies are consistent with the concept of the confounding influence of compensatory sympathoadrenal stimulation (absent in the *in vitro* heart preparations) in *in vivo* cardiovascular homeostasis during shock and sepsis (Fish *et al.*, 1985).

In late sepsis or following acute intravenous endotoxin administration, myocardial adrenergic responsiveness may be altered (Romanosky *et al.*, 1986; Shepherd *et al.*, 1986, 1987). These findings may relate to alterations in both α-

and β-adrenoceptors observed in other organs and cell types in endotoxemia and sepsis (Spitzer *et al.*, 1989). Romanosky *et al.* (1986) reported that isoproterenol increased mechanical work by hearts of endotoxin-treated rats ($LD_{50}$ 6 h), but not to the same level of performance as that of control hearts not given isoproterenol. Myocytes isolated from endotoxin-treated rats exhibited significantly blunted isoproterenol-stimulated accumulation of adenosine 3',5'-cyclic monophosphate (cAMP) when compared with myocytes from control rats (Shepherd *et al.*, 1987; Burns *et al.*, 1988; DeBlieux *et al.*, 1989; Spitzer *et al.*, 1989). Accumulation of cAMP in response to forskolin was similarly reduced (Shepherd *et al.*, 1987; Burns *et al.*, 1988). Binding studies using (±) [³H]-CGP 12177 suggested a 25 percent decrease in β-receptor density, with little effect on receptor affinity for radiolabeled antagonist (Shepherd *et al.*, 1987). Burns *et al.* (1988) reported that amrinone augmented cAMP levels fivefold and increased contractility in endotoxin-shocked rats. Interestingly, DeBlieux *et al.* (1989) reported that the reduced cAMP accumulation in response to isoproterenol and forskolin in endotoxin-treated rats may be prevented by exercise training. They proposed that training may maintain the integrity of the β-adrenergic receptor adenylyl cyclase system during endotoxin challenge *in vivo* (DeBlieux *et al.*, 1989).

## Diastolic properties of the heart after LPS and sepsis

In contrast to the expanding database corroborating a dysfunction of LV *systolic* dynamics during endotoxemia and septicemia, less is known about the influence of these syndromes on intrinsic *diastolic* cardiodynamics, as introduced above. Early studies in isovolumetric blood-perfused dog hearts indicated that global LV diastolic force increased after exposure to endotoxin, but this change was interpreted as a reflection of contractile failure rather than as a primary decrease in diastolic compliance (Elkins *et al.*, 1973). Hinshaw and co-workers (1974a) reported an increase in LV end-diastolic pressure and a decrease in LV $-dP/dt_{max}$ in pumping dog hearts exposed to endotoxemia. Numerous other studies have likewise indicated a reduction in LV $-dP/dt_{max}$ after LPS and sepsis (e.g. Abel and Beck, 1988; Abel, 1989; Adams *et al.*, 1985a; Parker *et al.*, 1990), indicating slowed LV myocardial relaxation during early diastole.

Although an increase in LV end-diastolic pressure and a decrease in LV $-dP/dt_{max}$ have been interpreted as endotoxin-mediated changes in LV diastolic compliance or stiffness, interpretations about LV chamber compliance and stiffness cannot be derived from pressure measurements alone (Glantz and Parmley, 1978; Lewis and Gotsman, 1980; Momomura *et al.*, 1988). Diastolic volume must be assessed along with diastolic pressure measurements before unique conclusions can be reached about diastolic pressure–volume relationships, i.e. compliance and stiffness (Glantz and Parmley, 1978; Lewis and Gotsman, 1980; Momomura *et al.*, 1988). Also, $-dP/dt_{max}$ is highly dependent on preload conditions, and it changes proportionately with changes in sarcomere length or other determinants that influence the magnitude of developed systolic pressure and $+dP/dt_{max}$

(Momomura *et al.*, 1988). Reductions in $-dP/dt_{max}$ can reflect nothing more than parallel changes in systolic function secondary to adjustments in cardiac loading conditions or inotropy. Thus, end-diastolic compliance and the rate of ventricular relaxation can be independent variables (Momomura *et al.*, 1988), and changes in one of these variables does not necessarily indicate changes in the other (Momomura *et al.*, 1988).

Left ventricular end-diastolic pressure–volume (compliance) relationships were measured in beating hearts isolated from unresuscitated guinea pigs 16–18 h after endotoxin (Adams *et al.*, 1985a). Results from this study suggested that intrinsic LV chamber stiffness was increased during endotoxemia, albeit these changes at 16–18 h after endotoxin did not achieve statistical significance (Adams *et al.*, 1985a). However, studies by Parker *et al.* (1990) with the guinea pig model indicated that LV chamber compliance was reduced significantly within 4 h after induction of endotoxemia, with this reduced compliance partially waning during the next 48 h (unpublished observations). Thus, in the absence of intravascular volume expansion, endotoxemia evoked an early reversible decrease in LV chamber compliance or distensibility.

Zhong *et al.* (1997a) re-examined LV chamber compliance of resuscitated and non-resuscitated endotoxemic guinea pigs. These studies demonstrated that volume resuscitation, although without effect on systolic dysfunction, significantly shifted left ventricular end-diastolic pressure–volume relationships of endotoxemic hearts to the right and thus reversed the endotoxin-meditated decrease in LV chamber compliance. As anticipated, resuscitation also significantly improved survival of LPS-exposed guinea pigs.

Hearts isolated from a septic rat model likewise indicated an early reduction in LV diastolic compliance (Field *et al.*, 1989), consistent with findings from the guinea pig endotoxin model (Parker *et al.*, 1990). However, even when the LV chamber undergoes dilatation after intravascular volume expansion in experimental peritonitis in dogs, normalized LV volume–strain analyses indicated an increase in diastolic stiffness (decreased compliance) of LV myocardium itself (Stahl *et al.*, 1990). Parrillo and co-workers (Cunnion and Parrillo, 1989a,b; Parrillo, 1989, 1990a; Snell and Parrillo, 1991) found that intravascular volume expansion enhanced LV diastolic compliance in survivors of sepsis, whereas LV compliance was apparently reduced in non-survivors. Thus, we would suggest that an early increase in LV diastolic stiffness may well signify a poor prognosis during sepsis, but that a subsequent decrease in LV stiffness (increase in compliance) owing to LV chamber dilatation signifies a beneficial response to intravascular volume resuscitation.

### *Isolated cell and subcellular preparations*

Considerable evidence from *in vivo* and *in vitro* experimental models exists documenting cardiac dysfunction in sepsis and following LPS treatment. More recent studies, utilizing isolated cardiac myocytes, have clearly localized the dysfunction to the muscle itself and provided a foundation for probing investigations into the cellular and subcellular mechanisms affected. Contractile function of myocytes isolated from hearts of LPS-treated guinea pigs (Brady, 1991; Brady et al., 1992; Rubin et al., 1994) and rabbits (Hung and Lew, 1993) or of rats subjected to cecal ligation and puncture (CLP) (Neviere et al., 1999) is significantly depressed compared with myocytes from sham control animals. These myocyte preparations exhibit uniform reductions in frequency-dependent cell shortening, as well as rates of shortening and relengthening which cannot be surmounted by increases in extracellular calcium availability (Hung and Lew, 1993; Rubin et al., 1994) or calcium channel agonists (Zhong et al., 1997b). The preponderance of evidence suggests contractile dysfunction in these models correlates with in vivo production of proinflammatory cytokines or mediators which are cardiodepressant (discussed below).

The ability of LPS itself to alter cardiac function directly is controversial. In vitro exposure of adult guinea pig ventricular myocytes to 100 µg ml$^{-1}$ LPS (E. coli) for 18 h had no effect on basal contractile function (Rubin et al., 1994). Contractile properties of adult rat ventricular myocytes also were unaffected by 24 h incubation in LPS (10 µg ml$^{-1}$; Salmonella typhimurium) independent of the presence of co-cultured LPS-treated or control endothelial cells (Ungureanu-Longrois et al., 1995a) or medium from LPS-conditioned pulmonary alveolar macrophage (Balligand et al., 1993). In contrast, direct depressant effects of LPS have been reported using cultured rat neonatal myocytes (Kinugawa et al., 1997a) and adult rat myocytes following 24 h incubation in LPS (Tao and McKenna, 1994). Apparent contradictions in these findings may be due to LPS tolerance of dissociated myocytes which results from LPS contamination of the enzyme solutions used in the dissociation process (Lew et al., 1997). Extensive depyrogenation of both dissociation enzymes and medium allowed Lew and co-workers to document a direct negative inotropic effect of LPS on adult rabbit ventricular myocytes (Lew et al., 1997; Yasuda and Lew, 1997a,b). However, the inotropic depression was small and decreased cell shortening from 12.9 percent in control to 11 percent in myocytes exposed to LPS for 6 h. This decrease represents a 15 percent change. In contrast, functional indices of myocytes isolated from in vivo endotoxin-treated guinea pigs were 45 percent of respective control values under similar stimulus conditions; 10 percent cell shortening of control myocytes; and 5.5 percent shortening of myocytes from LPS animals (Rubin et al., 1994). Balligand and co-workers used the limulus amebocyte lysate assay to assess LPS contamination of myocyte cell isolation solutions and reported that the level of LPS contamination had no effect on cyclic GMP levels of neonatal myocytes compared with myocytes isolated using "LPS-free" conditions. Cytokine treatment of the same cells readily increased cyclic GMP levels (Balligand et al., 1994). LPS also failed to alter inotropic responsiveness of intact cardiac tissues (Parker and Adams, 1979) which were not exposed to dissociation enzymes or culture medium. This issue remains controversial, however, as Starr and co-workers (1995) observed reduced contractility of feline papillary muscle following 70–

85 min of incubation in 40 $\mu$g ml$^{-1}$ LPS and Comstock and co-workers (1998) have identified both the protein and mRNA for CD14, a key cell membrane receptor for LPS, in neonatal and adult cardiac myocytes.

Independent of whether LPS either directly or through any of a multitude of proinflammatory mediators (discussed below) causes cardiac dysfunction, it is clear that a breakdown in the subcellular machinery of the cardiac excitation–contraction coupling process, particularly involving Ca$^{2+}$, occurs in experimental shock states. Evidence for Ca$^{2+}$-related functional abnormalities has been obtained using isolated heart muscle preparations, single cells and subcellular preparations of cardiac myofibrils, sarcoplasmic reticulum (SR), sarcolemma (SL), and mitochondria. An understanding of these interrelating dysfunctional processes can provide greater insight into possible pathophysiologic and mechanical alterations associated with myocardial failure in shock syndromes.

Various animal models of cardiac disease indicate that decreased Ca$^{2+}$ responsiveness of myofilament proteins can be a major contributing factor to depressed contractile function of the heart (Hofmann *et al.*, 1993, 1995; Gao *et al.*, 1995). Hess and colleagues (Bruni *et al.*, 1978; Hess, 1979; Hess and Krause, 1979, 1981; Krause *et al.*, 1980; Hess *et al.*, 1981a), in an intensive series of studies, demonstrated depressed myofibrillar ATPase activity from ventricular tissue in global myocardial ischemia, as well as in canine endotoxin shock. Augmenting venous return was found to prevent endotoxin-induced decreases in ATPase activity, suggesting a synergistic effect of low venous return in producing this effect (Soulsby *et al.*, 1978). In canine hemorrhagic shock, depressed myocardial contractility was associated with depression of myofibrillar ATPase activity characterized by decreased enzyme affinity for Ca$^{2+}$, as well as uncoupling of Ca$^{2+}$ transport from ATPase hydrolysis in the SR (Warner *et al.*, 1981). Similarly, in a rabbit model of early endotoxemia, intracellular free Ca$^{2+}$ of Langendorff perfused hearts, measured by fluorescence spectroscopy using Rhod-2, increased while contractile performance decreased (Takeuchi *et al.*, 1999), suggestive of reduced myofilament Ca$^{2+}$ sensitivity.

Powers *et al.* (1998) reported increased myofilament Ca$^{2+}$-dependent and Ca$^{2+}$-independent Mg$^{2+}$-ATPase activity of rat hearts following intraperitoneal injection of fecal material. These changes did not correlate with myofilament protein content nor with change in expression of myosin heavy chain isoforms. Furthermore, although Mg$^{2+}$-ATPase activity was increased in these preparations, Ca$^{2+}$ sensitivity of the reaction, reported as pCa$_{50}$, was not changed. Maximal Ca$^{2+}$-activated force of chemically skinned papillary muscle from endotoxemic rabbits was not different from controls at 4 h or 5 days after LPS injection, although myofilament Ca$^{2+}$ sensitivity was significantly decreased at 4 h (Tavernier *et al.*, 1998). Rigby *et al.* (1998) examined Ca$^{2+}$-dependent cell shortening of permeabilized ventricular myocytes as well as isometric tension of individual, chemically skinned ventricular myocytes from an *in vivo* guinea pig model of endotoxemia. They observed no effect of endotoxemia on myofilament Ca$^{2+}$ sensitivity, although membrane-intact myocytes from the same preparations exhibited clear decreases in contractility.

Maximal shortening, maximal tension and myofilament $Ca^{2+}$ sensitivity at either pH 7 or pH 6.6 did not differ between control and endotoxemic myocyte preparations. Differences in the animal model used, the route of administration of LPS or cecal content, the time point for measures or the choice of measurement instrument may impact these diverse and conflicting findings.

Multiple cardiac disease states present with abnormalities in intracellular $Ca^{2+}$ homeostasis, particularly increased diastolic $Ca^{2+}$ associated with "$Ca^{2+}$ overload" (Gwathmey *et al.*, 1987; Kihara *et al.*, 1989; Capasso *et al.*, 1993; Mewes and Ravens, 1994). The ability of calcium antagonists to prevent or ameliorate many of the systemic and metabolic derangements that occur with endotoxemia or sepsis (Sayeed, 1987; Hotchkiss and Karl, 1994) implicates $Ca^{2+}$ overload in the cardiac dysfunction of shock states. The role of $Ca^{2+}$ in inflammation and septic injury has been recently reviewed by Hotchkiss and Karl (1996) and Sayeed (1996). Increased diastolic $Ca^{2+}$ has been reported for some (Koshy *et al.*, 1997; Horton *et al.*, 1998; Takeuchi *et al.*, 1999), but not all (Zhong *et al.*, 1997a), experimental models of shock. $Ca^{2+}$ overload in many cardiac pathologies is associated with an inability of the SR to sequester and store $Ca^{2+}$. Several studies have evaluated $Ca^{2+}$ fluxes of SR vesicle preparations from hearts of septic or endotoxic rats (McDonough, 1988), guinea pigs (Kutsky and Parker, 1990), and dogs (Liu and Wu, 1991). Hess and colleagues reported that the canine endotoxin shock model was associated with depressed SR $Ca^{2+}$ uptake, as well as myofilament ATPase activity (Soulsby *et al.*, 1978; Hess, 1979; Hess *et al.*, 1980). Similarly, Wu and Liu (1991) reported decreased $V_{max}$ of $Ca^{2+}$ uptake into SR vesicles from a canine model of endotoxemia with no change in the $K_m$ for $Ca^{2+}$ or ATP. They speculated that decreased $Ca^{2+}$-ATPase activity in these preparations resulted from accelerated dephosphorylation of key SR proteins. Similar findings and conclusions were reached by Ji *et al.* (1995) for a rat model of CLP. The decreased SR $Ca^{2+}$-ATPase activity they observed in septic preparations could not be surmounted by addition of the catalytic subunit of protein kinase A, calmodulin, or protein kinase C, indicative of altered phosphorylation capacity.

McDonough (1988) also evaluated the capacity of the SR to take up $Ca^{2+}$, and measured $Ca^{2+}$-stimulated ATPase activity of SR vesicles from a hyperdynamic sepsis model of decreased cardiac function. In contrast to the previous studies of endotoxemia in dogs (Soulsby *et al.*, 1978; Hess, 1979; Hess *et al.*, 1980) and rats (McDonough *et al.*, 1986), McDonough (1988) reported that $Ca^{2+}$ uptake of SR from septic rats was not depressed, but in fact was increased compared with control SR. These results were consistent with those of Soulsby *et al.* (1978), which indicated SR function was normal in endotoxic dog hearts when venous return was maintained, i.e. a hyperdynamic model. Kutsky and Parker (1990) also reported no significant alterations in active $Ca^{2+}$ transport, $Ca^{2+}$-ATPase activity, or passive $Ca^{2+}$ efflux of SR membranes from a guinea pig endotoxin shock model. We have measured oxalate-supported $Ca^{2+}$ uptake in saponin-permeabilized myocytes from this same model by monitoring the rate of decline of indo-1 fluorescence following addition of 50 mM $CaCl_2$; uptake was increased in LPS compared with control

(Keller *et al.*, 1996) similar to the findings of McDonough (1988). However, functional measures of SR $Ca^{2+}$ uptake, such as post-rest recovery of contractile function (Keller *et al.*, 1996), do not implicate SR $Ca^{2+}$ uptake in the contractile depression reported for this model (Parker and Adams, 1981b; Parker, 1983; Adams *et al.*, 1985a; Miller and Parker, 1989; Rubin *et al.*, 1994). Similarly, post-rest contraction recovery and rapid cooling contractures of endotoxemic canine right ventricular trabeculae were not different from control (Jha *et al.*, 1993). Potential mechanisms for uncoupling of $Ca^{2+}$-ATPase activity and $Ca^{2+}$ sequestration in the guinea pig or rat model remain to be determined and may result from an inability to regulate either or both the phosphorylation state of key proteins [phospholamban, cyclic AMP-dependent protein kinase (PKA), phosphatase-1; Ji *et al.*, 1995; Yang *et al.*, 1995] or extracellular influences such as protease (Ji *et al.*, 1996) during the membrane isolation procedures. Alternatively, the data do not rule out the possibility that other influences (acidosis, toxins, ischemia, etc.) may be operative *in vivo* to alter indirectly $Ca^{2+}$ fluxes and cardiac performance.

Liu and Wu (1991) reported interesting data suggesting that $Ca^{2+}$-induced $Ca^{2+}$ release from either passively or actively loaded SR vesicles was decreased in a canine model of early endotoxemia independent of the presence of reduced SR $Ca^{2+}$ uptake. Maximal binding of [$^3$H]-ryanodine to cardiac SR from endotoxemic dog hearts was reduced, but neither the $S_{0.5}$ nor the Hill coefficient was affected. This group subsequently demonstrated that reduced [$^3$H]-ryanodine binding could be increased to control levels by addition of phosphatidylserine to the vesicle preparations suggestive of $PLA_2$ involvement (Wu and Liu, 1992). Using a similar canine model of early endotoxemia, SR $Ca^{2+}$ release of right ventricular trabeculae was assessed from functional measures of post-contractile amplitude and was found not to be different from that of control preparations (Jha *et al.*, 1993). However, mechanical restitution curves generated from functional measures of left ventricular $dP/dt$ for a rat model of endotoxemia does support a role for decreased SR $Ca^{2+}$ release (Hoshiai *et al.*, 1999). Clearly, the interaction and interdependence of SR $Ca^{2+}$ release and sarcolemma $Ca^{2+}$ flux make interpretation of functional measures difficult and do not rule out derangements in the SR $Ca^{2+}$ release channel as significant in shock-induced depression of myocardial contractility.

Although loss of sarcolemmal (SL) integrity has been observed in ischemia and shock models using morphometric techniques (Dhalla *et al.*, 1974; Rabinowitz *et al.*, 1975), precise correlations between SL dysfunction and cardiac depression remain uncertain. Bhagat *et al.* (1974, 1980) isolated cardiac fragments from guinea pigs subjected to *in vivo* endotoxin treatment; they reported reduced $^{45}Ca$ binding by a SL fraction but a lack of effect of this procedure on $^{45}Ca$ uptake by SR or mitochondrial fraction. Bhagat *et al.* (1974) suggested that endotoxin shock may act at the cell membrane of the myocardial fiber to reduce the amount of $Ca^{2+}$ released from superficial sites upon cellular depolarization. Parker and Adams (1981b) presented functional evidence suggesting that superficial $Ca^{2+}$ stores of the cardiac sarcolemma may be an important target site in the endotoxin-shocked guinea pig. Atrial muscles from shocked animals demonstrated increased sensitivity and prolonged recovery from the negative inotropic actions of $Mn^{2+}$ (thought to compete with $Ca^{2+}$ at outer SL sites), gentamicin (a SL $Ca^{2+}$ channel antagonist), and low $Ca^{2+}$ medium. However, companion studies with D-600, nifedipine, and slow $Ca^{2+}$ channel-activation techniques (Parker and Adams, 1981b) suggested $Ca^{2+}$ channels remained operative in this shock model. In contrast, Zhong et al. (1997b) used the whole-cell patch clamp method to examine L-type $Ca^{2+}$ current density more directly in guinea pig ventricular myocytes from this same in vivo model of endotoxemia. Their data indicate that L-type $Ca^{2+}$ channel activity is reduced in myocytes after in vivo endotoxin exposure (peak $I_{CaL}$: 3.5 ± 0.2 pA/pF, LPS; 6.1 ± 0.3 pA/pF, control). Reduced $Ca^{2+}$ currents of LPS myocytes could not be attributed to alterations in current–voltage relationships, steady-state activation or inactivation, or recovery from inactivation. The $Ca^{2+}$ channel agonist BayK 8644 increased $Ca^{2+}$ current density in both control and LPS myocytes, but currents of LPS cells remained significantly less than control at all BayK 8644 concentrations. These data suggest endotoxemia may reduce $Ca^{2+}$ channel numbers. In fact, decreased dihydropyridine binding to a crude SL preparation of endotoxemic rabbit hearts has been reported previously (Lew et al., 1996). However, Zhong et al. (1997b) were able to surmount depressed $Ca^{2+}$ currents, systolic $Ca^{2+}$ transients (measured by fura-2) and cell shortening with the β-adrenergic agonist isoproterenol. Thus, it appears as though $Ca^{2+}$ channel content is normal in guinea pig LPS myocytes, but that channels may exist in a gated mode less available for opening (Herzig et al., 1993; Hirano et al., 1994). Yang and co-workers (1996) presented evidence that cardiac dihydropyridine receptors can move between a distinct, light vesicle fraction and the SL in a rat CLP model, although movement between these pools appeared not to be phosphorylation dependent. Similar translocation of dihydropyridine receptors has been reported in ischemic myocardium (Zucchi et al., 1995) and may reflect a common pathway for cardiac dysfunctions involving sarcolemmal integrity.

The SL Na–Ca exchanger facilitates the transmembrane movement of $Ca^{2+}$ using the energy of an oppositely directed $Na^+$ gradient. The operation and direction of exchange can be affected by membrane potential and other interventions (Reeves and Hale, 1984). Alterations in Na–Ca exchange of the cardiac myocyte could potentially affect $Ca^{2+}$ regulation during both systole and diastole (Reeves, 1985), and the exchanger system has been proposed as a target during certain pathophysiologic insults such as ischemia, reperfusion injury, and endotoxin shock (Bershon et al., 1982; Liu and Xuan, 1986; Hale et al., 1989). Liu and Xuan (1986) reported that Na–Ca exchange in cardiac SL vesicles from endotoxin-shocked dogs exhibited decreased activity and altered stoichiometry from 3 $Na^+$ per $Ca^{2+}$ (Reeves and Hale, 1984) to 2 $Na^+$ per $Ca^{2+}$. In contrast, Hale et al. (1989) evaluated activity and stoichiometry of Na–Ca exchange using the thermodynamic approach of Reeves and Hale (1984). These studies suggested that cardiac SL Na–Ca exchange activity was not altered in canine endotoxin shock and that the exchange process remained electrogenic with a stoichiometry of 3 $Na^+$ per $Ca^{2+}$

(Hale *et al.*, 1989). These studies were supported by those of Kutsky and Parker (1990), with SL membrane vesicles prepared from a guinea pig endotoxin shock model. Calcium pump activity (energy-dependent $Ca^{2+}$ uptake) was similar in sarcolemma from control and shock animals, and no intrinsic alteration in the rate or equilibrium $Ca^{2+}$ concentration of Na–Ca exchange was observed. The electrogenic nature of the exchanger was maintained, suggesting that the stoichiometry was greater than 2 $Na^+$ per $Ca^{2+}$ (Kutsky and Parker, 1990), results supporting the findings of Hale *et al.* (1989). Because Na–Ca exchange and other $Ca^{2+}$-binding characteristics of the sarcolemma could be affected by changes in cardiac phospholipids, Hale *et al.* (1990) evaluated cardiac sarcolemmal phospholipid profiles of hearts isolated from a guinea pig endotoxin shock model characterized by marked functional depression of the LV myocardium and altered responsiveness to $Ca^{2+}$-dependent inotropic interventions acting at SL sites (Parker and Adams, 1981b; Parker, 1983). However, Hale *et al.* (1990) reported that cardiac SL phospholipid levels (measured by high-performance liquid chromatography) of phosphatidylethanolamine, phosphatidylcholine, and sphingomyelin were unaltered by endotoxemia when compared with sarcolemma from control subjects.

## Mediators of myocardial toxicity of LPS and sepsis

The etiologic mechanisms and pathways that couple complex systemic syndromes such as endotoxemia with intrinsic dysfunction of heart muscle remain elusive. A direct action of the endotoxin molecule itself to elicit the complex alterations in diastolic and systolic function seems unlikely. Rather, the endotoxemic syndrome affects the heart through more complex mechanistic pathways involving multiple mediators and mediator pathways. The multiplicity and temporal complexity of cellular mediator responses to an endotoxemic challenge has confounded efforts to ascribe causality to any single mediator or factor. Over the years, considerable effort has been directed at defining a role for circulating myocardial depressant peptides, endogenous opiates, hematologic factors, free radicals, eicosanoids, cytokines, and nitric oxide. Maldistribution of blood flow, either global or regional, has also received considerable attention (for complete compilation, see Parker and Adams, 1981a, 1985a; Parker and Jones, 1988; Cunnion and Parrillo, 1989a; Adams *et al.*, 1990; Parrillo, 1990a,b), but appears not to be a necessary prerequisite for the cardiodynamic complications of endotoxemia or sepsis (Cunnion *et al.*, 1986; McDonough *et al.*, 1986; Laughlin *et al.*, 1988; Cunnion and Parrillo, 1989a; Adams *et al.*, 1990; Parrillo, 1990a,b; Danner *et al.*, 1991; Snell and Parrillo, 1991). The reader is referred to Adams and colleagues (1990) for a comprehensive review of the role of myocardial ischemia in endotoxin syndromes. This review will focus on the role of autocrine and paracrine cellular "mediators" in eliciting the myocardial functional derangements associated with endotoxemia. Importantly, it is expected that developing and currently ongoing studies using selected knock-out mouse models and new molecular approaches (e.g. microarray genomic and proteomic analysis) will yield exciting new information in the near future regarding this issue.

### Circulating cardiodepressant toxins

The potential deleterious role of bloodborne substances which depress cardiac function in shock has been the basis of numerous publications for over two decades. One of the earliest described of these substances was designated myocardial depressant factor (MDF). This term was first used by Brand and Lefer (1966) and Baxter *et al.* (1966), working in independent laboratories, to describe the cardioinhibitory factors found in the plasma of cats in hemorrhagic shock and dogs in burn shock respectively. Since then, extensive studies have attempted to characterize the chemical and biologic properties of MDF, as well as other toxic factors purported to influence cardiac function in shock (Lefer, 1978; Parker and Adams, 1981a). For instance, contractile activity of cultured rat heart cells was shown to be depressed by sera from endotoxin-shocked rats (Carli *et al.*, 1981) or septic shock patients (Carli *et al.*, 1978, 1979). Indeed, cardioinhibitory substances have been reported to be present in endotoxin, hemorrhagic, cardiogenic, splanchnic ischemic, traumatic, and burn shock, and in many species including man, baboons, dogs, rats, cats, and guinea pigs. However, neither the chemical structure nor the precise myocardial cellular action of MDF has been identified.

The formation and subsequent release into the circulation of cardiotoxic factors in shock was postulated by many investigators to be intimately related to splanchnic ischemia (Wangensteen *et al.*, 1971; Beardsley and Lefer, 1974; Lefer and Spath, 1974; Lundgren *et al.*, 1976; Haglund and Lundgren, 1978; Lefer, 1979, 1987). Indeed, intestinal venous plasma obtained from animals experiencing simulated intestinal shock (Wangensteen *et al.*, 1971; Haglund and Lundgren, 1978) and splanchnic artery occlusion (Beardsley and Lefer, 1974) was shown to reduce contractility of isolated papillary muscles and perfused heart preparations. Systemic hypotension often develops as the shock state progresses and elicits hemodynamic processes which result in pancreatic and splanchnic hypoperfusion. Ischemia of the pancreas in shock was reported to be more intense than that in other splanchnic organs (Lefer and Spath, 1977), and resultant deleterious consequences of pancreatic hypoperfusion was suggested to play a major role in subsequent production of toxic factors (Lefer and Spath, 1977). Furthermore, in addition to its cardiotoxic effect, MDF was also thought to exert indirect positive feedback actions (coronary and splanchnic vasoconstriction, reticuloendothelial depression) which would further undermine circulatory dysfunction in shock.

Lefer (1987) reviewed the pathophysiology and biologic actions of MDF in shock, with particular relevance to direct and indirect interactions of MDF with other mediators. Foremost among the vasoconstrictor mediators that promote the formation or actions of MDF are believed to be eicosanoids and other lipids such as platelet-activating factor. All of the eicosanoids proposed are essentially free of direct negative inotropic activity at concentrations similar to those observed in shock (Lefer, 1987); platelet-activating factor, however, can exert direct depression of myocardial contractility (Lefer, 1987; Stahl and Lefer, 1987). As MDF is produced, its pathophysiologic effects may promote the continued production and actions of such lipid mediators. A variety of pharmacologic agents has been reported to prevent MDF formation and exert beneficial actions during shock, including angiotensin-converting enzyme inhibitors, angiotensin receptor antagonists, thromboxane antagonists, lipoxygenase inhibitors, leukotriene receptor antagonists, and calcium channel blockers (for a review, see Lefer 1987).

The findings described above are consistent with the hypothesis that circulating depressant factors are a common denominator producing cardiac depression in many forms of shock. However, none of these factors has been characterized in precise molecular terms, and it remains unknown whether they represent identical or unrelated substances (Lefer, 1978, 1979). The presence, and putative pathologic role, of these substances in shock has been questioned by other investigators (Hinshaw *et al.*, 1971a,b, 1972a,b, 1974a,b; Hinshaw, 1974; Archer *et al.*, 1975; Hess *et al.*, 1981a; Parker and Adams, 1981a; Archer, 1985). Certainly, the inability to isolate, purify, identify, and characterize fully a specific shock-induced cardiodepressant substance has played a principal role in the lack of general acceptance of the circulating cardiotoxic hypothesis in shock. Although a circulating myocardial depressant substance has been reported by Parrillo *et al.* (1985) in human septic shock, defining the relationship between such factors and prognosis will require better understanding of both its structure and function.

### *Free radical-induced myocardial injury*

Free radical interactions have been implicated in a large number of disease states, including inflammation, radiation injury, ischemia, and, more recently, circulatory shock. Much evidence indicates that irreversible cellular damage may be produced by the action of oxygen-derived radicals and intermediates such as superoxide anion, $O_2^-$; hydroxyl radical, OH; hydrogen peroxide, $H_2O_2$; and singlet oxygen (Del Maestro, 1980). Free radicals have been shown in a variety of tissues to produce endothelial damage (Sacks *et al.*, 1978; Kontos *et al.*, 1984), vasodilation (Rosenblum, 1983), epithelial lifting (Parks *et al.*, 1982), lysosomal disruption (Fong *et al.*, 1973), phospholipid membrane lysis (Mead, 1976; Lynch and Fridovich, 1978), damaged mitochondria (Del Maestro, 1980), increased vascular permeability (Demopoulos *et al.*, 1980), and disrupted $Ca^{2+}$ transport of cardiac sarcoplasmic reticulum (Hess *et al.*, 1981b; Manson and Hess, 1983). The role of these highly reactive activated metabolites of oxygen in the pathogenesis of myocardial ischemia and shock has been investigated in a number of model systems.

Oxygen radicals can be generated by a variety of biologic reactions. Most of these reactions result in the production of one- ($O_2^-$), two- ($H_2O_2$), or three-electron (OH·) reduction of oxygen. A group of cellular enzymes involved in catalyzing oxidation reactions (e.g. xanthine oxidase, glycolate oxidase) result in univalent or divalent reduction of $O_2$ (Del Maestro, 1980). Activation of polymorphonuclear leukocytes (PMNs) causes release of oxygen free radicals [via nicotinamide adenine dinucleotide phosphate (NADPH) oxidase], lysosomal enzymes, and arachidonic acid derivatives which are capable of generating oxygen free radicals (Del Maestro, 1980; Kuehl et al., 1980; Hess and Manson, 1983; Rowe et al., 1983). Free radicals produced by such systems are highly energetic and reactive; cellular viability and protection crucially depend on their effective removal and control. Under normal conditions, various endogenous enzymatic mechanisms (e.g. superoxide dismutase, catalase, peroxidase) and other scavenging processes effectively operate to remove oxygen radicals (Del Maestro, 1980). Imbalances in these interrelationships can produce profound biochemical alterations (Del Maestro, 1980). Numerous studies have provided evidence suggesting that free radical interactions may be involved in the damage observed in hypoxic and ischemic myocardium (Loschen et al., 1974; Del Maestro, 1980; Guarnieri et al., 1980; Kuehl et al., 1980; Hess et al., 1981b; Lefer et al., 1981; Hess and Manson, 1983; Manson and Hess, 1983; Rowe et al., 1983). Del Maestro (1980) suggested that, during partial ischemia and shock, free radicals are generated intracellularly, particularly in mitochondria. There is evidence that the heart mitochondrial electron-transfer system may function as a generator of superoxide radicals when all the components on the substrate side of cytochrome $c$ are reduced; these may produce cellular damage when scavenging mechanisms are reduced, ineffective, or overwhelmed (Del Maestro, 1980).

Specific alterations in cardiac sarcoplasmic reticulum produced by oxygen free radicals have been previously investigated (Hess et al., 1981b; Hess and Manson, 1983; Manson and Hess, 1983). Alterations in subcellular $Ca^{2+}$ fluxes of sarcoplasmic reticulum have been described by this group in shock and myocardial ischemia, and have been implicated in contributing to depressed cardiac contractility and irreversibility in shock. The addition of an oxygen free radical-generating system (xanthine–xanthine oxidase) to isolated sarcoplasmic reticulum produced severe depression of both $Ca^{2+}$ uptake velocity and $Ca^{2+}$-adenosine triphosphatase (ATP) activity (Inoue et al., 1998); the depressed $Ca^{2+}$ uptake velocity remained depressed in the presence of acidosis (pH 6.4). Importantly, mannitol, a scavenger of the hydroxyl radical, and superoxide dismutase (SOD) restored the depressed $Ca^{2+}$ uptake velocity. Manson and Hess (1983) reported evidence that free radicals produced by activated leukocytes similarly depressed $Ca^{2+}$ uptake rates, and, furthermore, that this effect was reduced by catalase or SOD plus catalase. These authors have presented the concept that, as endotoxin is known to activate complement and lead to the production of complement components (C5a), the resulting C5a-activated leukocytes could release free radicals and potentially lead to the loss of contractility in cardiac muscle observed in septic shock. In this regard, Lefer et al. (1981) reported that the free radical scavenger MK-447 improved myocardial contractility in myocardial ischemia and traumatic shock. Other studies have not provided support for beneficial actions of free radical scavengers in endotoxin shock models, and this area remains a contentious issue relative to the putative role of reactive oxygen species in the cardiac toxicity of LPS (Traber *et al.*, 1985; Laughlin *et al.*, 1988; Novotny *et al.*, 1988; Parker *et al.*, 1991).

### Endothelial and other mediators

A multitude of endogenously released, endothelium-dependent vasoconstrictor and vasodilator agents have been implicated in endotoxemia and septic states, including vasoactive lipids [leukotrienes, prostaglandins, thromboxanes, and platelet-activating factor (PAF); for reviews, see Altura *et al.*, 1983; Lefer, 1985; Traber *et al.*, 1985; Ball *et al.*, 1986; Feuerstein and Hallenbeck, 1987; Sprague *et al.*, 1989; Ayala and Chaudry, 1996] and, more recently, endothelium-derived relaxing (nitric oxide) and contracting (endothelin) factors. The effects of many of these agents on the vasculature and other organ systems have been extensively documented (Lefer, 1987; Crespo and Fernández-Gallardo, 1991; Ayala and Chaudry, 1996; DeFily *et al.*, 1996), and they exert actions that may intensify or prolong the shock state (Zingarelli *et al.*, 1992; Koltai *et al.*, 1993). Direct actions of endothelium-derived mediators on the myocardium, independent of vascular alterations, also have been documented with considerable emphasis over the last 10 years relative to the negative inotropic effects of nitric oxide. A comprehensive discussion of the role of nitric oxide in endotoxemia or septic shock is beyond the scope of the current discussion. Rather, this chapter will attempt to emphasize studies which relate endothelial mediators to alterations in cardiac calcium homeostasis.

The phospholipid mediator PAF is released from endothelial cells, as well as inflammatory cells in response to multiple immune stimuli, and appears to be a major therapeutic target in ischemia reperfusion and immune-mediated cardiovascular injury (Schoonderwoerd and Stam, 1992; Ayala and Chaudry, 1996; Oh, 1998). Infusion of PAF reduced cardiac output and contractility in anesthetized dogs (Gupta *et al.*, 1994; Tamura *et al.*, 1997) which could be blocked by the PAF antagonist CV-6209 (Gupta *et al.*, 1994). In isolated heart models, PAF has been shown to decrease contractile force and cause coronary constriction (Stahl and Lefer, 1987; Giessler *et al.*, 1995). Coronary artery constriction was prevented by the LTD$_4$ antagonist LY-171,883 (Stahl and Lefer, 1987) or indomethacin (Giessler *et al.*, 1995). These and other data suggest that PAF exerts effects on coronary function through release of additional vasoactive mediators. Interestingly, thromboxane and cyclooxygenase antagonists were less effective at blocking the negative inotropic response to PAF, suggesting PAF also may have direct effects on cardiac muscle. In fact, incubation of isolated adult or neonatal rat cardiac myocytes in PAF decreased contractile amplitude and velocity (Massey *et al.*, 1991; Delbridge *et al.*, 1994) and stimulated hydrolysis of inositol phospholipids (Massey *et al.*, 1991). Pietsch and co-workers (1998) further demonstrated that the PAF-elicited decrease in contractile amplitude of adult rat myocytes correlated with decreased intracellular $Ca^{2+}$ transients. The mechanism for PAF-induced changes in either contractility or cell [$Ca^{2+}$] may be complex, however, because PAF also stimulates L-type $Ca^{2+}$ currents of human cardiac myocytes (Bkaily *et al.*, 1996). Furthermore, the possibility remains that PAF exerts effects on cardiomyocytes via stimulated release of negative inotropic autocrine factors such as nitric oxide (Alloatti *et al.*, 1999) or additional lipid-derived mediators (Giessler *et al.*, 1995).

The role of PAF in endotoxemic/sepsis-induced cardiac failure has been difficult to evaluate because of the obvious multiplicity of PAF actions within multiple organ systems in conjunction with PAF-induced vascular control abnormalities. For example, although pretreatment with PAF receptor antagonists improved cardiovascular function of non-hypotensive endotoxemic pigs (Abu-Zidan and Walther, 1996) and increased cardiac output of endotoxin-treated rats (Ebara *et al.*, 1996), tachycardia was not improved (Ebara *et al.*, 1996). Furthermore, administration of PAF, either *in vivo* or *in vitro*, also failed to mimic the cardiovascular derangements associated with endotoxemia (Muñoz *et al.*, 1995; Wang *et al.*, 1997).

Without a doubt, the most renowned of the endothelial mediators significant in the pathogenesis of sepsis and shock is nitric oxide. Over the past decade, nitric oxide has been identified as a primary endothelium-derived relaxing factor, stimulating vascular smooth muscle relaxation. However, in addition to endothelial production of nitric oxide, it is now clear that multiple cells posses the ability to synthesize nitric oxide under physiologic or pathophysiologic conditions; these include immune cells (Klostergaard *et al.*, 1991; Förstermann *et al.*, 1992; Vanin *et al.*, 1993), smooth muscle (Koide *et al.*, 1993; Nunokawa *et al.*, 1993; Geng *et al.*, 1994), fibroblasts (Shindo *et al.*, 1994), neurons (Moreland, 1994), mesangial cells (Pfeilschifter *et al.*, 1992), and cardiac myocytes (for reviews, see Ungureanu-Longrois *et al.*, 1995b; Corda *et al.*, 1998; Parratt, 1998; Kojda and Kottenberg, 1999).

At least four isoforms of nitric oxide synthase (NOS), the enzyme responsible for nitric oxide production, have been identified (Pollock *et al.*, 1992; Förstermann *et al.*, 1993, 1994a,b; Nakane *et al.*, 1995), and multiple co-factors and regulatory sites have been defined. The physiologic and pathophysiologic significance of nitric oxide can be gleamed by the extensive number of reviews focused on this small molecule. As a starting point, the reader is directed to several recent reviews on this topic (Broillet, 1999; Fleming and Busse, 1999; Lane and Gross, 1999; Moncada, 1999; Murphy, 1999).

Changes in activity and expression of NOS isoforms, particularly induction of the $Ca^{2+}$-independent NOS isoform (iNOS) with corresponding elevations in synthesis of nitric oxide, is a hallmark of sepsis and endotoxemic shock states. Nitric oxide has profound effects on vascular reactivity and multiple organ function (Parratt, 1998; Kirkeboen and Strand, 1999; Symeonides and Balk, 1999; Titheradge, 1999), including that of the heart (for reviews, see Kojda and Kottenberg, 1999; Stoclet *et al.*, 1999). *In vivo*, endotoxemia stimulates expression of iNOS mRNA (Bateson *et al.*, 1996; Liu *et al.*, 1996; Nagasaki *et al.*, 1996) measured from ventricular extracts. Although these extracts also contained iNOS derived from endothelium and vascular smooth muscle (tissues which also express iNOS), iNOS expression was subsequently demonstrated in isolated adult rat ventricular myocytes following *in vitro* treatment with a cytokine cocktail of tumor necrosis factor-$\alpha$ (TNF-$\alpha$) and interleukin-1$\beta$ (IL-1$\beta$) (Schulz *et al.*, 1992; Balligand *et al.*, 1994). The time-course for expression of iNOS mRNA in these cells was 6 h after stimulation with the cytokine mixture (Balligand *et al.*, 1994). It is noteworthy that, in this same study, LPS itself was ineffective at induction of iNOS even when depyrogenated isolation conditions were employed. In contrast, LPS alone appears to be a very effective iNOS inducer in neonatal rat cardiac myocytes (Kinugawa *et al.*, 1997a,b). Using a porphyrinic microsensor, Balligand and co-workers (1994) were able to measure nitric oxide production from individual cytokine-stimulated adult rat cardiac myocytes following addition of L-arginine to the medium. Demonstration of NO production from these cells was a significant finding because induction of NOS mRNA by cytokine treatment does not always translate into functional NOS protein. Luss *et al.* (1997) demonstrated that dedifferentiated adult human cardiac myocytes were unable to translate mRNA for iNOS into protein even after 96 h of cytokine and LPS treatment.

The possibility that cardiac myocytes produce nitric oxide as a paracrine regulatory molecule during endotoxemia and sepsis prompted considerable investigation into the role of nitric oxide in shock-induced cardiac dysfunction. To be considered a mediator of endotoxin-induced negative inotropy, not only must nitric oxide synthesis be established but also nitric oxide itself should mimic the negative inotropy observed during endotoxemia. Moreover, inhibition of nitric oxide synthesis should restore normal function to the endotoxemic heart. In reference to the last point, in several cases cardiac production of nitric oxide has been inferred from data demonstrating improved function following treatment with NOS inhibitors. Brady *et al.* (1992) first demonstrated that the NOS inhibitor $N^{\omega}$–nitro-L-arginine methyl ester (L-NAME) improved contractile performance of ventricular myocytes isolated from *in vivo* endotoxin-treated guinea pigs. In this study, electrically stimulated myocytes from endotoxemic animals shortened 3 percent of cell length. This value increased to 4.3 percent following treatment of myocytes with L-NAME (100 $\mu$M). Control myocytes stimulated at the same frequency (0.5 Hz) shortened 5 percent of cell length. Using the same guinea pig model of endotoxemia, Decking *et al.* (1995) could not detect a beneficial effect of either L-NAME or $N$-G-monomethyl-L-arginine (L-NMMA) on left ventricular pressures (LVP) of Langendorff perfused hearts. Although NOS inhibition had no effect on ventricular function, both inhibitors significantly increased coronary resistance of both control and LPS hearts. Klabunde and Coston (1995) examined left ventricular function of rat hearts 6 h following administration of endotoxin and also observed no improvement in ventricular function with the NOS inhibitors, nitro-L-arginine or aminoguanidine even when the inhibitor was administered prior to endotoxin.

Keller and co-workers (1995) re-evaluated the ability of NOS inhibition to improve function of both isolated left atria and ventricular myocytes from the guinea pig model of endotoxemia also used by Decking *et al.* (1995) and Brady *et al.* (1992). In this study, NOS inhibition (L-NAME) did not improve depressed contractile tension of isolated left atria from endotoxemic animals at stimulation frequencies from 0.2 to 3.0 Hz, even when excess L-arginine was administered. Furthermore, in contrast to the results of Brady and co-workers (1992), neither L-NAME, L-NMMA, nor aminoguanidine (each at 100 μM) improved cell shortening of endotoxemic myocytes (LPS, 7.2 ± 2 percent; LPS + L-NAME, 6.9 ± 1 percent; LPS + L-NMMA, 6.8 ± 12; LPS + aminoguanidine, 7.5 ± 6 percent). NOS inhibitors were equally ineffective at changing control myocyte shortening, which remained near 11.8 ± 4 percent. Contradictions between these studies are difficult to reconcile as the only reported differences in methodology are the temperature at which the myocytes were studied (30°C in Brady *et al.*, 1992; 22°C in Keller *et al.*, 1995) and slight differences in enzymatic isolation. The higher temperature in the former study is reflected in the relatively small percent cell shortening of these myocytes (5 percent for controls) compared with studies conducted at room temperature (11 percent for controls).

Although NOS inhibitors were ineffective at improving contractile function of ventricular myocytes in the study by Keller *et al.* (1995), the β-adrenergic agonist isoproterenol significantly increased cell shortening such that differences between control and LPS myocytes were no longer evident when both groups were exposed to isoproterenol. The functional response of endotoxemic guinea pig myocytes to β-agonists argues against a role for nitric oxide in cardiac depression of this animal model. There is compelling evidence for nitric oxide inhibition of β-adrenergic receptor function from work with cytokine-treated myocytes (Balligand *et al.*, 1994), myocytes exposed to macrophage-conditioned medium (Balligand *et al.*, 1993; Joe *et al.*, 1998), myocytes co-cultured with cytokine-treated endothelial cells (Ungureanu-Longrois *et al.*, 1995a), and papillary muscle exposed to cytokines (Sun *et al.*, 1998). Although it appears that nitric oxide reduces the inotropic effectiveness of β-receptor stimulation in each of these studies, basal contractile activity was usually unaltered even after 24 h exposure to cytokine or conditioned medium (Balligand *et al.*, 1993; Ungureanu-Longrois *et al.*, 1995a).

Assuming that elevated levels of nitric oxide and/or cytokines are involved in the negative inotropic response of the endotoxemic myocardium, a significant literature has emerged relative to the mechanism of nitric oxide-induced changes in cell and subcellular function. Similar to its effect on vascular and other tissues (Bredt and Snyder, 1994; McDonald and Murad, 1996), nitric oxide appears to stimulate a soluble guanylyl cyclase in the myocardium, resulting in elevated levels of the second messenger cyclic GMP. Activation of soluble guanylyl cyclase has been interpreted from data demonstrating increased cyclic GMP in cardiac tissues or cells following treatment with nitric oxide donors (Flesch *et al.*, 1997), lipopolysaccharide (Shindo *et al.*, 1994), or cytokines (Schulz *et al.*, 1992; Shindo *et al.*, 1994). Furthermore, in some (Brady *et al.*, 1992) but not all (Keller *et al.*,

1995) studies, methylene blue, an inhibitor of soluble guanylyl cyclase, improved contractile function of myocytes from endotoxemic animals.

Although increases in cyclic GMP are highly correlated with increased nitric oxide production or use of nitric oxide donors, the connections between cyclic GMP and negative inotropic and chronotropic effects are less tightly associated. For example, cyclic GMP-dependent inhibition of $I_{CaL}$ remains controversial because of multiple cellular sites of cyclic GMP and protein kinase G action. Levi and co-workers (1994) enhanced guinea pig ventricular myocyte $I_{CaL}$ with 3-isobutyl-1-methylxanthine (IBMX), a phosphodiesterase inhibitor, and the enhancement could be reduced by including cyclic GMP in the pipette solution. Sodium nitroprusside also reduced the enhancement and its effect could be blocked by methylene blue, suggesting activation of a soluble guanylyl cyclase inhibited $I_{CaL}$. In this study, neither methylene blue nor sodium nitroprusside had any effect on basal $I_{CaL}$, suggesting dependence on prior activation by cAMP and PKA. Balligand *et al.* (1995) subsequently showed that NOS inhibitors could relieve muscarinic receptor inhibition of β-adrenergic receptor enhancement of $I_{CaL}$. These data are consistent with a negative inotropic effect of nitric oxide on β-adrenergic receptor actions with little or no effect on basal contractility.

More recently, Gallo *et al.* (1998) demonstrated a direct enhancement of $I_{CaL}$ by NOS inhibition in the absence of β-adrenergic receptor activation in guinea pig ventricular myocytes. Increased $I_{CaL}$ was blocked by pipette perfusion with cyclic GMP. In contrast, Vandecasteele and colleagues (1998) observed no effect of NOS inhibition on $I_{CaL}$ of human atrial myocytes. Furthermore, this study showed increased $I_{CaL}$ with the nitric oxide donor S-nitroso-*N*-acetylpenicillamine (SNAP), while inhibition of guanylyl cyclase failed to modify either β-adrenergic receptor stimulation of $I_{CaL}$ or muscarinic inhibition of the β-adrenergic receptor stimulation.

MacDonell and Diamond (1997) invoked muscarinic receptor-dependent negative inotropy of isoproterenol-treated ventricular strip but saw no change in cyclic GMP, suggesting that cyclic GMP is not necessary for this negative response. Along the same line, they induced large increases in cyclic GMP with sodium nitroprusside or atrial natriuretic peptide, but could not induce a negative inotropic response in either isoproterenol-perfused hearts or isolated myocytes. Controversy regarding the role of cyclic GMP as a mediator for nitric oxide actions is destined to continue because of the multiplicity of actions of cyclic GMP. Cyclic GMP not only activates protein kinase G, but also in many tissues, including the heart and vascular system, regulates the activity of cAMP-dependent phosphodiesterases (Fischmeister and Shrier, 1989; Mery *et al.*, 1993). Thus, it is possible that increases in cyclic GMP mediate effects on the heart through regulation of cyclic AMP-dependent protein kinase activity (Cornwell *et al.*, 1994).

Although the focus of nitric oxide research has been for the most part centered on its role as an activator of soluble guanylyl cyclase, it should be recognized that nitric oxide may alter cardiac function during shock states through other mechanisms. For example, nitric oxide inhibits neutrophil adhesion to both vascular endothelium and cytokine-stimulated cardiac myocytes, thus preventing the cardiotoxic effects associated with adhesion (Ohashi *et al.*, 1997). In addition, nitric oxide itself may have direct effects on signaling pathways which regulate $Ca^{2+}$ homeostasis and cell contraction (Vila-Petroff *et al.*, 1999). The nitric oxide donor SNAP inhibited L-type $Ca^{2+}$ channel currents in HEK293 cells (Hu *et al.*, 1997). Inhibition was not prevented by methylene blue nor mimicked by 8-Br-cyclic GMP, suggesting that inhibition was independent of cyclic GMP. Mechanisms suggested for such direct effects of nitric oxide include nitrosylation of tyrosine residues (Kooy *et al.*, 1997) or formation of peroxynitrite through combination with superoxide radical (Lopez *et al.*, 1997; Schulz *et al.*, 1997; Oyama *et al.*, 1998), both of which have been implicated in cardiac dysfunction including that associated with endotoxemia and inflammation. In spite of the plethora of information on nitric oxide, on cyclic GMP and on cellular targets of each, a clear understanding of their role in endotoxin- or sepsis-induced cardiac failure remains elusive. The multiplicity of actions of nitric oxide within the myocardium, both physiologic and pathophysiologic, as well as secondary interactions due to modulation of immune or vascular tissues should feed the research fires in this field for many decades to come.

## Conclusion and implications

Sufficient clinical and experimental data are now available to assemble a consensus that LV contraction–relaxation mechanisms intrinsic to heart muscle itself are indeed disordered during endotoxemic and septicemic syndromes. Evidence from studies with isolated hearts indicate that endotoxin-induced cardiodynamic changes present as reduced myocardial contractility (lowered isovolumic LV $+\mathrm{d}P/\mathrm{d}t_{max}$), impaired relaxation during early diastole (reduced isovolumic LV $-\mathrm{d}P/\mathrm{d}t_{max}$), reduced chamber compliance or distensibility during late diastole, and reduced LV stroke volume and cardiac output. In the intact subject, these changes would result in impaired filling of the ventricles during diastole as well as reduced ejection during systole.

Intrinsic cardiac dysfunction in shock may be masked in intact subjects by compensatory activation of endogenous cardiostimulants such as catecholamines or, also importantly, by therapeutic interventions. Indeed, intravascular volume expansion markedly alters manifestation of intrinsic systolic and diastolic defects during shock. Shock-induced dysfunctional hearts can still respond to increases in end-diastolic sarcomere length; intravascular volume loading can thereby provide the depressed heart with adequate preload to maintain stroke volume at near-normal values although ejection fraction can remain subnormal. Intravascular volume expansion evokes an apparent compensatory dilation of the heart during shock, thereby contributing to maintenance of stroke volume, although reduced ejection fractions still identify the intrinsically dysfunctional heart. Thus, *in situ* measurements either of stroke volume index or cardiac index alone may not accurately sample for altered heart function in septic shock patients.

Finally, clinical and experimental studies have indicated that inadequate myocardial blood flows are not necessary prerequisites for cardiac sequelae of endotoxemic and septicemic shock. Certainly, inadequate myocardial perfusion is likely to be an important confounding influence in those subsets of shock patients with pre-existing ischemic (coronary artery) heart disease. Also, when the systemic hypotensive state becomes severe enough to limit coronary vascular autoregulation, then myocardial malperfusion and ischemia may contribute to and exacerbate the cardiac changes already under way. Irrespective, the fact remains that direct or indirect evidence of cardiac mechanical dysfunction can develop in LPS and sepsis syndromes while total coronary blood flow, myocardial subendocardial/ subepicardial blood flow ratios, and LV concentrations of high-energy phosphates remain normal and adequate for the reduced workload imposed on the heart. The pathogenesis of intrinsic cardiac injury during endotoxemia and septicemia, although not requiring global myocardial ischemia as an obligatory etiologic factor, remains to be delineated. Recent development of exciting new molecular approaches (genomic and proteomic analysis in human patients and animal models) and technologic advances are likely to provide new insight into mediators and mechanisms underlying myocardial dysfunction in sepsis/shock states.

## References

Abel, F.L. 1989. Myocardial function in sepsis and endotoxin shock. *American Journal of Physiology* 257, R1265–R1281.

Abel, F.L. 1990. Does the heart fail in endotoxin shock? *Circulatory Shock* 30, 5–13.

Abel, F.L. and Beck, R.R. 1988. Canine peripheral vascular response to endotoxin shock at constant cardiac output. *Circulatory Shock* 2225, 267–274.

Abel, F.L. and Kessler, D.P. 1973. Myocardial performance in hemorrhagic shock in the dog and primate. *Circulation Research* 32, 492–500.

Abel, F.L., Sutherland, A.E., and Haleby, K. 1972. Comparative measurements of left-ventricular performance produced by rapid changes in blood volume in dogs. *Annals of Biomedical Engineering* 1, 9–22.

Abel, F.L., Kroesl, P, Redl, H., and Kropik, K. 2000. Myocardial depression after endotoxin in awake sheep. *Shock* 13, 11.

Abu-Zidan, F.M. and Walther, S. 1996. Platelet activating factor antagonism improves cardiovascular function in non-hypotensive sepsis in pigs. *European Journal of Surgery* 162, 499–504.

Adams, H.R., Baxter, C.R., Parker, J.L., and Watts, N.B. 1984. Contractile function and rhythmicity of cardiac preparations from *Escherichia coli* endotoxin-shocked guinea pigs. *Circulatory Shock* 13, 241–253.

Adams, H.R., Izenberg, S.D., and Baxter, C.R. 1985a. Adrenergic aspects of endotoxin shock. In: *Handbook of Endotoxin: Pathophysiology of Endotoxin*. Hindshaw, L.B. (ed.), pp. 145–172. Elsevier Press, Amsterdam.

Adams, H.R., Baxter, C.R., and Parker, J.L. 1985b. Reduction of intrinsic contractile reserves of the left ventricle by *Escherichia coli* endotoxin shock in guinea pigs. *Journal of Molecular and Cellular Cardiology* 17, 575–585.

Adams, H.R., Parker, J.L., and Laughlin, M.H. 1990. Intrinsic myocardial dysfunction during endotoxemia: dependent or independent of myocardial ischemia? *Circulatory Shock* 30, 63–76.

Alloatti, G., Penna, C., De Martino, A., *et al.* 1999. Role of nitric oxide and platelet-activating factor in cardiac alterations induced by tumor necrosis factor-alpha in the guinea-pig papillary muscle. *Cardiovascular Research* 41, 611–619.

Altura, B.M., Lefer, A.M., and Schumer, W. 1983. Role of prostaglandins and thromboxanes in shock states. In: *Handbook of Shock and Trauma*, Vol. 1. *Basic Science*. Altura, B.M., Lefer, A.M., and Schumer, W. (eds), pp. 355–376. Raven Press, New York.

Archer, L.T. 1985. Myocardial dysfunction in endotoxin and *E. coli*-induced shock: pathophysiological mechanisms. *Circulatory Shock* 15, 261–280.

Archer, L.T., Black, M.R., and Hinshaw, L.B. 1975. Myocardial failure with altered response to adrenaline in endotoxin shock. *British Journal of Pharmacology* 54, 145–155.

Archer, L.T., Benjamin, B.A., Beller-Todd, B.K., *et al.* 1982. Does LD$_{100}$ *E. coli* shock cause myocardial failure? *Circulatory Shock* 9, 7–16.

Ayala A. and Chaudry, I.H. 1996. Platelet activating factor and its role in trauma, shock, and sepsis. *New Horizons* 4, 265–275.

Ball, H.A., Cook, J.A., Wise, W.C., and Halushka, P.V. 1986. Role of thromboxane, prostaglandins, and leukotrienes in endotoxic and septic shock. *Intensive Care Medicine* 12, 116–126.

Balligand, J.-L., Ungureanu, D., Kelly, R.A., *et al.* 1993. Abnormal contractile function due to induction of nitric oxide synthesis in rat cardiac myocytes follows exposure to activated macrophage-conditioned medium. *Journal of Clinical Investigation* 91, 2314–2319.

Balligand, J.-L., Ungureanu-Longrois, D., Simmons, W.W., *et al.* 1994. Cytokine-inducible nitric oxide synthase (iNOS) expression in cardiac myocytes. Characterization and regulation of iNOS expression and detection of iNOS activity in single cardiac myocytes *in vitro*. *Journal of Biological Chemistry* 269, 27580–27588.

Balligand, J.-L., Kobzik, L., Han, X., *et al.* 1995. Nitric oxide-dependent parasympathetic signaling is due to activation of constitutive endothelial (type III) nitric oxide synthase in cardiac myocytes. *Journal of Biological Chemistry* 270, 14582–14586.

Barker, L.A., Winbery, S.L., Smith, L.W., and McDonough, K.H. 1989. Supersensitivity and changes in the active population of beta adrenoceptors in rat right atria in early sepsis. *Journal of Pharmacology and Experimental Therapeutics* 252, 675–682.

Bateson, A.N., Jakiwczyk, O.M., and Schulz, R. 1996. Rapid increase in inducible nitric oxide synthase gene expression in the heart during endotoxemia. *European Journal of Pharmacology* 303, 141–144.

Baxter, C.R., Cook, W.A., and Shires, G.T. 1966. Serum myocardial depressant factor of burn shock. *Surgical Forum* 17, 1–2.

Beardsley, A.C. and Lefer, A.M. 1974. Impairment of cardiac function after splanchnic artery occlusion shock. *Circulatory Shock* 1, 123–130.

Bell, H. and Thal, H. 1970. The peculiar hemodynamics of septic shock. *Postgraduate Medicine* 48, 106–118.

Bershon, M.M., Philipson, K.S., and Fukushima, J.Y. 1982. Sodium–calcium exchange and sarcolemmal enzymes in ischemic rabbit hearts. *American Journal of Physiology*, C288–C295.

Bhagat, B., Beaumont, M., Rawson, L., *et al.* 1974. Calcium metabolism and contractility of isolated cardiac muscle from endotoxin-treated guinea pig. In: *Recent Advances in Studies on Cardiac Structure and Metabolism*, Vol. 4. Dhalla, N.S. (ed.), pp. 305–328. University Park Press, Baltimore.

Bhagat, B., Rao, P.S., and Cavanagh, D. 1980. Contractility of endotoxic atria. In: *Advances in Myocardiology*, Vol. 2. Tajuddin, M., Bhatia, B., Siddiqui, H.H., and Rona, G. (eds), pp. 199–207. University Park Press, Baltimore.

Bkaily, G., Haddad, G., Jaalouk, D., *et al.* 1996. Modulation of $Ca^{2+}$ and $Na^+$ transport by taurine in heart and vascular smooth muscle. *Advances in Experimental Medicine and Biology* 403, 263–273.

Brady, A.J. 1991. Mechanical properties of isolated cardiac myocytes. *Physiological Reviews* 71, 413–428.

Brady, A.J.B., Poole-Wilson, P.A., Harding, S.E., and Warren, J.B. 1992. Nitric oxide production within cardiac myocytes reduces their contractility in endotoxemia. *American Journal of Physiology* 263, H1963–H1966.

Brand, E.D. and Lefer, A.M. 1966. Myocardial depressant factor in plasma from cats in irreversible postoligemic shock. *Proceedings of the Society for Experimental Biology and Medicine* 122, 200–203.

Bredt, D.S. and Snyder, S.H. 1994. Nitric oxide: A physiologic messenger molecule. *Annual Review of Biochemistry* 63, 175–195.

Brockman, S.K., Thomas, Jr., C.S. and Vasco, J.S. 1967. The effect of *Escherichia coli* endotoxin on the circulation. *Surgical Gynecology and Obstetrics* 125, 663–774.

Broillet, M.C. 1999. S-nitrosylation of proteins. *Cellular and Molecular Life Sciences* 55, 1036–1042.

Bruni, F.D., Komwatana, P., and Soulsbe, M.E. 1978. Endotoxin and myocardial failure: role of the myofibril. *American Journal of Physiology* 225, H150–H156.

Burns, A.H., Summer, W.R., Racey Burns, L.A., and Shepherd, R.E. 1988. Inotropic interactions of dichloroacetate with amrinone and ouabain in isolated hearts from endotoxin-shocked rats. *Journal of Cardiovascular Pharmacology* 11, 379–386.

Capasso, J.M., Li, P., and Anversa, P. 1993. Cytosolic calcium transients in myocytes isolated from rats with ischemic heart failure. *American Journal of Physiology* 265, H1953–H1964.

Carli, A., Auclair, M.C., and Bleichner, G. 1978. Inhibited response to isoproterenol and altered action potential of beating rat heart cells by human serum in septic shock. *Circulatory Shock* 5, 85–94.

Carli, A., Auclair, M.C., and Vernimmen, C. 1979. Reversal by calcium of rat heart cell dysfunction induced by human sera in septic shock. *Circulatory Shock* 6, 147–157.

Carli, A., Auclair, M.C., and Benassayag, C. 1981. Evidence for an early lipid soluble cardiodepressant factor in rat serum after a sublethal dose of endotoxin. *Circulatory Shock* 8, 301–312.

Cavanagh, D., Rao, P.S., and Sutton, D.M.C. 1970. Pathophysiology of endotoxin shock in the primate. *American Journal of Obstetrics and Gynecology* 108, 705–722.

Clowes, Jr., G.H.A. 1974. Pulmonary abnormalities in sepsis. *Surgical Clinics of North America* 54, 993–1002.

Clowes, Jr., G.H.A., O'Donnell, Jr., T.F., and Ryan, N.T. 1974. Energy metabolism in sepsis: treatment based on different patients in shock and high output stage. *Annals of Surgery* 179, 684–696.

Coalson, J.J., Hinshaw, L.B., and Guenter, C.A. 1975. Pathophysiologic responses of the sub-human primate in experimental septic shock. *Laboratory Investigation* 32, 561–569.

Coleman, B., Kallal, J.E., and Feigen, L.P. 1975. Myocardial performance during hemorrhagic shock in the pancreatectomized dog. *American Journal of Physiology* 228, 1462–1468.

Comstock, K.L., Krown, K.A., Page, M.T., *et al.* 1998. LPS-induced TNF-alpha release from and apoptosis in rat cardiomyocytes: obligatory role for CD14 in mediating the LPS response. *Journal of Molecular and Cellular Cardiology* 30, 2761–2775.

Corda, S., Mebazaa, A., Tavernier, B., *et al.*1998. Paracrine regulation of cardiac myocytes in normal and septic heart. *Journal of Critical Care* 13, 39–47.

Cornwell, T.L., Arnold, E., Boerth, N.J., and Lincoln, T.M. 1994. Inhibition of smooth muscle cell growth by nitric oxide and activation of cAMP-dependent protein kinase by cGMP. *American Journal of Physiology* 267, C1405–C1413.

Crespo, M.S. and Fernández-Gallardo, S. 1991. Pharmacological modulation of PAF: A therapeutic approach to endotoxin shock. *Journal of Lipid Mediators* 4, 127–144.

Cunnion, R.E. and Parrillo, J.E. 1989a. Myocardial dysfunction in sepsis: recent insights. *Chest* 95, 941–945.

Cunnion, R.E. and Parrillo, J.E. 1989b. Myocardial dysfunction in sepsis. *Critical Care Clinics* 5, 99–118.

Cunnion, R.E., Schaer, G.L., Parker, M.M., *et al.* 1986. The coronary circulation in human septic shock. *Circulation* 73, 637–644.

Danner, R.L., Elin, R.J., Hosseini, J.M., *et al.* 1991. Endotoxemia in human septic shock. *Chest* 99, 169–175.

David, D. and Rogel, S. 1976. Mechanical and humoral factors affecting cardiac function in shock. *Circulatory Shock* 3, 65–75.

DeBlieux, P.M.C., McDonough, K.H., Barbee, R.W., and Shepherd, R.E. 1989. Exercise training attenuates the myocardial dysfunction induced by endotoxin. *Journal of Applied Physiology* 66, 2805–2810.

Decking, U.K.M., Flesche, C.W., Gödecke, A., and Schrader, J. 1995. Endotoxin-induced contractile dysfunction in guinea pig hearts is not mediated by nitric oxide. *American Journal of Physiology* 268, H2460–H2465.

DeFily, D.V., Kuo, L., and Chilian, W.M. 1996. PAF attenuates endothelium-dependent coronary arteriolar vasodilation. *American Journal of Physiology* 270, H2094–H2099.

Delbridge, L.M., Stewart, A.G., Goulter, C.M., *et al.*1994. Platelet-activating factor and WEB-2086 directly modulate rat cardiomyocyte contractility. *Journal of Molecular and Cellular Cardiology* 26, 185–193.

Del Maestro, R.F. 1980. An approach to free radicals in medicine and biology. *Acta Physiologica Scandinavica* 492 (Suppl.), 153–168.

Demopoulos, H.B., Flamm, E.S., Pietronigro, D.D., *et al.* 1980. The free radical pathology and the microcirculation in the major central nervous system disorders. *Acta Physiologica Scandinavica* 492 (Suppl.), 91–119.

Dhainaut, J.F., Lanore, J.J., and de Gournay, J.M. 1988. Right ventricular dysfunction in patients with septic shock. *Intensive Care Medicine.* 14, 488–491.

Dhalla, N.S., Singh, J.N., and Fedelesova, M. 1974. Biochemical basis of heart function. XII. Sodium–potassium stimulated adenosine triphosphatase activity in the perfused rat heart made to fail by substrate lack. *Cardiovascular Research* 8, 227–236.

D'Orio, V., Mendes, P., Saad, G., and Marcelle, R. 1990. Accuracy in early prediction of prognosis of patients with septic shock by analysis of simple indices: prospective study. *Critical Care Medicine* 18, 1339–1345.

Ebara, T., Miura, K., Matsuura, T., *et al.*1996. Role of platelet-activating factor and prostanoids in hemodynamic changes in rat experimental endotoxic shock. *Japanese Journal of Pharmacology* 71, 247–253.

Elkins, R.C., McCurdy, J.R., and Brown, P.P. 1973. Effects of coronary perfusion pressure on myocardial performance during endotoxin shock. *Surgical Gynecology and Obstetrics.* 137, 991–996.

Feuerstein, G. and Hallenbeck, J.M. 1987. Prostaglandins, leukotrienes and platelet activating factor in shock. *Annual Review of Pharmacology and Toxicology* 27, 301–313.

Field, B.E., Rackow, E.C., Astiz, M.E., and Weil, M.H. 1989. Early systolic and diastolic dysfunction during sepsis in rats. *Journal of Critical Care* 4, 3–8.

Fink, M.P. 1991. Gastrointestinal mucosal injury in experimental models of shock, trauma, and sepsis. *Critical Care Medicine* 19, 627–641.

Fischmeister, R. and Shrier, A. 1989. Interactive effects of isoprenaline, forskolin and acetylcholin on $Ca^{2+}$ current in frog ventricular myocytes. *Journal of Physiology (London)* 417, 213–239.

Fish, R.E., Burns, A.H., Lang, C.H., and Spitzer, J.A. 1985. Myocardial dysfunction in a nonlethal, nonshock model of chronic endotoxemia. *Circulatory Shock* 16, 241–252.

Fleming, I. and Busse, R. 1999. NO: the primary EDRF. *Journal of Molecular and Cellular Cardiology* 31, 5–14.

Flesch, M., Kilter, H., Cremers, B., *et al.* 1997. Acute effects of nitric oxide and cyclic GMP on human myocardial contractility. *Journal of Pharmacology and Experimental Therapeutics* 281, 1340–1349.

Fong, K.L., McCay, P.B., Poyer, J.L., *et al.* 1973. Evidence that peroxidation of lysosomal membranes is initiated by hydroxyl free radicals produced during flavin enzyme activity. *Journal of Biological Chemistry* 248, 7792–7797.

Förstermann, U., Schmidt, H.H.H.W., Kohlhaas, K.L., and Murad, F. 1992. Induced RAW 264.7 macrophages express soluble and particulate nitric oxide synthase: inhibition by transforming growth factor-β. *European Journal of Pharmacology* 225, 161–165.

Förstermann, U., Pollock, J.S., and Nakane, M. 1993. Nitric oxide synthases in the cardiovascular system. *Trends in Cardiovascular Medicine* 3, 104–110.

Förstermann, U., Pollock, J.S., and Tracey, W.R. 1994a. Isoforms of nitric-oxide synthase: purification and regulation. *Methods in Enzymology* 233, 258–264.

Förstermann, U., Closs, E.I., Pollock, J.S., *et al.*1994b. Nitric oxide synthase isozymes: characterization, purification, molecular cloning, and functions. *Hypertension* 23, 1121–1131.

Gallo, M.P., Ghigo, D., Bosia, A., *et al.* 1998. Modulation of guinea-pig cardiac L-type calcium current by nitric oxide synthase inhibitors. *Journal of Physiology* 506, 639–651.

Gao, W.D., Atar, D., Back, P.H., and Marban, E. 1995. Relationship between intracellular calcium and contractile force in stunned myocardium: Direct evidence for decreased myofilament $Ca^{2+}$ responsiveness and altered diastolic function in intact ventricular muscle. *Circulation Research* 76, 1036–1048.

Geng, Y., Almqvist, M., and Hansson, G.K. 1994. cDNA cloning and expression of inducible nitric oxide synthase from rat vascular smooth muscle cells. *Biochimica et Biophysica Acta* 1218, 421–424.

Geocaris, T.V., Quebbeman, E., and Dewoskin, R. 1973. Effects of gram-negative endotoxemia on myocardial contractility in the awake primate. *Annals of Surgery* 178, 715–720.

Giessler, C., Ponicke, K., Steinborn, C., and Brodde, O.E. 1995. Effects of PAF on cardiac function and eicosanoid release in the isolated perfused rat heart: comparison between normotensive and spontaneously hypertensive rats. *Basic Research in Cardiology* 90, 337–347.

Glantz, S.A. and Parmley, W.W. 1978. Factors which affect the diastolic pressure–volume curve. *Circulation Research* 42, 171–180.

Goldfarb, R.D. 1982. Cardiac mechanical performance in circulatory shock: a critical review of methods and results. *Circulatory Shock* 9, 633–653.

Goldfarb, R.D. 1985. Evaluation of ventricular performance in shock. *Circulatory Shock* 15, 281–301.

Goldfarb, R.D., Tambolini, W., Wiener, S.M., and Weber, P.B. 1983. Canine left ventricular performance during $LD_{50}$ endotoxemia. *American Journal Physiology* 244, H370–H377.

Goldfarb, R.D., Nightingale, L.M., Kish, P., *et al.*1986. Left ventricular function during lethal and sublethal endotoxemia in swine. *American Journal Physiology* 251, H364–H373.

Goldfarb, R.D., Lee, K.J., and Dziuban, S.W. 1990. End-systolic elastance as an evaluation of myocardial function in shock. *Circulatory Shock* 30, 15–26.

Goodyer, A.V.N. 1967. Left ventricular function and tissue hypoxia in irreversible hemorrhagic and endotoxin shock. *American Journal Physiology* 228, 1462–1468.

Greenfield, L.J., Jackson, R.H., and Elkins, R.C. 1974. Cardiopulmonary effects of volume loading of primates in endotoxin shock. *Surgery* 76, 560–572.

Groeneveld, A.B.J., Bronsveld, W., and Thijs, L.G. 1986. Hemodynamic determinants of mortality in human septic shock. *Surgery* 99, 140.

Guarnieri, C., Flamigni, F., and Caldarera, C.M. 1980. Role of oxygen in the cellular damage induced by reoxygenation of hypoxic heart. *Journal of Molecular and Cellular Cardiology* 12, 797–808.

Gunnar, R.M., Loeb, H.S., and Winslow, E.J. 1973. Hemodynamic measurements in bacteremia and septic shock in man. *Journal of Infectious Diseases* 128, S295–S298.

Guntheroth, W.G., Kawabori, I., and Stevenson, J.G. 1978. Pulmonary vascular resistance and right ventricular function in canine endotoxin shock. *Proceedings of the Society for Experimental Biological Medicine* 157, 610–614.

Guntheroth, W.G., Jacky, P.J., Kawabori, I., *et al.* 1982. Left ventricular performance in endotoxin shock in dogs. *American Journal Physiology* 242, H172–H176.

Gupta, J.B., Prasad, M., Kalra, J., and Prasad, K. 1994. Platelet-activating-factor-induced changes in cardiovascular function and oxyradical status of myocardium in presence of the PAF antagonist CV-6209. *Angiology* 45, 25–36.

Gwathmey, J.K., Copelas, L., MacKinnon, R., *et al.* 1987. Abnormal intracellular calcium handling in myocardium from patients with end-stage heart failure. *Circulation Research* 61, 70–76.

Haglund, U. and Lundgren, O. 1978. Intestinal ischemia and shock factors. *Federation Proceedings* 37, 2729–2733.

Hale, C.C., Allert, J.A., Keller, R.S., *et al.*1989. Gram-negative endotoxemia: Effects on cardiac Na–Ca exchange and stoichiometry. *Circulatory Shock* 29, 133–142.

Hale, C.C., Novela, L., Adams, H.R., and Parker, J.L. 1990. Cardiac sarcolemma in endotoxin shock phospholipid profiles. *Circulatory Shock* 31, 15.

Hardaway, R.M. 1982. Pulmonary artery pressure versus pulmonary capillary wedge pressure and central venous pressure in shock. *Resuscitation* 10, 47–56.

Herzig, S., Patil, P., Neumann, J., *et al.* 1993. Mechanisms of β-adrenergic stimulation of cardiac Ca$^{2+}$ channels revealed by discrete-time Markov analysis of slow gating. *Biophysical Journal* 65, 1599–1612.

Hess, M.L. 1979. Concise review: subcellular function in the acutely failing myocardium. *Circulatory Shock* 6, 119–136.

Hess, M.L. and Krause, S.M. 1979. Myocardial subcellular function in shock. *Texas Reproductive Biology and Medicine* 39, 193–207.

Hess, M.L. and Krause, S.M. 1981. Contractile protein dysfunction as a determinant of depressed cardiac contractility during endotoxin shock. *Journal Molecular and Cellular Cardiology* 13, 715–723.

Hess, M.L. and Manson, N.H. 1983. The paradox of steroid therapy: inhibition of oxygen free radicals. *Circulatory Shock* 10, 1–5.

Hess, M.L., Krause, S.M., and Komwatana, P. 1980. Myocardial failure and excitation–contraction uncoupling in canine endotoxin shock: role of histamine and sarcoplasmic reticulum. *Circulatory Shock* 7, 277–287.

Hess, M.L., Hastillo, A., and Greenfield, L.J. 1981a. Spectrum of cardiovascular function during gram-negative sepsis. *Progress in Cardiovascular Disease* 23, 279–298.

Hess, M.L., Okabe, E., and Kontos, H.A. 1981b. Proton and free oxygen radical interaction with calcium transport system of cardiac sarcoplasmic reticulum. *Journal of Molecular and Cellular Cardiology* 13, 767–772.

Hinshaw, L.B. 1974. Role of the heart in the pathogenesis of endotoxin shock: a review of clinical findings and observations on animal species. *Journal of Surgical Research* 17, 134–145.

Hinshaw, L.B., Archer, L.T., and Greenfield, L.J. 1971a. Effects of endotoxin on myocardial hemodynamics, performance, and metabolism. *American Journal of Physiology* 221, 504–510.

Hinshaw, L.B., Greenfield, L.J., and Archer, L.T. 1971b. Effects of endotoxin on myocardial hemodynamics, performance, and metabolism during beta adrenergic blockade. *Proceedings of the Society for Experimental Biology and Medicine* 137, 1217–1224.

Hinshaw, L.B., Greenfield, L.J., and Owen, S.E. 1972a. Cardiac response to circulating factors in endotoxin shock. *American Journal of Physiology* 222, 1047–1053.

Hinshaw, L.B., Greenfield, L.J., and Owens, S.E. 1972b. Precipitation of cardiac failure in endotoxin shock. *Surgical Gynecology and Obstetrics* 135, 39–48.

Hinshaw, L.B., Archer, L.T., and Spitzer, J.J. 1974a. Myocardial function in shock. *American Journal of Physiology* 226, 357–366.

Hinshaw, L.B., Archer, L.T., and Black, M.R. 1974b. Effects of coronary hypotension and endotoxin on myocardial performance. *American Journal of Physiology* 227, 1051–1057.

Hirano, Y., Suzuki, K., Yamawake, N., and Hiraoka, M. 1994. Multiple kinetic effects of β-adrenergic stimulation on single cardiac L-type Ca channels. *American Journal of Physiology* 266, C1714–C1721.

Hofmann, P.A., Miller, W.P., and Moss, R.L. 1993. Altered calcium sensitivity of isometric tension in myocyte-sized preparations of porcine postischemic stunned myocardium. *Circulation Research* 72, 50–56.

Hofmann, P.A., Menon, V., and Gannaway, K.F. 1995. Effects of diabetes on isometric tension as a function of [Ca$^{2+}$] and pH in rat skinned cardiac myocytes. *American Journal of Physiology* 269, H1656–H1663.

Horton, J.W., White, J., and Maass, D. 1998. Protein kinase C inhibition improves ventricular function after thermal trauma. *Journal of Trauma – Injury, Infection and Critical Care* 44, 254–264.

Hoshiai, M., Hattan, N., Hirota, Y., *et al.* 1999. Impaired sarcoplasmic reticulum function in lipopolysaccharide-induced myocardial dysfunction demonstrated in whole heart. *Shock* 11, 362–366.

Hotchkiss, R.S. and Karl, I.E. 1994. Dantrolene ameliorates the metabolic hallmarks of sepsis in rats and improves survival in a mouse model of endotoxin. *Proceedings of the National Academy of Sciences of the United States of America* 91, 3039–3043.

Hotchkiss, R.S. and Karl, I.E. 1996. Calcium: A regulator of the inflammatory response in endotoxemia and sepsis. *New Horizons* 4, 58–71.

Hu, H., Chiamvimonvat, N., Yamagishi, T., and Marban, E. 1997. Direct inhibition of expressed cardiac L-type $Ca^{2+}$ channels by $S$-nitrosothiol nitric oxide donors. *Circulation Research* 81, 742–752.

Hung, J. and Lew, W.Y.W. 1993. Cellular mechanisms of endotoxin-induced myocardial depression in rabbits. *Circulation Research* 73, 125–134.

Inoue, N., Kawashima, S., Hirata, K.I., Rikitake, Y., Takeshita, S., Yamochi, W., Akita, H., and Yokoyama, M. 1998. Stretch force on vascular smooth muscle cells enhances oxidation of LDL via superoxide production. *American Journal of Physiology* 274, H1928–H1932.

Jardin, F., Brunney, D., Auvert, B., and Bourdarias, F.P. 1990. Sepsis-related cardiogenic shock. *Critical Care Medicine* 10, 1055–1060.

Jha, P., Jacobs, H., Bose, D., *et al.* 1993. Effects of *E. coli* sepsis and myocardial depressant factor on interval-force relations in dog ventricle. *American Journal of Physiology* 264, H1402–H1410.

Ji, Y., Dong, L.W., Wu, L.L., *et al.* 1995. Impaired calcium uptake by cardiac sarcoplasmic reticulum and its underlying mechanism during rat septic shock [Chinese]. *Acta Physiologica Sinica* 47, 336–342.

Ji, Y., Zhao, M., Qi, Y., *et al.* 1996. Effects of Arg–Gly–Asp–Ser on $Ca^{2+}$ transport of myocardial sarcoplasmic reticulum in rat septic shock. *Acta Pharmacologica Sinica* 17, 129–132.

Joe, E.K., Schussheim, A.E., Longrois, D., *et al.* 1998. Regulation of cardiac myocyte contractile function by inducible nitric oxide synthase (iNOS): Mechanisms of contractile depression by nitric oxide. *Journal of Molecular and Cellular Cardiology* 30, 303–315.

Keller, R.S., Jones, J.J., Kim, K.F., *et al.* 1995. Endotoxin-induced myocardial dysfunction: Is there a role for nitric oxide. *Shock* 4, 338–344.

Keller, R.S., Milanick, M.A., Adams, H.R., and Rubin, L.J. 1996. Enhanced cardiac sarcoplasmic reticulum $Ca^{2+}$ uptake in permeabilized myocytes from endotoxemic guinea pigs. *Shock* 5, 33.

Kihara, Y., Grossman, W., and Morgan, J.P. 1989. Direct measurement of changes in intracellular calcium transients during hypoxia, ischemia, and reperfusion of the intact mammalian heart. *Circulation Research* 65, 1029–1044.

Kimichi, A., Ellrodt, G., and Berman, D.S. 1984. Right ventricular performance in septic shock: a combined radionuclide and hemodynamic study. *Journal of the American College of Cardiology* 4, 945–951.

Kinugawa, K., Shimizu, T., Yao, A., *et al.* 1997. Transcriptional regulation of inducible nitric oxide synthase in cultured neonatal rat cardiac myocytes. *Circulation Research* 81, 921.

Kinugawa, K.I., Kohmoto, O., Yao, A., *et al.* 1997. Cardiac inducible nitric oxide synthase negatively modulates myocardial function in cultured rat myocytes. *American Journal of Physiology* 272, H35–H47.

Kirkeboen, K.A. and Strand, O.A. 1999. The role of nitric oxide in sepsis – an overview. *Acta Anaesthesiologica Scandinavica* 43, 275–288.

Klabunde, R.E. and Coston, A.F. 1995. Nitric oxide synthase inhibition does not prevent cardiac depression in endotoxic shock. *Shock* 3, 73–78.

Klostergaard, J., Leroux, M.E., and Hung, M.-C. 1991. Cellular models of macrophage tumoricidal effector mechanisms in vitro: Characterization of cytolytic responses to tumor necrosis factor and nitric oxide pathways in vitro. *Journal of Immunology* 147, 2802–2808.

Kober, P.M., Thomas, J., and Raymond, R.M. 1985. Increased myocardial contractility during endotoxin shock in dogs. *American Journal of Physiology* 249, H722.

Koide, M., Kawahara, Y., Tsuda, T., and Yokoyama, M. 1993. Cytokine-induced expression of an inducible type of nitric oxide synthase gene in cultured vascular smooth muscle cells. *FEBS Letters* 318, 213–217.

Kojda, G. and Kottenberg, K. 1999. Regulation of basal myocardial function by NO. *Cardiovascular Research* 41, 514–523.

Koltai, M., Hosford, D., and Braquet, P. 1993. PAF-induced amplification of mediator release in septic shock: Prevention or down regulation by PAF antagonists. *Journal of Lipid Mediators* 6, 183–198.

Kontos, H.A., Wei, E.P., Povlishock, J.T., *et al.* 1984. Oxygen radicals mediate the cerebral arteriolar dilation from arachidonate and bradykinin in cats. *Circulation Research* 55, 295–303.

Kooy, N.W., Lewis, S.J., Royall, J.A., *et al.* 1997. Extensive tyrosine nitration in human myocardial inflammation: evidence for the presence of peroxynitrite. *Critical Care Medicine* 25, 812–819.

Koshy, U.S., Burton, K.P., Le, T.H., and Horton, J.W. 1997. Altered ionic calcium and cell motion in ventricular myocytes after cutaneous thermal injury. *Journal of Surgical Research* 68, 133–138.

Krause, S.M., Kleinman, W., and Hess, M.L. 1980. Cardiogenic endotoxin shock: coronary flow and contractile protein dysfunction as determinants of depressed cardiac contractility. *Advances in Shock Research* 3, 105–116.

Krausz, M.M., Perel, A., and Eimerl, D. 1974. Cardiopulmonary effects of volume loading in patients in septic shock. *Surgical Clinics of North America* 54, 993–1002.

Kuehl, Jr., F.A., Humes, J.L., Ham, E.Z., *et al.* 1980. Inflammation: the role of peroxidase-derived products. In: *Advances in Prostaglandin and Thromboxane Research.* Samuelsson, B., Ramwell, P.W., and Paoletti, R. (eds), pp. 77–86. Raven Press, New York.

Kutsky, P. and Parker, J.L. 1990. Calcium fluxes in cardiac sarcolemma and sarcoplasmic reticulum isolated from endotoxin-shocked guinea pigs. *Circulatory Shock* 30, 349–364.

Lane, P. and Gross, S.S. 1999. Cell signaling by nitric oxide. *Seminars in Nephrology* 19, 215–229.

Laughlin, M.H., Smyk-Randall, E.M., Novotny, M.J., *et al.* 1988. Coronary blood flow and cardiac adenine nucleotides in *E. coli* endotoxemia in dogs: effects of oxygen radical scavengers. *Circulatory Shock* 25, 173–185.

Law, W.R., McLane, M.P., and Raymond, R.M. 1988. Substantiation of myocardial resistance to the inotropic action of insulin during endotoxin shock. *Circulatory Shock* 24, 237.

Lee, K.L., van der Zee, H., Dziuban, S.W., *et al.* 1988a. Left ventricular function during lethal and sublethal endotoxemia in swine. *American Journal of Physiology* 254, H324–H330.

Lee, K.L., Dziuban, S.W., van der Zee, H., *et al.* 1988b. Cardiac function and coronary flow in chronic endotoxemic pigs. *Proceedings of the Society Experimental Biology and Medicine* 189, 245–252.

Lefcoe, M.S., Sibbald, W.J., and Holliday, R.L. 1979. Wedged balloon catheter angiography in the critical care unit. *Critical Care Medicine* 7, 449–453.

Lefer, A.M. 1978. Properties of cardioinhibitory factors produced in shock. *Federation Proceedings* 37, 2734–2740.

Lefer, A.M. 1979. Mechanisms of cardiodepression in endotoxin shock. *Circulatory Shock* 1, 1–8.

Lefer, A.M. 1985. Eicosanoids as mediators of ischemia and shock. *Federation Proceedings* 44, 280.

Lefer, A.M. 1987. Interaction between myocardial depressant factor and vasoactive mediators with ischemia and shock. *American Journal Physiology* 252, R193–R205.

Lefer, A.M. and Spath, Jr., J.A. 1974. Pancreatic hypoperfusion and the production of a myocardial depressant factor in hemorrhagic shock. *Annals of Surgery* 179, 868–876.

Lefer, A.M. and Spath, Jr., J.A. 1977. Pharmacologic basis of the treatment of circulatory shock. In: *Cardiovascular Pharmacology*. Antonaccio, M.J. (ed.), pp. 377–428. Raven Press, New York.

Lefer, A.M., Araki, H., and Okamatsu, S. 1981. Beneficial actions of a free radical scavenger in traumatic shock and myocardial ischemia. *Circulatory Shock* 8, 273–282.

Levi, R.C., Alloatti, G., Penna, C., and Gallo, M.P. 1994. Guanylate-cyclase-mediated inhibition of cardiac $I_{Ca}$ by carbachol and sodium nitroprusside. *Pflügers Archive European Journal of Physiology* 426, 419–426.

Lew, W.Y.W., Yasuda, S., Yuan, T., and Hammond, H.K. 1996. Endotoxin-induced cardiac depression is associated with decreased cardiac dihydropyridine receptors in rabbits. *Journal of Molecular and Cellular Cardiology* 28, 1367–1371.

Lew, W.Y.W., Lee, M., Yasuda, S., and Bayna, E. 1997. Depyrogenation of digestive enzymes reduces lipopolysaccharide tolerance in isolated cardiac myocytes. *Journal of Molecular and Cellular Cardiology* 29, 1985–1990.

Lewis, B.S. and Gotsman, M.S. 1980. Current concepts of left ventricular relaxation and compliance. *American Heart Journal* 99, 101–112.

Liu, M-S. and Wu, L.-L. 1991. Reduction in the $Ca^{2+}$-induced $Ca^{2+}$ release from canine cardiac sarcoplasmic reticulum following endotoxin administration. *Biochemical and Biophysical Research Communications* 174, 1248–1254.

Liu, M-S. and Xuan, Y.T. 1986. Mechanisms of endotoxin-induced impairment in $Na^+$-$Ca^{2+}$ exchange in canine myocardium. *American Journal of Physiology* 251, R1078–R1085.

Liu, S.F., Adcock, I.M., Old, R.W., *et al.* 1996. Differential regulation of the constitutive and inducible nitric oxide synthase mRNA by lipopolysaccharide treatment *in vivo* in the rat. *Critical Care Medicine* 24, 1219–1225.

Lopez, B.L., Liu, G.L., Christopher, T.A., and Ma, X.L. 1997. Peroxynitrite, the product of nitric oxide and superoxide, causes myocardial injury in the isolated perfused rat heart. *Coronary Artery Disease* 8, 149–153.

Loschen, G., Azzi, A., Richter, C., *et al.* 1974. Superoxide radicals as precursor of mitochondrial hydrogen peroxide. *FEBS Letters* 43, 68–72.

Lundgren, O., Haglund, U., and Isaksson, O. 1976. Effects on myocardial contractility of blood-borne material released from feline small intestine in simulated shock. *Circulation Research* 8, 307–315.

Luss, H., Li, R., Shapiro, R., Tzeng, E., *et al.* 1997. Dedifferentiated human ventricular cardiac myocytes express inducible nitric oxide synthase mRNA in response to IL-1, TNF, IFN, and LPS. *Journal of Molecular and Cellular Cardiology* 29, 1153–1165.

Lynch, R.C. and Fridovich, I. 1978. Permeation of the erythrocyte stroma by superoxide radical. *Journal of Biological Chemistry* 253, 4699.

McDonald, L.J. and Murad, F. 1996. Nitric oxide and cyclic GMP signaling. *Proceedings of the Society for Experimental Biology and Medicine* 211, 1–6.

MacDonell, K.L. and Diamond, J. 1997. Cyclic GMP-dependent protein kinase activation in the absence of negative inotropic effects in the rat ventricle. *British Journal of Pharmacology* 122, 1425–1435.

McDonough, K.H. 1988. Calcium uptake by sarcoplasmic reticulum isolated from hearts of septic rats. *Circulatory Shock* 25, 291–297.

McDonough, K.H. and Lang, C.H. 1984. Depressed function of isolated hearts from hyperdynamic septic rats. *Circulatory Shock* 12, 241–251.

McDonough, K.H., Lang, C.H., and Spitzer, J.J. 1985a. Effects of cardiotropic agents on the myocardial dysfunction of hyperdynamic sepsis. *Circulatory Shock* 17, 1–19.

McDonough, K.H., Lang, C.H., and Spitzer, J.J. 1985b. The effect of hyperdynamic sepsis on myocardial performance. *Circulatory Shock* 15, 247–259.

McDonough, K.H., Henry, J.J., Lang, C.H., and Spitzer, J.J. 1986. Substrate utilization and high energy phosphate levels of hearts from hyperdynamic septic rats. *Circulatory Shock* 18, 161–170.

McDonough, K.H., Burke, E.C., and Smith, L.W. 1990. *In vitro* cardiac function in early sepsis. *Journal of Medicine* 21, 27–49.

Maclean, L.D. and Weil, M.H. 1956. Hypotension (shock) in dogs produced by *Escherichia coli* endotoxin. *Circulation Research* 4, 546–556.

McMichael, P., Thompson, M., Bryant, D., *et al.* 2000. iNOS activity and cardiac dysfunction in an endotoxin mouse model. *Shock* 13, 23.

Mammana, R.B., Hiro, S., Levitsky, S., *et al.* 1982. Inaccuracy of pulmonary capillary wedge pressure when compared to left atrial pressure in the early post-surgical period. *Journal of Thoracic Cardiovascular Surgery* 82, 420–425.

Manson, N.H. and Hess, M.L. 1983. Interaction of oxygen free radicals and cardiac sarcoplasmic reticulum: proposed role in the pathogenesis of endotoxin shock. *Circulatory Shock* 1, 205–213.

Massey, C.V., Kohout, T.A., Gaa, S.T., *et al.* 1991. Molecular and cellular actions of platelet-activating factor in rat heart cells. *Journal of Clinical Investigation* 88, 2106–2116.

Mead, J.R. 1976. Free radical mechanisms of lipid damage and consequences for cellular membranes. *Free Radical Biology* 1, 51–67.

Mery, P.F., Pavoine, C., Belhassen, L., *et al.* 1993. Nitric oxide regulates cardiac $Ca^{2+}$ current: involvement of cyclic GMP-inhibited and cyclic GMP stimulated phosphodiesterases through guanylyl cyclase activation. *Journal of Biological Chemistry* 268, 26286–26295.

Mewes, T. and Ravens, U. 1994. L-type calcium currents of human myocytes from ventricle of non-failing and failing hearts and from atrium. *Journal of Molecular and Cellular Cardiology* 26, 1307–1320.

Miller, H. and Parker, J.L. 1989. The guinea pig as a model in shock/trauma research. In: *Perspectives in Shock Research, Immunology, Mediators, and Models*, pp. 277–286. Alan R. Liss, New York.

Miller, T.H., Priano, L.L., and Jorgenson, J.H. 1977. Cardiorespiratory effects of *Pseudomonas* and *E. coli* endotoxins in the awake dog. *American Journal of Physiology* 232, H682–H689.

Momomura, S., Iizuka, M., Serizawa, T., and Sugimoto, T. 1988. Separation of rate of left ventricular relaxation from chamber stiffness in rats. *American Journal of Physiology* 225, H1468–H1475.

Moncada, S. 1999. Nitric oxide: discovery and impact on clinical medicine. *Journal of the Royal Society of Medicine* 92, 164–169.

Moreland, S. 1994. BQ-123, a selective endothelin $ET_A$ receptor antagonist. *Cardiovascular Drug Review* 12, 48–69.

Muñoz, H.R., Evans, R.D., Marsch, S.C.U., and Foëx, P. 1995. Platelet-activating factor (PAF) does not affect diastolic function in isolated rat hearts. *Cardiovascular Research* 30, 1028–1032.

Murphy, M.P. 1999. Nitric oxide and cell death. *Biochimica et Biophysica Acta* 1411, 401–414.

Nagasaki, A., Gotoh, T., Takeya, M., *et al.* 1996. Co-induction of nitric oxide synthase, argininosuccinate synthetase, and argininosuccinate lyase in lipopolysaccharide-treated rats. *Journal of Biological Chemistry* 271, 2658–2662.

Nakane, M., Pollock, J.S., Klinghofer, V., *et al.* 1995. Functional expression of three isoforms of human nitric oxide synthase in baculovirus-infected insect cells. *Biochemical and Biophysical Research Communications* 206, 511–517.

Natanson, C., Fink, M.P., Ballantyne, H.K., *et al.* 1986. Gram-negative bacteremia produces both severe systolic and diastolic cardiac dysfunction in a canine model that simulates human septic shock. *Journal of Clinical Investigation* 78, 259–270.

Natanson, C., Danner, R.L., Fink, M.P., *et al.* 1988. Cardiovascular performance with *E. coli* challenges in a canine model of human sepsis. *American Journal of Physiology* 254, H558–H569.

Natanson, C., Danner, R.L., and Elin, R.J. 1989. Role of endotoxemia in cardiovascular dysfunction and mortality. *Journal of Clinical Investigation* 83, 243–251.

Neviere, R.R., Cepinskas, G., Madorin, W.S., *et al.* 1999. LPS pretreatment ameliorates peritonitis-induced myocardial inflammation and dysfunction: role of myocytes. *American Journal of Physiology* 277, H885–H892.

Novotny, M.J., Laughlin, M.H., and Adams, H.R. 1988. Evidence for lack of importance of oxygen free radicals in *Escherichia coli* endotoxemia in dogs. *American Journal of Physiology* 254, H954–H962.

Nunokawa, Y., Ishida, N., and Tanaka, S. 1993. Cloning of inducible nitric oxide synthase in rat vascular smooth muscle cells. *Biochemical and Biophysical Research Communications* 191, 89–94.

Ognibene, F.P., Parker, M.M., Natanson, C., and Parrillo, J.E. 1988. Depressed left ventricular performance in response to volume infusion in patients with sepsis and septic shock. *Chest* 93, 903–910.

Oh, H.M. 1998. Emerging therapies for sepsis and septic shock. *Annals of the Academy of Medicine, Singapore* 27, 738–743.

Ohashi, Y., Kawashima, S., Hirata, K., *et al.* 1997. Nitric oxide inhibits neutrophil adhesion to cytokine-activated cardiac myocytes. *American Journal of Physiology* 272, H2807–H2814.

Oyama, J., Shimokawa, H., Momii, H., *et al.* 1998. Role of nitric oxide and peroxynitrite in the cytokine-induced sustained myocardial dysfunction in dogs in vivo. *Journal of Clinical Investigation* 101, 2207–2214.

Papadakis, E.J. and Abel, F.L. 1988. Left ventricular performance in canine endotoxin shock. *Circulatory Shock* 24, 123–131.

Parker, J.L. 1983. Contractile function of heart muscle isolated from endotoxin-shocked guinea pigs and rats. *Advances in Shock Research* 9, 133–145.

Parker, J.L. and Adams, H.R. 1979. Myocardial effects of endotoxin shock: Characterization of an isolated heart muscle model. *Advances in Shock Research* 2, 163–175.

Parker, J.L. and Adams, H.R. 1981a. Pathophysiology of the heart in shock. In: *Cardiac Toxicology*, Vol. 1. Balaza, T. (ed.), pp. 137–157. CRC Press, Boca Raton.

Parker, J.L. and Adams, H.R. 1981b. Myocardial dysfunction during endotoxin shock in the guinea pig. *American Journal of Physiology* 240, H954–H962.

Parker, J.L. and Adams, H.R. 1985a. Development of myocardial dysfunction in endotoxin shock. *American Journal of Physiology* 248, H818–H826.

Parker, J.L. and Adams, H.R. 1985b. Isolated cardiac preparations: models of intrinsic myocardial dysfunction in circulatory shock. *Circulatory Shock* 15, 227–245.

Parker, J.L. and Jamison, T.S. 1981. Dissimilarities of arterial and ventricular contractile dysfunction in endotoxin shock. *Circulatory Shock* 8, 224.

Parker, J.L. and Jones, C.E. 1988. The heart in shock. In: *Shock: the Reversible Step Toward Death*. Hardaway, R. (ed.), pp. 348–366. PSG Publishing, Littleton, MA.

Parker, J.L., Daily, C.S., and Adams, H.R. 1980. Effects of endotoxin shock on pause-induced inotropy in cardiac muscle. *Circulatory Shock* 7, 191.

Parker, J.L., Adams, H.R., and Defazio, P.L. 1984. Development of left ventricular dysfunction in endotoxin shock. *Federation Proceedings* 43, 325.

Parker, J.L., Keller, R.S., Behm, L.L., and Adams, H.R. 1990. Left ventricular dysfunction in early *E. coli* endotoxemia: Effects of naloxone. *American Journal of Physiology* 259, H504–H511.

Parker, J.L., Keller, R.S., DeFily, D.V., *et al.* 1991. Coronary vascular smooth muscle function in *E. coli* endotoxemia in dogs. *American Journal of Physiology* 260, H832–H841.

Parker, M.M., Shelhamer, J.H., Natanson, C., *et al.* 1987. Serial cardiovascular variables in survivors and nonsurvivors of human septic shock: Heart rate as an early predictor of prognosis. *Critical Care Medicine* 15, 923–929.

Parks, D.A., Bulkley, G.B., Granger, D.N., *et al.* 1982. Ischemic injury in the cat small intestine: role of superoxide radicals. *Gastroenterology* 82, 9–15.

Parratt, J.R. 1998. Nitric oxide in sepsis and endotoxemia. *Journal of Antimicrobial Chemotherapy* 41 (Suppl. A), 31–39.

Parrillo, J.E. 1989. The cardiovascular pathophysiology of sepsis. *Annual Review of Medicine* 40, 469–485.

Parrillo, J.E. 1990a. Myocardial depression during septic shock in humans. *Critical Care Medicine* 18, 1183–1184.

Parrillo, J.E. 1990b. Cardiovascular pattern during septic shock. *Annals of Internal Medicine* 113, 227–229.

Parrillo, J.E., Burch, C., Shelkamer, J.H., *et al.* 1985. A circulation myocardial depressant substance in humans with septic shock. *Journal of Clinical Investigation* 76, 1539–1553.

Pfeilschifter, J., Rob, P., Mülsch, A., Fandrey, J., *et al.* 1992. Interleukin 1β and tumour necrosis factor α induce a macrophage-type of nitric oxide synthase in rat renal mesangial cells. *European Journal of Biochemistry* 203, 251–255.

Pietsch, P., Hunger, T., Braun, M., *et al.* 1998. Effects of platelet-activating factor on intracellular $Ca^{2+}$ concentration and contractility in isolated cardiomyocytes. *Journal of Cardiovascular Pharmacology* 31, 758–763.

Pollock, J.S., Nakane, M., Förstermann, U., and Murad, F. 1992. Particulate and soluble bovine endothelial nitric oxide synthases are structurally similar proteins yet different from soluble brain nitric oxide synthase. *Journal of Cardiovascular Pharmacology* 20 (Suppl. 12), S50–S53.

Powers, F.M., Farias, S., Minami, H., *et al.* 1998. Cardiac myofilament protein function is altered during sepsis. *Journal of Molecular and Cellular Cardiology* 30, 967–978.

Priano, L.L., Wilson, R.D., and Traber, D.L. 1971. Cardiorespiratory alterations in unanesthetized dogs due to gram-negative bacterial endotoxin. *American Journal of Physiology* 220, 705–711.

Rabinowitz, B., Kligerman, M., and Parmley, W.W. 1975. Alterations in myocardial and plasma cyclic adenosine monophosphate in experimental myocardial ischemia. In: *The Cardiac Sarcoplasm.* Roy, P.E., and Harris, P. (eds), pp. 251–261. University Park Press, Baltimore.

Raetz, C.R.H., Ulevitch, R.J., Wright, S.D., *et al.* 1991. Gram-negative endotoxin: An extraordinary lipid with profound effects on eukaryotic signal transduction. *FASEB Journal* 5, 2652–2660.

Ravin, H.A., Rowley, D., Jenkins, C., and Fine, J. 1960. On the absorption of bacterial endotoxin from the gastrointestinal tract of the normal and shocked animal. *Journal of Experimental Medicine* 112, 783–792.

Raymond, R.M., King, N., Thomas, J.X., and Gordey, J. 1989. Differential effects of acute endotoxin shock on myocardial contractility and performance. In: *Perspectives in Shock Research: Metabolism, Immunology, Mediators, and Models,* pp. 123–129. Alan R. Liss, New York.

Reeves, J.P. 1985. The sarcolemmal sodium–calcium exchange system. In: *Current Topics in Membranes and Transport: Regulation of Calcium Transport Across Muscle Membranes.* Shamoo, A.E. (ed.), pp. 77–127. Academic Press, Orlando, FL.

Reeves, J.P. and Hale, C.C. 1984. The stoichiometry of the cardiac sodium–calcium exchange system. *Journal of Biological Chemistry* 259, 7733–7739.

Reinhart, K., Hannemann, L., and Kuss, B. 1990. Optimal oxygen delivery in critically ill patients. *Intensive Care Medicine.* 16, S149–S155.

Rigby, S.L., Hofmann, P.A., Zhong, J., *et al.* 1998. Endotoxemia-induced myocardial dysfunction is not associated with changes in myofilament $Ca^{2+}$ responsiveness. *American Journal of Physiology* 274, H580–H590.

Romanosky, A.J., Giaimo, M.E., Shepherd, R.E., and Burns, A.H. 1986. The effect of *in vivo* endotoxin on myocardial function in *vitro. Circulatory Shock* 19, 1–12.

Rosenblum, W.I. 1983. Effects of free radical generation on mouse pial arterioles: probable role of hydroxyl radicals. *American Journal of Physiology* 245, H139–H142.

Rothe, C.F. and Selkurt, E.E. 1964. Cardiac and peripheral failure in hemorrhagic shock in the dog. *American Journal of Physiology* 207, 203–214.

Rowe, G.T., Manson, N.H., Caplan, M., *et al.* 1983. Hydrogen peroxide and hydroxyl radical mediation of activated leucocyte depression of cardiac sarcoplasmic reticulum. *Circulation Research* 53, 584–591.

Rubin, L.J., Keller, R.S., Parker, J.L., and Adams, H.R. 1994. Contractile dysfunction of ventricular myocytes isolated from endotoxemic guinea pigs. *Shock* 2, 113–120.

Sacks, T., Moldow, C.F., Craddock, P.R., *et al.* 1978. Oxygen radicals mediate endothelial cell damage by complement-stimulated granulocytes. *Journal of Clinical Investigation.* 61, 1161–1167.

Sagawa, K. 1978. The ventricular pressure volume loop revisited. *Circulation Research* 43, 677–687.

Sayeed, M.M. 1987. Effect of diltiazem on altered cellular calcium regulation during endotoxin shock. *American Journal of Physiology* 253, R549–R554.

Sayeed, M.M. 1996. Alterations in calcium signaling and cellular responses in septic injury. *New Horizons* 4, 72–86.

Schneider, A.J., Teule, G.J.J., Groeneveld, A.B.J., *et al.* 1988. Bi-ventricular performance during volume loading in patients with early septic shock with emphasis on the right ventricle: a combined hemodynamic and radionuclide study. *American Heart Journal* 116, 103–112.

Schoonderwoerd, K. and Stam, H. 1992. Lipid metabolism of myocardial endothelial cells. *Molecular and Cellular Biochemistry* 116, 171–179.

Schulz, R., Nava, E., and Moncada, S. 1992. Induction and potential biological relevance of a $Ca^{2+}$-independent nitric oxide synthase in the myocardium. *British Journal of Pharmacology* 105, 575–580.

Schulz, R., Dodge, K.L., Lopaschuk, G.D., and Clanachan, A.S. 1997. Peroxynitrite impairs cardiac contractile function by decreasing cardiac efficiency. *American Journal of Physiology* 272, H1212–H1219.

Shepherd, R.E., McDonough, K.H., and Burn, A.H. 1986. Mechanism of cardiac dysfunction in hearts from endotoxin-treated rats. *Circulatory Shock* 19, 371–384.

Shepherd, R.E., Lang, C.H., and McDonough, K.H. 1987. Myocardial adrenergic responsiveness after lethal and nonlethal doses of endotoxin. *American Journal of Physiology* 252, H410–H416.

Shindo, T., Ikeda, U., Ohkawa, F., *et al.* 1994. Nitric oxide synthesis in rat cardiac myocytes and fibroblasts. *Life Sciences* 55, 1101–1108.

Shoemaker, W.C. 1976. Pathophysiology and therapy of shock states. In: *Handbook of Critical Care.* Berk, J.L., Sampliner, J.E., Artz, J.S., *et al.* (eds), pp. 205–224. Little Brown & Co, Boston, MA.

Siegel, J.H., Greenspan, M., and Del Guercio, R.R.M. 1967. Abnormal vascular tone, defective oxygen transport and myocardial failure in human septic shock. *Annals of Surgery* 165, 504–517.

Siegel, J.H., Goldwyn, R.M., and Del Guercio, L.R.M. 1971. Patterns of cardiovascular response in septic shock. In: *Septic Shock in Man.* Hershey, S.G., Del Guercio, L.R.M., and McConn, R. (eds), pp. 173–190. Little Brown & Co, Boston, MA.

Siegel, J.H., Farrell, E.J., and Goldwyn, R.M. 1972. Myocardial function in human septic shock states. In: *Shock in Low- and High-flow States.* Forscher, B.K., Lillehei, R.C., and Stubbs, S.S. (eds), pp. 250–262. Excerpta Medica, Amsterdam.

Smith, L.W. and McDonough, K.H. 1988. Inotropic sensitivity to β-adrenergic stimulation in early sepsis. *American Journal of Physiology* 251, H699–H703.

Smith, L.W., Winbery, S.L., Barker, L.A., and McDonough, K.H. 1986. Cardiac function and chronotropic sensitivity to β-adrenergic stimulation in sepsis. *American Journal of Physiology* 251, H405–H412.

Snell, R.J. and Parrillo, J.E. 1991. Cardiovascular dysfunction in septic shock. *Chest* 99, 1000–1009.

Snow, T.R., Dickey, D.T., Tapp, T., *et al*. 1990. Early myocardial dysfunction induced with endotoxin in rhesus monkeys. *Canadian Journal of Cardiology* 6, 130–136.

Snyder, J.V. 1984. Cardiac function in septic shock. *Letters Corrections* 879.

Solis, R.T. and Downing, S.E. 1966. Effects of *E. coli* endotoxemia on ventricular performance. *American Journal of Physiology*, 307–313.

Soulsby, M.E., Bruni, F.D., and Looney, T.J. 1978. Influence of endotoxin on myocardial calcium transport and the effect of augmented venous return. *Circulatory Shock* 5, 23–34.

Spitzer, J.A., Rodriquez de Turco, E.B., *et al.* 1989. Receptor changes in endotoxemia. In: *Perspectives in Shock Research: Metabolism, Immunology, Mediators, and Models*, pp. 95–106. Alan R. Liss, New York.

Sprague, R.S., Stephenson, A.H., Dahms, T.E., and Lonigro, A.J. 1989. Proposed role for leukotrienes in the pathophysiology of multiple systems organ failure. *Critical Care Medicine* 5, 315–329.

Stahl, G.L. and Lefer, A.M. 1987. Mechanisms of platelet-activating factor-induced cardiac depression in the isolated perfused rat heart. *Circulatory Shock* 23, 165–177.

Stahl, T.J., Alden, P.B., Ring, W.S., *et al*. 1990. Sepsis-induced diastolic dysfunction in chronic canine peritonitis. *American Journal of Physiology* 258, H625–H633.

Starr, R.G., Lader, A.S., Phillips, G.C., Stroman, C.E., and Abel, F.L. 1995. Direct action of endotoxin on cardiac muscle. *Shock* 3, 380–384.

Stoclet, J.C., Muller, B., Gyorgy, K., *et al*. 1999. The inducible nitric oxide synthase in vascular and cardiac tissue. *European Journal of Pharmacology* 375, 139–155.

Suffredini, A.F., Fromm, R.E., Parker, M.M., *et al*. 1989. The cardiovascular response of normal humans to the administration of endotoxin. *The New England Journal of Medicine* 321, 280–287.

Sun, X., Delbridge, L.M.D., and Dusting, G.J. 1998. Cardiodepressant effects of interferon-gamma and endotoxin reversed by inhibition of NO synthase 2 in rat myocardium. *Journal of Molecular and Cellular Cardiology* 30, 989–997.

Symeonides, S. and Balk, R.A. 1999. Nitric oxide in the pathogenesis of sepsis. *Infectious Disease Clinics of North America* 13, 449–463.

Takeuchi, K., Del Nido, P.J., Ibrahim, A.E., *et al*. 1999. Increased myocardial calcium cycling and reduced myofilament calcium sensitivity in early endotoxemia. *Surgery* 126, 231–238.

Tamura, T., Iwasaka, T., Takayama, Y., *et al*. 1997. Effects of platelet-activating factor on left ventricular performance in dogs. *Japanese Circulation Journal* 61, 180–188.

Tao, S. and McKenna, T.M. 1994. In vitro endotoxin exposure induces contractile dysfunction in adult rat cardiac myocytes. *American Journal of Physiology* 7, H1745–H1752.

Tavernier, B., Garrigue, D., Boulle, C., *et al.*1998. Myofilament calcium sensitivity is decreased in skinned cardiac fibers from endotoxin-treated rabbits. *Cardiovascular Research* 38, 472–479.

Titheradge, M.A. 1999. Nitric oxide in septic shock. *Biochimica et Biophysica Acta* 1411, 437–455.

Traber, D.L., Adams, T., Sziebert, L., *et al.* 1985. Potentiation of lung vascular response to endotoxin by superoxide dismutase. *Journal Applied Physiology* 58, 1005–1009.

Udhoji, V.N., and Weil, M.H. 1965. Hemodynamic and metabolic studies on shock associated with bacteremia. *Annals of Internal Medicine* 62, 966.

Ungureanu-Longrois, D., Balligand, J.-L., Simmons, W.W., *et al.* 1995a. Induction of nitric oxide synthase activity by cytokines in ventricular myocytes is necessary but not sufficient to decrease contractile responsiveness to β-adrenergic agonists. *Circulation Research* 77, 494–502.

Ungureanu-Longrois, D., Balligand, J.L., Kelly, R.A., and Smith, T.W. 1995b. Myocardial contractile dysfunction in the systemic inflammatory response syndrome: role of a cytokine-inducible nitric oxide synthase in cardiac myocytes. *Journal of Molecular and Cellular Cardiology* 27, 155–167.

Vandecasteele, G., Eschenhagen, T., and Fischmeister, R. 1998. Role of the NO-cGMP pathway in the muscarinic regulation of the L-type $Ca^{2+}$ current in human atrial myocytes. *Journal of Physiology* 506, 653–663.

Van Deventer, S.J.H., Ten Cate, J.W., and Ty Gat, G.N.J. 1988. Intestinal endotoxemia. *Gastroenterology* 94, 825–831.

Vanin, A.F., Mordvintcev, P.I., Hauschildt, S., and Mülsch, A. 1993. The relationship between L-arginine-dependent nitric oxide synthesis, nitrite release and dinitrosyl-iron complex formation by activated macrophages. *Biochimica et Biophysica Acta* 1177, 37–42.

Vila-Petroff, M.G., Younes, A., Egan, J., *et al.*. 1999. Activation of distinct cAMP-dependent and cGMP-dependent pathways by nitric oxide in cardiac myocytes. *Circulation Research* 84, 1020–1031.

Vincent, J.C., Reuse, C., Frank, N., *et al.* 1989. Right ventricular dysfunction in septic shock: assessment by measurements of right ventricular ejection fraction using the thermo dilution technique. *Acta Anaesthesiologica Scandinavica* 33, 34–38.

Vincent, J.L., Weil, M.H., and Puri, V. 1981. Circulatory shock associated with purulent peritonitis. *American Journal Surgery* 142, 262–270.

Walley, K.R. and Cooper, D.J. 1991. Diastolic stiffness impairs left ventricular function during hypovolemic shock in pigs. *American Journal of Physiology* 260, H702–H712.

Wang, S., Wright, G., Geng, W., and Wright, G.L. 1997. Retinol influences contractile function and exerts an anti-proliferative effect on vascular smooth muscle cells through an endothelium-dependent mechanism. *Pflügers Archive European Journal of Physiology* 434, 669–677.

Wangensteen, S.L., Geissinger, W.T., and Lovett, W.L. 1971. Relationship between splanchnic blood flow and a myocardial depressant factor in endotoxin shock. *Surgery* 69, 410–418.

Warner, M., Smith, J.M., and Eaton, R. 1981. The excitation–contraction coupling system of the myocardium in canine hemorrhagic shock. *Circulatory Shock* 8, 563–572.

Weil, M.H. and Nishijima, H. 1978. Cardiac output in bacterial shock. *American Journal of Medicine* 64, 920–922.

Weil, W.H., Maclean, L.D., and Visscher, M.B. 1956. Studies on the circulatory changes in the dog produced by endotoxin from gram-negative micro-organisms. *Journal of Clinical Investigation* 35, 1101–1198.

Weisel, R.D., Vito, L., and Dennis, R.C. 1977. Myocardial depression during sepsis. *American Journal of Surgery* 133, 512–521.

White, J., Horton, J., and Giroir, B. 2000. Transgenic model of I-κB over expression to examine the role of NF-κB in postburn myocardial contractile dysfunction. *Shock* 13, 23.

Wiggers, C.J. 1950. *Physiology of Shock*. The Commonwealth Fund/Harvard University Press, Cambridge, MA.

Wolff, S.M. and Bennett, J.V. 1974. Gram-negative rod bacteremia. *The New England Journal of Medicine* 291, 733–734.

Wu, L.-L. and Liu, M.-S. 1991. Impaired calcium uptake by cardiac sarcoplasmic reticulum and its underlying mechanism in endotoxin shock. *Molecular and Cellular Biochemistry* 108, 9–17.

Wu, L.-L. and Liu, M.-S. 1992. Altered ryanodine receptor of canine cardiac sarcoplasmic reticulum and its underlying mechanism in endotoxin shock. *Journal of Surgical Research* 53, 82–90.

Yang, Q., Wu, L.L., Tang, X., and Tang, C.S. 1995. Alteration of phospholamban phosphatase activity associated with cardiac sarcoplasmic reticulum during sepsis in rats [in Chinese]. *Acta Physiologica Sinica* 47, 357–365.

Yang, Q., Tang, X., Dong, L.W., and Tang, C.S. 1996. Changes in the calcium channels in rat cardia cells during sepsis [Chinese]. *Acta Physiologica Sinica* 48, 141–148.

Yasuda, S. and Lew, W.Y. 1997a. Lipopolysaccharide depresses cardiac contractility and β-adrenergic contractile response by decreasing myofilament response to $Ca^{2+}$ in cardiac myocytes. *Circulation Research* 81, 1011–1020.

Yasuda, S. and Lew, W.Y.W. 1997b. Endothelin-1 ameliorates contractile depression by lipopolysaccharide in cardiac myocytes. *American Journal of Physiology* 273, H1403–H1407.

Zhong, J., Adams, H.R., and Rubin, L.J. 1997a. Cytosolic $Ca^{2+}$ concentration and contraction–relaxation properties of ventricular myocytes from *Escherichia coli* endotoxemic guinea pigs: Effect of fluid resuscitation. *Shock* 7, 383–388.

Zhong, J., Hwang, T.C., Adams, H.R., and Rubin, L.J. 1997b. Reduced L-type calcium current in ventricular myocytes from endotoxemic guinea pigs. *American Journal of Physiology* 273, H2312–H2324.

Zingarelli, B., Squadrito, F., Ioculano, M., *et al.* 1992. Platelet activating factor interaction with tumor necrosis factor and myocardial depressant factor in splanchnic artery occlusion shock. *European Journal of Pharmacology*. 222, 13–19.

Zucchi, R., Ronca-Testoni, S., Yu, G.Y., *et al.* 1995. Are dihydropyridine receptors downregulated in the ischemic myocardium? *Cardiovascular Research* 30, 769–774.

# 9

# CATECHOLAMINE-INDUCED CARDIOMYOPATHY

*Naranjan S. Dhalla,\* Hideki Sasaki,\* Seibu Mochizuki,†
Ken S. Dhalla,\* Xueliang Liu,\* and Vijayan Elimban\**

*\*Institute of Cardiovascular Sciences, St. Boniface General
Hospital Research Centre, and Department of Physiology, Faculty
of Medicine, University of Manitoba, Winnipeg, Canada; and
†Department of Internal Medicine, Jikei University School of
Medicine, Tokyo, Japan*

## Introduction

The sympathoadrenal system consists of the sympathetic nervous system with cholinergic preganglionic and adrenergic post-ganglionic nerves and the adrenal medulla. The hormones of the sympathoadrenal system, while not necessary for life, are required for adaptation to acute and chronic stress. Catecholamines, such as epinephrine (adrenaline), norepinephrine (noradrenaline), and dopamine, are major elements in the response to severe stress. Isoproterenol is a synthetic catecholamine and is well known as a non-selective β-adrenergic receptor agonist. Low concentrations of catecholamines exert positive inotropic action on the myocardium, and thus are considered to be beneficial in regulating heart function. On the other hand, not only high concentrations of catecholamines but also low concentrations of catecholamines over a prolonged period produce deleterious effects on the cardiovascular system. It has been known for many years that epinephrine, norepinephrine, and isoproterenol can cause cardiac hypertrophy and/ or myocardial lesions.[1-4] These myocardial lesions had been considered to represent "catecholamine-induced myocardial cell damage," "catecholamine-induced myocarditis," or "myocardial infarction," and are now designated "catecholamine-induced cardiomyopathy."

Catecholamines are known to produce a wide variety of direct and indirect pharmacologic actions on cardiovascular hemodynamics and metabolism. As a consequence of these complex effects, it has been difficult to determine whether catecholamines exert a direct toxic influence on the myocardium, or whether myocardial cell damage is in some way secondary to other actions of catecholamines.[4-10] Several mechanisms, such as cardiovascular hemodynamic and metabolic changes, alterations in the sarcolemmal permeability, formation of oxidation products of catecholamines, and accumulation of catecholamine metabolites during the monoamine oxidase reaction, have been suggested to explain the pathogenesis of catecholamine-induced cardiomyopathy.[11–22] However, because none of these mechanisms has yet been clearly implicated, an attempt has been made in this review to formulate a unifying concept regarding the pathophysiology and clinical significance of catecholamine-induced cardiomyopathy.

## Cardiotoxicity of catecholamines

### *Epinephrine-induced cardiomyopathy*

It was first reported in 1905 that epinephrine caused cardiac lesions.[1] The epinephrine-induced lesions were visible to the naked eye and occurred in about 60 percent of the studied animals; microscopic examination revealed further lesions in a still larger percentage. It was subsequently reported that injection of sparteine sulfate or caffeine sodium benzoate followed by epinephrine provided an easy and certain method of producing myocardial lesions,[23–26] whereas sparteine sulfate alone did not produce myocardial lesions.[27] Not only relatively high dose levels of epinephrine but also a continuous infusion of epinephrine for 120–289 h, at a rate considered to be well below the maximum physiologic rate of secretion by the adrenal gland, was found to cause small endocardial lesions in the left ventricle.[28]

### *Norepinephrine-induced cardiomyopathy*

The hypertension resulting from norepinephrine infusion could not be maintained in the course of a study on the effects of a prolonged infusion of norepinephrine.[29] Furthermore, norepinephrine did not increase the survival rate of dogs in hemorrhagic shock.[30] As a consequence of these findings, the concept that norepinephrine may cause cardiac lesions appeared in the literature.[31,32] Thus, it was found that norepinephrine caused focal myocarditis in association with subendocardial and subepicardial hemorrhages. A series of experiments with both epinephrine and norepinephrine proved that epinephrine, norepinephrine, or both caused extensive lesions of the myocardium.[33] In a quantitative study on the pathologic effects of norepinephrine, it was found that dosages which may be considered physiologic, and indeed harmless, when administered for short periods of time might become lethal after prolonged infusion.[34] Thus, the duration of infusion appears to be an important factor in determining whether a particular dose of norepinephrine is likely to produce myocardial lesions. In addition to myocardial cell damage, norepinephrine was also demonstrated to produce derangements of metabolic processes in the heart. For example, a fatty degeneration of the myocardium under the influence of high doses of norepinephrine was reported.[35] In subsequent studies,[36,37] remarkable similarities were found in heart triglyceride content and serum enzyme levels after large doses of epinephrine and norepinephrine as well as after myocardial infarction produced by coronary artery occlusion.

### Isoproterenol-induced cardiomyopathy

It was discovered that relatively low and non-lethal doses of isoproterenol can cause severe myocardial necrosis.[4,38] Although the $LD_{50}$ of isoproterenol in rats was reported to be 680 mg kg$^{-1}$, doses as low as 0.02 mg kg$^{-1}$ produced microscopic focal necrotic lesions. The severity of myocardial damage was closely related to the dosage of isoproterenol used and varied from focal lesions affecting single cells to massive infarcts involving large portions of the left ventricle. Isoproterenol-induced myocardial lesions were generally found to be localized in the apex as well as the left ventricular subendocardium, and were observed less frequently in the papillary muscle and the right ventricle. Isoproterenol was also found to produce apical lesions and disseminated focal necrosis;[39] however, these lesions were frequently fatal and the median lethal dosage was much lower. In poikilothermic hearts (frog, turtle), isoproterenol-induced myocardial lesions were localized in the inner spongious musculature, which has no vascular supply,[40] thus indicating that these changes may not be the result of myocardial ischemia.

### Comparison of the cardiotoxic effects of different catecholamines

The lesions caused by epinephrine, norepinephrine, and isoproterenol were qualitatively similar, but the lesions which were seen after isoproterenol treatment were more severe than those produced by epinephrine or norepinephrine.[41,42] The median lethal doses of isoproterenol, epinephrine, and norepinephrine were found to be 581 mg kg$^{-1}$, 6.1 mg kg$^{-1}$, and 8.6 mg kg$^{-1}$ respectively.[42] In fact, isoproterenol was found to be twenty-nine to seventy-two times more potent in producing myocardial lesions of equal severity than epinephrine or norepinephrine. In the clinical setting, myocardial lesions similar to those produced by catecholamine injections have also been reported in patients with pheochromocytoma,[3,43–45] subarachnoid hemorrhage and various other intracranial lesions,[46–49] as well as following electrical stimulation of the stellate ganglion[50,51] or hypothalamus[52] in experimental animals. These studies not only demonstrate that catecholamines are capable of producing myocardial necrosis but also suggest that myocardial cell damage seen in patients may be the result of high levels of circulating catecholamines for a prolonged period. However, reversible catecholamine-induced cardiomyopathy has also been reported.[53–57]

## Characteristics of catecholamine-induced cardiomyopathy

Although a number of long-term studies have been conducted on the development and healing of catecholamine-induced myocardial lesions, the present discussion will be limited to early events, i.e. less than 48 h after the injection of catecholamines for the production of myocardial necrosis.

271

## *Ultrastructural changes*

Table 9.1 shows the time-course of ultrastructural changes following isoproterenol injections in rats, as reported previously.[48,58–62] It has been observed that there is no correlation between mitochondrial damage and disruption of myofilaments seen by 10 min after the isoproterenol injection: normal appearing mitochondria being found among fragmented filaments, and swollen mitochondria with ruptured cristae and electron-dense deposits among apparently undamaged sarcomeres.[59–63] Within 30–60 min, there also occurs a spectrum of damage to the contractile filaments, ranging from irregular bands of greater or less than normal density in sarcomeres of irregular length to fusion of sarcomeres into confluent masses and granular disintegration of the myofilaments.[58–61] Comparison of the effects of norepinephrine and epinephrine with isoproterenol has shown that the effects of these three agents are qualitatively identical at the cellular level,[61–66] with the exception that glycogen depletion[61,64] and fat deposition[66] were much more extensive with epinephrine than with isoproterenol or norepinephrine. Similar alterations following isoproterenol administration in monkeys have also been reported.[11]

From the foregoing discussion, it appears that alterations of the contractile filaments begin with irregularities in length and misalignment of the sarcomeres which are usually associated with an increased thickness and density of the Z-band. Contracture ensues, with the Z-bands becoming indistinct, and actin and myosin filaments can no longer be distinguished. Granular disintegration of the sarcomeres follows, with the appearance of large empty spaces within the muscle cells, and this fragmentation likely contributes to swelling of the cell. The tubular elements and mitochondria commence swelling very soon after catecholamine injection, and the mitochondrial matrix is subsequently decreased in electron

*Table 9.1* Ultrastructural changes in catecholamine-induced cardiomyopathy

| Time after isoproterenol injection | Findings |
| --- | --- |
| A  Within 4–6 min | Disorientation of myofilament, irregular sarcomere length, occasional regions of contracture, rupture of myofilaments and slight dilatation of sarcoplasmic reticulum |
| B  Within 10 min | Swelling of mitochondria, occasional occurrence of electron-dense bodies and disorganization as well as fragmentation of myofibrils |
| C  Within 30–60 min | Electron-dense granular deposits in mitochondria, numerous lipid droplets, margination of nuclear chromatin, disappearance of glycogen granules and swelling as well as disruption of transverse and longitudinal tubules |
| D  Within 1–24 h | Interstitial and intercellular edema, extensive inflammation, herniation of cellular discs, and extensive vacuolization |

density. However, it is pointed out that swelling of the transverse tubules and sarcoplasmic reticulum is not as consistent a finding as the mitochondrial swelling and may not be evident with certain fixatives. Following norepinephrine injection, the T-system is dilated and much more extensively branched than in normal animals. Rupture of the cristae and deposition of electron-dense material in mitochondria represent the final stage in the disruption of these organelles. Accumulation of lipid droplets and disappearance of glycogen granules is not usually evident until these other changes have occurred to some degree and are probably due to well-known metabolic effects of catecholamines. Herniation of intercalated discs and vacuolization are probably secondary to the swelling and disruption of subcellular organelles and the disintegration of myofilaments.

## Histologic and histochemical changes

Histologic changes in catecholamine-induced cardiomyopathy are generally characterized by degeneration and necrosis of myocardial fiber, accumulation of inflammatory cells such as leukocytes, interstitial edema, lipid droplet (fat deposition), and endocardial hemorrhage. Table 9.2 shows the time-course of histologic changes following isoproterenol injection in rats, as reported previously.[4,10,11,39,61,63,65,67,68] Interstitial edema is usually associated with subendocardial and subepicardial hemorrhages following administration of catecholamines and is characteristically present in damaged areas of the

*Table 9.2* Histological changes in catecholamine-induced cardiomyopathy

| Time after isoproterenol injection | Findings |
|---|---|
| A   Within 10 min | Darkly stained contraction band in thin sections from Araldite-embedded ventricular pieces |
| B   Within 2–6 h | Focal myocardial degeneration, including loss of striations with sarcoplasmic smudging, lipid accumulation, margination of nuclear chromatin and increased cytoplasmic eosinophilia, capillary dilatation, interstitial edema, subendocardial and subepicardial hemorrhage, opacity and fuchsinorrhagia of the muscle fiber, myocytolysis, vacuolization and aggregation of lymphomononuclear cells |
| C   Within 12–24 h[a] | Fibers with highly eosinophilic cytoplasm (mottled appearance); fibers show swelling, fragmentation and hyalinization; fibers are homogeneous, strongly eosinophilic, peroxidase acid–Schiff (PAS) positive, stain pink or deep red with Cason's trichrome and exhibit fat deposition (lipid droplet) |

Note
a Changes similar to these have also been reported within 4–5 h after norepinephrine injection.

myocardium, even after 72 h.[4,14,39,61,63,67] Interstitial edema and inflammation are much more prominent following epinephrine or norepinephrine injections, even though isoproterenol is more potent in producing cellular damage.[14,61] Accordingly, it has been suggested that edema and inflammation result from mechanisms different from those causing necrotic tissue damage during the development of catecholamine-induced cardiomyopathy. Histochemical alterations subsequent to administration of lesion-producing doses of catecholamines have also been reported in detail.[61,62,64,66] A marked loss of glycogen, as visualized by periodic acid–Schiff (PAS) reaction, is seen within 30 min, and is most marked following epinephrine administration. Accumulation of PAS-positive material is seen at 1 h and in an increasing number of fibers over the next 24 h. This is associated with loss of normal striations and appearance of clear vacuoles. A metachromatic substance is usually observed in areas of interstitial edema and inflammation.

All three catecholamines have been shown to produce biphasic changes in the activities of different oxidative enzymes (Table 9.3). There is a rapid increase in the activities of enzymes; this is evident within 5 min in various individual fibers followed by a gradual decline in the activities during 6–12 h. Certain areas of the myocardium having markedly diminished oxidative enzyme activities are interspersed with fibers of normal activities. Decline in oxidative enzyme activities of certain fibers progresses until frank necrosis is evident and there is complete loss of the activities. In each case, the degree of change of the enzyme activities is proportional to the normal level of activity of the enzyme involved. Cytochrome oxidase activity is unchanged until evidence of early necrosis is seen after 6–

*Table 9.3* Biochemical changes in catecholamine-induced cardiomyopathy

| | | |
|---|---|---|
| A | Cardiac oxidative enzymes | Biphasic ($\uparrow\downarrow$) changes in succinic dehydrogenase, NAD diaphorase, lactic dehydrogenase, isocitric dehydrogenase, malic dehydrogenase, β-hydroxybutyric dehydrogenase, α-glycerophosphate dehyrogenase, glutamic dehydrogenase, and ethanol dehydrogenase |
| B | Blood (serum) contents | Glucose $\uparrow$, TG $\uparrow$, non-esterified fatty acid $\uparrow$, cholesterol ~, total protein $\downarrow$, aldosterone $\uparrow$, glucocorticoid $\downarrow$, total steroid $\downarrow$, GOT/AST $\uparrow$, GPT $\uparrow$, LDH $\uparrow$, CPK $\uparrow$ |
| C | Myocardial contents | Glycogen $\downarrow$ then $\uparrow$, lactate $\downarrow$, non-esterified fatty acid $\downarrow$, TG $\uparrow$, free fatty acids ~ (LV, epi), phospholipids ~ (LV, epi), TG uptake $\uparrow$, TG synthesis from acetate or palmitate ~, hexosamine $\uparrow$ (iso), mucopolysaccharide $\uparrow$ (iso), GOT activity $\downarrow$ (iso), LDH activity $\downarrow$ (iso), ratio of H/M isozyme $\downarrow$ |

Note
$\uparrow$, increase; ~, no change; $\downarrow$, decrease; iso, by isoproterenol; epi, by epinephrine; TG, triglyceride; GOT, glutamate–oxalacetate transferase; AST, aspartate amino transferase; GPT, glutamate–pyruvate transferase; LDH, lactate dehydrogenase; CPK, creatine phosphokinase; LV, left ventricle.

12 h, at which time the activity of this enzyme decreases as well. An increased number of lipid droplets is observed at 30 min. Fatty change is more evident in the endocardial region than elsewhere and has been reported by Ferrans et al.[61] to be least apparent with epinephrine; this is in direct contradiction to the findings of Lehr et al.[66] The reason for this discrepancy in these results is not clear; however, fibers which contain large lipid droplets show decreased activities of the oxidative enzymes, including cytochrome oxidase. Furthermore, all three catecholamines cause a slight increase in the staining of cytoplasm for lysosomal esterase activity.[66] It has been reported that ATPase and acid phosphatase were also increased in norepinephrine-induced cardiomyopathy.[68]

### Biochemical changes

Following catecholamine administration, the coronary blood flow, myocardial oxygen uptake, and cardiac respiratory quotient are increased.[69] Table 9.3 shows some biochemical changes in catecholamine-induced cardiomyopathy.[15,69–78] Glycogen content of the heart decreased rapidly after an injection of isoproterenol and then rose above control level during the subsequent 5 h.[73] Serum glutamate–oxaloacetate transaminase (GOT), aspartate aminotransferase (AST), glutamate–pyruvate transaminase (GPT), lactate dehydrogenase (LDH), and creatine phosphokinase (CPK) were all greatly elevated during the acute phase of necrotization following catecholamine administration.[69,71,72,74] There was no significant increase in the contents of free fatty acids or phospholipids in the left ventricle, whereas there was a significant increase in the triglyceride (TG) content of every layer of the left ventricular wall following epinephrine infusion; the greatest increase in triglyceride content occurred in the endocardium.[13] Furthermore, increased TG uptake and unchanged TG synthesis from acetate or palmitate are consistent with the appearance of numerous lipid droplets reported in histologic and ultrastructural studies.[75] The myocardial content of hexosamines became greatly elevated within 24 h after an injection of isoproterenol, and this increase in mucopolysaccharide could not be attributed to fibroblasts or other infiltrating cells.[76] Cardiac AST and GOT activities decreased in a time- and dose-dependent manner following isoproterenol injection.[77] Such a decrease in the enzyme activities correlated well with the occurrence and severity of macroscopic lesions. Total cardiac LDH activity also fell after isoproterenol injection;[78] this depression of activity was of long duration, lasting several days, and appeared to be due to a decrease in the H/M ratio of its isoenzymes. These findings are consistent with the loss of enzymes from the heart, as reflected by an increase in plasma concentrations of transaminases and LDH.

It has been reported that a single, large subcutaneous dose of epinephrine, norepinephrine, or isoproterenol produced uncoupling of oxidative phosphorylation in rat heart mitochondria;[22] however, these catecholamines did not affect normal rat heart mitochondria under in vitro conditions. A reduced respiratory control index of heart mitochondria 24 h after isoproterenol injection has also been reported.[79,80] The results of several studies on cardiac adenine nucleotides following isoproterenol injection in rats are somewhat contradictory. A decrease in the levels of all adenine nucleotides has been reported,[81] but no change in the relative amounts of ATP, ADP, and AMP was evident. On the other hand, a decrease in ATP and creatine phosphate (CrP) levels and a decrease in both ATP/ADP and ATP/AMP ratios without any significant difference in the levels of ADP, AMP, glycogen, lactate, pyruvate, lactate–pyruvate ratio, TG, cholesterol, or phospholipids have been reported.[82] Studies of this sort are difficult to evaluate; first, because the results are expressed in terms of gram wet heart weight, which increases because of a large increase in extracellular fluid volume following catecholamine administration,[82,83] and second because the scattered portions of the myocardium undergoing necrotic change are "diluted" within a very large mass of cardiac tissue which has been affected only slightly or not at all. When both ATP and CrP stores of the myocardium were decreased upon injecting catecholamines, it was evident that the high-energy phosphate stores in the heart were depressed;[84,85] a large increase in the orthophosphate content of the myocardium was also observed. These results suggest lowering of the energy state of myocardium as a result of high doses of catecholamines, and this change appears to be at least partly due to an impairment in the process of energy production. On the other hand, relatively little information regarding changes in the process of energy utilization during catecholamine-induced myocardial cell damage is available in the literature. In this regard, it has found that myosin extracted from rat hearts following isoproterenol injections contained a large component consisting of a stable aggregated form of myosin,[86,87] whereas only the monomeric form of myosin was extracted from control animals. The first phase of aggregation involved a low polymer, probably a dimer, and the aggregated form of myosin did not possess any ATPase activity; there was no evidence of proteolytic damage to the myosin. It has been reported that injection of a lesion-producing dose of isoproterenol caused an elevation of cardiac myofibrillar ATPase activity and decreased high-energy phosphate stores.[88] However, studies in our laboratory[89] did not reveal any change in myofibrillar $Ca^{2+}$-stimulated ATPase while the basal ATPase activity was depressed. Thus, it appears that further investigations are needed for a meaningful conclusion regarding changes in the process of energy utilization in hearts of animals treated with toxic doses of catecholamines to be drawn.

### Electrolyte changes

#### Tissue cation contents

Table 9.4 shows electrolyte changes in catecholamine-induced cardio-myopathy.[65,66,84,85,90,91] The sodium content of the myocardium did not change until about 24 h, at which time it was increased; this may be a reflection of an increased interstitial fluid volume.[65,66,90,91] On the other hand, alterations of myocardial potassium content are less certain. Although a transient loss of myocardial

*Table 9.4* Electrolyte changes on catecholamine-induced cardiomyopathy

| Time after the injection | Electrolyte changes |
|---|---|
| A Changes in tissue cation content | |
| 3–24 h | Mg ↓, phosphate ↓ |
| 6 h | Ca ↑, Ca uptake ↑ (iso) (six- to sevenfold) |
| 24 h | Na ~ or ↑ |
| B Serum levels of electrolytes | |
| 3 h | Mg ↑ (iso), Na ↓ (iso), Ca ↓ (iso) |
| 7 h | Mg to control K ↑, Na ↓, Ca ↓ |
| 24 h | All of electrolytes to normal with the exception of Ca |

Note
↑, increase; ~, no change; ↓, decrease; iso, by isoproterenol.

potassium has been frequently reported,[83,92–94] this is a short-term phenomenon not lasting more than 1–5 min and may be a result of the increased frequency of contraction.[95] In this regard, it has been reported that norepinephrine causes a dose-dependent uptake of potassium.[96] In studies concerned with the cardiotoxicity of epinephrine, both an increase[66] and a decrease[13] in the potassium content of the myocardium have been reported. A decrease in myocardial potassium content following isoproterenol injection has been also reported.[79] As mentioned previously, myocardial content determinations are complicated both by the increase in interstitial fluid volume which accompanies necrosis and by the admixture of necrotic and normal fibers which characterizes "multifocal disseminated" necrosis.

### Serum levels of electrolytes

By 24 h, all serum electrolyte levels returned to normal with the exception of calcium, which remained slightly low. It has been reported that, after an initial period of uptake of potassium and phosphate, loss of these ions from the left ventricle was evident.[69] Thus, serum electrolyte measurements appear to confirm the loss of magnesium and phosphate from the heart and the uptake of calcium as early, important events in the etiology of catecholamine-induced necrosis. As both net increases and decreases of myocardial and serum potassium have been found at different times, it is possible that potassium may be taken up by more or less undamaged myocardial cells while it is being released from fibers undergoing necrotic changes.

### Membrane changes

By virtue of their ability to regulate $Ca^{2+}$ movements in the myocardial cell, different membrane systems such as sarcolemma, sarcoplasmic reticulum, and mitochondria are considered to determine the status of heart function in health and disease.[97–100] Accordingly, alterations in sarcoplasmic reticular, mitochondrial, and sarcolemmal membranes were observed in myocardium from animals treated with high doses of catecholamines.[101,102] To investigate the role of these membrane changes in the development of contractile dysfunction and myocardial cell damage due to catecholamines, rats were injected intraperitoneally with high doses of isoproterenol (40 mg kg$^{-1}$) and the hearts were removed after 3, 9, or 24 h.[89,103–109] The cardiac hypertrophy as measured by the heart–body weight ratio and depression in contractile function were seen at 9 and 24 h, whereas varying degrees of myocardial cell damage occurred within 3–24 h of isoproterenol injection (Table 9.5). Alterations in heart membranes were evident from the fact that phospholipid contents in sarcolemma and mitochondria were increased at 3 and 9 h, whereas the sarcoplasmic reticular phospholipid contents increased at 3, 9, and 24 h after injection of isoproterenol. It was interesting to observe that phospholipid *N*-methylation, which has been shown to modulate the $Ca^{2+}$ transport activities,[104] exhibited an increase at 3 h and a decrease at 24 h in both sarcolemma and sarcoplasmic reticulum, whereas no changes were observed in mitochondria (Table 9.5). These studies[89,103–105] suggest that changes in heart membranes during the development of catecholamine-induced cardiomyopathy are of crucial importance in determining the functional and structural status of the myocardium.

An analysis of results described in various investigations[89,106–108] revealed that the activities of the sarcolemmal $Ca^{2+}$ pump (ATP-dependent $Ca^{2+}$ uptake and $Ca^{2+}$-stimulated ATPase), which is concerned with the removal of $Ca^{2+}$ from the cytoplasm, were increased at 3 h and decreased at 24 h after isoproterenol injection (Table 9.6). On the other hand, $Na^+$-dependent $Ca^{2+}$ uptake, unlike the $Na^+$-induced $Ca^{2+}$ release, was decreased at 3, 9, and 24 h after isoproterenol administration.

*Table 9.5* Contractile function, structure and membrane phospholipid changes in myocardium at different times of injecting high doses of isoproterenol (40 mg kg$^{-1}$, i.p.) in rats

|  | *Time after isoproterenol injection* | | |
|---|---|---|---|
|  | *3 h* | *9 h* | *24 h* |
| Heart/body weight ratio | No change | Increase | Increase |
| Contractile force development | No change | Decrease | Decrease |
| Myocardial cell damage | Slight | Moderate | Severe |
| Sarcolemmal phospholipid contents | Increase | Increase | No change |
| Sarcoplasmic reticular phospholipid contents | Increase | Increase | Increase |
| Mitochondrial phospholipid contents | Increase | Increase | No change |
| Sarcolemmal phospholipid methylation | Increase | No change | Decrease |
| Sarcoplasmic reticular phospholipid methylation | Increase | No change | Decrease |
| Mitochondrial phospholipid methylation | No change | No change | No change |

Note
The information in this table is taken from papers by Dhalla *et al.*,[89,105] Panagia *et al.*,[103] and Okumura *et al.*[104]

*Table 9.6* Sarcolemmal changes in myocardium at different times of injecting high doses of isoproterenol (40 mg kg$^{-1}$, i.p.) in rats

|  | Time after isoproterenol injection | | |
|---|---|---|---|
|  | *3 h* | *9 h* | *24 h* |
| ATP-dependent Ca$^{2+}$ uptake | Increase | No change | Decrease |
| Ca$^{2+}$-stimulated ATPase | Increase | No change | Decrease |
| Na$^+$-dependent Ca$^{2+}$ uptake | Decrease | Decrease | Decrease |
| Na$^+$-induced Ca$^{2+}$ release | No change | No change | No change |
| ATP-independent Ca$^{2+}$ binding | No change | Increase | Increase |
| Sialic acid content | No change | Increase | Increase |
| Nitrendipine binding | No change | No change | No change |
| Na$^+$/K$^+$-ATPase | No change | No change | No change |
| Ca$^{2+}$/Mg$^{2+}$-ecto-ATPase | No change | No change | No change |

Note

The information in this table is taken from papers by Dhalla *et al.*,[89] Panagia *et al.*,[108] and Makino *et al.*[106,107]

The sarcolemmal ATP-independent Ca$^{2+}$ binding, which is considered to reflect the status of superficial stores of Ca$^{2+}$ at the cell membrane, and sarcolemmal sialic acid residues, which bind Ca$^{2+}$, were increased at 9 and 24 h (Table 9.6). All these sarcolemmal alterations were not associated with any changes in the nitrendipine binding (an index of Ca$^{2+}$ channels), Na$^+$,K$^+$-ATPase (an index of the Na$^+$ pump), and Ca$^{2+}$,Mg$^{2+}$-ecto-ATPase (an index of the Ca$^{2+}$-gating mechanism). An early increase in the sarcolemmal Ca$^{2+}$ pump may help the cell to remove Ca$^{2+}$, whereas depressed Na$^+$/Ca$^{2+}$ exchange can be seen to contribute toward the occurrence of intracellular Ca$^{2+}$ overload. Likewise, an increase in the entry of Ca$^{2+}$ from the elevated sarcolemmal superficial Ca$^{2+}$ stores as well as the depressed sarcolemmal Ca$^{2+}$ pump may contribute toward the occurrence of intracellular Ca$^{2+}$ overload at a late stage of catecholamine-induced cardiomyopathy.

It is now well known that relaxation of the cardiac muscle is mainly determined by the activity of the Ca$^{2+}$ pump located in the sarcoplasmic reticulum, whereas the interaction of Ca$^{2+}$ with myofibrils determines the ability of the myocardium to contract. On the other hand, mitochondria, which are primarily concerned with the production of ATP, are also known to accumulate Ca$^{2+}$ in order to lower the intracellular concentration of Ca$^{2+}$ under pathologic conditions. Data from different studies,[80,103,105] as summarized in Table 9.7, indicate biphasic changes in the sarcoplasmic reticular Ca$^{2+}$ pump (ATP-dependent Ca$^{2+}$ uptake and Ca$^{2+}$-stimulated ATPase) activities during the development of catecholamine-induced cardiomyopathy. Mitochondrial Ca$^{2+}$ uptake, unlike mitochondrial ATPase activity, was increased at 9 and 24 h after isoproterenol injection. Although no change in myofibrillar Ca$^{2+}$-stimulated ATPase activity was apparent, the myofibrillar Mg$^{2+}$-ATPase activity was depressed at 9 and 24 h after isoproterenol injection (Table 9.7). Time-dependent changes in the adrenergic receptor mechanisms,[109] which are also concerned with the regulation of Ca$^{2+}$ movements in myocardium, were also seen during the development of catecholamine-induced cardiomyopathy (Table 9.8). In particular, the number of β-adrenergic receptors was decreased at 9 h, whereas the number of α-adrenergic receptors was decreased at 24 h after isoproterenol injection. The basal adenylyl cyclase activities were not changed, whereas stimulation of adenylyl cyclase by epinephrine was depressed at 3 and 9 h. Activation of adenylyl cyclase by a non-hydrolyzable analog of guanine nucleotide [Gpp(NH)p] and NaF was decreased at 3, 9, and 24 h after isoproterenol injection (Table 9.8). These results suggest that subcellular mechanisms concerned with the regulation of $Ca^{2+}$ movements are altered in catecholamine-induced cardiomyopathy.

In summary, it appears that some of the changes in heart membranes are adaptive in nature whereas others contribute toward the pathogenesis of myocardial cell damage and contractile dysfunction. The early increase in sarcolemmal and sarcoplasmic reticular $Ca^{2+}$ pump mechanisms as well as late changes in mitochondrial $Ca^{2+}$ uptake seems to help the myocardial cell in lowering the

*Table 9.7* Subcellular alterations in myocardium at different times of injecting high doses of isoproterenol (40 mg kg⁻¹; i.p.) in rats

|  | *Time after isoproterenol injection* | | |
|---|---|---|---|
|  | *3 h* | *9 h* | *24 h* |
| Sarcoplasmic reticular $Ca^{2+}$ uptake | Increase | No change | Decrease |
| Sarcoplasmic reticular $Ca^{2+}$-stimulated ATPase | Increase | No change | Decrease |
| Mitochondrial $Ca^{2+}$ uptake | No change | Increase | Increase |
| Mitochondrial ATPase | No change | No change | No change |
| Myofibrillar $Ca^{2+}$-stimulated ATPase | No change | No change | No change |
| Myofibrillar $Mg^{2+}$-ATPase | No change | Decrease | Decrease |

Note
The information in this table was taken from papers by Dhalla *et al.*[89,105] and Panagia *et al.*[103]

*Table 9.8* Changes in adrenergic receptor mechanisms in myocardium at different times of injecting high doses of isoproterenol (40 mg kg⁻¹; i.p.) in rats

|  | *Time after isoproterenol injection* | | |
|---|---|---|---|
|  | *3 h* | *9 h* | *24 h* |
| β-Adrenergic receptors | No change | Decrease | No change |
| α-Adrenergic receptors | No change | No change | Decrease |
| Adenylyl cyclase activity | No change | No change | No change |
| Epinephrine-stimulated adenylyl cyclase | Decrease | Decrease | No change |
| Gpp(NH)p-stimulated adenylyl cyclase | Decrease | Decrease | Decrease |
| NaF-stimulated adenylyl cyclase | Decrease | Decrease | Decrease |

Note
The information in this table is taken from Corder *et al.*[109]

intracellular concentration of $Ca^{2+}$. On the other hand, the early depression in sarcolemmal $Na^+/Ca^{2+}$ exchange and late decrease in sarcolemmal and sarcoplasmic reticular $Ca^{2+}$ pump may lead to the development of intracellular $Ca^{2+}$ overload. This change may result in the redistribution and activation of lysosomal enzymes[110] and in other mechanisms for the disruption of the myocardial cell as a result of high levels of circulating catecholamines.

### Coronary spasm and catecholamines

Under a wide variety of stressful conditions, in which circulating levels of catecholamines are markedly elevated, occurrence of coronary spasm and arrhythmia has been well recognized.[111] In fact, coronary spasm is considered to result in arrhythmia, myocardial ischemia, and myocardial cell damage as a result of catecholamines. To understand the mechanisms of coronary spasm, changes in coronary resistance were monitored upon infusion of norepinephrine in the isolated perfused rat heart preparations.[112] A biphasic change in coronary resistance was evident; however, when norepinephrine infusion was carried out in the presence of a β-adrenergic blocking agent, propranolol, only a marked increase in coronary resistance (coronary spasm) was evident. This coronary spasm was dependent upon the extracellular concentration of $Ca^{2+}$ and was prevented by α-adrenergic blocking agents as well as $Ca^{2+}$ antagonists.[112] On the other hand, indomethacin and acetylsalicylic acid, which interfere with prostaglandin metabolism, did not modify the norepinephrine-induced coronary spasm.[112] In another set of experiments, intravenous injection of epinephrine in rats was found to elicit varying degrees of arrhythmia depending upon the time and dose of the hormone.[113,114] Pretreatment of animals with vitamin E, reducing agent (cysteine), or oxygen free radical scavenger (superoxide dismutase) was found to reduce markedly the incidence of arrhythmia due to epinephrine. These results indicate the importance of free radicals in the generation of cardiotoxic effects of high concentrations of catecholamines.

## Interventions on catecholamine-induced cardiomyopathy

### Pharmacologic interventions

#### Monoamine oxidase inhibitors

Table 9.9 shows the effects of different types of drugs, including monoamine oxidase inhibitors (MAOIs), on catecholamine-induced cardiomyopathy. MAOIs of the hydrazine type have been found to decrease the incidence and severity of myocardial lesions following catecholamine administration[73,79,115–119] and to antagonize increases in myocardial water, sodium, and chloride as well as loss of potassium.[79] The hydrazine-type inhibitors investigated include isocarboxazide, iproniazide, pivaloylbanzhydrazine, and phenylzine. On the other hand, the non-

*Table 9.9* The effects of drugs on catecholamine-induced cardiomyopathy

| | Drugs | Effects |
|---|---|---|
| A Monoamine oxidase inhibitors | | |
| a Hydrazine type | Isocarboxazide | Decrease |
| | Iproniazide | Decrease |
| | Pivaloylbanzhydrazine | Decrease |
| | Phenylzine | Decrease |
| b Non-hydrazine type | Tranilcypromine | No change |
| | Pargyline | No change |
| | R05-707 | No change or decrease (iso) |
| | E-250 | Decrease |
| B β-Adrenergic blocking agents | Popranolol | Decrease (iso) |
| | Pronethalol | Decrease or no change (iso, epi, nor) |
| | Dicloroisoproterenol | Decrease (iso) |
| C α-Adrenergic blocking agents | Azapetine | Decrease (phe, epi, nor) No change (iso) |
| | Phentolamine | Decrease (phe, epi, nor) No change (iso) |
| | Diberanamine | Decrease (phe, epi, nor) No change (iso) |
| | Dihydroergocryptin | Decrease (phe, epi, nor) No change (iso) |
| | Phenoxybenzamine | Decrease (phe, epi, nor) No change (iso) |
| | Tolazoline | Decrease (phe, epi, nor) No change (iso) |
| D Post-ganglionic blockers | Guanethidine | No change (iso) |
| | Isocaramidine | No change (iso) |
| | Reserpine | No change (iso) |
| | Pyrogallol | No change (iso) |
| | Serotonin + nialimide | Decrease |
| E Calcium channel blocker | Verapamil | Decrease (iso) |
| | D600 | Decrease (iso) |
| | Phenylamine | Decrease (iso) |
| | Vascoril | Decrease (iso) |
| | Diltiazem | Decrease (iso) |
| | Clentiazem | Decrease (epi) |
| F Angiotensin-converting enzyme inhibitor | Captopril | Decrease |
| G Antiarrhythmic drug | Propafenone | Decrease (epi) |

Note
Decrease, decrease in the severity of myocardial lesion; no change, no change of the severity of myocardial lesion; iso, isoproterenol; epi, epinephrine; nor, norepinephrine; phe, phenylephrine.

hydrazine type MAOIs such as tranylcypromine, pargyline, and RO5-707 have been reported by some workers to be ineffective,[73,118,119] although a reduction of the severity of isoproterenol-induced lesions with pargyline and another non-hydrazine MAOI identified as E-250 has been reported.[120] It was also found that hydrazine-type inhibition is long-lasting whereas tranylcypromine is a competitive blocker with an intensive but transient effect, and thus the inhibition produced by the non-hydrazine type drugs may be of insufficient duration to afford protection.[121]

### β-Adrenergic blocking agents

The β-receptor-blocking compounds propranolol, pronethalol, and dichloro-isoproterenol were found to reduce the incidence and severity of myocardial lesions induced by isoproterenol.[90,91,115,122–124] While some investigators[78] have reported that pronethalol was ineffective, others[77] have reported that pronethalol afforded some protection against the loss of myocardial AST activity caused by epinephrine, norepinephrine and high doses of isoproterenol but potentiated the loss of AST activity with moderate lesion-producing doses of isoproterenol. Propranolol has also been found to ameliorate or to prevent completely electrolyte shifts (increased myocardial $Ca^{2+}$) associated with the isoproterenol-induced necrosis,[91,122] thus producing an apparent dichotomy between the occurrence of lesions and electrolyte shifts as less severe myocardial lesions were still seen. In view of the proportion of the ventricle not undergoing necrotic damage in these experiments, it is difficult to know whether the alterations of electrolytes are truly and completely prevented. It has been reported that propranolol reduced the amount by which myocardial ATP declined following the isoproterenol-induced damage.[125] Propranolol appears to have a more selective action on endocardial versus mid-myocardial or epicardiac changes in metabolism due to catecholamines.[126] One can thus conclude that the β-adrenergic blocking agents are capable of modifying certain cardiotoxic effects of catecholamines.

### α-Adrenergic blocking agents

The α-adrenergic blocking compounds such as azapetine, phentolamine, dibenamine, dihydroergocryptin, phenoxybenzamine, and tolazoline were ineffective against isoproterenol,[73,78,123,124,127] but reduced somewhat the incidence and severity of lesions caused by α-receptor agonists such as phenylephrine,[90,127] epinephrine,[78,90,127,128] and norepinephrine.[78,127] The α-blockers also ameliorated the loss of myocardial AST and LDH activities as well as the shift of electrolytes caused by epinephrine and norepinephrine.[66,78,129] These agents were usually more effective against epinephrine lesions when used in combination with a β-blocker.[66,90,127] It should be pointed out that isoproterenol has been shown to reduce the endogenous norepinephrine stores from the nerve endings,[130] and it is possible that endogenously released norepinephrine may also be participating in producing the cardiotoxic effects when animals are injected with isoproterenol.

## Post-ganglionic blockers and others

The post-ganglionic blocker guanethidine has been reported to be ineffective[73,124] or to increase the severity[120] of necrosis caused by isoproterenol. Isocaramidine, another post-ganglionic blocker, has also been found to have no effect on the isoproterenol-induced necrosis.[73] Reserpine, which is known to decrease catecholamine stores, has been reported to be without effect[73,119] or to increase the severity[120,121] of isoproterenol-induced lesions. Pyrogallol, a catechol-*O*-methyl transferase inhibitor, increased the severity of lesions.[121] Serotonin and nialimide administered together reduced the severity and incidence of myocardial lesions.[131] Other drugs which were found to influence the production of lesions by isoproterenol are the vasodilators, such as sodium nitrite, aminophylline, dipyridamole, and hexobenzine, and the psychosedative drugs, such as chlorpromazine, chlordiazepoxide, meprobamate, amitriptyline, and creatinol *O*-phosphate, as well as antioxidants, such as zinc.[73,132–134] In this regard, it is worth mentioning that most of these drugs are not specific with respect to their site of action and conclusions drawn from such studies should be interpreted with some caution. Inhibition of lipolysis by nicotinic acid or β-pyridyl carbonyl decreased the amount by which isoproterenol infusion increased the myocardial oxygen consumption.[135] Chronic administration of nicotine in high doses tended to increase the severity and incidence of lesions produced by isoproterenol.[136]

## Calcium channel blockers

The calcium channel blockers verapamil, D-600, phenylamine, and vascoril reduced the severity of lesions and prevented the decrease in high-energy phosphate stores and accumulation of calcium by the myocardium caused by isoproterenol injections.[84,85,137] Another $Ca^{2+}$ antagonist, diltiazem, also prevented the isoproterenol-induced changes in myocardial high-energy phosphate stores in rats.[138] Furthermore, it has been reported that clentiazem prevented epinephrine-induced myocardial lesions in addition to reducing the mortality.[139]

## Angiotensin-converting enzyme inhibitors and anti-arrhythmic drugs

It has been reported that trandolapril prevented both cardiac hypertrophy and increased the angiotensin II content by isoproterenol.[140] It has also been reported that captopril attenuated cardiomyopathy associated with phenochromo-cytoma.[141,142] Myocardial accumulation of propafenone, an antiarrhythmic drug, was reduced in areas of extensive necrosis in norepinephrine-induced cardio-myopathy.[143]

## Hormonal, electrolyte, and metabolic interventions

Table 9.10 shows the effects of hormonal, electrolyte, and metabolic interventions

*Table 9.10* Hormonal, electrolytic, and metabolic interventions in catecholamine-induced cardiomyopathy

|  | *Effects* |
|---|---|
| **A Steroids** | |
| Deoxycorticosterone | Increase |
| 9-α-Fluorocortisol | Increase |
| Estrone | Increase |
| Testosterone | Increase |
| Estrogen | No change |
| Progesterone | No change |
| Glucocorticoids | No change |
| Cortisone | No change |
| **B Thyroid hormones** | |
| Thyroxine, hyperthyroidism | Increase |
| Thyroidectomy, thiouracil, propylthiouracil | Decrease |
| Anthracitic agents (dihydrotachysterol, calfenil) | Increase |
| Thyrocalcitonin | Decrease |
| **C Electrolytes** | |
| Low serum $Ca^{2+}$ concentration | Decrease |
| $NaHPO_4$ | Increase |
| High-sodium, low-potassium diets | Increase |
| Low-sodium, high-potassium diets | Decrease |
| Administration of KCl, $MgCl_2$, $NH_4Cl$ | Decrease |
| Low plasma $Mg^{2+}$, $K^+$, $H^+$ concentrations | Increase |
| Administration of $K^+ + Mg^{2+}$-aspartate | Decrease |
| **D Others** | |
| Glucose, lactate, pyruvate | No change |
| Sex, breed | No change |
| Increased body weight, excess body fat | Increase |
| Starvation, restricted food intake | Decrease |
| Previous myocardial damage | Decrease |
| Previous isoproterenol injection | Decrease |
| Coronary arteriosclerosis | Decrease |
| Cardiac hypertrophy, simultaneous hypoxia | Increase |
| Higher ambient temperature | Increase |
| High altitude acclimation, hyperbaric oxygen | Decrease |
| Isolation stress, cold exposure | Increase |

Note
Increase, increased the severity of myocardial lesion; decrease, decreased the severity of myocardial lesion; no change, no change in the severity of myocardial lesion.

on catecholamine-induced cardiomyopathy. The mineralocorticoids, such as deoxycorticosterone and 9α-fluorocortisol, increased the severity of myocardial lesions,[38,85,115,116,144] the level of $Ca^{2+}$ accumulation,[84,85] and the depletion of high-energy phosphate[85] caused by isoproterenol. Administration of KCl, $MgCl_2$, or $NH_4Cl$ reduced the severity of lesions[67,85,145] and protected against the electrolyte shifts and reduction of the high-energy phosphate store.[75,85,145] On the other hand, when plasma $Mg^{2+}$, $K^+$, and $H^+$ concentrations were low, the isoproterenol-induced lesions were potentiated.[146] Administration of $K^+/Mg^{2+}$-aspartate together with isoproterenol has also been found to prevent or reduce the changes in myofibrillar ATPase activity, $Ca^{2+}$ accumulation by mitochondria and microsomes, and high-energy phosphates stores,[88] in addition to decreasing the severity of ultrastructural damage in the myocardium.[147] Calciferol and another antirachitic agent, dihydrotachysterol, increased the severity of necrotic lesions, as did $Na_2HPO_4$.[84,85,115] The increased severity of the lesions was associated with a further increase in $Ca^{2+}$ uptake and a greater fall of high-energy phosphate stores in the heart. Likewise, thyrocalcitonin as well as reduction of plasma calcium with EDTA decreased the extent of both lesions and electrolyte shifts.[85]

The severity of myocardial damage due to catecholamines was increased with increased body weight and excess body fat.[115,116,148,149] The severity of lesions did increase with age, but this is probably an indirect effect as a consequence of an increase in body weight with age.[150] It has also been reported that the pattern of catecholamine-induced cardiomyopathy may not be uniform, but instead may depend strictly on the stage of cardiac growth.[40] Previous myocardial damage markedly reduced the severity of lesions produced by high doses of isoproterenol;[151–153] this protective effect disappeared with time and did not result from necrosis of the extracardiac tissue. A higher ambient temperature also potentiated the necrotic effect of isoproterenol, possibly as a result of the increased work load on the heart during thermoregulatory vasodilation[154] as well as changes in the $Ca^{2+}$ transport mechanisms.[101] Isolation stress or cold exposure both increased the severity of isoproterenol-induced lesion and electrolyte shifts,[115,116,148,155,156] although this may be an indirect result of increased mineralocorticoid production which occurs under these conditions.[155–157]

Thus, it appears that factors which increase the work load on the heart, increase the metabolic rate, interfere with oxygen supply to myocardial cells, favor the electrolyte change, or favor mobilization of lipids aggravate the necrotic influence of catecholamines. On the other hand, factors which block the stimulatory effects of catecholamines, thereby reducing cardiac work, or otherwise reduce myocardial metabolic rate, aid in the supply of oxygen to the myocardium, limit the mobilization of lipids, or counteract the ionic shifts and reduce the severity of necrotic changes. In particular, interventions which promote the occurrence of intracellular $Ca^{2+}$ overload have been shown to aggravate and those which reduce the intracellular $Ca^{2+}$ overload have been reported to prevent the catecholamine-induced cardiotoxicity. Although the protective effect of MAOI compounds is still enigmatic, it is clear from the above discussion that an imbalance among oxygen availability and work, the metabolism of lipids, and the alteration of electrolyte balance are all crucial factors contributing to the etiology of catecholamine lesions. The evidence available in the existing literature does not permit the identification of a single molecular lesion which can be considered responsible for the pathogenesis of myocardial necrosis due to catecholamines.

# Mechanisms of catecholamine-induced cardiomyopathy

It has, for the most part, been assumed that cardiac cell necrosis following administration of catecholamines is due to a defect in the supply of energy for the maintenance of essential cellular processes. Various theories have been proposed to suggest the cause of the energy deficiency and the nature of the irreversible step following decreased energy availability. The major hypotheses include:

1  a relative cardiac hypoxemia caused by increased cardiac work and myocardial oxygen demands, aggravated by hypotension in the case of isoproterenol;[10,39]
2  coronary arterial vasoconstriction (spasm) causing endocardial ischemia;[7,8]
3  inadequate perfusion of the endocardium due to impaired venous drainage of the heart;[158]
4  hypoxia due to direct oxygen wasting effects of catecholamines or their oxidation products;[21]
5  interference with mitochondrial oxidative phosphorylation by free fatty acids;[135,159]
6  occurrence of intracellular $Ca^{2+}$ overload as a result of massive calcium influx;[85]
7  formation of adrenochromes and other oxidation products including oxyradicals;[105,112,114]
8  potassium depletion,[160] and altered permeability of the myocardial cell membrane through elevation of plasma non-esterified free fatty acids;[161]
9  depletion of intracellular magnesium required for many ATP-dependent enzymatic processes;[90,145]

This section is devoted to discussion of different mechanisms which have been suggested to explain the cardiotoxic effects of catecholamines.

## *Relative hypoxia and hemodynamic changes*

Figure 9.1 shows the concept of relative cardiac hypoxemia and hemodynamic changes which have been shown to occur as a consequence of an injection of isoproterenol. It was found that both high and low doses of isoproterenol increased heart rate similarly, but the cardiac lesion-producing doses of isoproterenol resulted in a fall in blood pressure. It was suggested that the fall in aortic blood pressure was of such a degree that a reduced coronary flow could be inferred. It was further postulated that the necrotic lesions are the ischemic infarcts due to a decreased coronary flow during a time when both amplitude and frequency of cardiac contractions are increased. Thus, the greater cardiotoxicity of isoproterenol than epinephrine or norepinephrine was attributed to the dramatic hypotension. Various factors, such as previous myocardial damage, previous isoproterenol injections, or activation of metabolic processes were considered to provide cardiac muscle cells with an enhanced adaptation to withstand the increased oxygen demand and relative hypoxia produced by isoproterenol.[162] On the other hand, it was found

287

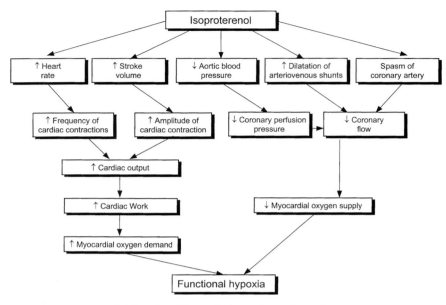

*Figure 9. 1* Myocardial functional hypoxia due to isoproterenol.

that mephenteramine, DL-ephedrine, and D-amphetamine produced lesions in less than 50 percent of animals, although these agents increase blood pressure while ephedrine and amphetamine have a positive inotropic effect.[14] Accordingly, it was suggested that drugs with both positive inotropic and chronotropic actions may not produce cardiac lesions. In fact, methoxamine, which has no positive inotropic effect, was found to produce cardiac lesions. In another study,[15] the hemodynamic effects of "pharmacologic" and "lesion-producing" doses of sympathomimetics were compared. It was found that lesion-producing doses of isoproterenol decreased aortic flow and heart rate compared with pharmacologic doses, but these were still above the control values. Stroke work was greater with lesion-producing doses than with pharmacologic doses, but the mean aortic pressure, which determines the coronary perfusion pressure, was not reduced by the lesion-producing doses of isoproterenol. Thus, there is evidence of impaired function of the myocardium, but the hemodynamic change does not appear adequate to produce insufficient myocardial perfusion. As a result of these findings, it was suggested that the effects of isoproterenol were due to some direct action on the myocardial cell and not solely to the hemodynamic effects. Furthermore, the coronary flow could not have been greatly reduced by isoproterenol because the blood pressure remained above that in shock and the cardiac output was increased;[11] thus, it was concluded that hypotension is non-essential for the production of cardiac necrosis by isoproterenol. This view was supported by the finding that verapamil was effective in protecting the heart from isoproterenol-induced necrosis, even though blood pressure fell almost twice as much when verapamil was administered together with isoproterenol as it did following administration of isoproterenol alone.[163]

## Coronary spasms and hemodynamic effects

Another hypothesis closely related to that of coronary insufficiency of hemodynamic origin is that of a relative ischemia resulting from coronary vascular changes. It was found that isoproterenol changed the distribution of uniform coronary flow in endomyocardium.[7] These results suggested that dilatation of arteriovenous shunts might be responsible for the endocardial ischemia because coronary flow is usually increased with isoproterenol. On the other hand, a marked occlusion of coronary vessels was observed in 69 percent of animals at 30 min and in 33 percent of animals at 60 min, but practically no occlusion was seen at 24 h after isoproterenol injection.[164] It was thought that these results were caused by spasm of the coronary vessels. Changes in peripheral resistance due to catecholamines were also important because it was possible to reproduce essentially similar pathologic changes by surgical occlusion of the efferent vessels.[158] On this basis, it was suggested that impairment of venous drainage via venospasm largely accounts for the adverse effects of sympathomimetic amines.

The occurrence of coronary arterial or venous spasms is of course only conjectural, and a somewhat simpler explanation of the impaired perfusion of the endocardium can be inferred from certain other studies of the circulation in the heart. Blood flow to the left ventricular subendocardial muscle has been suggested to be compromised during systole and to occur mainly during diastole because intramyocardial compressive force is greatest in this region.[165,166] Furthermore, it has been shown[167] that when aortic diastolic pressure was lowered or diastole shortened (by pacing) and myocardial oxygen demands simultaneously raised, myocardial performance was found to be impaired. Scintillation counting of the distribution of $^{141}$Ce-, $^{85}$Sr-, or $^{46}$Sc-labeled microspheres was used to determine the coronary flow distribution during isoproterenol infusion.[168] When isoproterenol was infused at a rate which failed to maintain the increase in contractile force, it was found that subendocardial flow fell by 35 percent whereas subepicardial flow increased by 19 percent. Thus, although spasm of coronary arteries and/or veins may well occur, it is possible that increased cardiac activity, reduced aortic pressure, and greatly decreased diastole could also be responsible for an underperfusion of the endocardium.

A serious challenge to the concept of impaired ventricular perfusion as the primary cause of necrosis was presented by using the $^{85}$Kr clearance method to study perfusion of the ventricle during epinephrine infusion.[13] Evidence of myocardial necrosis was obtained by 75 min after the start of epinephrine infusion, but $^{85}$Kr clearance studies showed no difference in the rate of clearance from inner, middle, and outer layers of the left ventricle in either the control or epinephrine-treated hearts. Thus, there was no evidence for ischemia of subendocardial tissue as a causal factor in the epinephrine-induced necrosis. On the other hand, a decreased passage of the trace substance horseradish peroxidase from the capillaries to the myocardial interstitium was observed in a study in which isoproterenol was infused at a low concentration.[5] Thus, this controversy still remained to be resolved. The hypothesis that the vascular factors are the primary cause of necrotic lesions was also tested using the turtle heart as a unique model in which perfusion of the endocardium was not vascular.[12] In the turtle heart, the internal spongy musculature is supplied by diffusion from the ventricular lumen via intertrabecular spaces, whereas the outer compact layer is supplied by the coronary artery branching off the aorta. Isoproterenol injections were found to produce necrotic lesions in the spongy layer of the turtle heart, which does not support the concept that isoproterenol-induced cardiac necrosis is due to a vascular mechanism.

## *Metabolic effects*

Figure 9.2 shows the concept involving metabolic and hemodynamic changes in the development of catecholamine-induced cardiomyopathy. It was pointed out that the catecholamine-induced myocardial necrosis must be considered to be of a mixed pathogenesis involving both direct metabolic actions in the cardiac muscle as well as factors secondary to vascular and hemodynamic effects.[169] Although cardiac lesions induced by epinephrine, methoxamine, and isoproterenol are indistinguishable with respect to both distribution and histologic characteristics, it would appear that the methoxamine-induced lesion is a typical secondary cardiomyopathy. On the other hand, cardiac lesions due to epinephrine and isoproterenol are of a mixed type in which both hypoxia secondary to vascular and hemodynamic effects as well as direct metabolic effects in the heart muscle have a role in their development. It is not, then, unreasonable to regard vascular and hemodynamic effects as complicating factors which greatly aggravate some more direct toxic influence of catecholamines on myocardial cells. Accordingly, it can be readily understood how a reduction in the extent and severity of catecholamine-induced lesions is brought about by interventions which specifically block the peripheral vascular change, prevent the positive inotropic and chronotropic effects of these drugs on the heart, or which improve the delivery of oxygen to the myocardium.

Many years ago, Raab[21] attributed the cardiotoxic actions of catecholamines to their oxygen-wasting effect. According to him:

> The most conspicuous reaction of myocardial metabolism to the administration of epinephrine is an intense enhancement of local oxygen consumption which, in certain dosages, by far exceeds the demand of simultaneously increased myocardial muscular work and which is only partially compensated by a simultaneous increase of coronary blood flow. In this respect, adrenaline is able, so to speak, to mimic the anoxiating

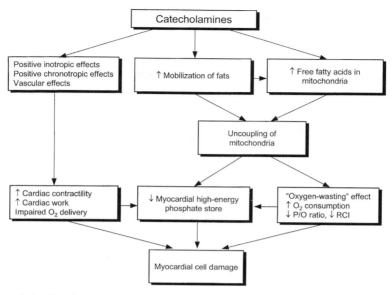

*Figure 9.2.* Cardiac function and lipid mobilization in catecholamine-induced cardiomyopathy.

effects of coronary insufficiency in the absence of any real coronary anomaly. It should be emphasized, however, that the tissue anoxia resulting from the administration of adrenaline is probably not caused by epinephrine itself but by an oxidation product of adrenaline (Bruno Kisch's omega), which acts as an oxidation catalyst even in very high dilutions. It was found that identical electrocardiographic changes occurred during cardiac sympathetic nerve stimulation, electrically induced muscular exercise, or intravenous injection of norepinephrine or epinephrine when coronary artery dilatability is impaired and during exogenous anoxia or partial occlusion of the coronary arteries.[170] This was taken as evidence that the increased $O_2$ consumption caused by catecholamines produced a relative hypoxia if coronary flow could not be sufficiently increased.

A crucial point in the concept of the "oxygen-wasting" effect concerns the origin of the increased $O_2$ consumption with catecholamines – whether it is due to a decreased efficiency of oxygen utilization or an increased oxygen demand. It was found that the oxygen consumption of resting papillary muscle was not increased by catecholamines even in concentrations ten times higher than those effective in stimulating $O_2$ consumption of contracting papillary muscle;[171] this study concluded that the increased $O_2$ consumption of the intact heart following administration of epinephrine or norepinephrine is secondary to the increased contractility. On the other hand, it was reported that a low dose of norepinephrine exerted a maximal inotropic effect with little or no increase in $O_2$ consumption whereas larger doses had no further inotropic effect but did increase $O_2$ consumption, indicating that it is excessive catecholamine concentrations which cause "oxygen wasting."[172] It was observed that the increase in $O_2$ consumption of the potassium-arrested heart caused by catecholamines was 5–20 percent of that found in the beating heart;[173] this study concluded that most, but not all, of the increased $O_2$ consumption was secondary to hemodynamic alterations and increased cardiac work. In a similar comparison of the effects of epinephrine on $O_2$ consumption in beating and arrested hearts, it was found that about one-third of the increment in $O_2$ consumption in beating hearts was accounted for by a metabolic effect dissociable from the increased work.[174] Furthermore, it was reported that this effect could be blocked by dichloroisoproterenol but not by phentolamine.[175] From these studies, it is evident that catecholamines can cause an increase in $O_2$ consumption that is not related to increased cardiac work or activity and the concept of decreased efficiency or "oxygen wasting" is therefore justified. Furthermore, it has been suggested that this "oxygen-wasting" effect was actually due to an oxidation product of epinephrine,[21] and one such oxidation product, adrenochrome, was shown to uncouple mitochondria.[176] The uncoupling of mitochondria by adrenochrome was antagonized by glutathione in high concentration, probably as a result of a direct reduction of adrenochrome because the characteristic red color of adrenochrome was lost when glutathione was added in the presence or absence of mitochondria whereas oxidized glutathione did not affect this uncoupling by adrenochrome.

It was found that the P/O ratio (the ratio between added ADP and consumed oxygen) of heart mitochondria by norepinephrine, epinephrine, or isoproterenol was significantly low.[22] Respiratory control index (RCI) and state III respiration ($QO_2$) were similar to control, but unfortunately the control RCI values in these experiments were very low. A good relationship between elevation of myocardial catecholamine content and depression of the P/O ratio in mitochondria was observed. Whereas propranolol pretreatment enhanced the increase in myocardial catecholamines and caused a more marked depression of mitochondrial P/O ratios, dibenzyline inhibited both the increase in catecholamine contents and the decrease in the mitochondrial P/O ratio. Reserpine pretreatment caused a depletion of myocardial catecholamines and prevented the depression of the mitochondrial P/O ratio. As catecholamines under *in vitro* conditions did not effect the P/O ratio of heart mitochondria at a concentration of $10^{-3}$ M, it was concluded that this was not a direct action of the catecholamine on the mitochondria, but instead adrenochrome or one of its metabolites might be responsible for the observed effect.[22] Experiments on the oxidative phosphorylation of heart mitochondria from isoproterenol-treated rats revealed that the RCI was reduced without affecting the P/O ratio.[79] It is not possible to draw any definite conclusions from these studies with respect to the effects of catecholamines on mitochondrial respiration, although uncoupling of oxidative phosphorylation is certainly indicated and would explain both the "oxygen-wasting" effect and the depletion of myocardial high-energy phosphate stores caused by large doses of catecholamines.

Having found that heart mitochondria from catecholamine-treated rats were uncoupled, the level of free fatty acids in the mitochondria was determined because free fatty acids are known to uncouple mitochondria.[22] No difference in mitochondrial free fatty acid content or composition was found, and it was concluded that the observed uncoupling may not be due to the accumulation of fatty acids. Furthermore, ephedrine, which produced no significant changes in plasma non-esterified free fatty acids, was observed to cause cardiac lesions.[161] Nevertheless, it was found that inhibition of lipolysis by nicotinic acid, β-pyridyl carbonyl, or high plasma glucose concentrations during infusion of isoproterenol could substantially reduce the increase in myocardial oxygen consumption, possibly by preventing an uncoupling action of high intracellular concentrations of free fatty acid in the heart following catecholamine administration.[135] A casual relationship between the increase in plasma free fatty acids following norepinephrine administration and the occurrence of cardiac lesions has also been postulated.[159] The evidence fails to implicate elevated levels of free fatty acids as primary agents in mitochondrial uncoupling following administration of catecholamines. But it was suggested that metabolism of free fatty acids in some way aggravates the cardiotoxic effects of catecholamines[135] as well as the correlation of severity of lesions with the amount of body fat.[115]

### *Electrolyte shifts and intercellular $Ca^{2+}$ overload*

Figure 9.3 shows the concept of electrolyte shifts in the genesis of catecholamine-induced cardiomyopathy. In view of the close relationship between electrolyte shifts and the occurrence of necrotic lesions, it has been suggested that changes in myocardial electrolyte contents initiated by altered cationic transfer ability of myocardial cells at the plasma membrane and subcellular membrane sites by catecholamines contribute to irreversible failure of cell function.[90] The critical step in the pathogenesis of irreversible damage was the loss of cellular magnesium in particular.[145] In this regard, it was pointed out that $Mg^{2+}$ is an important prosthetic or activator cation participating in the function of many enzymes involved in phosphate transfer reactions, including utilization of ATP. Unfortunately, this mechanism cannot be considered adequate to explain the reduction of high-energy phosphate content in the myocardium,[85] because interference with energy utilization would have the opposite effect. On the other hand, $Mg^{2+}$ is reported to cause a decrease in the respiration-supported uptake of $Ca^{2+}$ by isolated heart mitochondria,[177] and could thus be important in regulating the mitochondrial function in terms of oxidative phosphorylation versus $Ca^{2+}$ uptake. It has been similarly argued that it is the derangement of myocardial electrolyte balance, specifically the loss of $K^+$ and $Mg^{2+}$ ions from the myocardium, which is the central mechanism in a variety of cardiomyopathies.[160] But this derangement of electrolyte balance was considered to be secondary to an inadequate supply of energy for transmembrane cation pumps required for the maintenance of electrolyte equilibrium which occurs with oxygen deficiency or impaired energy production.

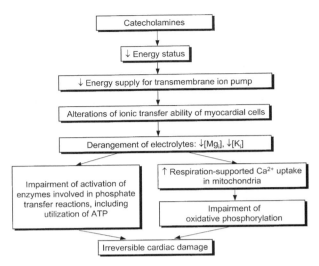

*Figure 9.3.* Energy status and electrolyte shifts in catecholamine-induced cardiomyopathy.

It has also been suggested that electrolyte shifts are an important component in the development of irreversible damage produced by both direct and indirect pathogenic mechanisms and that myocardial resistance is related to the ability of the heart to maintain a normal electrolyte balance in the face of potentially cardiotoxic episodes.[169]

Figure 9.4 shows the involvement of intercellular $Ca^{2+}$ overload in the pathogenesis of catecholamine-induced cardiomyopathy. It was observed that the isoproterenol-induced necrosis and decline in high-energy phosphates were associated with a six- to sevenfold increase in the rate of radioactive $Ca^{2+}$ uptake and a doubling of net myocardial calcium content.[85] This finding suggested that isoproterenol causes a greatly increased influx of $Ca^{2+}$, which overloads the cardiomyocytes. It was postulated that the intracellular $Ca^{2+}$ overload initiates a high-energy phosphate deficiency by excessive activation of $Ca^{2+}$-dependent ATPases and by impairing mitochondrial oxidative phosphorylation. When high-energy phosphate exhaustion reaches a critical level, fiber necrosis results. This hypothesis attempts to explain why myocardium is sensitized to isoproterenol-induced necrosis by factors, such as $9\alpha$-fluorocortisol acetate, dihydrotachysterol, $NaH_2PO_4$, high extracellular $Ca^{2+}$, or increased blood pH, that favor intracellular $Ca^{2+}$ overload. Consistent with this hypothesis, K and Mg salts, low extracellular calcium, thyrocalcitonin, low blood pH, or specific blockers of transmembrane $Ca^{2+}$ fluxes protect the heart against isoproterenol, presumably by preventing calcium overload. In support of the central role for $Ca^{2+}$ in the pathogenesis of catecholamine-induced necrosis is the observation that spontaneous necrotization of cardiac tissue in myopathic hamsters, which exhibit high levels of circulating catecholamines, is prevented by treatment with the calcium channel blocker

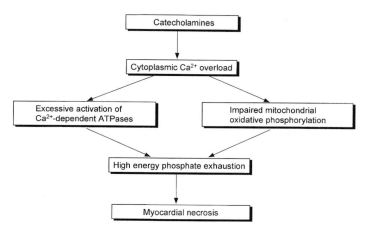

*Figure 9.4.* Intracellular $Ca^{2+}$ overload in catecholamine-induced cardiomyopathy.

verapamil.[178,179] Also, necrosis of skeletal muscle fibers can be induced through mechanical injury of the cell membrane, permitting $Ca^{2+}$ influx, which can be prevented by elimination of $Ca^{2+}$ from the Ringer solution or by an outward electric current that blocks $Ca^{2+}$ influx.[180] Unfortunately, there is no direct evidence that it is in fact $Ca^{2+}$ which produces the decline of high-energy phosphate in the hearts of animals given isoproterenol, and a causal relationship has not yet been established. Furthermore, it has been found that myocardial $Ca^{2+}$ content increased upon increasing the dose of isoproterenol in the range 0.1–10 μg/kg, but did not increase further with higher dose levels required to produce myocardial lesions.[122] Thus, it was suggested that the inotropic response to catecholamines is related to $Ca^{2+}$ entry but that the necrosis may be due to some other factor, possibly including the intracellular metabolism of $Ca^{2+}$. It was also shown that propranolol could completely block the increase in $Ca^{2+}$ content of the myocardium but would only reduce the incidence of lesions rather than preventing them. Nonetheless, the dramatic modification of necrosis by factors influencing transmembrane calcium fluxes clearly suggests the involvement of $Ca^{2+}$ at some level in the etiology of necrosis caused by catecholamines.[122]

Figure 9.5 shows the concept involving monoamine oxidase (MAO) and other oxidation processes in the development of catecholamine-induced cardiomyopathy. On the basis of coincidence of localization of isoproterenol-induced myocardial lesions and the highest myocardial MAO activity, it has been suggested that the accumulation of products metabolically formed during deamination of catecholamines may be the cause of necrosis in the heart.[121] It is further pointed out that the lower sensitivity to isoproterenol may be caused by the lesser MAO activity in the hearts of young rats compared with the older rats. These observations, as well as the protective effect of MAOIs, do not appear to be consistent with the hypothesis of intracellular $Ca^{2+}$ overload. Likewise, no specific explanation has

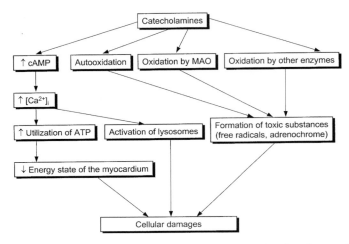

*Figure 9.5.* Increase in cyclic AMP and oxidation of catecholamines in catecholamine-induced cardiomyopathy. MAO, monamine oxidase.

been offered for the changes in contractile proteins which are seen to occur in catecholamine-induced necrotic lesions except for the suggestion that a direct interaction of catecholamine or some metabolite with the heavy meromyosin region of the myosin molecule is involved.[87] It is possible that MAOIs may reduce the oxidation of catecholamines and thus decrease the formation of toxic substances such as free radicals and adrenochrome and subsequent myocardial necrosis. It may very well be that lysosomes[110] are activated because of intracellular $Ca^{2+}$ overload, and this may produce cellular damage due to catecholamines. Furthermore, catecholamines are known to increase markedly the concentration of cyclic AMP in the heart, and it is likely that this agent in high concentrations may represent an important factor for causing catecholamine-induced myocardial necrosis in association with changes due to the oxidation products of catecholamines (Figure 9.5).

In summary, the majority of the factors found to influence the severity of catecholamine-induced lesions can be understood in terms of their effects on hemodynamic factors, delivery of oxygen to the myocardium, electrolyte balance, metabolism of calcium, and mobilization of lipids. It would thus appear that hemodynamic and coronary vascular factors contribute significantly to the severity of myocardial damage following catecholamine administration, but that some primary pathogenic mechanism acting directly on the myocardial cell is probably involved as well. Furthermore, it is clear that the exhaustion of the high-energy phosphate store and disruption of electrolyte balance are crucial events in the etiology of irreversible cell damage. Although mobilization of lipids and the occurrence of intracellular $Ca^{2+}$ overload may be involved, the nature of the direct pathogenic influence following injection of catecholamines is yet unknown. Some of the possible mechanisms which have been proposed to explain the cardiotoxic effects of catecholamines are given in Table 9.11.

### Adrenochrome and related oxidation products

The oxidation products of epinephrine, adrenochrome, and adrenolutin, have been identified in the heart, skeletal muscle, liver, brain, and kidney of rabbits[181–183] by paper chromatography and by their fluorescence properties. In addition to the spontaneous oxidation of epinephrine to adrenochrome by an autocatalytic process,[184] adrenochrome is enzymatically formed in mammalian tissues. These enzymes include tyrosinases[185–190] and polyphenol oxidases from various sources,[190–194] particularly in guinea pig and rat muscles.[194] Other enzyme systems shown actively to convert epinephrine to adrenochrome are xanthine oxidase,[195] leukocyte myeloperoxidase,[196,197] heart muscle cytochrome $c$ oxidase,[198–200] cyanide-insensitive system present in the heart and skeletal muscle,[201] cytochrome-indophenol oxidase system present in all tissues,[201,202] and an unidentified enzyme in the cat salivary gland.[203] The oxidation of epinephrine has also been reported to be catalyzed by cytochrome $c$ and methemoglobin,[204] which stabilizes the formation of adrenochrome in the presence of bicarbonate buffer regardless of the oxidizing system used[205] and has been reported to occur in blood.[206,207] Recently, a method for the measurement of adrenolutin in plasma has been developed by using reverse-phase high-performance liquid chromatography.[208] Much of the work in the literature dealing with the physiologic and pharmacologic effects of the oxidation

*Table 9.11* Possible mechanisms for cardiotoxic effects of high levels of circulating catecholamines

| | | | |
|---|---|---|---|
| 1 | Functional hypoxia | a | Increased cardiac work |
| | | b | Excessive demand for $O_2$ |
| 2 | Coronary insufficiency | a | Coronary spasm |
| | | b | Hemodynamic effects |
| 3 | Increased membrane permeability | a | Electrolyte shift |
| | | b | Loss of intracellular contents |
| 4 | Decreased levels of high-energy phosphate stores | a | Excessive hydrolysis of ATP |
| | | b | Uncoupling of mitochondrial oxidative phosphorylation |
| 5 | Alterations in lipid metabolism | a | Increased lipolysis |
| | | b | Increased accumulation of fatty acids |
| 6 | Intracellular $Ca^{2+}$ overload | a | Excessive $Ca^{2+}$ entry and intracellular release |
| | | b | Depressed $Ca^{2+}$ efflux and intracellular uptake |
| 7 | Oxidative stress | a | Formation of free radicals |
| | | b | Formation of adrenochrome |

products of epinephrine was carried out before the structure of adrenochrome was known and has been discussed in a review on this subject.[209] Furthermore, in view of the inherent instability of adrenochrome in solution, one cannot be certain whether the specific effects or the absence of certain effects can truly be considered as an accurate assessment of the adrenochrome activity. Nevertheless, it is well worth reviewing the broad spectrum of physiologic activities which have been attributed to adrenochrome or at least to some closely related products of adrenochrome.

Table 9.12 shows the effects of adrenochrome, adrenoxyl, and oxidized epinephrine. Oxidized epinephrine solutions have been found to inhibit cardiac inotropism and chronotropism[186,187,191,210–212] and to increase rather than decrease the tone of rabbit intestinal strips.[213] Adrenochrome has been reported to increase blood pressure,[214,215] to be effective as a vasoconstrictor,[216] to be a powerful hemostatic agent, and to diminish the capillary permeability.[217,218] Adrenochrome has frequently been reported to reduce blood sugar levels and potentiate the effects of insulin and has been described as an anti-insulinase,[209,219] although this claim has been disputed.[220] Administration of adrenochrome either by injection or by feeding has been reported to increase oxygen consumption in humans and guinea pigs[221,222] as well as tissue oxygen consumption *in vitro*.[223,224] On the other hand, some workers have observed that adrenochrome may stimulate, inhibit, or have

*Table 9.12* Effects of adrenochrome, adrenoxyl, and oxidized epinephrine

| A Adrenochrome | | Blood pressure $\uparrow$, vasoconstriction, powerful hemostatic agents, capillary permeability $\downarrow$, blood sugar $\downarrow$ (anti-insulinase), $O_2$ consumption $\uparrow$ (?), oxygen uptake $\sim$ or $\downarrow$, lactic acid production $\downarrow$, uncoupling of mitochondria oxidation phosphorylation, P/O ratio $\downarrow$, pyruvate oxidation > succinate oxidation |
|---|---|---|
| B Adrenoxyl | | Mitochondrial $K^+$ $\downarrow$, ATPase activity $\downarrow$, alteration of P/O ratio |
| Adrenochrome | (Inhibition) | Glucose phosphorylation, glycolysis, hexokinase, phosphofructokinase |
| | (Stimulation) | Glycogen synthesis, hexose monophosphate shunt |
| Adrenochrome + Adrenoxyl | (Inhibition) | Myosin ATPase activity |
| Adrenochrome + oxidized epinephrine | (Inhibition) | Monoamine oxidase, the enzyme alkaline phosphatase |
| Adrenochrome + Adrenoxyl | | Antimitotic activity $\downarrow$, coenzyme A $\downarrow$, antihistaminic effect $\downarrow$, mitochondrial material $\uparrow$ |

no effect on tissue oxygen consumption depending upon the metabolic substrate utilized[225] or the adrenochrome concentration.[226] Reports are also available to show that adrenochrome did not affect the oxygen uptake in rat muscle[227] but inhibited oxygen uptake and lactic acid production in dog heart slices.[228]

Adrenochrome has been observed to uncouple mitochondrial oxidative phosphorylation and depress P/O ratios.[176,229,230] It has been suggested that adrenochrome may act as a hydrogen carrier between substrate and molecular oxygen with the formation of water and regeneration of adrenochrome after each cycle.[229] Adrenochrome was also reported to be much more effective in inhibiting pyruvate oxidation than succinate oxidation.[230] Adrenoxyl, a closely related epinephrine oxidation product, has been found to lower mitochondrial potassium content, to decrease mitochondrial ATPase activity, and to alter the mitochondrial P/O ratio.[231] Adrenochrome also inhibited hexokinase and phosphofructokinase, thus inhibiting glucose phosphorylation and glycolysis while stimulating glycogen synthesis[201,232–235] and the hexose monophosphate shunt.[236,237] Adrenochrome and adrenoxyl have both been found to be inhibitors of myosin ATPase activity in the heart and smooth muscle.[238–241] Adrenochrome and oxidized epinephrine solutions were also observed to inhibit monoamine oxidase in a variety of tissues[242–244] and alkaline phosphatase activity.[245] It was thought that inhibition of different enzymes is due at least partly to the reversible oxidation of sulfhydryl groups in the enzymes.[240,242] Other effects attributed to adrenochrome and adrenoxyl include antimitotic activity,[246] reduction of coenzyme A levels in heart, kidneys, and brain,[247] antihistaminic properties,[209] and an increase in mitochondrial material of cultured cells.[248] Thus, it can be appreciated that adrenochrome is a highly reactive molecule chemically. It not only is capable of oxidizing protein sulfhydryl groups but also is a dynamic catalyst for the deamination of a variety of amines and amino acids.[249–253] Furthermore, it is capable of functioning as an oxidative hydrogen carrier acting upon either metabolic substrates[229] or NADP[+237] and thus altering or disrupting essential metabolic pathways. The metabolism of adrenochrome and related epinephrine oxidation products has been studied in rabbits, cats, and dogs.[254–256] Adrenochrome injected into rabbits rapidly disappeared from the blood, transformed to adrenolutin in the liver and then removed from the system via the kidney.[254] Most of the adrenochrome was excreted in the urine as adrenolutin (both free and conjugated), or in the form of a fluorescent brown pigment, while a small amount was excreted unchanged. In cats and dogs, approximately 70 percent was excreted in the form of a variety of adrenochrome reduction products and other indoles.[255] An unstable yellow pigment has been observed in the urine of rats after the injection of $^{14}$C-labeled adrenochrome.[257]

In view of the foregoing discussion, it can be appreciated that there is evidence both for the presence of and for the formation of adrenochrome in mammalian tissues. Furthermore, adrenochrome has been shown to be capable of producing a wide variety of metabolic changes by interfering with numerous enzyme systems. Thus, adrenochrome and/or other catecholamine oxidation products may be regarded as possible candidates which are involved in toxic manifestation occurring in conjunction with catecholamine excess or altered catecholamine metabolism. The injection of catecholamine into animals can be conceived to result in the formation of oxidation products such as adrenochrome in the circulating blood as well as in the myocardial cell. The accumulation of these oxidation products in myocardium could then directly or indirectly, acting by themselves or in conjunction with other effects of catecholamines, initiate processes leading to myocardial necrosis. Accordingly, experiments were undertaken to understand the problem of whether or not catecholamines, their oxidation products, or their metabolites are indeed capable of a direct toxic influence on the heart. For this purpose, the isolated perfused rat heart preparation was used as this appears to be an ideal model for several reasons. These include elimination of hemodynamic factors, neural mechanisms, availability of exogenous lipids, and other physiologic parameters which tend to complicate the production of heart lesions in the intact animals. In addition, changes in contractile events can be monitored concomitantly and the heart can be readily fixed at a desired time for ultrastructural examination. Fresh isoproterenol, oxidized isoproterenol, fresh epinephrine, adrenochrome, and various metabolites of epinephrine were used for investigating changes in ultrastructure and contractile functions of the isolated perfused rat hearts. In addition to studying the time-course and dose–responses to the cardiotoxic agents, attempts were made to elucidate the mechanisms subserving the functional and morphologic alterations. The hearts were perfused in the absence or presence of the cardiotoxic substance with media of different cationic compositions or containing various pharmacologic agents which are known to influence the catecholamine-induced myocardial necrosis *in vivo*.

When the isolated rat hearts were perfused with high concentrations of isoproterenol for 1 h, no depression in contractile activity or myocardial cell damage was evident.[258] These observations were confirmed by other investigators.[259] On the other hand, perfusion of the isolated hearts with oxidized isoproterenol produced dramatic cardiac contractile, morphologic, and subcellular alterations.[258,260] Toxic effects of isoproterenol on cultured cardiac muscle cells were also shown to be the result of its oxidation.[261] In fact, the contractile dysfunction and myocardial cell damage in the isolated perfused rat hearts due to adrenochrome were shown to depend upon its concentration as well as time of perfusion.[262] Various pharmacologic agents and cations, which prevent the occurrence of intracellular $Ca^{2+}$ overload, were observed to reduce the cardiac contractile failure and cell damage due to adrenochrome.[263,264] Adrenochrome was suggested to affect $Ca^{2+}$ movements in the myocardial cell as a result of its action on the sarcolemmal, sarcoplasmic reticular and mitochondrial membranes.[265–268] In fact, adrenochrome was found to be accumulated in the myocardium and localized at different subcellular organelles.[268,269] Adrenochrome was also shown to be a potent coronary artery constrictor in the isolated rat heart preparations.[270] Although administration of adrenochrome to rats was found to induce arrhythmia, myocardial cell damage and heart dysfunction under *in vivo* conditions,[271–273] oxidation products other than adrenochrome have also been suggested to be involved in the genesis of catecholamine-induced cardiotoxicity.[274]

Because the oxidation of catecholamines results in the formation of aminochromes (such as adrenochrome) and free radicals, it is possible that free radicals may also be involved in the development of catecholamine-induced cardiotoxicity. Pretreatment of rats with vitamin E, a well-known free radical scavenger, was found to prevent the isoproterenol-induced arrhythmia, lipid peroxidation, myocardial cell damage and loss of high-energy phosphates, whereas vitamin E deficiency was shown to increase the sensitivity of animals to the cardiotoxic actions of isoproterenol.[114,275,276] Other antioxidants such as ascorbic acid and sodium bisulfate were also shown to prevent the cytotoxic effects of isoproterenol in cultured rat myocardial cells.[277–279] Exercise training, which is considered to increase the antioxidant reserve, has also been reported to decrease the myocardial cell damage caused by catecholamines.[280,281] It is therefore likely that antioxidant therapy may prove highly beneficial in preventing the cardiovascular problems under stressful conditions in which the circulating levels of catecholamines are elevated markedly. In this regard, it should be pointed out that oxygen free radials have been shown to exert cardiotoxic effects such as myocardial cell damage, contractile failure, subcellular alterations, and intracellular $Ca^{2+}$ overload.[282–290] Thus, it appears that the generation of oxyradicals, in addition to the formation of aminochromes, may play an important role in the pathogenesis of cardiotoxicity under conditions associated with high levels of circulating catecholamines. A scheme indicating the involvement of both free radicals and adrenochrome in the development of catecholamine-induced arrhythmia, coronary spasm, contractile failure, and myocardial cell damage is depicted in Figure 9.6.

## Summary and conclusions

It is well known that massive amounts of catecholamines are released from the sympathetic nerve endings and adrenal medulla under stressful situations. Initially, these hormones produce beneficial effects on the cardiovascular system to meet the energy demands of various organs in the body, and their actions on the heart are primarily mediated through the stimulation of β-adrenergic receptors–G protein–adenylate cyclase–cyclic AMP system in the myocardium. However, prolonged exposure of the heart to high levels of catecholamines results in coronary spasm, arrhythmia, contractile dysfunction, cell damage, and myocardial necrosis. Different pharmacologic, hormonal, and metabolic interventions, which are known to reduce the occurrence of intracellular $Ca^{2+}$ overload, have been shown to prevent the cardiotoxic actions of catecholamines, whereas interventions that promote the development of intracellular $Ca^{2+}$ overload attenuate the catecholamine-induced cardiomyopathy. Several mechanisms such as relative hypoxia, hemodynamic alterations, coronary insufficiency, changes in lipid mobilization and energy metabolism, electrolyte imbalance, and membrane alterations have been suggested to explain the cardiotoxic effects of high concentrations of catecholamines. Recent

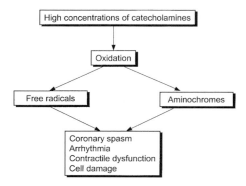

*Figure 9.6.* Schematic representation of the mechanism for the genesis of cardiotoxic effects of high concentrations of catecholamines.

studies have shown that oxidation of catecholamines results in the formation of highly toxic substances such as aminochromes (e.g. adrenochrome) and free radicals, which then, by virtue of their actions on different types of heart membranes, cause intracellular $Ca^{2+}$ overload and myocardial cell damage. Hemodynamic and metabolic actions of catecholamines may aggravate toxic effects of the oxidation products of catecholamines. Thus, it appears that antioxidant therapy in combination with some $Ca^{2+}$ antagonists and/or metabolic intervention may be most effective in preventing the catecholamine-induced cardiomyopathy.

## Acknowledgments

The work reported in this article was supported by a grant from the Medical Research Council of Canada (MRC Group in Experimental Cardiology). N.S.D. holds the MRC/PMAC Chair in Cardiovascular Research, supported by Merck Frosst, Canada.

## References

1. Ziegler K. 1905. Uber die Wirkung intravenoser Adrenalin injection auf das Gefasssystem und ihre Beziehungen zur Arterisclerose. *Beitr Path Anat Allg Path* 38: 229–254.
2. Pearce RM. 1906. Experimental myocarditis: A study of the histological changes following intravenous injections of adrenaline. *J Exp Med* 8: 400–409.
3. Szakacs JE, Cannon A. 1958. L-Norepinephrine myocarditis. *Am J Clin Pathol* 30: 425–430.
4. Rona G, Chappel CI, Balazs T, Gaudry R. 1959. An infarct-like myocardial lesion and other toxic manifestations produced by isoproterenol in the rat. *Arch Pathol* 67: 443–455.

5. Boutet M, Huttner I, Rona G. 1973. Aspect microcirculatoire des lesions myocardiques provoquees par l'infusion de catecholamines. Etude Ultra structural a l'aide de traceurs de diffusion. I. Isoproterenol. *Pathol Biol* 21: 811–825.

6. Boutet M, Huttner I, Rona G. Aspect microcirculatoire des lesions myocardiques provoquees par l'infusion de catecholamines. 1974. Etude Ultra structural a l'aide traceurs de diffusion. II. Norepinephrine. *Pathol Biol* 22: 377–387.

7. Handforth CP. 1962. Isoproterenol-induced myocardial infarction in animals. *Arch Pathol* 73: 161–165.

8. Handforth CP. 1962. Myocardial infarction and necrotizing arteritis in hamsters produced by isoproterenol (Isuprel). *Med Serv J Can* 18: 506–512.

9. Rona G, Boutet M, Hutter I, Peters H. 1973. Pathogenesis of isoproterenol induced myocardial alterations: Functional and morphological correlates. In *Recent Advances in Studies on Cardiac Structure and Metabolism*, Vol. 3. Dhalla NS (ed.), pp. 507–525. Baltimore: University Park Press.

10. Rona G, Kahn DS, Chappel CI. 1963. Studies on infarct-like myocardial necrosis produced by isoproterenol: A review. *Rev Can Biol* 22: 241–255.

11. Maruffo CA. 1967. Fine structural study of myocardial changes induced by isoproterenol in Rhesus monkeys (Macaca mulatta). *Am J Pathol* 50: 27–37.

12. Ostadal B, Rychterova V, Poupa O. 1968. Isoproterenol-induced acute experimental cardiac necrosis in the turtle. *Am Heart J* 76: 645–649.

13. Regan TJ, Markov A, Kahn MI, Jesrani MJ, Oldewurtel HA, Ettinger PO. 1972. Myocardial ion and lipid exchanges during ischemia and catecholamine induced necrosis: Relation to regional blood flow. In *Recent Advances in Studies in Cardiac Structure and Metabolism*, Vol. 1. Bajusz E, Rona G (eds), pp. 656–664. Baltimore: University Park Press.

14. Rosenblum I, Wohl A, Stein AA. 1965. Studies in cardiac necrosis. I. Production of cardiac lesions with sympathomimetic amines. *Toxicol Appl Pharmacol* 7: 1–8.

15. Rosenblum I, Wohl A, Stein AA. 1965. Studies in cardiac necrosis. II. Cardiovascular effects of sympathomimetic amines producing cardiac lesions. *Toxicol Appl Pharmacol* 7: 9–17.

16. Bhagat B, Sullivan JM, Fisher VW, Nadel EM, Dhalla NS. 1978. cAMP activity and isoproterenol-induced myocardial injury in rats. In *Recent Advances in Studies on Cardiac Structure and Metabolism*, Vol. 12. Kobayashi T, Ito Y, Rona G (eds), pp. 465–470. Baltimore: University Park Press.

17. Todd GL, Baroldi G, Pieper GM, Clayton FC, Eliot RS. 1985. Experimental catecholamine-induced myocardial necrosis. I. Morphology, quantification and regional distribution of acute contraction band lesions. *J Mol Cell Cardiol* 17: 317–338.

18. Todd GL, Baroldi G, Pieper GM, Clayton FC, Elliot RS. 1985. Experimental catecholamine-induced myocardial necrosis. II. Temperal development of isoproterenol-induced contraction band lesions correlated with ECG, hemodynamic and biochemical changes. *J Mol Cell Cardiol* 17: 647–656.

19. Boutet M, Huttner I, Rona G. 1976. Permeability alterations of sarcolemmal membrane in catecholamine-induced cardiac muscle cell injury. *Lab Invest* 34: 482–488.

20. Todd GL, Cullan GE, Cullan GM. 1980. Isoproterenol-induced myocardial necrosis and membrane permeability alterations in the isolated perfused rabbit heart. *Exp Mol Pathol* 33: 43–54.

21. Raab W. 1943. Pathogenic significance of adrenalin and related substances in heart muscle. *Exp Med Surg* 1: 188–225.
22. Sobel B, Jequier E, Sjoerdsma A, Lovenberg W. 1966. Effect of catecholamines and adrenergic blocking agents on oxidative phosphorylation in rat heart mitochondria. *Circ Res* 19: 1050–1061.
23. Fleisher MS, Loeb L. 1909. Experimental myocarditis. *Arch Int Med* 3: 78–91.
24. Fleisher MS, Loeb L. 1909. The later stages of experimental myocarditis. *J Am Med Assoc* 53: 1561–1571.
25. Fleisher MS, Loeb L. 1909. Uber experimentelle Myocarditis. *Centr Allg Path Path Anat* 20: 104–106.
26. Fleisher MS, Loeb L. 1910. Further investigations in experimental myocarditis. *Arch Int Med* 6: 427–438.
27. Christian HA, Smith RM, Walker IC. 1911. Experimental cardiorenal disease. *Arch Int Med* 8: 468–551.
28. Samson PC. 1932. Tissue changes following continuous intravenous injection of epinephrine hydrochloride into dogs. *Arch Pathol* 13: 745–755.
29. Blacket RB, Pickering GW, Wilson GM. 1950. The effects of prolonged infusion of noradrenaline and adrenaline on arterial pressure of rabbit. *Clin Sci* 9: 247–257.
30. Catchpole BN, Hacket DB, Simeone FA. 1955. Coronary and peripheral blood flow in experimental hemorrhagic hypotension treated with ʟ-norepinephrine. *Ann Surg* 142: 372–380.
31. Hackel DB, Catchpole BN. 1958. Pathologic and electrocardiographic effects of hemorrhagic shock in dogs treated with ʟ-norepinephrine. *Lab Invest* 7: 358–368.
32. Vishnevskaya OP. 1956. Reflex mechanisms in the pathogenesis of adrenaline myocarditis. *Bull Exp Biol Med* 41: 27–31.
33. Nahas GG, Brunson JG, King WM, Cavert HM. 1958. Functional and morphological changes in heart lung preparations following administration of adrenal hormones. *Am J Pathol* 34: 717–729.
34. Szakacs JE, Mehlman B. 1960. Pathologic change induced by ʟ-norepinephrine. Quantitative aspects. *Am J Cardiol* 5: 619–627.
35. Maling HM, Highman B. 1958. Exaggerated ventricular arrhythmia and myocardial fatty changes after large doses of norepinephrine and epinephrine in unanesthetized dogs. *Am J Physiol* 194: 590–596.
36. Highman B, Maling HM, Thompson EC. 1959. Serum transaminase and alkaline phosphate levels after large doses of norepinephrine and epinephrine in dogs. *Am J Physiol* 196: 436–440.
37. Maling HM, Highman B, Thompson EC. 1960. Some similar effects after large doses of catecholamine and myocardial infarction in dogs. *Am J Cardiol* 5: 628–633.
38. Chappel CI, Rona G, Balazs T, Gaudry R. 1959. Severe myocardial necrosis produced by isoproterenol in the rat. *Arch Int Pharmacodyn* 122: 123–128.
39. Rona G, Zsoter T, Chappel C, Gaudry R. 1959. Myocardial lesions, circulatory and electrocardiographic changes produced by isoproterenol in the dog. *Rev Can Biol* 18: 83–94.
40. Ostadal B, Pelouch V, Ostadalova I, Novakova O. 1995. Structural and biochemical remodeling in catecholamine-induced cardiomyopathy: comparative and ontogenetic aspects. *Mol Cell Biochem* 147: 83–88.
41. Ostadal B, Muller E. 1966. Histochemical studies on the experimental heart infarction in the rat. *Naunyn-Schmiedebergs Arch Pharmok Exp Pathol* 254: 439–447.

42. Chappel CI, Rona G, Balazs, Gaudry R. 1959. Comparison of cardiotoxic actions of certain sympathomimetic amines. *Can J Biochem Physiol* 37: 35–42.
43. Kline IK. 1961. Myocardial alterations associated with pheochromocytoma. *Am J Pathol* 38: 539–551.
44. Szakacs JE, Dimmette RM, Cowart Jr., EC. 1959. Pathologic implication of the catecholamines, epinephrine and norepinephrine. *US Armed Forces Med J* 10: 908–925.
45. van Vliet PD, Burchell HB, Titus JL. 1966. Focal myocarditis associated with pheochromocytoma. *N Engl J Med* 274: 1102–1108.
46. Connor RCR. 1969. Focal myocytolysis and fuchsinophilic degeneration of the myocardium of patients dying with various brain lesions. *Ann NY Acad Sci* 156: 261–270.
47. Greenhoot JH, Reichenbach DD. 1969. Cardiac injury and subarachnoid hemorrhage. A clinical, pathological and physiological correlation. *J Neurosurg* 30: 521–526.
48. Reichenbach DD, Benditt EP. 1970. Catecholamines and cardiomyopathy: The pathogenesis and potential importance of myofibrillar degeneration. *Hum Pathol* 1: 125–150.
49. Smith RP, Tomlinson BE. 1954. Subendocardial hemorrhages associated with intracranial lesions. *J Pathol Bacteriol* 68: 327–334.
50. Kaye MP, McDonald RH, Randall WC. 1961. Systolic hypertension and subendocardial hemorrhages produced by electrical stimulation of the stellate ganglion. *Circ Res* 9: 1164–1170.
51. Klouda MA, Brynjolfson G. 1969. Cardiotoxic effects of electrical stimulation of the stellate ganglia. *Ann NY Acad Sci* 156: 271–279.
52. Melville KI, Garvey HL, Sluster HE, Knaack J. 1969. Central nervous system stimulation and cardiac ischemic change in monkeys. *Ann NY Acad Sci* 156: 241–260.
53. Wood R, Commerford PJ, Rose AG, Tooke A. 1991. Reversible catecholamine-induced cardiomyopathy. *Am Heart J* 121: 610–613.
54. Hicks RJ, Wood B, Kalff V, Anderson ST, Kelly MJ. 1991. Normalization of left ventricular ejection fraction following resection of pheochromocytoma in a patient with dilated cardiomyopathy. *Clin Nucl Med* 16: 413–416.
55. Hamada N, Akamatsu A, Joh T. 1993. A case of phlochromocytoma complicated acute renal failure and cardiomyopathy. *Jpn Circ J* 57: 84–90.
56. Elian D, Harpaz D, Sucher E, Kaplinsky E, Motro M, Vered Z. 1993. Reversible catecholamine-induced cardiomyopathy presenting as acute pulmonary edema in a patient with pheochromocytoma. *Cardiology* 83: 118–120.
57. Powers FM, Pifarre R, Thomas Jr., JX. 1994. Ventricular dysfunction in norepinephrine-induced cardiomyopathy. *Circ Shock* 43: 122–129.
58. Bloom S, Cancilla PA. 1969. Myocytolysis and mitochondrial calcification in rat myocardium after low doses of isoproterenol. *Am J Pathol* 54: 373–391.
59. Csapa Z, Dusek J, Rona G. 1972. Early alterations of cardiac muscle cells in isoproterenol induced necrosis. *Arch Pathol* 93: 356–365.
60. Kutsuna F. 1972. Electron microscopic studies on isoproterenol-induced myocardial lesions in rats. *Jpn Heart J* 13: 168–175.
61. Ferrans VJ, Hibbs RG, Walsh JJ, Burch GE. 1969. Histochemical and electron microscopic studies on the cardiac necrosis produced by sympathomimetic agents. *Ann NY Acad Sci* 156: 309–332.

62. Ferrans VJ, Hibbs RG, Black WC, Weilbaecher DG. 1964. Isoproterenol-induced myocardial necrosis. A histochemical and electron microscopic study. *Am Heart J* 68: 71–90.
63. Ferrans VJ, Hibbs RG, Cipriano PR, Buja LM. 1972. Histochemical and electron microscopic studies of norepinephrine-induced myocardial necrosis in rats. In *Recent Advances in Studies on Cardiac Structure and Metabolism*, Vol. 1. Bajusz E, Rona G (eds), pp. 495–525. Baltimore: University Park Press.
64. Ferrans VJ, Hibbs RG, Weiley HS, Weilbaecher DG, Walsh JJ, Burch GE. 1970. A histochemical and electron microscopic study of epinephrine-induced myocardial necrosis. *J Mol Cell Cardiol* 1: 11–22.
65. Lehr D. 1972. Healing of myocardial necrosis caused by sympathomimetic amines. In *Recent Advances in Studies on Cardiac Structure and Metabolism*, Vol. 1. Bajusz E, Rona G (eds), pp. 526–550. Baltimore: University Park Press.
66. Lehr D, Krukowshi M, Chau R. 1969. Acute myocardial injury produced by sympathomimetic amines. *Israel J Med Sci* 5: 519–524.
67. Schenk EA, Moss AJ. 1966. Cardiovascular effects of sustained norepinephrine infusions. II. Morphology. *Circ Res* 18: 605–615.
68. Khullar M, Datta BN, Wahi PL, Chakravarti RN. 1989. Catecholamine-induced experimental cardiomyopathy – a histopathological, histochemical and ultrastructural study. *Indian Heart J* 41: 307–313.
69. Regan TJ, Moschos CB, Lehan PH, Oldewurtel HA, Hellems HK. 1966. Lipid and carbohydrate metabolism of myocardium during the biphasic inotropic response to epinephrine. *Circ Res* 19: 307–316.
70. Wexler BC, Judd JT, Kittinger GW. 1968. Myocardial necrosis induced by isoproterenol in rats: Changes in serum protein, lipoprotein, lipids and glucose during active necrosis and repair in arteriosclerotic and nonarteriosclerotic animals. *Angiology* 19: 665–682.
71. Wexler BC, Judd JT, Lutmer RF, Saroff J. 1972. Pathophysiologic change in arteriosclerotic and nonarteriosclerotic rats following isoproterenol-induced myocardial infarction. In *Recent Advances in Studies on Cardiac Structure and Metabolism*, Vol. 1. Bajusz E, Rona G (eds), pp. 463–472. Baltimore: University Park Press.
72. Wexler BC, Kittinger GW. 1963. Myocardial necrosis in rats: Serum enzymes, adrenal steroid and histopathological alterations. *Circ Res* 13: 159–171.
73. Zbinden G, Moe RA. 1969. Pharmacological studies on heart muscle lesions induced by isoproterenol. *Ann NY Acad Sci* 156: 294–308.
74. Wexler BC. 1970. Serum creatine phosphokinase activity following isoproterenol-induced myocardial infarction in male and female rats with and without arteriosclerosis. *Am Heart J* 79: 69–79.
75. Regan TJ, Passannante AJ, Oldewurtel HA, Burke WM, Ettinger PO. 1968. Metabolism of $^{14}$C labeled triglycerides by the myocardium during injury induced by norepinephrine. *Circulation* 38 (Suppl. VI): 162.
76. Judd JT, Wexler BC. 1969. Myocardial connective tissue metabolism in response to injury: Histological and chemical studies of mucopolysaccharides and collagen in rat hearts after isoproterenol-induced infarction. *Circ Res* 25: 201–214.
77. Wenzel DG, Chau RYP. 1966. Dose–time effect of isoproterenol on aspartate amino-transferase and necrosis of the rat heart. *Toxicol Appl Pharmacol* 8: 460–463.

78. Wenzel DG, Lyon JP. 1967. Sympathomimetic amines and heart lactic dehydrogenase isoenzymes. *Toxicol Appl Pharmacol* 11: 215–228.
79. Stanton HC, Schwartz A. 1967. Effects of hydrazine monoamine oxidase inhibitor (phenelzine) on isoproterenol-induced myocardiopathies in the rat. *J Pharmacol Exp Ther* 157: 649–658.
80. Vorbeck ML, Malewski EF, Erhart LS, Martin AP. 1975. Membrane phospholipid metabolism in the isoproterenol-induced cardiomyopathy of the rat. In *Recent Advances in Studies on Cardiac Structure and Metabolism*, Vol. 6. Fleckenstein A, Rona G (eds), pp. 175–181. Baltimore: University Park Press.
81. Hattori E, Yatsaki K, Miyozaki T, Nakamura M. 1969. Adenine nucleotides of myocardium from rats treated with isoproterenol and/or Mg- or K-deficiency. *Jpn Heart J* 10: 218–224.
82. Kako K. 1965. Biochemical changes in the rat myocardium induced by isoproterenol. *Can J Physiol Pharmacol* 43: 541–549.
83. Robertson WVB, Peyser P. 1951. Changes in water and electrolytes of cardiac muscle following epinephrine. *Am J Physiol* 166: 277–283.
84. Fleckenstien A. 1971. Specific inhibitors and promoters of calcium action in the excitation–contraction coupling of heart muscle and their role in the prevention or production of myocardial lesions. In *Calcium and the Heart*. Harris P, Opie LH (eds), pp. 135–188. London: Academic Press.
85. Fleckenstein A, Janke J, Doering HJ. 1974. Myocardial fiber necrosis due to intracellular Ca-overload. A new principle in cardiac pathophysiology. In *Recent Advances in Studies on Cardiac Structure and Metabolism*, Vol. 4. Dhalla NS (ed.), pp. 563–580. Baltimore: University Park Press.
86. Pelouch V, Deyl Z, Poupa O. 1968. Experimental cardiac necrosis in terms of myosin aggregation. *Physiol Bohemoslov* 17: 480–488.
87. Pelouch V, Deyl Z, Poupa O. 1970. Myosin aggregation in cardiac necrosis induced by isoproterenol in rats. *Physiol Bohemoslov* 19: 9–13.
88. Fedelesova M, Ziegelhoffer A, Luknarova O, Kostolansky S. 1975. Prevention by $K^+$, $Mg^{2+}$-aspartate of isoproterenol-induced metabolic changes in myocardium. In *Recent Advances in Studies on Cardiac Structure and Metabolism*, Vol. 6. Fleckenstein A, Rona G (eds), pp. 59–73. Baltimore: University Park Press.
89. Dhalla NS, Dzurba A, Pierce GN, Tregaskis MG, Panagia V, Beamish RE. 1983. Membrane changes in myocardium during catecholamine-induced pathological hypertrophy. In *Perspectives in Cardiovascular Research*, Vol. 7. Alpert NR (ed.), pp. 527–534. New York: Raven Press.
90. Lehr D. 1969. Tissue electrolyte alteration in disseminated myocardial necrosis. *Ann NY Acad Sci* 156: 344–378.
91. Lehr D, Krukowski M, Colon R. 1966. Correlation of myocardial and renal necrosis with tissue electrolyte changes. *J Am Med Assoc* 197: 105–112.
92. Melville KI, Korol B. 1958. Cardiac drug responses and potassium shifts. Studies on the interrelated effects of drugs on coronary flow, heart action and cardiac potassium movement. *Am J Cardiol* 2: 81–94.
93. Melville KI, Korol B. 1958. Cardiac drug responses and potassium shifts. Studies on the interrelated effect of drugs on coronary flow, heart action and cardiac potassium movement. *Am J Cardiol* 2: 189–199.
94. Nasmyth PA. 1957. The effect of corticosteroids on the isolated mammalian heart and its response to adrenaline. *J Physiol* 139: 323–336.

95. Langer GA. 1968. Ion fluxes in cardiac excitation and contraction and their relation to myocardial contractility. *Physiol Rev* 48: 708–757.

96. Daggett WM, Mansfield PB, Sarnoff SJ. 1964. Myocardial $K^+$ changes resulting from inotropic agents. *Fed Proc* 23: 357.

97. Dhalla NS, Ziegelhoffer A, Harrow JAC. 1977. Regulation role of membrane systems in heart function. *Can J Physiol Pharmacol* 55: 1211–1234.

98. Dhalla NS, Das PK, Sharma GP. 1978. Subcellular basis of cardiac contractile failure. *J Mol Cell Cardiol* 10: 363–385.

99. Dhalla NS, Pierce GN, Panagia V, Singal PK, Beamish RE. 1982. Calcium movements in relation to heart function. *Basic Res Cardiol* 77: 117–139.

100. Dhalla NS, Dixon IMC, Beamish RE. 1991. Biochemical basis of heart function and contractile failure. *J Appl Cardiol* 6: 7–30.

101. Varley KG, Dhalla NS. 1973. Excitation–contraction coupling in heart. XII. Subcellular calcium transport in isoproterenol-induced myocardial necrosis. *Exp Mol Pathol* 19: 94–105.

102. Fedelesova M, Dzurba A, Ziegelhoffer A. 1974. Effect of isoproterenol on the activity of $Na^+$-$K^+$ adenosine triphosphatase from dog heart. *Biochem Pharmacol* 23: 2887–2893.

103. Panagia V, Pierce GN, Dhalla KS, Ganguly PK, Beamish RE, Dhalla NS. 1985. Adaptive changes in subcellular calcium transport during catecholamine-induced cardiomyopathy. *J Mol Cell Cardiol* 17: 411–420.

104. Okumura K, Panagia V, Beamish RE, Dhalla NS. 1987. Biphasic changes in the sarcolemmal phosphatidylethanolamine N-methylation in catecholamine-induced cardiomyopathy. *J Mol Cell Cardiol* 19: 357–366.

105. Dhalla NS, Ganguly PK, Panagia V, Beamish RE. 1987. Catecholamine-induced cardiomyopathy: Alterations in $Ca^{2+}$ transport systems. In *Pathogenesis of Myocarditis and Cardiomyopathy*. Kawai C, Abelman WH (eds), pp. 135–147. Tokyo: University of Tokyo Press.

106. Makino N, Dhruvarajan R, Elimban V, Beamish RE, Dhalla NS. 1985. Alterations of sarcolemmal $Na^+$-$Ca^{2+}$ exchange in catecholamine-induced cardiomyopathy. *Can J Cardiol* 1: 225–232.

107. Makino N, Jasmin G, Beamish RE, Dhalla NS. 1985. Sarcolemmal $Na^+$-$Ca^{2+}$ exchange during the development of genetically determined cardiomyopathy. *Biochem Biophys Res Commun* 133: 491–497.

108. Panagia V, Elimban V, Heyliger CE, Tregaskis M, Beamish RE, Dhalla NS. 1985. Sarcolemmal alterations during catecholamine induced cardiomyopathy. In *Pathogenesis of Stress-induced Heart Disease*. Beamish RE, Panagia V, Dhalla NS (eds), pp. 121–131. Boston: Martinus Nijhoff.

109. Corder DW, Heyliger CE, Beamish RE, Dhalla NS. 1984. Defect in the adrenergic receptor–adenylate cyclase system during development of catecholamine-induced cardiomyopathy. *Am Heart J* 107: 537–542.

110. Roman S, Kutryk MJB, Beamish RE, Dhalla NS. 1985. Lysosomal changes during the development of catecholamine-induced cardiomyopathy. In *Pathogenesis of Stress-induced Heart Disease*. Beamish RE, Panagia V, Dhalla NS (eds), pp. 270–280. Boston: Martinus Nijhoff.

111. Selye H. 1961. *The Pluicausal Cardiopathies*. Springfield, IL: Charles C Thomas.

112. Beamish RE, Dhalla NS. 1985. Involvement of catecholamines in coronary spasm under stressful conditions. In *Stress and Heart Disease*. Beamish RE, Singal PK, Dhalla NS (eds), pp. 129–141. Boston: Martinus Nijhoff.

113. Lown B. 1982. Clinical management of ventricular arrhythmias. *Hosp Pract* 17: 73–86.

114. Singal PK, Kapur N, Beamish RE, Das PK, Dhalla NS. 1985. Antioxidant protection against epinephrine-induced arrhythmias. In *Stress and Heart Disease*. Beamish RE, Singal PK, Dhalla NS (eds), pp. 190–201. Boston: Martinus Nijhoff.

115. Kahn DS, Rona G, Chappel CI. 1969. Isoproterenol-induced cardiac necrosis. *Ann NY Acad Sci* 156: 285–293.

116. Rona G, Chappel CI, Kahn DS. 1963. The significance of factors modifying the development of isoproterenol-induced myocardial necrosis. *Am Heart J* 66: 389–395.

117. Zbinden G. 1960. Inhibition of experimental myocardial necrosis by the monoamine oxidase inhibitor isocarboxazid (Marplan). *Am Heart J* 60: 450–453.

118. Zbinden G. 1961. Effects of anoxia and amine oxidase inhibitors on myocardial necrosis induced by isoproterenol. *Fed Proc* 20: 128.

119. Zbinden G, Bagdon RE. 1963. Isoproterenol-induced heart necrosis, an experimental model for the study of angina pectoris and myocardial infarct. *Rev Can Biol* 22: 257–263.

120. Leszkovsky GP, Gal G. 1967. Observations on isoprenaline-induced myocardial necroses. *J Pharm Pharmacol* 19: 226–230.

121. Muller E. Histochemical studies on the experimental heart infarction in the rat. *Naunyn-Schmiedebergs Arch Pharmok Exp Pathol* 1966; 254: 439–447.

122. Bloom S, Davis D. 1974. Isoproterenol myocytolysis and myocardial calcium. In *Myocardial Biology: Recent Advances in Studies on Cardiac Structure and Metabolism*, Vol. 4. Dhalla NS (ed.), pp. 581–590. Baltimore: University Park Press.

123. Dorigotti L, Gaetani M, Glasser AH, Turollia E. 1969. Competitive antagonism of isoproterenol-induced cardiac necrosis by β-adrenoreceptor blocking agents. *J Pharm Pharmacol* 21: 188–191.

124. Mehes G, Rajkovits K, Papp G. 1966. Effect of various types of sympatholytics on isoproterenol-induced myocardial lesions. *Acta Physiol Acad Sci Hung* 29: 75–85.

125. Kako K. 1966. The effect of beta-adrenergic blocking agent on biochemical changes in isoproterenol-induced myocardial necrosis. *Can J Physiol Pharmacol* 44: 678–682.

126. Pieper GM, Clayton FC, Todd GL, Eliot RS. 1979. Temporal changes in endocardial energy metabolism following propranolol and the metabolic basis for protection against isoprenaline cardiotoxicity. *Cardiovasc Res* 13: 207–214.

127. Mehes G, Papp G, Rajkovits K. 1967. Effect of adrenergic- and β-receptor blocking drugs on the myocardial lesions induced by sympathomimetic amines. *Acta Physiol Acad Sci Hung* 32: 175–184.

128. Waters LL, deSuto-Nagy GI. 1950. Lesions of the coronary arteries and great vessels of the dog following injection of adrenaline. Their prevention by Dibenamine. *Science* 111: 634–635.

129. Wenzel DG, Chau RY. 1966. Effect of adrenergic blocking agents on reduction of myocardial aspartate-amino transferase activity by sympathomimetics. *Toxicol Appl Pharmacol* 9: 514–520.

130. Dhalla NS, Balasubramanian V, Goldman J. 1971. Biochemical basis of heart function. III. Influence of isoproterenol on the norepinephrine stores in the rat heart. *Can J Physiol Pharmacol* 49: 302–311.

131. Bajusz E, Jasmin G. 1962. Protective action of serotonin against certain chemically and surgically induced cardiac necroses. *Rev Can Biol* 21: 51–62.

132. Okumura K, Ogawa K, Satake T. 1983. Pretreatment with chlorpromazine prevents phospholipid degradation and creatine kinase depletion in isoproterenol-induced myocardial damage in rats. *J Cardiovasc Pharmacol* 5: 983–988.

133. Godfraind T, Strubois X. 1979. The prevention by creatinol O-phosphate of myocardial lesions evoked by isoprenaline. *Arch Int Pharmacodyn Ther* 237: 288–297.

134. Singal PK, Dhillon KS, Beamish RE, Dhalla NS. 1981. Protective effects of zinc against catecholamine-induced myocardial changes. Electrocardiographic and ultrastructural studies. *Lab Invest* 44: 426–433.

135. Mjos DD. 1971. Effect of inhibition of lipolysis on myocardial oxygen consumption in the presence of isoproterenol. *J Clin Invest* 50: 1869–1873.

136. Wenzel DG, Stark LG. 1966. Effect of nicotine on cardiac necrosis induced by isoproterenol. *Am Heart J* 71: 368–370.

137. Sigel H, Janke J, Fleckenstein A. 1975. Restriction of isoproterenol-induced myocardial Ca uptake and necrotization by a new Ca-antagonistic compound (ethyl-4(3,4,5-trimethoxycinnamoyl) piperazinyl acetate (Vascoril). In *Recent Advances in Studies on Cardiac Structure and Metabolism*, Vol. 6. Fleckenstein A, Rona G (eds), pp. 121–126. Baltimore: University Park Press.

138. Takeo S, Takenaka F. 1977. Effects of diltizen on high-energy phosphate content reduced by isoproterenol in rat myocardium. *Arch Int Pharmacodyn Ther* 228: 205–212.

139. Deisher TA, Narita H, Zera P, Ginsburg R, Bristow MR, Billingham ME, Fowler MB, Hoffman BB. 1993. Protective effect of clentiazem against epinephrine-induced cardiac injury in rats. *J Pharmacol Exp Ther* 266: 262–269.

140. Nagano M, Higaki J, Nakamura F, Higashimori K, Nagano N, Mikami H, Ogihara T. 1992. Role of cardiac angiotensin II in isoproterenol-induced left ventricular hypertrophy. *Hypertension* 19: 708–712.

141. Hu ZW, Billingham M, Tuck M, Hoffman BB. 1990. Captopril improves hypertension and cardiomyopathy in rats with pheochromocytoma. *Hypertension* 15: 210–215.

142. Salathe M, Weiss P, Ritz R. 1992. Rapid reversal of heart failure in a patient with phaeochromocytoma and catecholamine-induced cardiomyopathy who was treated with captopril. *Br Heart J* 68: 527–528.

143. Gillis AM, Lester WM, Keashly R. 1991. Propafenone disposition and pharmacodynamic in normal and norepinephrine-induced cardiomyopathic rabbit hearts. *J Pharmacol Exp Ther* 258: 722–727.

144. Rona G, Chappel CI, Gaudry R. 1961. Effect of dietary sodium and potassium content on myocardial necrosis elicited by isoproterenol. *Lab Invest* 10: 892–897.

145. Lehr D, Chau R, Kaplan J. 1972. Prevention of experimental myocardial necrosis by electrolyte solutions. In *Recent Advances in Studies on Cardiac Structure and Metabolism*, Vol. 1. Bajusz B, Rona G (eds), pp. 684–698. Baltimore: University Park Press.

146. Janke J, Fleckenstein A, Hein B, Leder O, Sigel H. 1975. Prevention of myocardial Ca overload and necrotization by Mg and K salts or acidosis. In *Recent Advances in Studies on Cardiac Structure and Metabolism*, Vol. 6. Fleckenstein A, Rona G (eds), pp. 33–42. Baltimore: University Park Press.

147. Slezak J, Tribulova N. 1975. Morphological changes after combined administration of isoproterenol and $K^+$-$Mg^{2+}$-aspartate as a physiological $Ca^{2+}$ antagonist. In *Recent Advances in Studies on Cardiac Structure and Metabolism*, Vol. 6. Fleckenstein A, Rona G (eds), pp. 75–84. Baltimore: University Park Press.

148. Balazs T. 1972. Cardiotoxicity of isoproterenol in experimental animals. Influence of stress, obesity, and repeated dosing. In *Recent Advances in Studies on Cardiac Structure and Metabolism*, Vol. 1. Bajusz B, Rona G (eds), pp. 770–778. Baltimore: University Park Press.

149. Balazs T, Sahasrabudhe MR, Grice HC. 1962. The influence of excess body fat on cardiotoxicity of isoproterenol rats. *Toxicol Appl Pharmacol* 4: 613–620.

150. Rona G, Chappel CI, Balazs T, Gaudry R. 1959. The effect of breed, age and sex on myocardial necrosis produced by isoproterenol in the rat. *J Gerontol* 14: 169–173.

151. Dusek J, Rona G, Kahn DS. 1970. Myocardial resistance. A study of its development against toxic doses of isoproterenol. *Arch Pathol* 89: 79–83.

152. Dusek J, Rona G, Kahn DS. 1971. Myocardial resistance to isoprenaline in rats: Variations with time. *J Pathol* 105: 279–282.

153. Selye H, Veilleux R, Grasso S. 1960. Protection by coronary ligation against isoproterenol-induced myocardial necrosis. *Proc Soc Exp Biol Med* 104: 343–345.

154. Faltova E, Poupa P. 1969. Temperature and experimental acute cardiac necrosis. *Can J Physiol Pharmacol* 47: 295–299.

155. Balazs T, Murphy JG, Grice HC. 1962. The influence of environmental changes on the cardiotoxicity of isoprenaline in rats. *J Pharm Pharmacol* 14: 750–755.

156. Raab W, Bajusz E, Kimura H, Henlich HC. 1968. Isolation, stress, myocardial electrolytes and epinephrine cardiotoxicity in rats. *Proc Soc Exp Biol Med* 127: 142–147.

157. Hatch AM, Wiberg GS, Zawidzka Z, Cann M, Airth JM, Grice GC. 1965. Isolation syndrome in the rat. *Toxicol Appl Pharmacol* 7: 737–745.

158. Jasmin G. 1966. Morphologic effects of vasoactive drugs. *Can J Physiol Pharmacol* 44: 367–372.

159. Hoak JC, Warner ED, Connor WE. 1969. New concept of levarterenol-induced acute myocardial ischemic injury. *Arch Pathol* 87: 332–338.

160. Raab W. 1969. Myocardial electrolyte derangement: Crucial feature of plusicausal, so-called coronary, heart disease. *Ann NY Acad Sci* 147: 627–686.

161. Rosenblum I, Wohl A, Stein A. 1965. Studies in cardiac necrosis. III. Metabolic effects of sympathomimetic amines producing cardiac lesions. *Toxicol Appl Pharmacol* 7: 344–351.

162. Rona G, Dusek J. 1972. Studies on the mechanism of increased myocardial resistance. In *Recent Advances in Studies on Cardiac Structure and Metabolism*, Vol. 1. Bajusz E, Rona G (eds), pp. 422–429. Baltimore: University Park Press.

163. Strubelt O, Siegers CP. Role of cardiovascular and ionic changes in pathogenesis and prevention of isoprenaline-induced cardiac necrosis. Pathophysiology and morphology of myocardial cell alteration. In: Fleckenstein A, Rona G (eds). *Recent Advances in Studies on Cardiac Structure and Metabolism*, Baltimore: University Park Press, 1975; 6: 135–142.

164. Ostadal B, Poupa O. 1967. Occlusion of coronary vessels after administration of isoprenoline, adrenalin and noradrenalin. *Physiol Bohemoslov* 16: 116–119.

165. Brandi G, McGregor M. 1969. Intramural pressure in the left ventricle of the dog. *Cardiovasc Res* 3: 472–475.

166. Cutarelli R, Levy MN. 1963. Intraventricular pressure and the distribution of coronary blood flow. *Circ Res* 12: 322–327.

167. Buckberg GD, Fixler DE, Archie JP, Hoffmann JIE. 1972. Experimental subendocardial ischemia in dogs with normal coronary arteries. *Circ Res* 30: 67–81.

168. Buckberg GD, Ross G. 1973. Effects of isoprenaline on coronary blood flow: Its distribution and myocardial performance. *Cardiovasc Res* 7: 429–437.

169. Bajusz E. 1975. The terminal electrolyte-shift mechanism in heart necrosis: Its significance in the pathogenesis and prevention of necrotizing cardiomyopathies. In *Electrolytes and Cardiovascular Diseases*. Bajusz E (ed.). Basle: S. Karger.

170. Raab W, van Lith P, Lepeschkin E, Herrlich HC. 1962. Catecholamine-induced myocardial hypoxia in the presence of impaired coronary dilatability independent of external cardiac work. *Am J Cardiol* 9: 455–470.

171. Lee KS, Yu DH. 1964. Effects of epinephrine on metabolism and contraction of cat papillary muscle. *Am J Physiol* 206: 525–530.

172. Wesifeldt ML, Gilmore JP. 1964. Apparent dissociation of the inotropic and $O_2$ consumption effects of norepinephrine. *Fed Proc* 23: 357.

173. Klocke FJ, Kaiser GA, Ross Jr., J, Braunwald E. 1965. Mechanism of increase of myocardial oxygen uptake produced by catecholamines. *Am J Physiol* 209: 913–918.

174. Challoner DR, Steinberg D. 1965. Metabolic effect of epinephrine on the $QO_2$ of the arrested isolated perfused rat heart. *Nature* 205: 602–603.

175. Hauge A, Oye I. 1966. The action of adrenaline in cardiac muscle. II. Effect on oxygen consumption in the asystolic perfused rat heart. *Acta Physiol Scand* 68: 295–303.

176. Park JH, Meriwether BP, Park CR, Mudd SH, Lipmann F. 1956. Glutathione and ethylenediamine-tetraacetate antagonism of uncoupling of oxidative phosphorylation. *Biochim Biophys Acta* 22: 403–404.

177. Sordahl LA, Sliver BB. 1975. Pathological accumulation of calcium by mitochondria: Modulation by magnesium. In *Recent Advances in Studies on Cardiac Structure and Metabolism*, Vol. 6. Fleckenstein A, Rona G (eds), pp. 85–93. Baltimore: University Park Press.

178. Lossnitzer K, Janke J, Hein B, Stauch M, Fleckenstein A. 1975. Disturbed myocardial calcium metabolism: A possible pathogenetic factor in the hereditary cardiomyopathy of the Syrian hamster. In *Recent Advances in Studies on Cardiac Structure and Metabolism*, Vol. 6. Fleckenstein A, Rona G (eds), pp. 207–217. Baltimore: University Park Press.

179. Jasmin G, Bajusz E. 1975. Prevention of myocardial degeneration in hamsters with hereditary cardiomyopathy. In *Recent Advances in Studies on Cardiac Structure and Metabolism*, Vol. 6. Fleckenstein A, Rona G (eds), pp. 219–229. Baltimore: University Park Press.

180. Fleckenstein A, Janke J, Doering HJ, Leder O. 1975. Key role of Ca in the production of noncoronarogenic myocardial necroses. In *Recent Advances in Studies on Cardiac Structure and Metabolism*, Vol. 6. Fleckenstein A, Rona G (eds), pp. 21–32. Baltimore: University Park Press.

181. Osinskaya VO. 1964. Catecholamines and compounds with the properties of their oxidation products in the animal organism. In *Adrenalin: Noradrenalin*. Regulyatsii: Akad Nauk SSSR, Lab Neiro-Gumoralin, 118–123 (*Chem Abstr* 1965; 63: 869).

182. Osinskaya VO. 1957. Adrenalin and noradrenalin metabolism in animal tissues. *Biokhimiya* 22: 537–545 (*Chem Abstr* 1958; 52: 2211).

183. Utevskii AM, Osinskaya VO. 1955. The nature, properties and significance of fluorescing substances formed in the processes of adrenaline and noradrenaline oxidation. *Ukr Biokhim Zh* 27: 401–406 (*Chem Abstr* 1956; 50: 1948).

184. Kisch B. 1930. Die autokatalyse der adrenalinoxydation. *Biochem Z* 220: 84–91.

185. Okagawa M, Ichitsubo H. 1935. Oxidation and reduction of adrenaline in the body. *Proc Jpn Pharmacol Soc* 9: 155.

186. Heirman P. 1937. L'adrenoxine, adrenaline oxydee inhibitrice. *C R Soc Biol* 126: 1264–1266.

187. Heirman P. 1937. Action de la tyrosinase sur l'oxidation et les effets cardiaques de l'adrenaline et de la tyramine. *C R Soc Biol* 124: 1250–1251.

188. Hogeboom GH, Adams MH. 1942. Mammalian tyrosinase and dopa oxidase. *J Biol Chem* 145: 272–279.

189. Mason HS. 1947. The chemistry of melanin. II. The oxidation of dihydroxyphenylalanine by mammalian dopa oxidase. *J Biol Chem* 168: 433–438.

190. von Euler US. 1956. *Noradrenaline – Chemistry, Physiology, Pharmacology and Clinical Aspects*. Springfield, IL: Charles C. Thomas.

191. Heirman P. 1938. Modifications of the cardiac action of adrenaline in the course of its oxidation by phenolases. *Arch Intern Physiol* 46: 404–415.

192. Blaschko H, Schlossman H. 1940. The inactivation of adrenaline by phenolases. *J Physiol* 98: 130–140.

193. Derouaux G. 1943. The in vitro oxidation of adrenaline and other diphenol amines by phenol oxidase. *Arch Intern Pharmacodyn Ther* 69: 205–234.

194. Wajzer J. 1946. Oxydation de l'adrenaline. *Bull Soc Chim Biol* 28: 341–345.

195. Valerno DM, McCormack JJ. 1971. Xanthine oxidase-mediated oxidation of epinephrine. *Biochem Pharmacol* 20: 47–55.

196. Vercauteren R. 1951. Sur la cytochimie des granulocytes eosinophiles. *Bull Soc Chim Biol* 33: 522–525.

197. Odajima T. 1971. Myeloperoxidase of the leukocyte of normal blood. II. Oxidation–reduction reaction mechanism of the myeloperoxidase. *Biochim Biophys Acta* 235: 52–60.

198. Philpot FJ. 1940. Inhibition of adrenaline oxidation by local anaesthetics. *J Physiol* 97: 301–307.

199. Slater EC. 1949. The measurement of the cytochrome oxidase activity of enzyme preparations. *Biochem J* 44: 305–318.

200. Iisalo E, Rekkarinen A. 1958. Enzyme action on adrenaline and noradrenaline. Studies on heart muscle *in vitro*. *Acta Pharmacol Toxicol* 15: 157–174.

201. Green DE, Richter D. 1937. Adrenaline and adrenochrome. *Biochem J* 31: 596–616.

202. Bacq ZM. 1949. Metabolism of adrenaline. *Pharmacol Rev* 1: 1–26.

203. Axelrod J. 1964. Enzymic oxidation of epinephrine to adrenochrome by the salivary gland. *Biochim Biophys Acta* 85: 247–254.

204. Falk JE. 1949. The formation of hydrogen carriers by haemitin-catalyzed peroxidations. *Biochem J* 44: 369–373.

205. Chaix P, Pallaget C. 1952. Comparative characteristics of the oxidation of adrenaline and noradrenaline. *Congr Int Biochim Resumes Commun, 2nd Congr, Paris* 54 (*Chem Abstr* 1954; 48: 12851).

206. Chikano M, Kominami M. 1929. Uber die spaltung des adrenalins im serum. *Biochem Z* 205: 176–179.

207. Hoffer A. 1957. Adrenochrome and adrenolutin and their relationship to mental disease. In *Psychotropic Drugs*. Garattini S, Ghetti V (eds), pp. 10–25. Amsterdam: Elsevier.

208. Dhalla KS, Ganguly PK, Rupp H, Beamish RE, Dhalla NS. 1989. Measurement of adrenoleutin as an oxidation product of catecholamines in plasma. *Mol Cell Biochem* 87: 85–92.

209. Osmond H, Hoffer A. 1959. Schizophrenia: A new approach continued. *J Mental Sci* 105: 653–673.

210. Schweitzer A. 1931. Comparative investigations of the action of p-benzo-quinone and omega on the function of the frog heart. *Arch Ges Physiol* 228: 568–585.

211. Sanders E. 1939. The inhibiting effect of oxidized adrenalin. *Arch Exp Pathol Pharmakol* 193: 572–575.

212. Webb WR, Dodds RP, Unal MO, Karow AM, Cook WA, Daniel CR. 1966. Suspended animation of the heart with metabolic inhibitors. Effect of magnesium sulfate or fluoride and adrenochrome in rats. *Ann Surg* 164: 343–350.

213. Yen T. 1930. The reversal of the effect of adrenaline upon the rabbit intestine and the toad limb vessels. *Tohoku J Exp Med* 14: 415–465.

214. Raab W, Lepeschkin E. 1950. Pressor and cardiac effects of adrenochrome (omega) in the atropinized cat. *Exp Med Surg* 8: 319–329.

215. Titaev AA. 1964. Relation of some metabolites to the sympathetic nervous system in newborn animals. *Chem Abstr* 60: 8438.

216. Green S, Mazur A, Shorr E. 1956. Mechanism of catalytic oxidation of adrenalin by ferritin. *J Biol Chem* 220: 237–255.

217. Parrot JL. 1949. Decrease of capillary permeability under the influence of adrenochrome. *C R Soc Biol* 143: 819–822 (*Chem Abstr* 1950; 44: 5008).

218. Lecomte J, Fischer P. 1951. The effect of trihydroxy-1-methylindole on bleeding time and capillary permeability. *Arch Int Pharmacodyn Ther* 87: 225–231.

219. Marquordt P. 1944. The pharmacology and chemistry of the adrenochromes. *Z Ges Exp Med* 114: 112–126 (*Chem Abstr* 1950; 44: 2657).

220. Snyder FH, Leva E, Oberst FW. 1947. An evaluation of adrenochrome and iodoadrenochrome based on blood-sugar levels in rabbits. *J Am Pharm Assoc* 36: 253–255.

221. Kaulla KNV. 1949. Uber die beeinflussung des $O_2$ – Verbrauches durch adrenochrom beim meerschweinchen. *Biochem Z* 319: 453–456.

222. Parrot JL, Cara M. 1951. Action of adrenochrome on oxygen consumption of man and guinea pig. *C R Soc Biol* 145: 1829–2862 (*Chem Abstr* 1952; 46: 10415).

223. Kisch B. 1930. Katalytische wirkungen oxydierten adrenalins. *Klin Wochenschr* 9: 1062–1064.

224. Gaisinska MY, Utevskii AM. 1962. Effect of catecholamines on oxidative processes under normal conditions and in experimental hypertension. *Ukr Biokhim Zh* 34: 237–242 (*Chem Abstr* 1962; 57: 3986).

225. Radsma W, Golterman HL. 1954. Influence of adrenaline and adrenochrome on oxygen consumption of liver homogenates. *Biochim Biophys Acta* 13: 80–86.

226. Kisch B, Leibowitz J. 1930. Die beeinflussung der gewebsatmung der omega und durch chinon. *Biochem Z* 220: 97–116.
227. Issekutz Jr., B, Lichtneckert I, Hetenyi Jr., G, Bedo M. 1950. Metabolic effects of noradrenaline and adrenochrome. *Arch Int Pharmacodyn Ther* 84: 376–384.
228. Itasaka K. 1958. Tissue respiration and substrate utilization of heart muscle slices. *Fukuoka Igaku Zasshi* 49: 3347–3367 (*Chem Abstr* 1959; 53: 7436).
229. Wieland O, Suyter M. 1956. Der stoffwechselwirkung des adrenochroms. *Klin Wochenschr* 34: 647–648.
230. Krall AR, Siegel GJ, Goznaski DM, Wagner FL. 1964. Adrenochrome inhibition of oxidative phosphorylation by rat brain mitochondria. *Biochem Pharmacol* 12: 1519–1525.
231. Sudovtsov VE. 1969. Effect of adrenoxyl on the oxidative phosphorylation and potassium and sodium permeability of mitochondria. In *Mitokhondrii, Bioklium*, Vol. 4. Severin SE (ed.), Moscow: Funkts, Sist Kletochnykh Organell, Mater, Simp, pp. 83–88 (*Chem Abstr* 1971; 74: 2436).
232. Wajzer J. 1946. Effect pasteur du muscle de grenouille et adrenochrome. *Bull Soc Chim Biol* 28: 345–349.
233. Wajzer J. 1947. Synthese dur glycogene en presence d'adrenochrome. *Bull Soc Chim Biol* 29: 237–239.
234. Meyerhof O, Randall LO. 1948. Inhibitory effects of adrenochrome on cell metabolism. *Arch Biochem* 17: 171–182.
235. Walaas E, Walaas O, Jervell K. 1952. Action of adrenochrome on glucose phosphorylation in the rat diaphragm. *Congr Intern Biochim Resumes Commun 2nd Congr Paris*, p. 67 (*Chem Abstr* 1955; 49: 5632).
236. Pastan I, Herring B, Johnson P, Field JB. 1962. Mechanisms by which adrenaline stimulates glucose oxidation in the thyroid. *J Biol Chem* 237: 287–290.
237. Dumont JE, Hupka S. 1962. Action of neuromimetic amines on the metabolism of thyroid incubated *in vitro*. *C R Soc Biol* 156: 1942–1946 (*Chem Abstr* 1963; 59: 5434).
238. Dickens F, Glock GE. 1951. Mechanism of oxidative inhibition of myosin. *Biochim Biophys Acta* 7: 578–584.
239. Inchiosa Jr., MA, Van Demark NL. 1958. Influence of oxidation products of adrenaline on adenosinetriphosphatase activity of a uterine muscle preparation. *Proc Soc Exp Biol Med* 97: 595–597.
240. Denisov VM. 1964. Effect of the oxidation products of catecholamines on the ATPase activity of myosin. *Ukr Biokhim Zh* 36: 711–717 (*Chem Abstr* 1965; 62: 2930).
241. Denisov VM, Rukavishnikova SM. 1968. Influence of adrenoxyl on the activity of heart adenosine-triphosphatase and phosphorylase. *Ukr Biokhim Zh* 40: 384–387 (*Chem Abstr* 1968; 69: 105000).
242. Friedenwald JS, Heniz H. 1942. Inactivation of amine oxidase by enzymatic oxidative products of catechol and adrenaline. *J Biol Chem* 146: 411–419.
243. Usdin VR, Su X, Usdin E. 1961. Effects of psychotropic compounds on enzyme systems. II. *In vitro* inhibition of monoamine oxidase (MAO). *Proc Soc Exp Biol Med* 108: 461–463.
244. Petryanik VD. 1971. Effect of adrenochrome and vikasol on monoamine oxidase of some rabbit organs. *Ukr Biokhim Zh* 43: 225–228 (*Chem Abstr* 1971; 75: 47117).
245. Anderson AB. 1961. Inhibition of alkaline phosphatase by adrenaline and related dihydroxyphenols and quinones. *Biochim Biophys Acta* 54: 110–114.

246. Heacock RA. 1959. The chemistry of adrenochrome and related compounds. *Chem Rev* 59: 181–237.
247. Shebeko GS. 1970. Effect of adrenaline and adrenoxyl on the level of coenzyme A in some organs of albino rats. *Ukr Biokhim Zh* 42: 596–599 (*Chem Abstr* 1971; 74: 72333).
248. Frederick J. 1958. Cytologic studies on the normal mitochondria and those submitted to experimental procedures in living cells cultured in vitro. *Arch Biol* 69: 167–349.
249. Blix G. 1929. Adrenaline as an oxidation catalyzer. Oxidative deamination of amino acids by some means of adrenaline or some simple hydroxygenzenes. *Skand Arch Physiol* 56: 131–172.
250. Kisch B, Leibowitz J. 1930. Die omegakatalyze der oxydativen glykokollspaltung. *Biochem Z* 220: 370–377.
251. Kisch B. 1931. Die omegakatalyze der oxydativen glykokollspaltung. Neue untersuchungen. *Biochem Z* 236: 380–386.
252. Kisch B. 1932. O-Chinone als fermentmodell. II. Mitteilung: Versuche mit verschiedened substraten. *Biochem Z* 244: 440–450.
253. Aberhalden E, Baertich E. 1937. Deamination of glycine by "omega" (adrenaline oxidation product). *Fermentforschung* 15: 342–347 (*Chem Abstr* 1938; 32: 3431).
254. Fischer P, Landtsheer L. 1950. The metabolism of adrenochrome and trihydroxy-methylindole in the rabbit. *Experientia* 6: 305–306.
255. Fischer P, Lecomte J. 1951. Metabolisme de l'adrenochrome, de ses produits de reuction et du trihydroxy-N-methylindol chez le lapin, le chat et le chien. *Bull Soc Chim Biol* 33: 569–600.
256. Noval JJ, Sohler A, Stackhouse SP, Bryan AC. 1962. Metabolism of adrenochrome in experimental animals. *Biochem Pharmacol* 11: 467–473.
257. Schayer RW, Smiley RL. 1953. The metabolism of epinephrine containing isotropic carbon. III. *J Biol Chem* 202: 425–430.
258. Yates JC, Dhalla NS. 1975. Induction of necrosis and failure in the isolated perfused rat heart with oxidized isoproterenol. *J Mol Cell Cardiol* 7: 807–816.
259. Steen EM, Noronha-Dutra AA, Woolf N. 1982. The response of isolated rat heart cells to cardiotoxic concentrations of isoprenaline. *J Pathol* 137: 167–176.
260. Dhalla NS, Yates JC, Lee SL, Singh A. 1978. Functional and subcellular changes in the isolated rat heart perfused with oxidized isoproterenol. J Mol Cell Cardiol 10: 31–41.
261. Severin S, Sartore S, Schiaffino S. 1977. Direct toxic effects of isoproterenol on cultured muscle cells. *Experientia* 33: 1489–1490.
262. Yates JC, Beamish RE, Dhalla NS. 1981. Ventricular dysfunction and necrosis produced by adrenochrome metabolite of epinephrine: relation to pathogenesis of catecholamine cardiomyopathy. *Am Heart J* 102: 210–221.
263. Yates JC, Taam GML, Singal PK, Beamish RE, Dhalla NS. 1980. Protection against adrenochrome-induced myocardial damage by various pharmacological interventions. *Br J Exp Pathol* 61: 242–255.
264. Yates JC, Taam GML, Singal PK, Beamish RE, Dhalla NS. 1980. Modification of adrenochrome-induced cardiac contractile failure and cell damage by changes in cation concentrations. *Lab Invest* 43: 316–326.
265. Takeo S, Fliegel L, Beamish RE, Dhalla NS. 1980. Effects of adrenochrome on rat heart sarcolemmal ATPase activities. *Biochem Pharmacol* 29: 559–564.

266. Takeo S, Taam GML, Beamish RE, Dhalla NS. 1980. Effects of adrenochrome on calcium accumulating and adenosine triphosphate activities of the rat heart microsomes. *J Pharmacol Exp Ther* 214: 688–693.
267. Takeo S, Taam GML, Beamish RE, Dhalla NS. 1981. Effect of adrenochrome on calcium accumulation by heart mitochondria. *Biochem Pharmacol* 30: 157–163.
268. Taam GML, Takeo S, Ziegelhoffer A, Singal PK, Beamish RE, Dhalla NS. 1986. Effect of adrenochrome on adenine nucleotides and mitochondrial oxidative phosphorylation in rat heart. *Can J Cardiol* 2: 88–93.
269. Fliegel L, Takeo S, Beamish RE, Dhalla NS. 1985. Adrenochrome uptake and subcellular distribution in the isolated perfused rat heart. *Can J Cardiol* 1: 122–127.
270. Karmazyn M, Beamish RE, Fliegel L, Dhalla NS. 1981. Adrenochrome-induced coronary artery constriction in the rat heart. *J Pharmacol Exp Ther* 219: 225–230.
271. Singal PK, Dhillon KS, Beamish RE, Dhalla NS. 1982. Myocardial cell damage and cardiovascular changes due to I.V. infusion of adrenochrome in rats. *Br J Exp Pathol* 63: 167–176.
272. Beamish RE, Dhillon KS, Singal PK, Dhalla NS. 1981. Protective effect of sulfinpyrazone against catecholamine metabolite adrenochrome-induced arrhythmias. *Am Heart J* 102: 149–152.
273. Beamish RE, Singal PK, Dhillon KS, Karmazyn M, Kapur N, Dhalla NS. 1981. Effects of sulfinpyrazone on adrenochrome-induced changes in the rat heart. In *Effects of Platelet-active Drugs on the Cardiovascular System.* Hirsch J, Steele PP, Verrier RL (eds), pp. 131–146. Denver: University of Colorado.
274. Singal PK, Yates JC, Beamish RE, Dhalla NS. 1981. Influence of reducing agents on adrenochrome-induced changes in the heart. *Arch Pathol Lab Med* 105: 664–669.
275. Singal PK, Kapur N, Dhillon KS, Beamish RE, Dhalla NS. 1982. Role of free radials in catecholamine-induced cardiomyopathy. *Can J Physiol Pharmacol* 60: 1390–1397.
276. Singal PK, Beamish RE, Dhalla NS. 1983. Potential oxidative pathways of catecholamines in the formation of lipid peroxides and genesis of heart disease. In *Myocardial Injury.* Spitzer JJ (ed.), pp. 391–401. Plenum Publishing Corporation.
277. Ramos K, Acosta D. 1983. Prevention by L(−)ascorbic acid of isoproterenol induced cardiotoxicity in primary culture of rat myocytes. *Toxicology* 26: 81–90.
278. Ramos K, Combs AB, Acosta D. 1983. Cytotoxicity of isoproterenol to cultured heart cells: effects of antioxidants on modifying membrane damage. *Toxicol Appl Pharmacol* 70: 317–323.
279. Acosta D, Combs AB, Ramos K. 1984. Attenuation by antioxidants of $Na^+/K^+$ ATPase inhibition by toxic concentrations of isoproterenol in cultured rat myocardial cells. *J Mol Cell Cardiol* 16: 281–284.
280. Rupp H, Bukhari AR, Jacob R. 1983. Modulation of catecholamine synthesizing and degrading enzymes by swimming and emotional excitation in the rat. In *Cardiac Adaptation to Hemodynamic Overload, Training and Stress.* Jacob R (ed.), pp. 267–273. Berlin: Steinkopff Verlag.
281. Mitova M, Bednarik B, Cerny E, Foukal T, Dratky J, Popousek F. 1983. Influence of physical exertion on early isoproterenol-induced heart injury. *Basic Res Cardiol* 78: 131–139.
282. Burton KP, McCord JM, Ghai G. 1984. Myocardial alterations due to free radical generation. *Am J Physiol* 246: H1776–H1783.

283. Blaustein AS, Schine L, Brooks WW, Fanburg BL, Bing OHL. 1986. Influence of exogenously generated oxidant species on myocardial function. *Am J Physiol* 250: H595–H599.

284. Gupta M, Singal PK. 1989. Time course of structure, function and metabolic changes due to an exogenous source of oxygen metabolites in rat heart. *Can J Physiol Pharmacol* 67: 1549–1559.

285. Kaneko M, Beamish RE, Dhalla NS. 1989. Depression of heart sarcolemmal $Ca^{2+}$-pump activity by oxygen free radicals. *Am J Physiol* 256: H368–H374.

286. Rowe GT, Manson NH, Caplan M, Hess ML. 1983. Hydrogen peroxide and hydroxyl radical mediation of activated leukocyte depression of cardiac sarcoplasmic reticulum: Participation of cyclooxygenase pathway. *Circ Res* 53: 584–591.

287. Hata T, Kaneko M, Beamish RE, Dhalla NS. 1991. Influence of oxygen free radicals on heart sarcolemmal $Na^+$-$Ca^{2+}$ exchange. *Coronary Artery Dis* 2: 397–407.

288. Kaneko M, Hayashi H, Kobayashi A, Yamazaki N, Dhalla NS. 1991. Stunned myocardium and oxygen free radicals – sarcolemmal membrane damage due to oxygen free radicals. *Jpn Circ J* 55: 885–892.

289. Matsubara T, Dhalla NS. 1996. Effect of oxygen free radicals on cardiac contractile activity and sarcolemmal $Na^+$-$Ca^{2+}$ exchange. *J Cardiovasc Pharmacol Ther* 1: 211–218.

290. Matsubara T, Dhalla NS. 1996. Relationship between mechanical dysfunction and depression of sarcolemmal $Ca^{2+}$-pump activity in hearts perfused with oxygen free radicals. *Mol Cell Biochem* 160/161: 179–185.

# 10

# CARDIOVASCULAR EFFECTS OF CENTRALLY ACTING DRUGS

*Kenneth A. Skau and Gary Gudelsky*

*University of Cincinnati College of Pharmacy,
Cincinnati, OH, USA*

Most of the major classes of drugs for the treatment of central nervous system (CNS) disorders are relatively free from cardiovascular toxicologic effects. The exceptions to this are tricyclic antidepressants and licit and illicit psychostimulants, e.g. amphetamines, cocaine.

The cardiovascular effects of centrally acting drugs may be a direct result from an action of the agent on cardiac tissue or an indirect effect that results from an interaction of the drug with central and peripheral neurotransmitter systems. Many CNS-acting drugs affect noradrenergic and cholinergic mechanisms that regulate cardiac function.

This chapter will review the adverse cardiovascular effects of a number of drugs whose primary site of action is the central nervous system.

## Antidepressant agents

Tricyclic antidepressants have been in use for the treatment of depression for almost 40 years. In therapeutic doses, these agents are relatively free of adverse cardiovascular effects, with the exception of orthostatic hypotension. In some instances, mild tachycardia is also observed, which is most likely the consequence of the combined inhibition of reuptake of norepinephrine and blockade of cholinergic receptors.

A common adverse effect of tricyclic antidepressants is postural, or orthostatic, hypotension. The mechanism of orthostatic hypotension induced by tricyclic antidepressants is unknown, although the response often is attributed to $\alpha_1$-adrenergic receptor blockade. This adverse cardiovascular effect is best documented for imipramine, but it is also shared by desmethylimipramine and amitriptyline; the incidence of orthostatic hypotension is less for nortriptyline (Muller *et al.*, 1961; Freyschuss *et al.*, 1970; Roose *et al.*, 1986; Glassman *et al.*, 1987).

Tricyclic antidepressants also have been reported to produce abnormalities in electrocardiographic tracings (Burrows *et al.*, 1976; Kantor *et al.*, 1978). On the basis of numerous studies, it appears that tricyclic antidepressant drugs impair intraventricular conduction velocity.

In contrast to relatively mild effects of tricyclic antidepressants at therapeutic doses, severe adverse cardiovascular effects have occurred in people taking overdoses of these drugs. Fatalities from overdoses of tricyclics have often been the result of heart block and/or arrhythmias (Williams and Sherter, 1971). Although tricyclics exert quinidine-like antiarrhythmic activity at therapeutic doses (Glassman and Bigger, 1981), fatal doses of these drugs have been shown to produce marked conduction defects and subsequent ventricular arrhythmias (Langou *et al.*, 1980).

While the incidence of cardiovascular effects associated with toxic, as well as therapeutic, levels of tricyclic antidepressants has been significant, there appears to be little or no adverse cardiovascular effect associated with the use of newer antidepressant drugs, such as bupropion (Farid *et al.*, 1983; Wenger *et al.*, 1983), and the selective serotonin reuptake inhibitors, e.g. fluoxetine (Baldessarini, 1996).

## Antipsychotic agents

The most prominent adverse cardiovascular effect associated with the use of antipsychotic agents is orthostatic hypotension (Stimmel, 1996). This effect is more often associated with low-potency phenothiazines of the aliphatic type (e.g. chlorpromazine) and piperidine type (e.g. thioridazine). Orthostatic hypotension in response to these agents is generally believed to result from the blockade of $\alpha_1$-adrenergic receptors.

Phenothiazine antipsychotics also have been reported to exert negative inotropic effects on the heart (Landmark, 1971). The ability of thioridazine to exert antagonist effects on calcium channels might account for the negative inotropic effects of this drug (Gould *et al.*, 1984).

There also is evidence of electrocardiographic abnormalities associated with the use of phenothiazine-type antipsychotics (Desautels *et al.*, 1964; Schoonmaker *et al.*, 1966). As noted by Buckley *et al.* (1995), defects in cardiac conduction and cardiotoxicity are more prevalent for thioridazine than for other antipsychotic agents. The cardiotoxicity associated with overdose of thioridazine is manifested by conduction defects resulting in ventricular arrhythmias and atrioventricular block (Giles and Modlin, 1968; Kemper *et al.*, 1983). Although thioridazine has been suggested to inactivate fast sodium channels and decrease potassium efflux within the heart (Landmark *et al.*, 1972; Arita and Surawicz, 1973), it is unclear whether these effects mediate thioridazine-induced cardiotoxicity (Hale and Poklis, 1986).

## Stimulants

### *Cocaine*

Cocaine can induce cardiac toxicity through at least two mechanisms: indirectly by altering catecholamine uptake and directly by altering ion fluxes. Cardiac toxicity of cocaine is complicated by metabolism of this drug (Inaba *et al.*, 1978). Cocaine is initially metabolized into three substances:

1. Norcocaine is produced through cytochrome P450 metabolism in the liver.
2. Benzoylecognine has been reported to occur spontaneously in the blood, but recent evidence indicates that the rate of hydrolysis of cocaine to benzoylecognine is too fast to be spontaneous (Isenschmid *et al.*, 1989) and is probably due to a liver carboxyesterase.
3. Ecognine methyl ester is produced through enzymatic hydrolysis by butyrylcholinesterase.

In addition, each of these metabolites may be further metabolized, producing ecognine, norecognine methyl ester, benzoylnorecognine and norecognine. The cardiac toxicity of these metabolic products is not well understood. Furthermore, when cocaine is used with alcohol, cocaethylene is produced and may also be cardiotoxic. There have been some suggestions that a subset of the population that is homozygous for an atypical form of butyrylcholinesterase has a reduced metabolism of cocaine and possible enhanced toxicity (Jatlow *et al.*, 1979).

Cocaine acts indirectly by blocking reuptake of catecholamines. In cardiac tissue, this means inhibition of reuptake of norepinephrine from the cardioaccelerator nerves (Billman, 1990). The result is a predictable response from excess adrenergic stimulation and includes increased heart rate and myocardial oxygen demand. In susceptible individuals, this may lead to arrhythmias, including sinus tachycardia, premature ventricular contractions, ventricular tachycardia, fibrillation, and asystole (Bauman *et al.*, 1994). The increased oxygen demand may result in myocardial infarction (Cregler and Mark, 1986). Vasoconstriction, as a consequence of increased norepinephrine, may exacerbate any of these symptoms. Moreover, toxic levels of cocaine have been shown to reduce vagal tone (Newlin, 1995) and inhibit muscarinic $M_2$ receptors of the heart, an action that would reduce the normal vagus-induced slowing of heart rate (Sharkey *et al.*, 1988). Those at risk include people with pre-existing coronary artery disease because of predictable increase in heart rate, systolic blood pressure, and myocardial oxygen demand.

In addition to the indirect effects, cocaine is a local anesthetic and may reduce myocardial contractility. Cocaine has been shown to block sodium influx, potassium efflux (Przywara and Dambach, 1989: Das, 1993), and calcium influx (Kimura *et al.*, 1992) in myocytes. The blockade of these channels can result in arrhythmias. Although the dose of cocaine necessary to produce ion channel block is generally considered to be higher than the dose necessary to produce the inhibition of catecholamine uptake, and, therefore, the euphoric effects, there are two factors that need to be considered. First, the usual way of abusing cocaine is through nasal snorting of cocaine crystals or smoking of crack or freebase cocaine. This will result in a high concentration of cocaine to the heart as the blood flow of the lungs drains directly to the heart. The heart, therefore, is subjected to a higher concentration of cocaine than are other tissues. Second, tolerance develops to the euphoric effects but not the local anesthetic effects. Thus, as an abuser becomes tolerant, he/she will increase the dose to acquire the euphoria and will increase the risk of local anesthetic effects.

An additional complication of cocaine on the heart is the production of ischemia, perhaps as a complication of both the indirect and direct effects. Recently, it has been demonstrated that cocaine (in rats) can cause reversible and irreversible cardiac changes as a consequence of reactive oxygen intermediates that produce ischemia and reperfusion injury. Increased cardiac levels of malonaldehyde, glutathione and superoxide dismutase along with reduced levels of ATP and glutathione peroxidase and transferase suggested oxidative stress as a major contributor to cardiac toxicity (Devi and Chan, 1999)

Chronic cocaine use has been reported to produce cardiomyopathies such as left ventricular hypertrophy (Virmani *et al.*, 1988; Brickner *et al.*, 1991). Although the molecular mechanisms of this myopathy are not understood in humans, an investigation in rats showed alterations of mRNAs associated with atrial natriuretic factor, collagens, and myosin heavy chains. These alterations were similar to those found in mechanically induced ventricular hypertrophy (Besse *et al.*, 1997).

In laboratory animals, cocaine, when administered to conscious animals, typically produces an increase in heart rate (Hale *et al.*, 1989; Stambler *et al.*, 1993); isolated heart preparations, such as the Langendorff preparation (Simkhovich *et al.*, 1994) or isolated working heart preparation (K. A. Skau, unpublished observations), exhibit reduced cardiac rate from cocaine administration, probably because of the lack of sympathetic nerve input and predominance of local anesthetic effect. Direct toxic effects of cocaine on cardiac contractility have been noted in cultured cardiomyocytes (Qiu and Morgan, 1993), an effect that may be related to block of calcium channels (Yuan and Acosta, 1994). The last investigators also found that lower cocaine doses impair sodium–calcium exchange, which might lead to a positive inotropic effect.

As stated above, the metabolites of cocaine also have potential to produce cardiac toxicity. Norcocaine is produced in relatively small amounts and probably has little effect. However, of significant concern is cocaethylene, which is produced when cocaine and ethanol are consumed together. Cocaethylene produces cardiovascular effects similar to cocaine (McCance *et al.*, 1995).

In summary, cocaine and its metabolites can produce effects on heart function through at least three mechanisms: (1) cocaine inhibits uptake of catecholamines, which can increase heart rate and force and increase oxygen demand; (2) ion channel block can result in depressed cardiac contractility; (3) inhibition of vagal tone and muscarinic receptors can increase heart rate. The net effect of cocaine on heart function is complex and will depend on pre-existing conditions, metabolism of cocaine, and the dose administered.

### *Amphetamines*

Amphetamines have been associated with myocardial infarctions probably through reflex effects on blood pressure (Ragland *et al.*, 1993). There is no convincing evidence that they directly affect the heart.

# Depressants

## *Benzodiazepines*

There are virtually no references to cardiac abnormalities that can be attributed to benzodiazepines, even in overdose situations.

## *Barbiturates*

Barbiturates, especially those used as general anesthetics, can increase the incidence of ventricular arrhythmias by depressing the function of potassium channels. This effect is most often observed when combined with epinephrine and halothane (Pancrazio *et al.*, 1993). These authors showed a slightly prolonged action potential but also a reduced time to threshold which resulted in the proarrhythmic effect. Ikemoto (1977) and Frankl and Poole-Wilson (1981) have demonstrated that barbiturates reduce the calcium channel current and reduce cardiac contractility.

Barbiturates may exert a direct depressant effect on isolated heart tissue, but the doses appear to be far in excess of those compatible with life (Mark, 1971).

## *Non-barbiturate depressants*

Chloral hydrate overdose causes some arrhythmias, probably by sensitizing the heart to catecholamines. Both supraventricular and ventricular tachyarrhythmias have been observed (Gustafson *et al.*, 1977; Boyer and Glasser, 1980). The mechanisms involved have not been explored, but these authors express the view that the arrhythmias are likely caused by metabolites rather than the chloral hydrate itself.

# Anticonvulsants

Phenytoin has been reported to produce arrhythmias, especially when given intravenously (Barron, 1976), although Browne and LeDuc (1995) state that there is no definitive study showing this effect. Phenytoin has been shown to block L-type calcium channels in cardiac tissue, although the implications of this finding are not clear (Rivet *et al.*, 1990)

Carbamazepine has been shown to produce bradycardia (Herzberg, 1978) and complete heart block (Hamilton, 1978), especially in elderly patients. Kasarskis *et al.* (1992) report that at massive overdose there may be a sinus tachycardia. The heart block is probably due to conduction deficits (Beerman *et al.*, 1975; Boesen *et al.*, 1983; Kasarskis *et al.*, 1992) involving prolonged conduction and reduced rate of phase 4 depolarization (Steiner *et al.*, 1970).

# References

Arita, M. and Surawicz, B. 1973. Electrophysiologic effects of phenothiazines on canine cardiac fibers. *Journal of Pharmacology and Experimental Therapeutics* 184: 619–630.

Baldessarini, R.J. 1996. Drugs and the treatment of psychiatric disorders. In *Goodman and Gilman's The Pharmacological Basis of Therapeutics*. Hardman, J., Limbird, L., Molinoff, P., and Ruddon, R. (eds), pp. 431–459. McGraw-Hill, New York.

Barron, S. 1976. Cardiac arrhythmias after small i.v. dose of phenytoin (letter). *New England Journal of Medicine* 295: 678.

Bauman, J., Grawe, J., Winecoff, A., and Hariman, R. 1994. Cocaine-related sudden cardiac death: A hypothesis correlating basic science and clinical observations. *Journal of Clinical Pharmacology* 34: 902–911.

Beerman, B., Edhag, O., and Vallin, H. 1975. Advanced heart block aggravated by carbamazepine. *British Heart Journal* 37: 668–671.

Besse, S., Assayar, P., Latour, C., Janmot, C., Robert, V., Delcayre, C., Nahas, G., and Swynghedauw, B. 1997. Molecular characteristics of cocaine-induced cardiomyopathy in rats. *European Journal of Pharmacology* 338: 123–129.

Billman, G.E. 1990. Mechanisms responsible for the cardiotoxic effects of cocaine. *FASEB Journal* 4: 2469–2475.

Boesen, F., Anderson, E., Jensen, E., and Ladefoged, S. 1983. Cardiac conduction disturbances during carbamazepine therapy. *Acta Neurologica Scandinavica* 68: 49–52.

Boyer, K. and Glasser, P. 1980. Chloral hydrate overdose and cardiac arrhythmias. *Chest* 77: 232–235.

Brickner, M.E., Willard, J.E., Eichhorn, E.J., Black, J., and Grayburn, P.A. 1991. Increased left ventricular mass and wall thickness associated with chronic cocaine abuse. *Circulation* 84: 1130–1135.

Browne, T. and LeDuc, B. 1995. Phenytoin. Chemistry and biotransformation. In *Antiepileptic Drugs*, 4th edn. Levy, R., Mattson, R., and Meldrum, B. (eds), pp. 283–300. Raven Press, New York.

Buckley, N., Med, B., Whyte, I., and On, A.H. 1995. Cardiotoxicity more common in thioridazine overdose than with other neuroleptics. *Clinical Toxicology* 33: 199–204.

Burrows, G.D., Vohra, J., Hunt, D., Sloman, J., Scoggins, B., and Davies, B. 1976. Cardiac effects of different tricyclic antidepressant drugs. *British Journal of Psychiatry* 129: 335–341.

Cregler, L.L. and Mark, H. 1986. Medical complications of cocaine abuse. *New England Journal of Medicine* 315: 1495–1500.

Das, G. 1993. Cardiovascular effects of cocaine abuse. *International Journal of Clinical Pharmacology and Therapeutic Toxicology* 31: 521–528.

Desautels, S., Filteau, C., St.-Jean, A. 1964. Ventricular tachycardia associated with administration of thioridazine hydrochloride (Mellaril): a report of a case with a favorable outcome. *Canadian Medical Association Journal* 90: 1030–1031.

Devi, B. and Chan, A. 1999. Effect of cocaine on cardiac biochemical functions. *Journal of Cardiovascular Pharmacology* 33: 1–6.

Farid, F., Wenger, T., Tsai, S., Singh, B., and Stern, W. 1983. Use of bupropion in patients who exhibit orthostatic hypotension on tricyclic antidepressants. *Journal of Clinical Psychiatry* 44: 170–173.

Frankl, W. and Poole-Wilson, P. 1981. Effects of thiopental on tension development, action potential, and exchange of calcium and potassium in rabbit ventricular myocardium. *Journal of Cardiovascular Pharmacology* 3: 554–565.

Freyschuss, U., Sjoqvist, F., Tuck, D., and Asberg, M. 1970. Circulatory effects in man of nortriptyline, a tricyclic antidepressant drug. *Pharmacologia Clinica* 2: 68–71.

Giles, T.D. and Modlin, R.K. 1968. Death associated with ventricular arrhythmia and thioridazine hydrochloride. *Journal of the American Medical Association* 205: 98–100.

Glassman, A.H. and Bigger, J.T. 1981. Cardiovascular effects of therapeutic doses of tricyclic antidepressants: a review. *Archives of General Psychiatry* 38: 815–825.

Glassman, A.H., Roose, S.P., Giardina, E-G., and Bigger, J.T. 1987. Cardiovascular effects of tricyclic antidepressants. In *Psychopharmacology: The Third Generation of Progress.* Meltzer, H.Y. (ed.), pp. 1437–1442. Raven Press, New York.

Gould, R.J., Murphy, K., Reynolds, I., and Snyder, S.H. 1984. Calcium channel blockade: possible explanation for thioridazine's peripheral side effects. *American Journal of Psychiatry* 141: 352–357.

Gustafson, A., Svensson, S., and Ugander, L. 1977. Cardiac arrhythmias in chloral hydrate poisoning. *Acta Medica Scandinavica* 201: 227–230.

Hale, P.W. and Poklis, A. 1986. Cardiotoxicity of thioridazine and two stereoisomeric forms of thioridazine 5-sulfoxide in the isolated perfused rat heart. *Toxicology and Pharmacology* 86: 44–55.

Hale, S., Lehmann, M., and Kloner, R. 1989. Electrocardiographic abnormalities after acute administration of cocaine in the rat. *American Journal of Cardiology* 63: 1529–1530.

Hamilton. D. 1978. Carbamazepine and heart block (letter). *Lancet* I: 1365.

Herzberg, L. 1978. Carbamazepine and bradycardia (letter). *Lancet* I: 1097–1098.

Ikemoto, Y. 1977. Reduction by thiopental of the slow-channel-mediated action potential of canine papillary muscle. *Pflügers Archives* 372: 285–286.

Inaba, T., Stewart, D.J., and Kalow, W. 1978. Metabolism of cocaine in man. *Clinical Pharmacology and Therapeutics* 23: 547–552,.

Isenschmid, D., Levine, B., and Caplan, Y. 1989. A comprehensive study of the stability of cocaine and its metabolites. *Journal of Analytical Toxicology* 13: 250–256.

Jatlow, P., Barash, P., Van Dyke, C., Radding, J., and Byck, R. 1979. Cocaine and succinylcholine sensitivity: A new caution. *Anesthesia and Analgesia* 58: 235–238.

Kantor, S.J., Glassman, A.H., Bigger, J.T., Perel, J.M., and Giardina, E.G. 1978. The cardiac effects of therapeutic plasma concentrations of imipramine. *American Journal of Psychiatry* 135: 534–538.

Kasarskis, E., Kuo, C-S., Berger, R., and Nelson, K. 1992. Carbamazepine-induced cardiac dysfunction. Characterization of two distinct clinical syndromes. *Archives of Internal Medicine* 152: 186–191.

Kemper, A.J., Dunlap, R., and Pietro, D.A. 1983. Thioridazine-induced torsade de pointes. Successful therapy with isoproterenol. *Journal of the American Medical Association* 249: 2931–2934.

Kimura, S., Bassett, A.L., Xi, H., and Myerburg, R.J. 1992. Early afterdepolarizations and triggered activity induced by cocaine. *Circulation* 85: 2227–2235.

Landmark, K. 1971. The actions of promazine and thioridazine in isolated rat atria. 1. Effects on automaticity, mechanical performance, refractoriness and excitability. *European Journal of Pharmacology* 16: 1–7.

Landmark, K., Haffner, J., and Setekleiv, J. 1972. Reduction in $^{42}$K-efflux from rat atria by promazine and thioridazine. *Acta Pharmacologica et Toxicologica* 31: 54–64.

Langou, R.A., Van Dyke, C., Tahan, S.R., and Cohen, L.S. 1980. Cardiovascular manifestations of tricyclic antidepressant overdose. *American Heart Journal* 100: 458–464.

McCance, E., Price, L., Kosten, T., and Jatlow, P. 1995. Cocaethylene: Pharmacology, physiology and behavioral effects in humans. *Journal of Pharmacology and Experimental Therapeutics* 274: 215–223.

Mark, L. 1971. Mode of action of acute toxic effects of barbiturates. In *Acute Barbiturate Poisoning*. Matthew, H. (ed.). Excerpta Medica, Amsterdam.

Muller, O.F., Goodman, N., and Bellet, S. 1961. The hypotensive effect of imipramine hydrochloride in patients with cardiovascular disease. *Clinical Pharmacology and Therapeutics* 2: 300–307.

Newlin, D. 1995. Effect of cocaine on vagal tone: A common factors approach. *Drug and Alcohol Dependence* 37: 211–216.

Pancrazio. J., Frazer, M., and Lynch, C. 1993. Barbiturate anesthetics depress the resting K$^+$ conductance of myocardium. *Journal of Pharmacology and Experimental Therapeutics* 265: 358–365.

Przywara, D.A. and Dambach, G.E. 1989. Direct actions of cocaine on cardiac cellular electrical activity. *Circulation Research* 65: 185–192.

Qiu, Z., and Morgan, J. 1993. Differential effects of cocaine and cocaethylene on intracellular Ca$^{2+}$ and myocardial contraction in myocytes. *British Journal of Pharmacology* 109: 293–298.

Ragland, A., Ismail, Y., and Arsura, E. 1993. Myocardial infarction after amphetamine use. *American Heart Journal* 125: 247–249.

Rivet, M., Bois, P., Cognard, C., and Raymond, G. 1990. Phenytoin preferentially inhibits L-type calcium currents in whole-cell patch-clamped cardiac and skeletal muscle cells. *Cell Calcium* 11: 581–588.

Roose, S.P., Glassman, A.H., Giardina, E.G., Johnson, L., Walsh, B., Woodring, S., and Bigger, J.T. 1986. Nortriptyline in depressed patients with left ventricular impairment. *Journal American Medical Association* 256: 3253–3257.

Schoonmaker, F.W., Osteen, R.T., and Greenfield, J.C. 1966. Thioridazine (Mellaril)-induced ventricular tachycardia controlled with an artificial pacemaker. *Annals of Internal Medicine* 65: 1076–1079.

Sharkey, J., Ritz, M., Schenden, J.A., Hanson, R.C., and Kuhar, M.J. 1988. Cocaine inhibits muscarinic cholinergic receptors in heart and brain. *Journal of Pharmacology and Experimental Therapeutics* 246: 1048–1052.

Simkhovich, B., Kloner, R., Alker, K., and Giaconi, J. 1994. Time course of direct cardiotoxic effects of high cocaine concentration in isolated rabbit heart. *Journal of Cardiovascular Pharmacology* 23: 509–516.

Stambler, B., Komamura, K., Ihara, T., and Shannon, R. 1993. Acute intravenous cocaine causes transient depression followed by enhanced left ventricular function in conscious dogs. *Circulation* 87: 1687–1697.

Steiner, C., Wit, A., Weiss, M., and Damato, A. 1970. The antiarrhythmic actions of carbamazepine (Tegretol). *Journal of Pharmacology and Experimental Therapeutics* 173: 323–335.

Stimmel, G.L. 1996. Schizophrenia. In *Textbook of Therapeutics: Drug and Disease Management*. Herfindal, T. and Gourley, D. (eds), pp. 1117–1131. Williams and Wilkins, Baltimore, MD.

Virmani, R., Robinowitz, M., Smialek, J.E., and Smyth, D.F. 1988. Cardiovascular effects of cocaine. An autopsy study of 40 patients. *American Heart Journal* 115: 1068–1076.

Wenger, T., Cohn, J., and Bustrack, J. 1983. Comparison of the effects of bupropion and amitriptyline on cardiac conduction in depressed patients. *Journal of Clinical Psychiatry* 44: 5 174–175.

Williams, R.B. and Sherter, C. 1971. Cardiac complications of tricyclic antidepressant therapy. *Annals of Internal Medicine* 74: 395–398.

Yuan, C. and Acosta, D. 1994. Inhibitory effect of cocaine on calcium mobilization in cultured rat myocardial cells. *Journal of Molecular and Cell Cardiology* 26: 1415–1419.

# 11

# TOXINS THAT AFFECT ION CHANNELS, PUMPS, AND EXCHANGERS

*N. Sperelakis, M. Sunagawa, M. Nakamura,*
*H. Yokoshiki, and T. Seki*

*Department of Molecular and Cellular Physiology, College of*
*Medicine, University of Cincinnati, Cincinnati, OH, USA*

## Introduction

Many of the toxins in the environment that are derived from plant and animal sources or are made by mankind affect the ion channels, ion pumps, and ion exchangers of the cell membrane and/or the membranes of the endoplasmic reticulum (ER) or sarcoplasmic reticulum (SR). Many drugs used for therapy are also toxic, especially at higher concentrations. Ion channels especially are targets for a number of different toxins and drugs. Although much of the basic data elucidating mechanisms of action have been obtained on neurons, there also are considerable data on the cardiovascular systems, e.g. heart muscle and vascular smooth muscle (VSM) cells. As a general rule (with a few notable exceptions), the actions of toxins and drugs are similar in all excitable membranes, whether they be from nerve, skeletal muscle, heart, or smooth muscle in both vertebrates and invertebrates. Because there are so many toxins, and because of space and time limitations, this chapter will focus on only some of them, particularly on some of the major cardiotoxins.

The reader is referred to a recent textbook of cell physiology for the molecular structure of the various types of ion channels, pumps, and exchangers (Sperelakis, 1998a). This information is not presented here because of space limitations. Major changes have been made to the organization and content of our chapter since the publication of the previous edition (Sperelakis, 1992).

## Target ion channels

### Fast Na channels

At least six neurotoxin receptor sites have been identified by direct radiotoxin binding on the rat brain $Na^+$ channel (see Table 11.1). Receptor site 1 binds the water-soluble heterocyclic guanidines such as tetrodotoxin (TTX) and saxitoxin (STX). These toxins inhibit $Na^+$ conductance by binding to and occluding the extracellular opening of the ion pore. Lipid-soluble alkaloid toxins that bind at receptor site 2, such as batrachotoxin (BTX), grayanotoxin (GTX), and veratridine, cause persistent activation of the channel at the resting membrane potential by blocking $Na^+$ channel inactivation (inhibiting closing of the I-gate) and shifting the voltage dependence of channel activation to more negative membrane potentials. Receptor site 3 binds $\alpha$-scorpion toxins and sea anemone toxins that inhibit $Na^+$ channel inactivation. They also enhance persistent activation of $Na^+$ channels by lipid-soluble toxins acting at receptor site 2; their affinity to receptor site 3 is reduced by depolarization. $\beta$-Scorpion toxins bind to receptor site 4 and shift the voltage dependence of $Na^+$ channel activation. The hydrophobic polyether

Table 11.1 Various toxins affecting $Na^+$ channels

| Site | Toxins | Characteristics of toxins | Source | Actions |
|------|--------|---------------------------|--------|---------|
| 1 | Tetrodotoxin | Guanidinium group | Puffer fish | Blockade |
|   | Saxitoxin | Guanidinium group | Shellfish | Blockade |
| 2 | Veratridine | Lipophilic alkaloid | | Persistent activation |
|   | Aconitine (ajacine, delphinine, delphisine, deltaline, heteratisine, lappaconitine, N-deacetyl-lappaconitine) | Diterpenoid | Plant | Persistent activation |
|   | Batrachotoxin | Lipophilic alkaloid | Frog skin | Persistent activation |
|   | Grayanotoxins | Lipophilic alkaloid | Plant | Persistent activation |
|   | Pumiliotoxin-B | Lipophilic alkaloid | Frog skin | |
| 3 | $\alpha$-Scorpion toxins | Peptide | Scorpion | Delayed inactivation |
|   | $\delta$-Atracotoxins | Peptide | Spider | |
|   | Sea anemone toxin | Peptide | Sea anemone | Delayed inactivation |
| 4 | $\beta$-Scorpion toxins | Peptide | Scorpion | Shifts voltage dependence of activation |
| 5 | Brevetoxin-B | Polyether | Dinoflagellate | Shifts voltage dependence of activation |
|   | Ciguatoxin | Polyether | Fish | Depolarizes |
| 6 | $\delta$-Conotoxins | Peptide | Shellfish | Inhibits inactivation |

toxins brevetoxin (PbTx) and ciguatoxin bind to receptor site 5 and shift the activation to more negative membrane potentials. Receptor site 6 binds the δ-conotoxin (δ-TxVI) that inhibits Na⁺ channel inactivation in mollusk neurons but binds with high affinity to both mollusk and rat brain Na⁺ channels (reviewed in Blumenthal, 1998).

*Binding site 1*

TTX acts on the outer surface of the membrane channel (Narahashi *et al.*, 1964). The TTX molecule contains a guanidinium group that is required for activity, and it is generally believed that the positively charged guanidinium group sticks into the mouth of the fast Na⁺ channel (binding to a negative charge near the selectivity filter of the channel) and acts like a plug to block physically the passage of Na⁺ ions through the channel. The channel gates (A and I) are not blocked by TTX because the gating current is unaffected by TTX (Armstrong and Bezanilla, 1974). However, some studies suggest that TTX may block by binding to a site adjacent to the mouth of the channel ("receptor") and producing a conformational change in the channel protein.

Saxitoxin (STX) is present in the Alaska butter clam (*Saxidomas giganteus*) and in a dinoflagellate parasite (*Gonyoulax catanella*) (Narahashi, 1974). STX is chemically different from TTX, containing two guanidinium groups, but has an action nearly identical to that of TTX. One major difference is that washout of STX occurs faster than for TTX.

The TTX sensitivity of the fast Na⁺ channels (in rat papillary muscle) increases when the membrane is partly depolarized, i.e. there is a voltage dependence of TTX block (Baer *et al.*, 1976). However, others report that there is no voltage dependence for the steady-state TTX block of the fast Na⁺ current (Colatsky and Gadsby, 1980; Cohen *et al.*, 1981).

Binding studies on cultured heart cells from neonatal rats showed presence of both high-affinity ($K_d$ = 1.6 nM) and low-affinity ($K_d$ = 130 nM) binding sites, the number of low-affinity binding sites being forty-five times greater than the high-affinity sites (Renaud *et al.*, 1983). Although both high-affinity and low-affinity binding sites coexist in mammalian heart cells, the Na⁺ channels with low affinity for TTX predominate (Narahashi *et al.*, 1964). TTX binding is inhibited at acid pH, half inhibition occurring at pH 6.2 (Lombet *et al.*, 1981). The relevant ionizable group on the Na⁺ channel may be a carboxylate. Monovalent and divalent cations displace TTX binding in the sequence: guanidinium⁺ > Tl⁺ > NH₄⁺ > Li⁺ > Na⁺ > K⁺ > Rb⁺ > Cs⁺ > Mg²⁺ ($K_d$ = 1.3 mM) > Ca²⁺ ($K_d$ = 3.2 mM) (Renaud and Lazdunski, 1988). Photoactivatable TTX derivatives have been prepared that can irreversibly bind to and block the fast Na⁺ channel upon irradiation (Chicheportiche *et al.*, 1979).

## Binding site 2

Veratridine is a $Na^+$ channel toxin that exerts a powerful positive inotropic effect and prolongs the action potential duration in the heart (Brill and Wasserstrom, 1986). Veratridine (50 $\mu M$) induces long-lasting openings of the channels (from guinea pig ventricle) with two different single-channel conductances of 7.6 and 3.0 pS (Sunami et al., 1993).

Single-channel recordings have shown that batrachotoxin (BTX) greatly prolongs the mean open time of the channels (Narahashi, 1986). BTX strangely reduces the single-channel current amplitude, thus suggesting a second effect, such as slower activation. After exposure to BTX, channel openings are observed (at large negative potentials at which no opening normally occurs). In the BTX-poisoned membrane of the neuroblastoma cell, there are two separate groups of $Na^+$ channels, one exhibiting normal characteristics and the other exhibiting prolonged openings and reduced amplitude (Narahashi, 1986).

The properties of BTX-modified Na channels in heart are qualitatively similar to those in nerve, but quantitative differences do exist. In the heart, the shift of the conductance–voltage curve for the modified channel is less pronounced, the maximal activation rate of modified channels is considerably slower, and the inactivation of the channels is slower (Huang et al., 1987).

Extracts of the plant Aconitum sp. (Ranunculaceae) are used in traditional Chinese medicine predominantly as anti-inflammatory and analgesic agents. For analgesia, aconitine is as potent as morphine but is not habit-forming (Gutser et al., 1998). Aconitine is a highly toxic diterpenoid alkaloid that is known to suppress the inactivation of voltage-dependent $Na^+$ channels by binding to neurotoxin binding site 2 on the $\alpha$-subunit of the channel protein. A use-dependent inhibition of neuronal activity occurs with these alkaloids (Ameri, 1998).

Eight N-oxides of the norditerpenoid alkaloids (aconitine, ajacine, delphinine, delphisine, deltaline, heteratisine, lappaconitine, and N-deacetyllappaconitine) have been reported previously (Bai and Pelletier, 1995). Aconitine and 3-acetylaconitine have similar potencies (in rat hippocampal synaptosomes), with $EC_{50}$ values of about 230 nM (Seitz and Ameri, 1998).

The alkaloid pumiliotoxin-B (PTX-B), extracted from the skin of the frog Dendrobates pumilio, activates $Na^+$ channels by interacting with a site that is allosterically coupled to other sites on the $Na^+$ channel, namely two scorpion toxin sites and the brevetoxin site. PTX-B interacts with a part of the alkaloid-binding domain that is shared by aconitine (but not by batrachotoxin or veratridine), whereas aconitine interacts with a part of the domain shared by PTX-B and by batrachotoxin/veratridine (Gusovsky et al., 1992).

Grayanotoxins (GTXs) are known to produce cardiac tachyarrhythmias. GTXs induce a persistent increase in the membrane permeability to $Na^+$ ions (Yakehiro et al., 1993). At a GTX concentration of 100 $\mu M$ (at +20 mV), 64 percent of the $Na^+$ channel population is modified (Yakehiro et al., 1997). 3$\beta$-OH, 5$\beta$-OH, and 6$\beta$-OH groups of the GTX molecule make contact with the Na channel by hydrogen bonding and with the remainder of the molecule by hydrophobic binding to the channel (Yakehiro *et al.*, 1993). α-Dihydrograyanotoxin-II (GTX) modifies the channel (of squid giant axons) to generate a sustained inward current ($EC_{50}$ of 10 μM), but only when the membrane is depolarized. The activation–voltage relationship for the sustained $Na^+$ current is greatly shifted in the hyperpolarizing direction (compared with that for peak $Na^+$ current).

### Binding site 3

δ-Atracotoxins from the venom of Australian funnel web spiders are a unique group of peptide toxins that slow $Na^+$ current inactivation in a manner similar to that of α-scorpion toxins and they bind to the same receptor site (Little *et al.*, 1998).

Sea anemone toxin (ATX-II) is a polypeptide toxin isolated from the sea anemone *Anemonia sulcata*. ATX-II binds to the same site on the $Na^+$ channel as scorpion toxins (Lawrence and Catterall, 1981). Sea anemone toxins slow the Na channel inactivation process, inducing a sustained Na current during a depolarizing pulse. The binding of these toxins markedly decreases with depolarization (Warashina *et al.*, 1988).

### Binding site 4

The scorpion toxins can be divided into (1) "long-chain toxins" (60–70 amino acid residues cross-linked by four disulfide bridges) that affect exclusively voltage-dependent $Na^+$ channels of excitable cells; (2) "short-chain toxins" (30–40 amino acid residues cross-linked by three disulfide bridges) that block several types of $K^+$ channels (Legros and Martin-Eauclaire, 1997).

Scorpion neurotoxins, which bind to and modulate $Na^+$ channels, have been divided into two groups: the α-toxins and β-toxins. α-Scorpion toxins bind to neurotoxin receptor site 3 (Nicholson *et al.*, 1996). The β-toxin class includes the groups of excitatory and depressant toxins, which differ in their mode of action and are highly specific against insects (Oren *et al.*, 1998). β-Scorpion toxins negatively shift voltage dependence of activation and enhance closed state inactivation; they bind to receptor site 4, which requires glycine 845 (Gly-845) in the S3–S4 loop at the extracellular end of the S4 segment in domain II of the α-subunit (Cestele *et al.*, 1998).

### Binding site 5

Brevetoxin-B (GbTX-B), a cyclic polyether purified from the marine dinoflagellate *Gymnodinium breve* (involved in "red tide"), produces positive inotropic and arrhythmogenic effects on isolated rat and guinea pig cardiac preparations at concentrations between $1.25 \times 10^{-8}$ and $1.87 \times 10^{-7}$ M (Rodgers *et al.*, 1984). Brevetoxins act as $Na^+$ channel activators and bind to receptor site 5. This site is located on the α-subunit of the Na$^+$ channel, and peptide segments in domain IV of that subunit are important in brevetoxin binding (Catterall *et al.*, 1992). Brevetoxin-3 (*Ptychodiscus brevis* toxin 3; Pbtx-3) shifts steady-state activation to negative potentials at the single-channel level without major effects on the time-course of macroscopic current activation or decay. Single-channel open times are prolonged. Under the influence of the toxin, Na$^+$ channel openings could be observed even at maintained depolarization (Schreibmayer and Jeglitsch, 1992).

Ciguatera is a disease caused by ciguatoxin, another Na$^+$ channel agonist (opener). Ciguatera poisoning is the most common fish poisoning encountered in man (Cameron *et al.*, 1991). The ciguatoxins are lipid-soluble polyether compounds which have some structural and biochemical features in common with the brevetoxins (Lewis, 1992). The affinity of ciguatoxin for the Na$^+$ channel is at least twenty to fifty times higher than that of brevetoxin. Both toxins act at the same binding site on the Na$^+$ channel (Lombet *et al.*, 1987).

In isolated parasympathetic neurons from neonatal rat intracardiac ganglia, bath application of 1–10 nM of the marine neurotoxin ciguatoxin-1 causes gradual membrane depolarization and tonic action potential firing. Action potential firing ceases when depolarization becomes larger. In cell-attached membrane patches, 1–10 nM in the patch pipette markedly increases the opening probability of single TTX-sensitive Na$^+$ channels (at various depolarizing voltage steps), but does not alter the unitary conductance or reversal potential. Under steady-state conditions (at hyperpolarized membrane potentials), ciguatoxin-1 causes spontaneous opening of single Na$^+$ channels, which do not inactivate. Ciguatoxin-1 increases neuronal excitability by shifting the voltage of activation of TTX-sensitive Na$^+$ channels to more negative potentials (Hogg *et al.*, 1998).

### Binding site 6

μ-Conotoxin is a blocker of Na$_f$ channels and is a competitive inhibitor of STX binding to Na$^+$ channels of muscle (but not nerve). μ-Conotoxin is a twenty-two-residue hydroxyproline-containing peptide that is tightly cross-linked by three disulfide bonds. The binding of μ-conotoxin varies with membrane potential (unlike TTX and STX). Na channels that are TTX/STX resistant (i.e. cardiac) are also resistant to μ-conotoxins (Fainzibler *et al.*, 1994, 1995).

### Other binding sites

DPI 201–106 {4-[3-(4-diphenylmethyl-1-piperazinyl)-2-hydroxypropoxy]-1 H-indole-2-carbonitrile} is a cardiotonic agent which prolongs the open state of the cardiac Na$^+$ channel. This agent slows the rate of Na$^+$ channel inactivation (but has no effect on inactivation) (Krafte *et al.*, 1991). The differential voltage dependencies of these two effects suggest two different binding sites (Kohlhardt *et al.*, 1987).

## Ca²⁺ channels

### Fast T type

T-type (transient or short lasting) $Ca^{2+}$ currents are known to play roles in growth, genetic hypertension, cardiac hypertrophy, and cardiac rhythm. Some excitable tissues such as the heart (mainly pacemaker cells) and smooth muscle possess low-threshold T-type $Ca^{2+}$ channels. These channels rapidly inactivate, are blocked by nickel ($Ni^{2+}$) (low concentration), have low conductance (< 10 pS), and have similar $Ca^{2+}$ and barium ($Ba^{2+}$) permeabilities. $Ca^{2+}$ antagonist drugs have almost no effect on the T-type $Ca^{2+}$ channel.

Mibefradil (Ro 40-5967) is a novel non-dihydropyridine $Ca^{2+}$ antagonist (the tetralol derivatives) that selectively blocks the T-type $Ca^{2+}$ channel (Kobrin *et al.*, 1998). This drug is structurally and pharmacologically different from traditional $Ca^{2+}$ antagonists. Although mibefradil has anti-ischemic properties (such as relaxation of VSM) and produces a slight reduction in heart rate, it does not have significant negative inotropic action at therapeutic concentrations (Ernst and Kelly, 1998).

Flunarizine blocks the T-type current of guinea pig ventricular myocytes in a use-dependent manner, and the block can be relieved by hyperpolarizing pulses (Tytgat *et al.*, 1988). The L-type current is also blocked by flunarizine in a use-dependent manner.

Zonisamide, a new antiepileptic drug, substantially reduces T-type $Ca^{2+}$ current of cultured neuroblastoma cells of human origin (NB-I) and shifts the inactivation curve (~20 mV negative) (Kito *et al.*, 1996). It was suggested that zonisamide shifts the channels toward the inactivation state, allowing fewer channels to open during membrane depolarization.

Amiloride, a $K^+$-sparing diuretic and inhibitor of the Na–H exchanger, also blocks the low-threshold $Ca^{2+}$ channel in mouse neuroblastoma cells and chick dorsal root ganglion neurons (Tang *et al.*, 1988).

### Slow L type

The L-type (long-lasting) $Ca^{2+}$ channels are very important in excitation–contraction (E–C) coupling. They are present in all types of excitable cells and in some non-excitable cells. Their single-channel conductance is over double that of the T-type channels (e.g. 20–25 pS), and their permeability to $Ba^{2+}$ is greater than that for $Ca^{2+}$. These $Ca_L$ channels are blocked by the various $Ca^{2+}$ antagonist drugs, such as verapamil, nifedipine, diltiazem, and bepridil, and are opened by the $Ca^{2+}$ agonist drugs (e.g. the dihydropyridine BayK 8644). They are more sensitive to block by acidosis, and they require ATP binding for activity. The $Ca_L$ channels are stimulated by phosphorylation ($\alpha_{1C}$ subunit) by cAMP/PKA and are inhibited by phosphorylation by cGMP/PKG (protein kinase G) (Sperelakis, 1998b). There are many toxins and alkaloids which affect $Ca_L$ channel activity (see Table 11.2).

*Table 11.2*  Various toxins inhibit Ca$^{2+}$ channels

| Toxins | Characteristics of toxins | Source | Actions |
|---|---|---|---|
| ω-Conotoxin GVIA | Peptide | Fish-hunting marine snail | Blockade |
| ω-Agatoxin-IIIA | Peptide | Funnel web spider | Blockade |
| Calcicludine | Polypeptide | African green mamba | Blockade |
| Calciseptine | Polypeptide | Black mamba | Blockade |
| FTX | Polyamine | Spider | Blockade |
| Taicatoxin | Protein | Australian taipan snake | Blockade |
| Rotundium | Alkaloid | Plant | Blockade |
| Liriodenine | Alkaloid | Plant | Blockade |
| Aporphine | Alkaloid | Plant | Blockade |

The peptide ω-agatoxin-IIIA (ω-Aga-IIIA) from venom of the funnel web spider *Agelenopsis aperta* blocks L-type and N-type Ca$^{2+}$ channels with equal high potency (IC$_{50}$ < 1 nM). ω-Aga-IIIA blocks atrial Ca$_L$ channels over 100-fold more potently than ω-Aga-IIIB or ω-Aga-IIID (Ertel *et al.*, 1994).

Calcicludine (CaC) is a 60-amino-acid polypeptide from the venom of *Dendroaspis angusticeps*. It is structurally homologous to the Kunitz-type protease inhibitor, to dendrotoxins (which block K$^+$ channels), and to the protease inhibitor domain of the amyloid beta protein (that accumulates in Alzheimer's disease). CaC blocks most of the high-threshold Ca$^{2+}$ channels (e.g. L type) in the range 10–100 nM. In rat cerebellar granule neurons in primary culture, the IC$_{50}$ value for CaC block of Ca$_L$ channels is 0.2 nM (Schweitz *et al.*, 1994).

The ω-conotoxin GVIA, a 27-amino-acid peptide from the venom of the marine snail *Conus geographus*, is a Ca$^{2+}$ channel antagonist (Sauviat, 1997). Calciseptine and FS2 are 60-amino-acid polypeptides, isolated from venom of the black mamba (*Dendroaspis polylepis polylepis*), that block Ca$_L$ channels (Kini *et al.*, 1998).

A polyamine component of *Agelenopsis aperta* spider venom designated FTX is a selective antagonist of P-type Ca$^{2+}$ channels in the mammalian brain. Natural FTX and synthesized polyamine FTX-3.3 (sFTX-3.3) block Ca$_L$ channels with similar potencies (Norris *et al.*, 1996).

Taicatoxin, isolated from the venom of the Australian taipan snake *Oxyuranus scutellatus*, is a specific blocker of Ca$_L$ channels in heart (Doorty *et al.*, 1997). It is composed of three different molecular entities: (1) an α-neurotoxin-like peptide of molecular weight 8000; (2) a neurotoxic phospholipase of molecular weight 16 000; and (3) a serine protease inhibitor of molecular weight 7000. They are linked by non-covalent bonds, at an approximate stoichiometry of 1:1:4. The block occurs at a site that is accessible extracellularly but not intracellularly. This drug is selective for Ca$_L$ channels, does not affect single-channel conductance, but changes channel gating; it is voltage dependent, with higher affinity for inactivated channels (Possani *et al.*, 1992).

L-Tetrahydropalmatine (Rotundium) is an alkaloid from *Corydalis turtschaninovii*. Rotundium has a potent antiarrhythmic effect as a class IV antiarrhythmic agent (blocking the $Ca^{2+}$ channel) (Wang *et al.*, 1993). Liriodenine, an aporphine alkaloid isolated from the plant *Fissistigma glaucescens*, decreases the $Ca_L$ currents in rat heart (Chang *et al.*, 1996).

Cadmium ($Cd^{2+}$) (100–500 µM) is used commonly to block $Ca_L$ channels completely (Hobai *et al.*, 1997a). External $Cd^{2+}$ shortens the mean open time of single channels. In contrast, $Cd^{2+}$ applied internally (in inside-out patches) does not affect the mean open time or mean unitary current (Huang *et al.*, 1989). In cultured 17-day-old embryonic chick heart cells, $Na^+$ and $Ca^{2+}$ currents were blocked by 3 mM $Co^{2+}$ (Josephson and Sperelakis, 1990).

EGIS-7229 {5-chlor-4-[*N*-(3,4-dimethoxy-phenyl-ethyl)-amino-propylamino]-3 (2H)-pyridazinone fumarate}, a novel antiarrhythmic agent, blocks $I_K$ in cardiac muscle at low concentrations, but at higher concentrations also inhibits $Ca^{2+}$ and $Na^+$ currents (Pankucsi *et al.*, 1997). NE-10064 (Azimilide) is a new selective blocker of the slowly activating component of the delayed rectifier ($I_{ks}$) (Fermini *et al.*, 1995). NE-10064 also inhibits $I_{Ca}$ in a use-dependent fashion.

Salicylaldoxime [2-(OH)$C_6H_4$CH=NOH] reduces the slow inward $Ca^{2+}$ currents in isolated rat ventricular myocytes (Karhu *et al.*, 1995). $Ba^{2+}$ currents ($I_{Ba}$) through a human wild-type $Ca_L$ channel complex (i.e. $\alpha_{1C}$, $\alpha_2$-$\delta$ and $\beta_{1b}$) are inhibited by 2,3-butanedione monoxime (BDM, DAM), a chemical phosphatase (with an $IC_{50}$ of 16 µM) that dephosphorylates the $Ca_L$ channel. BDM may produce direct channel block (Allen *et al.*, 1998).

Ethanol consumption is often accompanied by an increase in both cardiac and vascular dysfunction, and acetaldehyde is a metabolic product (via alcohol dehydrogenase). Acetaldehyde (30 mM) causes a progressive decline in inward $Ca_L$ current, beginning within 4 min (Morales *et al.*, 1997).

Ethaverine is a derivative of papaverine used in the treatment of peripheral vascular disease and is thought to cause vasodilation by reducing [Ca]$_i$ in VSM cells. Ethaverine (on either side of the channel) causes a reduction in channel opening probability ($EC_{50}$ of 1 µM). In addition, ethaverine causes a reduction in the unitary current amplitude in single channels, indicating reduction in the channel conductance. Because ethaverine is structurally related to verapamil, it may act by binding to the verapamil binding site on $Ca_L$ channels (Wang and Rosenberg, 1991).

### K+ channels

#### General

4-Aminopyridine (4-AP), tetraethylammonium (TEA), and $Ba^{2+}$ ions have been widely used to block $K^+$ channels in a variety of tissues, such as heart, VSM, skeletal muscles, and neurons. Use of such blocking agents helps to clarify the physiologic roles of the various types of $K^+$ channels. In VSM, relatively selective inhibition of voltage-dependent $K^+$ ($K_v$) channels, large-conductance $Ca^{2+}$-activated $K^+$ ($B_{K_{Ca}}$) channels, and inward rectifier $K^+$ ($K_{ir}$) channels can be achieved by extracellular application of 4-AP (0.2–1 mM), TEA (0.2 mM), and low concentration of $Ba^{2+}$ (2 µM) respectively (Nelson and Quayle, 1995; Brayden, 1996).

On the other hand, many peptidyl $K^+$ channel toxins have been purified from venom of scorpions, snakes, sea anemones, honeybees, and spiders since the discovery of noxiustoxin (NxTX) in 1982. In 1985, charybdotoxin (ChTX), which has been most extensively studied, was identified from the scorpion *Leiurus quinquestriatus* var. *hebraeus* (Garcia *et al.*, 1997). Nuclear magnetic resonance techniques elucidated the three-dimensional structure of ChTX, which yields an α-helical region that is linked by disulfide bonds to a three-strand antiparallel β-sheet (Lambert *et al.*, 1990; Bontems *et al.*, 1991, 1992). Three disulfide bridges (linking Cys-7 to Cys-28, Cys-13 to Cys-33, and Cys-17 to Cys-35) would make the peptide have a very rigid structure. These major features are conserved among $K^+$ channel toxins from scorpion venom (Table 11.3). During the last decade, the great advance in molecular biology, combined with electrophysiology, has allowed elucidation of the molecular structures of $K^+$ channels, which consist of diverse channel subunits. The mechanisms by which ChTX inhibits *Shaker* $K^+$ channels (i.e. Kv1 subfamily) have been well examined. ChTX is thought to bind to the sequences joining S5 and S6 segments, i.e. the P (pore forming) region. One face of the β-sheet interacts with the channel, whereas the α-helical region does not make direct contact with it (Garcia *et al.*, 1997; Blumenthal, 1998).

The following factors promote the great diversity of $K^+$ channels. These include (1) many isoforms of channel subunits (α-subunit) are present (including alternatively spliced forms); (2) the general structure of the channels is a tetrameric assembly of such subunits (except for two-pore background $K^+$ channel, which is thought to be composed of two subunits; Kim *et al.*, 1998); and (3) auxiliary subunits (β-subunit), which include the sulfonylurea receptor (SUR) in ATP-sensitive $K^+$ ($K_{ATP}$) channels, greatly modify the function, as well as the kinetics, of the channels. In addition, the heteromeric assembly of these subunits may form the native $K^+$ channels (Garcia *et al.*, 1997; Tseng, 1999). For example, the Kv1.3–Kv1.2 heteromultimeric channel is thought to be present as a delayed rectifier $K^+$ channel in neurons (Garcia *et al.*, 1997), and Kv4.2 and Kv4.3 may form a heteromultimeric channel to yield some transient outward current ($I_{to}$) in rat hearts (Tseng, 1999). Furthermore, in rat neonatal ventricular cells, it has been suggested that a small population of $K_{ATP}$ channels may be constructed with a heteromeric assembly of SUR1 and SUR2 (Yokoshiki et al., 1999). Tissue (as well as species) differences in the distribution of $K^+$ channel subunits also contribute to the diversity of $K^+$ channels, and therefore to distinct responses to $K^+$ channel toxins in various tissues.

In the following section, the major $K^+$ channel toxins are briefly mentioned, with emphasis on the molecular clones which construct individual $K^+$ channels. There are several excellent review papers which cover not only peptidyl toxins

*Table 11.3* Summary of representative K$^+$ channel toxins and their target K$^+$ channel clones

| Group | K$^+$ channel toxin | Origin of venom | Target K$^+$ channel clone |
|---|---|---|---|
| I | ChTX | Scorpion | Kv1.3, Kv1.2, $B_{K_{Ca}}$ |
| | Lq2 | Scorpion | Kir1.1(ROMK1)[a] |
| | NxTX | Scorpion | Kv1.3, Kv1.2 |
| | MgTX | Scorpion | Kv1.3, Kv1.2 |
| | AgTX | Scorpion | Kv1.1, Kv1.3, Kv1.6 |
| | KTX | Scorpion | Kv1.3 |
| | IbTX | Scorpion | $B_{K_{Ca}}$ |
| | LbTX | Scorpion | $B_{K_{Ca}}$ |
| II | DTX | Snake | Kv1.1, Kv1.2, Kv1.6 |
| | AsKC | Sea anemone | Kv1.2 (weak) |
| III | ShK | Sea anemone | Kv1.3 |
| | AsKS | Sea anemone | Kv1.3, Kv1.2 |
| IV | HaTX | Spider | Kv2.1, Kv4.2[b] |
| | HpTX | Spider | Kv4.2[c] |
| | PaTX | Spider | Kv4.2, Kv4.3[d] |
| V | BDS-I | Sea anemone | Kv3.4[e] |
| VI | Apamine | Honeybee | SK1($S_{K_{Ca}}$) |
| | ScTX (LeTX) | Scorpion | $S_{K_{Ca}}$ |
| | PO5 | Scorpion | $S_{K_{Ca}}$ |

Notes

a  Effect of Lq2 on Kv1 subfamily has not been tested well.

b  Effect on Kv4.3 was not examined (Swartz and MacKinnon, 1995).

c  Effect on Kv4.3 and Kv2.1 was not examined (Sanguinetti *et al.*, 1997).

d  No effects on Kv1.1, Kv1.2, Kv1.3, Kv1.4, Kv1.5, Kv3.1, Kv3.2, Kv3.4, human egg-related gene (*HERG*), KvLQT1, Kir2.1(IRK1) and TWIK-related K$^+$ channel (TREK-1) were confirmed. Kv2.1 and Kv2.2 were only slightly inhibited (Diochot *et al.*, 1999).

e  No effects on Kv1.2, Kv1.3, Kv1.4, Kv1.5, Kv2.2, Kv4.2, Kv4.3, and Kir2.1 were confirmed. Kv3.1 and Kv3.2 were only slightly inhibited (Diochot *et al.*, 1998).

ShK, a polypeptide from *Stichodactyla helianthus*; LeTX, leiurotoxin; $B_{K_{Ca}}$, large-conductance Ca$^{2+}$-activated K$^+$ channel; $S_{K_{Ca}}$, small-conductance Ca$^{2+}$-activated K$^+$ channel.

but also non-peptidyl blockers and modulators (e.g. see Garcia *et al.*, 1997; Blumenthal, 1998).

## Delayed rectifier K$^+$ channels

As summarized in Table 11.3, K$^+$ channel toxins can be classified into six groups based on sequence homology (especially of Cys residues) and specificity. The peptidyl K$^+$ channel toxins from scorpion venom have a structure similar to ChTX in terms of the disulfide bonds between Cys residues. Most of them, including ChTX, NxTX, margatoxin (MgTX), and kaliotoxin (KTX), inhibit Kv1.3 and/or Kv1.2 channels (Garcia *et al.*, 1997). Agitoxin (AgTX) is known to be the most potent inhibitor of the Kv1.3 channel, and also inhibits the Kv1.1 and Kv1.6 channels (Garcia *et al.*, 1994, 1997). α-Dendrotoxin (DTX), which was purified from snake venom, possesses amino acid sequences longer than those of the ChTX group. The structural homology was identified in kalicludine (AsKC), a peptide purified from sea anemone (*Anemonia sulcata*) venom (Schweitz *et al.*, 1995). DTX inhibits Kv1.1, Kv1.2, and Kv1.6 channels, whereas AsKC is a weak inhibitor of Kv1.2. Another $K^+$ channel toxin from sea anemone venom, kaliseptine (AsKS), is composed of thirty-six amino acids, which indicates some similarity in length to the ChTX group (Schweitz *et al.*, 1995). AsKS inhibits Kv1.3 and Kv1.2 channels. When these *Shaker* $K^+$ channel subunits (Kv1.1, Kv1.2, Kv1.3, and Kv1.6) are expressed in neurons, they yield delayed rectifier $K^+$ currents.

In contrast, the major component of delayed rectifier $K^+$ currents in smooth muscle cells may be produced through Kv1.5 channels (Adda *et al.*, 1996). A specific toxin against Kv1.5 is not available now, but a relatively low concentration (~50 µM) of 4-AP is a relatively selective inhibitor of the Kv1.5 channel (Wang *et al.*, 1993).

In heart, (non-inactivating) delayed rectifier-type $K^+$ currents are composed of at least three $K^+$ currents: (1) a slowly activating delayed rectifier ($I_{Ks}$); (2) a rapidly activating delayed rectifier ($I_{Kr}$); and (3) an ultra-rapidly activating delayed rectifier ($I_{Kur}$) (Roden and George, 1997). Non-inactivating background $K^+$ current, which was designated as $I_{Kp}$ (Backs and Marban, 1993), may also contribute to delayed rectifier $K^+$ currents. The Kv1.5 channel is thought to form a $I_{Kur}$ channel, which is dominant in atrium compared with ventricle. However, assembly of recently cloned $K^+$ channel subunits (other than *Shaker* $K^+$ channel) would construct the $K^+$ channels responsible for $I_{Ks}$, $I_{Kr}$, and $I_{Kp}$ (Table 11.4). Although there are no specific peptidyl toxins for these $K^+$ channels now, the major action of class III antiarrhythmic drugs (such as E-4031 and D-sotalol) is to inhibit $I_{Kr}$ (Sanguinetti and Jurkiewicz, 1990). The chromanol derivative 293B is currently used as a specific $I_{Ks}$ blocker (Busch *et al.*, 1996).

*Transient outward current*

Among *Shaker* $K^+$ channel subunits, only the Kv1.4 channel produces a $K^+$ current which exhibits fast activation and rapid inactivation, i.e. such as A-type current. In neurons, the Kv1.4 channel is present, but a specific toxin has not been found yet. The Kv3.3 and Kv3.4 channels, *Shaw* (Kv3) subfamily, are A-type channels and are expressed in neurons. Blood-depressing substance-I (BDS-I), purified from venom of sea anemone, inhibits the Kv3.4 channel very specifically (Diochot *et al.*, 1998).

In heart, A-type ($K^+$) channel current is generally called transient outward current ($I_{to}$). $I_{to}$ is divided into two classes: (1) $Ca^{2+}$-insensitive $I_{to}$ ($I_{to1}$) and (2) $Ca^{2+}$-sensitive $I_{to}$ ($I_{to2}$). As the latter is believed actually to be a $Cl^-$ current, for simplicity we will use the term $I_{to}$ to designate the former in this chapter. *Shal* (Kv4) $K^+$ channels (Kv4.1, Kv4.2, and Kv4.3) exhibit $I_{to}$-type $K^+$ currents, and $I_{to}$

*Table 11.4* Proposed molecular clones and inhibitors of voltage-dependent K⁺ channel (S4 superfamily) currents in heart

| K⁺ current | K⁺ channel clone | Blocker | Peptidyl toxin |
|---|---|---|---|
| $I_{Ks}$ | KvLQT1 + minK | Chromanol 293B | |
| $I_{Kr}$ | HERG[a] | E-4031, dofetilide | |
| $I_{Kur}$ | Kv1.5 | Low 4-AP (e.g. 50 μM) | |
| $I_{to}$ (rat, ferret) | Kv4.2, Kv4.3 | High 4-AP (e.g., 3 mM) | HaTX,[b] HpTX,[b] PaTX |
| $I_{to}$ (human, canine) | Kv4.3 | High 4-AP | PaTX |

Notes

a  As in the case of $I_{Ks}$, the $I_{Kr}$ channel (HERG) was also regulated by minK, a regulatory subunit (McDonald *et al.*, 1997).

b  Effects of HaTX and HpTX on Kv4.3 were not tested (Swartz and MacKinnon, 1995; Sanguinetti *et al.*, 1997).

A recent study demonstrated that MiRP-1 (minK-related peptide-1), rather than minK, contributes to $I_{Kr}$; therefore, it is now thought that cardiac $I_{Kr}$ channels consist of HERG and MiRP1 (Abbott *et al.*, 1999).

in heart is thought to be composed of Kv4.3 and Kv4.2 channels. However, the regional and species difference is one of the characteristics of $I_{to}$. For example, $I_{to}$ in the epicardium of ferret and rat ventricle is greater than that in endocardium and is suggested to be composed of both Kv4.2 and Kv4.3 channels. On the other hand, a significant contribution of the Kv1.4 channel is proposed in endocardial $I_{to}$ of ferret (and probably rat) ventricle as well as rabbit atrium (Tseng, 1999; Wang *et al.*, 1999). In human (and probably canine) heart, the Kv4.3 (not Kv4.2) channel plays a major role in $I_{to}$ (Kääb *et al.*, 1998; Wang *et al.*, 1999).

Hanatoxin (HaTX), heteropodatoxin (HpTX), and phrixotoxin (PaTX) are peptidyl toxins purified from spider venom (Table 11.3). They inhibit the Kv4 subfamily (Swartz and MacKinnon, 1995; Diochot *et al.*, 1999), e.g. the Kv4.2 channel can be blocked. Among them, PaTX is a very specific inhibitor of Kv4.2 and Kv4.3 channels, without any effect on other $I_{to}$-type K⁺ channel subunits, i.e. Kv1.4, Kv3.4 (Diochot *et al.*, 1999).

In addition to Kv4.2, HaTX inhibits Kv2.1 channel (called *drk1* as a rat clone) (Swartz and MacKinnon, 1995). In contrast to ChTX, AgTX, and DTX [which bind to the linker between S5 and S6 (pore-region)], the HaTX binding sites are thought to be residues near the outer edges of S3 and S4 (Swartz and MacKinnon, 1997).

## Ca²⁺-activated K⁺ channels

Ca²⁺-activated K⁺ channels are generally divided into three classes: (1) large conductance ($B_{K_{Ca}}$) (200–300 pS), (2) intermediate conductance ($I_{K_{Ca}}$) (20–60 pS), and (3) small conductance ($S_{K_{Ca}}$) (10–15 pS) (Brayden, 1996). The $B_{K_{Ca}}$ (*slo*;

*slowpoke* subfamily) channel is abundant in neurons, skeletal muscles, and smooth muscles (Rudy, 1988; Brayden, 1996), but is not present in heart. ChTX is widely used to inhibit $Bk_{Ca}$ channels, although it also affects Kv1.3 and Kv1.2 channels. Specific inhibitors of $Bk_{Ca}$ channels include iberiotoxin (IbTX) and probably limbatustoxin (LbTX), both of which were purified from scorpion venom (Garcia *et al.*, 1997). IbTX inhibits ChTX binding to bovine aortic smooth muscle non-competitively (Galvez *et al.*, 1990), consistent with it having a distinct binding site (Blumenthal, 1998). The Kv1.3 channel is not inhibited by IbTX. As the presence of auxiliary (β) subunits increases the $Ca^{2+}$ sensitivity of the $K_{Ca}$ channels, stimulation by dehydrosoyasaponin-I (DHS-I), a non-peptidyl activator of $Bk_{Ca}$ channels, was much more pronounced when the β-subunit was present (McManus *et al.*, 1995). The conformational change of the channel due to the β-subunit might endow the DHS-I sensitivity.

Apamin, a honeybee toxin, is often used as a specific inhibitor of $Sk_{Ca}$ channels in neurons, skeletal muscles, and smooth muscles. In fact, the rat $Sk1$ (rSk1) channel (recently cloned from rat brain) was highly sensitive to apamin (Köhler *et al.*, 1996). Both rSk1 and hSk1 (human) are $Ca^{2+}$-activated, voltage-independent $K^+$ channels (similar to the neuronal $Sk_{Ca}$ channel) which contribute to after-hyperpolarization. However, a novel $Sk_{Ca}$ channel clone (hSk4), which was abundant in placenta but not in brain, was blocked by ChTX, whereas it was resistant to apamin (Joiner *et al.*, 1997). Two scorpion toxins, scyllatoxin (ScTX) (which is identical to leiurotoxin; LeTX) and PO5, have binding properties similar to those of apamin and are thought to inhibit $Sk_{Ca}$ channels (Garcia *et al.*, 1997).

The $K_{Ca}$ channel (intermediate) cloned recently from human pancreas was designated as h*I*κ1 (Ishii *et al.*, 1997). It exhibits a unique pharmacologic property, i.e. ChTX inhibited h*I*κ1, but both IbTX and apamin failed to block.

### Inward rectifier K⁺ channels

Lq2, purified from scorpion venom, should belong to the toxin group that mainly inhibits *Shaker* K⁺ channels (Table 11.3), although the effect of Lq2 on these channels is not well tested (Garcia *et al.*, 1997). However, an inward rectifier K⁺ ($K_{ir}$) channel subunit, ROMK1 (Kir1.1), which is expressed in kidney and neurons, was inhibited by Lq2 (Lu and MacKinnon, 1997).

The ATP-sensitive K⁺ ($K_{ATP}$) channel is composed of a Kir channel subunit (Kir6.2 or Kir6.1) and a sulfonylurea receptor (SUR) subunit (Yokoshiki *et al.*, 1998). No specific peptidyl toxin against the $K_{ATP}$ channel has been identified yet. However, sulfonylurea compounds, such as glibenclamide and tolbutamide, specifically inhibit $K_{ATP}$ channels when used at low concentration (e.g. less than 1 μM glibenclamide). Nucleotide-binding folds (NBFs) in the SUR subunit probably play an essential role for such inhibition (Ueda *et al.*, 1999). Similarly, stimulation of $K_{ATP}$ channels by K⁺ channel-opening drugs (KCOs) (e.g. diazoxide) also requires NBFs in the SUR subunit. PNU-99963 is a structural analog of P1075, which is one of the KCO drugs. However, PNU99963 is a strong inhibitor of $K_{ATP}$

channels in VSM because it inhibited vascular relaxation produced by several KCOs (pinacidil, cromakalim, and minoxidil) (Khan *et al.*, 1997). Thus, a common mechanism may be involved in inhibition by sulfonylurea compounds and stimulation by KCOs.

Truncation of Kir6.2 in either the last twenty-six or thirty-six amino acids of the COOH terminus (Kir6.2ΔC26, Kir6.2ΔC36) allowed the $K_{ATP}$ channel to exhibit activity in the absence of the SUR subunit (Tucker *et al.*, 1997). Phentolamine (which contains an imidazoline moiety) inhibited Kir6.2ΔC26, a functioning $K_{ATP}$ channel (without the SUR subunit) (Proks and Ashcroft, 1997). Therefore, phentolamine may directly act on the Kir6.2 subunit, but not on the SUR subunit, to inhibit the $K_{ATP}$ channel.

### Hyperpolarization-activated channels

The hyperpolarization-activated channels ($I_h$ or $I_f$), which generate an inward depolarizing current (primarily Na+ influx), are present in certain pacemaker cells, including cardiac nodal (SA) cells and Purkinje fibers. It is thought these $I_h$ channels are more important to pacemaker activity in Purkinje fibers than in SA nodal cells. These channels are blocked by cesium ions (Cs+) (3 mM) and by certain drugs such as alinidine, zatebradine, falipamil (Van Bogaert and Goethals, 1987; Goethals *et al.*, 1993), ZD-7288 (Gasparini and DiFrancesco, 1997), DK-AH-268 (Janigro *et al.*, 1997), and THA (9-amino-1,2,3,4-tetrahydroacridine) (DiFrancesco *et al.*, 1991). Some of these drugs block the $I_h$ channel in a use-dependent manner (e.g. open-channel blocker) (e.g. zatebradine and falipamil), and some block in a voltage-independent manner (e.g. THA). The site of block by zatebradine may be within the middle pore region of the channel (DiFrancesco, 1994).

### Non-selective cation channels

Non-selective cation channels are found in many diverse cell types and are an entry path for $Ca^{2+}$ (Poronnik *et al.*, 1991). Efonidipine, a dihydropyridine derivative which inhibits the $Ca_L$ channels of carotid artery VSM, also blocks voltage-dependent non-selective cation currents in VSM cells (Matsuoka *et al.*, 1997). Diphenylamine-2-carboxylate (DPC), which blocks the inwardly rectifying K+ channel in isolated turtle colon cells, also blocks the non-selective cation channel (Richards and Dawson, 1993). Its analog, 4′-methyl-DPC, is also effective in blocking non-selective cation channels (Poronnik *et al.*, 1992). DPC causes a reduction (~50 percent) in the rate of rise in $[Ca]_i$ following a step increase in $[Ca]_o$ in cells (ST885) which contain large numbers of non-selective cation channels (Poronnik *et al.*, 1991).

Flufenamic acid is a blocker of the $Ca^{2+}$-activated non-selective cation channels (25 pS) (Poronnik *et al.*, 1992). Flufenamic acid and mefenamic acid rapidly produce reversible channel block, with an $IC_{50}$ of 10 μM (Jung *et al.*, 1992).

Flufenamic acid ($10^{-4}$ M) reduced the $NP_o$ (number of channels times the probability of opening) of non-selective cation channels by 35 percent at depolarizing voltages and by 80 percent at hyperpolarizing voltages (in M-1 mouse cortical collecting duct cells) (Korbmacher et al., 1995).

Capsaicin, the main pungent ingredient in "hot" chili peppers, elicits a sensation of burning pain by activating sensory neurons. Capsaicin activates the non-selective cation channel in sensory neurons (Caterina et al., 1997). This allows $Na^+$, $Ca^{2+}$, and $K^+$ ions to flow down their electrochemical gradients and depolarize.

Gadolinium (10 μM) potently blocks the non-selective cation channel in cells of the blood–brain barrier (Popp et al., 1993). The non-selective cation channel isolated from a mouse insulin-secreting beta-cell line is completely blocked by $La^{3+}$ (Suzuki et al., 1998). $La^{3+}$ or $Cd^{2+}$ (1 nM) completely blocks the non-selective cation channel in cultured aortic VSM cells (A7r5) (Nakajima et al., 1995).

### Stretch-activated channels

Mechanosensitive or stretch-activated channels (SACs) respond to membrane stress by changes in open probability. SACs can be divided into channels that are (1) selectively permeable to anions (e.g. $Cl^-$); (2) selectively permeable to cations (e.g. $Na^+$, $K^+$, $Ca^{2+}$); or (3) selectively permeable to $K^+$. All SACs are blocked by gadolinium ($Gd^{3+}$) and $La^{3+}$ ($IC_{50}$ ~10–20 μM). Most of these channels in non-excitable cells are also blocked by amiloride (Nilius, 1998). Aluminofluoride (AF) increases (reversibly) SAC activity in isolated toad gastric smooth muscle cells; the mechanism of AF-induced activation of SACs remains unclear (Hisada et al., 1993).

In heart cells, five distinct types of SACs were demonstrated in cell-attached patches. Four channels have linear conductances of about 25, 50, 100, and 200 pS, and the other type of channel is an inward rectifier of 25 pS (at 0 mV) (with 140 mM $K^+$ in the pipette). The 100-pS and 200-pS channels are $K^+$ selective, whereas the others pass all alkali metal cations and $Ca^{2+}$ ions. All five types are blocked by 20 μM $Gd^{3+}$. Additionally, the 25-pS linear channel is blocked by Grammostola spatulata spider venom (and even by TTX and diltiazem).

There are two kinds of stretch-activated channel openings in guinea pig gastric smooth muscle cells: (1) a short-lasting and small opening (OS) and (2) a long-lasting and large opening (OL), with conductances of 33 and 53 pS respectively. Both OS and OL are blocked by 100 μM $Gd^{3+}$ in the pipette (Yamamoto and Suzuki, 1996).

Ionic mechanisms underlying the enhancement of cardiac pacemaking activity by mechanical stretch is unknown. A stretch causes a shortening of spontaneous cycle length in rabbit isolated sinoatrial (SA) node. As the positive chronotropic response to mechanical stretch is reduced by 4,4'-dinitrostilbene-2,2'-disulfonic acid (DNDS), 4-acetamido-4'-isothiocyanatostilbene-2,2'-disulfonic acid (SITS), or 4,4'-dinitrostilbene-2,2'-disulfonic acid (DIDS), stretch-activated $Cl^-$ channels may be involved in the stretch-induced enhancement of pacemaking activity in

SA node (Hagiwara *et al.*, 1992; Arai *et al.*, 1996). Transient diastolic stretch of the left ventricle elicits arrhythmias, which are inhibited by $Gd^{3+}$. Thus, SACs are involved in stretch-induced arrhythmias. This mechanism of arrhythmogenesis may be particularly important in patients with dilated left ventricles (Hansen *et al.*, 1991; Stacy *et al.*, 1992).

Since a stretch causes a large increase in $[Ca^{2+}]_i$ in isolated ventricular cells because of activation of SACs, it could contribute to cardiac contracture and perhaps to stretch-induced hypertrophy (Ruknudin *et al.*, 1993; Hu and Sachs, 1996; Tatsukawa *et al.*, 1997). The aminoglycoside antibiotic streptomycin (40 µM) prevents the increase in $[Ca]_i$ induced by stretch (Gannier *et al.*, 1994).

SACs are involved in regulation of cardiac cell volume. The cell swelling induced by hypo-osmotic stress is reduced by $Gd^{3+}$ in isolated rabbit ventricular myocytes. Omitting bath $Ca^{2+}$ does not alter cell volume under hypo-osmotic conditions, suggesting stretch-activated $Ca^{2+}$ influx is not important in regulating cell volume (Suleymanian *et al.*, 1995).

SAC cation channels exist in VSM cells, and their opening causes $Na^+$ and $Ca^{2+}$ influx and membrane depolarization. In cell-attached recording, suction applied to the recording pipette to produce membrane stretch evokes single SAC currents (conductance of 32 pS), which are blocked by $Gd^{3+}$ (Ohya *et al.*, 1998). In addition, a stretch causes increase in $Ca^{2+}$ influx, which is mediated by a pathway sensitive to $Gd^{3+}$ (and verapamil). The stretch-induced increase in $Ca^{2+}$ influx may play a role in regulating vascular tone (Bialecki *et al.*, 1992). $Gd^{3+}$-sensitive SACs are the mechanoelectrical transducers in baroreceptors (in carotid artery and aortic arch) (Sullivan *et al.*, 1997).

There are non-selective cation SACs and $K^+$-selective SACs in rat aortic endothelial cells. The non-selective channel shows a permeability ratio for $Na^+$, $K^+$, and $Ca^{2+}$ of 1:0.95:0.23 and is completely blocked by 50 µM $Gd^{3+}$. The $K^+$-selective channel is selectively permeable to $K^+$, with a $K^+/Na^+$ permeability ratio of 10.9:1. As the channels are capable of acting as mechanosensors in endothelial cells, alterations of channel properties could contribute to hypertension (Hoyer *et al.*, 1997).

## Cl⁻ channels

### Types of Cl⁻ channels in cardiovascular tissues

In heart, although Cl⁻ ions are almost passively distributed in accordance with the resting membrane potential, transient net movement of Cl⁻ ions across the membrane does influence $E_m$; for example, washout of Cl⁻ produces a transient depolarization, and reintroduction of Cl⁻ produces a hyperpolarization (Sperelakis, 1995). Because activation of the Cl⁻ current can cause shortening of the action potential (AP) duration, the cardiac Cl⁻ channel has physiologic significance in regulating AP duration (Harvey *et al.*, 1990). The expression of cAMP-activated Cl⁻ channels $[I_{Cl(cAMP)}]$, which are known to be an isoform of the cystic fibrosis transmembrane conductance regulator (CFTR), was found in guinea pig ventricular myocytes (Bahinski *et al.*, 1989; Harvey and Hume, 1989). In addition, at least five different Cl⁻ channels have been reported in heart (Ackerman and Clapham, 1993), including swelling-activated Cl⁻ [$I_{Cl(vol)}$] channels (Sorota, 1992; Tseng, 1992; Zhang *et al.*, 1993), Ca²⁺-activated Cl⁻ channels [$I_{Cl(Ca)}$] (Zygmunt and Gibbons, 1991; Collier *et al.*, 1996), PKC-activated Cl⁻ channels (Walsh and Long, 1994; Collier and Hume, 1995), and ATP-activated Cl⁻ channels (Matsuura and Ehara, 1992; Kaneda *et al.*, 1994; Levesque and Hume, 1995). The pharmacologic properties of these channels are somewhat distinct. For example, $I_{Cl(cAMP)}$ is sensitive to anthracene-9-carboxylic acid (9-AC) and acrylaminobenzoates [e.g. diphenylamine-2-carboxilic acid (DPC) and 5-nitro-2-(3-phenylpropylamino)-benzoic acid (NPPB)], but not to stilbene derivatives (e.g. SITS and DIDS) (Harvey *et al.*, 1990; Harvey, 1993; Vandenberg *et al.*, 1994; Walsh and Wang, 1996). On the other hand, $I_{Cl(vol)}$ and $I_{Cl(Ca)}$ are inhibited by DIDS (Sorota, 1994; Vandenberg *et al.*, 1994).

In VSM cells, [Cl]$_i$ is much higher (~30 mM) than the value of 12.5 mM predicted from passive distribution. The elevated [Cl]$_i$ in VSM cells could be due to an exchanger carrier or to a co-transporter (Sperelakis, 1998c). At least four distinct pathways contribute to Cl⁻ homeostasis in VSM cells: (1) Na⁺/K⁺/Cl⁻ co-transport; (2) Na⁺-dependent Cl⁻/HCO$_3$⁻ exchanger; (3) Na⁺-independent Cl⁻/HCO$_3$⁻ exchanger; and (4) conductive Cl⁻ channels (White *et al.*, 1995). The presence of Ca²⁺-dependent and Ca²⁺-independent Cl⁻ channels have been reported. $I_{Cl(Ca)}$ channels are activated during agonist stimulation and may produce depolarization (because $E_{Cl}$ is less negative than the resting $E_m$) (Byrne and Large, 1988; Amédée *et al.*, 1990; Droogmans *et al.*, 1991; Klöckner and Isenberg, 1991). Ca²⁺-independent Cl⁻ current was recorded in A7r5 VSM cells, and these channels are voltage dependent (Soejima and Kokubun, 1988). Loop diuretics, such as furosemide and bumetanide, block Cl⁻ influx in VSM cells, suggesting that the co-transporter plays an important role in maintaining basal [Cl]$_i$ (Gerstheimer *et al.*, 1987). DIDS reduces Cl⁻ efflux by approximately 30–60 percent in VSM cells (McMahon and Jones, 1988).

High-conductance anion channels activated by depolarization, volume, and [Ca]$_i$ have been described in endothelial cells (Nilius *et al.*, 1996). Additionally, two types of outwardly rectifying Cl⁻ channels were found in endothelium: volume-activated channels and Ca²⁺-activated channels (Nilius *et al.*, 1997).

## Voltage-dependent Cl⁻ channels

The unitary conductance of the voltage-dependent Cl⁻ channels ranges from 5 to 450 pS. Cl⁻ channels are blocked by various agents, including SITS, DIDS, NPPB, DPC, and 9-AC. In addition, hyperpolarization-activated inwardly rectifying Cl⁻ currents (likely CIC-2) are blocked by DIDS, NPPB, and 9-AC (SITS and niflumic acid are ineffective) (Clark *et al.*, 1998).

## Ca²⁺-activated Cl⁻ channels

Inhibition of $I_{Cl(Ca)}$ in *Xenopus* oocytes by NPPB is voltage dependent (Wu and Hamil, 1993). DIDS, SITS, 3′,5-dichlorodiphenylamine-2-carboxylate (DCDPG), niflumic acid, and flufenamic acid reduce the peak amplitude of Cl⁻ tail currents (neuronal). Furosemide (0.5–1 mM) and 9-AC (0.2–0.3 mM) inhibit $I_{Cl(Ca)}$ in VSM cells (Amédée *et al.*, 1990; Hogg *et al.*, 1994). Picrotoxin inhibits γ-amino butyric acid (GABA)-activated Cl⁻ conductances and also inhibits $I_{Cl(Ca)}$ (caffeine stimulated) in neurons (Akaike and Sadoshima, 1989). Argiotoxin-636, which is isolated from orb web spiders (*Argiope lobata*), inhibits $I_{Cl(Ca)}$ (in cultured DRG neurons) (Scott *et al.*, 1995). Argiotoxin-636 contains an Arg amino acid residue and the guanidino functional group at one end of the toxin may act as a Ca²⁺ ion "look-alike," thus enabling the toxin to interact with Ca²⁺ binding sites and thereby disrupt activation of the Cl⁻ channel by Ca²⁺. The ubiquitous polyamine spermine (at 1 mM) may modulate $I_{Cl(Ca)}$; it accelerates the decay of Cl⁻ tail currents (Scott *et al.*, 1995).

## cAMP-dependent Cl⁻ channels

The stilbene derivatives DNDS, DIDS, and SITS block certain Cl⁻ channels, including epithelial outwardly rectifying Cl⁻ channels, but do not block epithelial CFTR Cl⁻ channels. In cardiac myocytes, high concentrations of DNDS or SITS irreversibly diminish Cl⁻ current elicited by isoproterenol (Iso) (Bahinski *et al.*, 1989). In contrast, there is no effect of DNDS on isoproterenol-elicited Cl⁻ conductance in cardiac myocytes; SITS and DIDS enhance the Iso-stimulation of the β-adrenoceptor (Harvey, 1993). 9-AC (200 µM) greatly reduces Iso-evoked Cl⁻ conductance in cardiac myocytes (Levesque *et al.*, 1993).

Reports of effects of arylaminobenzoates such as NPPB and DPC on CFTR channels are varied. NPPB strongly reduces cardiac PKA-regulated Cl⁻ current, and epithelial CFTR Cl⁻ current in pancreatic cells (Gray *et al.*, 1993). DPC greatly decreases PKA-regulated Cl⁻ current in guinea pig ventricular myocytes (Walsh, 1994), whereas no effect was found on forskolin-induced Cl⁻ (Hwang *et al.*, 1992). Interestingly, sulfonylureas, such as the $K_{ATP}$ channel blockers (glibenclamide and tolbutamide) and $K_{ATP}$ channel openers (diazoxide and minoxidil), inhibit PKA-regulated Cl⁻ current in 3T3 cells expressing CFTR Cl⁻ channels and in guinea pig ventricular myocytes (Sheppard and Welsh, 1992; Holevinsky *et al.*, 1994; Yamazaki and Hume, 1997). Glibenclamide and tolbutamide are open-channel blockers of CFTR Cl⁻ channels in transfected mouse L cells (Vengralik *et al.*, 1994). In cardiac myocytes, PKA-regulated Cl⁻ current is blocked by glibenclamide (Tominaga *et al.*, 1994).

## Swelling-activated Cl⁻ channels

The molecular entity responsible for swelling-activated Cl⁻ current $[I_{Cl(vol)}]$ in cardiac myocytes has been recently identified as CIC-3, and it is also present in colonic smooth muscle cells (Dick *et al.*, 1998). The classic Cl channel blockers, such as DIDS, SITS, 9-AC, *N*-phenylanthranilic acid (NPA), IAA-94, NPA and MK-196, have a low affinity for the $Cl_{vol}$ channel. Substances such as NPPB, flufenamic acid, and niflumic acid block $Cl_{vol}$. Quinine and quinidine, which are known to block K channels, also inhibit $I_{Cl(vol)}$. The phenol derivative gossypol (isolated from the cotton wool extract) also blocks $Cl_{vol}$ of endothelial cells (Szück *et al.*, 1996).

Inhibitors of $PLA_2$ (such as cyclosporine A) also block $I_{Cl(vol)}$ (Nilius *et al.*, 1996). Lipoxygenase/cytochrome P450 blockers (e.g. ketoconazole) block $I_{Cl(vol)}$. The block of $I_{Cl(vol)}$ by extracellularly applied unsaturated fatty acids (arachidonic acid, linoleic acid, linolenic acid) may be due to a direct inhibition, rather than an interference with the proposed activation mechanism. The block of $I_{Cl(vol)}$ by the anti-estrogen tamoxifen (used in the treatment of breast cancer) correlates with its inhibitory effects on the proliferation of endothelial cells (Nilius *et al.*, 1994). Divalent cations [such as zinc ($Zn^{2+}$), $Mg^{2+}$, $Ca^{2+}$, $Ba^{2+}$] and trivalent cations (such as $Gd^{3+}$ and $La^{3+}$) not only reduce the amplitude of $I_{Cl(vol)}$ but also accelerate inactivation of the current. Molecular biologic studies of the $pI_{Cln}$ protein, a putative candidate for the $Cl_{vol}$ channel, demonstrates an extracellular nucleotide-binding site that may interfere with volume-activated Cl⁻ channels. Extracellular nucleotides inhibit $I_{Cl(vol)}$. The reader is referred to several reviews (Hoffmann and Dunham, 1995; Strange and Jackson, 1995; Valverde *et al.*, 1995; Nilius *et al.*, 1996).

### *Neurotransmitter-activated Cl⁻ channels*

There are several compounds that enhance neurotransmitter-activated $I_{Cl}$: senktide, heavy metals [e.g. lead (Pb) and mercury (Hg)], diazepam, and allopregnanolone. Senktide (3 µM), a neurokinin-3 receptor agonist, causes an inward current, which is inhibited by niflumic acid and mefenamic acid (Bertrand and Galligan, 1994). In neurons of *Helix pomatia*, lead actually potentiates the glutamate-evoked Cl⁻ current, and so may be another possible site of action of lead (Salanki *et al.*, 1994). $Hg^{2+}$ causes a dramatic increase (up to 300 percent) in the acetylcholine- and carbachol-induced Cl⁻ current in neurons of *Aplysia* (the effect was only partly reversible). The toxic actions of $Hg^{2+}$ on synaptic transmission at both pre- and post-synaptic sites could be important factors in the mechanism of $Hg^{2+}$ toxicity (Gyori *et al.*, 1994). Benzodiazepine, diazepam, and the steroid derivative allopregnanolone greatly potentiate GABA-induced Cl⁻ currents in oocytes injected with synaptosomes (Sanna *et al.*, 1998).

There are many Cl channel blockers, including insecticides and natural toxins, which mostly target the GABA-gated Cl channels. The insecticide–channel interactions that have been studied most extensively are pyrethroid actions on the voltage-gated $Na^+$ channel and cyclodiene/lindane actions on the $GABA_A$ receptor–

Cl⁻ channel complex. Most insecticides act on the Na⁺ channel and the GABA system. Pyrethroids also act on the voltage-gated Cl⁻ channels. Pyrethroids are divided into two groups: type I, not having a cyano group in the $\alpha$ position, and type II, having such a group. Type II pyrethroids deltamethrin and cypermethrin significantly decrease $Cl_v$ channel activity, whereas the type I pyrethroid cismethrin has only a slight effect. Deltamethrin blocks $I_{Cl(vol)}$ (conductance of 340 pS), whereas $I_{Cl(Ca)}$ (conductance of 225 pS) is not affected. Actions on $I_{Cl(vol)}$ are likely to contribute significantly to type II pyrethroid toxicity (Ray *et al.*, 1997). Cyclodienes and lindane exert a dual action on the $GABA_A$ system, an initial transient stimulation being followed by a suppression. The stimulation requires the presence of the $\gamma_2$-subunit (Narahashi, 1996). Blockage of the GABA-gated Cl channel by cyclodienes attenuates inhibitory synapses, which leads to hyperexcitation of the central nervous system, convulsions, and death. Although actions on the GABA-gated Cl channel can explain most of the effects of these compounds, the involvement of other types of Cl⁻ channels cannot be excluded (Bloomquist, 1993).

A polypeptide isolated from Leiurus venom and designated as chlorotoxin contains thirty-seven amino acid residues cross-linked by four disulfide bonds. Chlorotoxin displays no sequence homology to toxins from the same venom that target Na⁺ or K⁺ channels, but is highly homologous to the scorpion insectotoxins derived from *Buthus eupeus* venom (DeBin *et al.*, 1993). Interestingly, chlorotoxin blocks Cl⁻ conductance (with an affinity in the low $\mu M$ range), only when applied inside. The insectotoxins may also target the insect post-synaptic glutamate receptor. Chlorotoxin contains a small three-stranded $\beta$-sheet packed against a single $\alpha$-helix (Lippens *et al.*, 1995). The folding of the chlorotoxin molecule is similar to that of charybdotoxin, despite the lack of significant sequence homology between these two proteins.

Picrotoxin, which is isolated from the seed of *Anamirta cocculus*, consists of picrotoxinin and picrotin, with a ratio of 1:1. Picrotoxin inhibits the GABA response in lobster cardiac ganglion (Kerrison and Freschi, 1992). Avermectins, a group of broad-spectrum antiparasitic antibiotics, are derivative of pentacyclic sixteen-member lactones related to the milbemycines from *Streptomyces avermilitis*. Avermectin $B_{1a/b}$ (abamectin) activates GABA-gated Cl channels, thereby suppressing neuronal activity, resulting in ataxia, paralysis, and death (Bloomquist, 1993). Maitotoxin (MTX), which is a 3424-Da polyether marine toxin obtained from the marine dinoflagellate *Gambier toxicus*, activates voltage-independent Cl⁻ conductance in GH4C1 cells. This may promote the sequence of ionic events leading to activation of $Ca_L$ channels and massive $Ca^{2+}$ entry (Young *et al.*, 1995). MTX also increases the amplitude of $I_{Cl(Ca)}$ in *Xenopus* oocytes (Martinez *et al.*, 1999).

# Target pumps and exchangers

## *Na/K pump*

### *General*

The intracellular ion concentrations are maintained differently from those in the extracellular fluid by active ion transport mechanisms that expend metabolic energy to push specific ions against their concentration or electrochemical gradients. These ion pumps are located in the cell membrane at the cell surface and probably also in the transverse tubular membrane. The major ion pump is the Na/K-linked pump, which pumps $Na^+$ out of the cell against its electrochemical gradient while simultaneously pumping $K^+$ in against its electrochemical gradient. The coupling of $Na^+$ and $K^+$ pumping is obligatory, for in zero $[K]_0$ the $Na^+$ can no longer be pumped out. The driving mechanism for the Na/K pump is a membrane ATPase, the Na/K-ATPase, which spans across the membrane and requires both $Na^+$ and $K^+$ ions for activation. This enzyme also requires $Mg^{2+}$ for activity. ATP, $Mg^{2+}$, and $Na^+$ are thus required at the inner surface of the membrane, and $K^+$ is required at the outer surface. A phosphorylated intermediate of the Na/K-ATPase occurs in the transport cycle, its phosphorylation being $Na^+$ dependent and its dephosphorylation being $K^+$ dependent (for references, see Sperelakis, 1967). The pump enzyme usually drives three $Na^+$ ions in and two $K^+$ ions out for each ATP molecule hydrolyzed. The rate of Na/K pumping in myocardial cells must change with the heart rate to maintain the intracellular ion concentrations relatively constant. The Na/K-ATPase is specifically inhibited by vanadate ions and by the cardiac glycosides (digitalis drugs) acting on the outer surface. The pump enzyme is also inhibited by sulfhydryl reagents (such as *N*-ethylmaleimide, mercurial diuretics, and ethacrynic acid), thus indicating that the SH groups are crucial for activity.

### *Cardiac glycosides*

The cardiac glycosides increase the maximal force generated and the rate at which the force is developed. The major specific action of the cardiac glycosides is the inhibition of the Na/K-ATPase and Na/K pump of all types of cells, vertebrate and invertebrate. Although there is some degree of variability from tissue to tissue with respect to the dose–response curves, in general 50 percent inhibition of the enzyme occurs at $10^{-7}$ to $10^{-6}$ M ouabain.

The therapeutic effect of digitalis on cardiac contractility is presumably due to partial inhibition of the Na/K pump, thus causing an elevation in $[Na]_i$, which, in turn, produces a steady-state elevation of $[Ca]_i$ because of the Na/Ca exchange system. The elevation in $[Ca]_i$ may allow the SR to load more with $Ca^{2+}$ for a greater release in subsequent beats. That is, there may be a shift in $Ca^{2+}$ balance so that more $Ca^{2+}$ is retained by the myocardial cells (Schwartz *et al.*, 1975). The toxic effect of the cardiac glycosides is presumably the result of a greater degree of inhibition of the Na/K pump that causes the ionic gradients to run down too far and cause $Ca^{2+}$ overload. An ouabain-like steroid is used as a part of venom in some animals, e.g. bufagenin and bufatalin in toads.

Release of catecholamines from nerve terminals, another effect of the cardiac glycosides (which may be mediated by inhibition of the Na/K pump and elevation of $[Ca]_i$), could contribute to their overall cardiotoxicity and arrhythmogenesis.

### Vanadate and amiodarone

The vanadate ion ($VO_4^{3-}$), a known inhibitor of the Na/K-ATPase (see Table 11.5), exerts a positive inotropic effect in ventricular (papillary) muscle (Borchard *et al.*, 1979). In cultured chick heart (ventricular) cells, vanadate (0.5 mM) produced repetitive firing of spikes on a lengthened plateau (P. Jourdon and N. Sperelakis, unpublished observations).

Amiodarone has been shown to affect cell membrane physicochemical properties. Amiodarone has no effect on the voltage dependence of the pump or on the affinity of the pump for extracellular $K^+$ (Gray *et al.*, 1998). Exposure of cardiomyocytes to amiodarone reduces the apparent $Na^+$ affinity of the Na/K pump. An amiodarone-induced inhibition of the hyperpolarizing Na/K pump current may contribute to the action potential prolongation.

### Doxorubicin, maitotoxin, and VX

Doxorubicin (Adriamycin) is a highly effective cancer chemotherapeutic drug, but its clinical utility is limited by its cardiotoxicity. Doxorubicin is a potent inhibitor of ion pumps. Doxorubicinol, the major metabolite of doxorubicin, is up to ten times more potent than doxorubicin itself at inhibiting isometric contraction of the rabbit papillary muscle. Doxorubicinol, but not doxorubicin, also increases

*Table 11.5* Summary of some toxins that inhibit the Na/K-ATPase/pump of SL

| Name | Action | $IC_{50}$ concentration | Reference |
|---|---|---|---|
| Ouabain | Inhibition | ~20 μM | Evangeline *et al.* (1993) |
| $Na_3VO_4$ | Inhibition | 0.5–0.75 μM | Borchard *et al.* (1979) |
| Amiodarone | Inhibition | nr | Gray *et al.* (1998) |
| Doxorubicinol | Inhibition | < 10 μM | Boucek *et al.* (1987) |
| Maitotoxin | Inhibition | nr | Legrand *et al.* (1982) |
| VX | Inhibition (isoforms α1 and α2) | 100 μM (75% inhibition[a]) | Robineau *et al.* (1991) |

Notes
a The value is measured when both isoforms are inhibited.
nr, not reported.

resting tension of isolated cardiac muscle, indicative of incomplete relaxation between contractions. Doxorubicinol is a potent inhibitor of the Na/K-ATPase of cardiac sarcolemma. Doxorubicinol also is a potent inhibitor of $Ca^{2+}$-ATPase activity of SR (from canine heart and rabbit skeletal muscle). Thus, doxorubicinol is a potent inhibitor of several key cationic pumps that directly or indirectly regulate intracellular $Ca^{2+}$, $Na^+$, and $K^+$ ion concentrations. These observations are important to understanding the cardiotoxicity produced by doxorubicin (Boucek *et al.*, 1987).

One mechanism for the positive inotropic effect of maitotoxin may involve inhibition of the Na/K-ATPase (Bengmann and Nechay, 1982), which would lead to an enhanced $[Ca]_i$ (via the Na/Ca exchange mechanism). In the whole animal, maitotoxin produces arrhythmias and tachycardias leading to fibrillation and cardiac arrest (Legrand *et al.*, 1982), perhaps like the cardiac glycosides, producing release of catecholamines.

Organophosphorous cholinesterase inhibitor (serine specific) compounds such as VX provoke digitalis-like ventricular arrhythmias. VX inhibits the two cardiac Na/K-ATPase isoforms ($\alpha 1$ and $\alpha 2$). Digitalis selectively inhibits the $\alpha 1$ isoform (Robineau *et al.*, 1991).

### *Ca pumps*

#### *General*

The myocardial cell membrane exerts tight control over the contractile machinery by regulating the amount of $Ca^{2+}$ influx during the cardiac action potential. The $Ca^{2+}$ entering across the cell membrane brings about the further release of $Ca^{2+}$ from the internal $Ca^{2+}$ stores within the SR, thereby elevating $[Ca]_i$ to the level necessary to activate the myofilaments. The steps in this overall control process compose excitation–contraction coupling (or electromechanical coupling). Relaxation of the heart is produced by lowering $[Ca]_i$ as a result of resequestration of $Ca^{2+}$ by the SR Ca-ATPase/pump and by extrusion of $Ca^{2+}$ across the cell membrane (by Na/Ca exchanger and by a sarcolemmal Ca-ATPase/pump).

The SR membrane contains a $Ca^{2+}$-ATPase that actively pumps two $Ca^{2+}$ ions from the myoplasm into the SR lumen at the expense of one ATP. This pump ATPase is capable of pumping down the $[Ca]_i$ to less than $10^{-7}$ M. The Ca-ATPase is regulated by an associated low molecular weight protein, phospholamban. (Phospholamban is not associated with the sarcolemmal Ca-ATPase.) Phospholamban is phosphorylated by cyclic AMP-dependent protein kinase (PKA) and, when phosphorylated, stimulates the Ca-ATPase and $Ca^{2+}$ pumping by a process of disinhibition. The sequestration of $Ca^{2+}$ by the SR is essential for muscle relaxation. (The mitochondria also actively take up $Ca^{2+}$ almost to the same degree as the SR, but this $Ca^{2+}$ pool probably does not play an important role in normal excitation–contraction coupling.)

The sympathetic neurotransmitter (norepinephrine) activates the $\beta$-adrenergic receptor and stimulates the A-cyclase (via G coupling protein) to elevate cAMP and activate PKA. The β-agonists are positive inotropic by several mechanisms, including phosphorylation of phospholamban (and derepression of the SR Ca pump) and phosphorylation of the $Ca_L$ channels (which stimulates their activity and hence $Ca^{2+}$ influx). Methylxanthines, such as caffeine and theophylline, are positive inotropic by inhibiting the phosphodiesterase (PDE) that destroys cAMP. Toxic concentrations of caffeine activate the $Ca^{2+}$-release channels of the SR and cause a sustained, large elevation of $[Ca]_i$ and resultant contracture. Quinidine toxicity may depress contraction of cardiac muscle by inhibiting the Ca-ATPase of the SR (Fuchs *et al.*, 1968) (see Table 11.6).

Elevation of $[Ca]_i$ allows the SR to load more with $Ca^{2+}$ for a greater release in subsequent beats, i.e. there may be a shift in $Ca^{2+}$ balance so that more $Ca^{2+}$ is retained within the myocardial cells. Thus, the therapeutic action of digitalis is to make more $Ca^{2+}$ available to the myofilaments (Schwartz *et al.*, 1975). However, a greater $Ca^{2+}$ overload produces a number of deleterious functional and morphologic changes. The rundown of the $Na^+$ and $K^+$ gradients leads to partial depolarization and all of its repercussions. In addition, overloading the SR with $Ca^{2+}$ causes uncontrolled, spontaneous $Ca^{2+}$ release, resulting in delayed after-depolarizations (DADs) and triggered arrhythmias. The cardiac glycosides also could have an internal site of action that may contribute to their therapeutic or toxic actions on the heart. For example, the SR was shown histochemically to have some ouabain-sensitive ATPase activity (Forbes and Sperelakis, 1972), and the glycosides are known to be able to penetrate intracellularly.

## Volvatoxin A

Volvatoxin A, a cardiotoxic protein from a species of mushroom (*Volvariella volvacea*), causes cardiac arrest in systole. The toxin is composed of two subunits

*Table 11.6* Summary of some toxins that inhibit the Ca-ATPase/pump in SR or SL

| Name | Action | $IC_{50}$ concentration | Reference |
|------|--------|------------------------|-----------|
| Quinidine | Inhibition (SR) | 10–100 μM | Fuchs *et al.* (1968) |
| Cobra cardiotoxin | Inhibition (SR) | 10–50 μg ml$^{-1}$ | Nayler *et al.* (1976) |
| Thapsigargin | Inhibition (SR) | 10–100 μM | Thastrup (1990) |
| CPA | Inhibition (SR) | 10 μM (98% inhibition) | Agata *et al.* (1993) |
| Carboxyeosin and eosin | Inhibition (SL) | 1 μM | Bassani *et al.* (1995); Gatto *et al.* (1995) |
| Doxorubicinol | Inhibition (SR) | < 9 μM | Boucek *et al.* (1987) |
| Volvatoxin-A | Makes the SR membrane leaky | 10–50 μg ml$^{-1}$ | Fassold *et al.* (1976) |
| LPC | $Ca^{2+}$ release from SR | 2.5–10 μM | Yu *et al.* (1998) |

Note
LPC, lysophosphatidylcholine; eosin, tetrabromofluorescein; CPA, cyclopiazonic acid.

(in a ratio of 1:3), one with a molecular weight of 50 000 and one of 24 000, and their amino acid compositions have been determined (Lin *et al.*, 1973). The mechanism of action of this toxin is to make the SR membrane leaky to $Ca^{2+}$ ions so that the SR cannot adequately sequester the myoplasmic $Ca^{2+}$ (Table 11.6) (Fassold *et al.*, 1976). The Ca-ATPase of the SR (or the sarcolemmal Na/K-ATPase activity) was not inhibited. The toxin also alters the ultrastructure of the mitochondria and inhibits their ability to accumulate $Ca^{2+}$. These findings can explain why the toxin increases the diastolic resting tension of cardiac muscle because of the predicted rise in $[Ca]_i$, causing Ca overload. The metabolic impairment of the mitochondria would contribute to the $Ca^{2+}$ overload.

### Cobra venom cardiotoxin

Two toxins isolated from the venom of the Indian cobra (*Naja nigricollis*) are polypeptides; one is a neurotoxin and the other is a cardiotoxin (Tazieff-Depierre *et al.*, 1969; Lee, 1972). The cardiotoxin has a molecular weight of about 6500 (60–62 amino acids) and causes systolic arrest. The cobra cardiotoxin depresses $Ca^{2+}$ accumulation by cardiac SR (Table 11.6) (Nayler *et al.*, 1976). This effect is due to inhibition of the Ca-ATPase and to release of sequestered $Ca^{2+}$, i.e. the SR membrane becomes more leaky. Thereby, the toxin causes an elevated $[Ca]_i$ and all the consequences of $Ca^{2+}$ overload (Nayler *et al.*, 1976). The toxin also depresses $Ca^{2+}$ accumulation by isolated mitochondria and causes ultrastructural damage, including disruption of the cell membrane, vacuolated mitochondria, disrupted myofibrils, and contracture bands. Thus, the mode of action of the cobra cardiotoxin is quite different from volvatoxin-A, although both toxins have an effect on the SR (Nayler *et al.*, 1976).

### Lysophosphatidylcholine, thapsigargin, cyclopiazonic acid, and eosin

Lysophosphatidylcholine (LPC) increases $[Ca]_i$ in the heart; however, the mechanism responsible for this increase is not clear. The increase in $[Ca]_i$ induced by LPC depends both on increased $Ca^{2+}$ influx from the extracellular space via the $Ca_L$ channels and on $Ca^{2+}$ release from the SR stores. LPC may also affect the Na/Ca exchanger (see below) (Yu *et al.*, 1998).

Thapsigargin is a chemical compound isolated from *Thapsia garganica* that has a molecular weight of 650 (Patkar *et al.*, 1979). Thapsigargin inhibits the Ca-ATPase/pump of the SR, thereby depressing contraction (Thastrup, 1990). Cyclopiazonic acid (CPA), a mycotoxin from *Aspergillus* and *Penicillium*, has been described as a highly selective inhibitor of $Ca^{2+}$-ATPase in the SR in skeletal and smooth muscles. Thus, CPA exerts negative inotropic effects on adult myocardium (minimum effects on neonatal), probably through inhibition of SR function (Agata *et al.*, 1993).

Eosin (tetrabromofluorescein) and carboxyeosin are potent inhibitors of the cardiac sarcolemmal Ca pump. In contrast, eosin does not inhibit the cardiac Na/ Ca exchanger (see below). Thus, eosin can effectively eliminate the Ca pump-mediated transport of $Ca^{2+}$ ions, leaving intact the Na/Ca exchange mechanism. Hence, eosin can be used to determine the roles played by the two pathways in Ca homeostasis (Bassani *et al.*, 1995; Gatto *et al.*, 1995).

## Na/Ca exchanger

### General

The Na/Ca exchanger exchanges one internal $Ca^{2+}$ ion for three external $Na^+$ ions via a membrane carrier molecule; therefore, it is an electrogenic exchange, producing a net current. Thus, the exchanger contributes to the resting membrane potential ($E_m$) and its reversal potential ($E_{Na/Ca}$) changes during the cardiac action potential (AP). As the $E_m$ is more negative than the $E_{Na/Ca}$ during the period of rest between action potentials, this indicates that the exchanger will mediate $Ca^{2+}$ efflux during these periods (i.e. the forward mode). At the beginning of the AP, however, there is a brief period during which the AP is more positive than $E_{Na/Ca}$. During this period, the exchanger theoretically mediates Ca influx (i.e. reverse mode), which would contribute to the activation of cardiac contraction.

The Na/Ca exchanger protein contains a large cytoplasmic region (calmodulin-binding site), which acts as an autoinhibitory domain. The peptide, named XIP, corresponding to the amino acid sequence of this inhibitory domain, inhibits the Na/Ca exchanger (Xu *et al.*, 1997). However, XIP also inhibits the $Ca^{2+}$-ATPases in both SR and SL. Because the C-terminal Arg–Phe–$CONH_2$ is found to be critical for pharmacologic inhibition, a number of positively charged hexapeptides (two Arg, two Phe, and two Cys) are produced. One of these potent inhibitory peptides is FRCRCFa, which inhibits the exchanger of intact cardiac cells (only when applied intracellularly) (Hobai *et al.*, 1997b) (see Table 11.7).

Taurine has recently been shown to protect against ischemia and heart failure. Taurine has non-specific actions on various ion channels and exchanger systems. Taurine was reported to stimulate indirectly the inward Na/Ca exchanger current (forward mode) in atrial cells (rabbit) via release of $Ca^{2+}$ from the SR (Earm *et al.*, 1993). There is no direct effect on the Na/Ca exchanger of rat ventricular cells (Sperelakis *et al.*, 1996). Taurine may directly and indirectly help to regulate the $[Ca]_i$ level by several mechanisms, including modulation of the activity of the $Ca_L$ channels, regulation of the activity of the $Na^+$ channels (Satoh and Sperelakis, 1998), and by bidirectional $Na^+$/taurine co-transport (Chapman *et al.*, 1993), i.e. when $[Na]_i$ becomes elevated during ischemia, the Na/taurate efflux lowers $[Na]_i$ at the expense of loss of the normally high intracellular taurine concentration (e.g. 10 mM). Thus, taurine serves to protect heart cells against ischemia, and under various pathologic conditions the taurine level of the heart is markedly lowered.

Heavy metal ions such as $Ni^{2+}$, $Mn^{2+}$, and $Cd^{2+}$ are known to inhibit the Na/Ca

*Table 11.7* Summary of some toxins that inhibit the Na/Ca exchange of SL

| Name | Action | $IC_{50}$ concentration | Reference |
|---|---|---|---|
| XIP | Inhibition | 1.7–17 µM | Xu *et al.* (1997) |
| $Cd^{2+}$ | Inhibition | 320 µM ($K_d$) | Hobai (1996) |
| KB-R7943 | Inhibition | 17 µM | Watano and Kimura (1998); Nakamura *et al.* (1998) |
| FRCRCFa | Inhibition | 0.01–1 µM[a] | Hobai *et al.* (1997b) |

Note
a  The concentration of FRCRCFa in the pipette.

exchanger current, but they also inhibit $Ca_L$ channels and K channels (Kimura *et al.*, 1987; Hobai *et al.*, 1997a). Amiloride derivatives, which inhibit the Na/H exchanger (and Na⁺ channels) with a high affinity, also inhibit the Na/Ca exchanger.

### Sea anemone toxins

A series of neurotoxins was isolated from the sea anemone (*Anemonia sulcata*). One of these toxins (ATX-II) has been purified and sequenced. ATX-II is a small polypeptide containing forty-seven amino acids (molecular weight of about 50 000) and is cross-linked by three disulfide bridges; the molecule is positively charged (at pH 7.4). It has potent effects on many excitable membranes, including those of nerve and cardiac muscle.

In cultured embryonic chick hearts, ATX-II greatly increases both $Ca^{2+}$ uptake and Na⁺ uptake. The effects of ATX-II are synergistic with those of veratridine, subthreshold doses of both agents causing pronounced effects. The positive inotropic effect of ATX-II may be due to a pronounced slowing of Na⁺ channel inactivation (see Na⁺ channel section), thereby causing an increased $[Na]_i$ (and thereby $[Ca]_i$ via the Na/Ca exchanger system). Slowing of Na⁺ channel inactivation is produced by inhibition of the kinetic movement of the inactivation gate (I-gate) of the channel. Likewise, other compounds [aconitine, GTX-I (grayanotoxin) and BTX (batrachotoxin)], which greatly increase Na⁺ influx by the same mechanism (i.e. slowing of Na⁺ channel inactivation), also have a positive inotropic effect on heart muscle.

### Other toxins

Toxicosis by monensin, a Na⁺-selective ionophore, induces skeletal muscle and cardiac muscle necrosis. A monensin-induced Na⁺ influx causes $Ca^{2+}$ overload in the cytoplasm of cells (even non-excitable cells), probably via the Na/Ca exchanger system (Shier and DuBourdieu, 1992). The monensin-induced $Ca^{2+}$ overload can be prevented when $pH_0$ is acidified, suggesting that the Na/H exchanger is also involved.

KB-R7943 {2-[2-[4-(4-nitrobenzyloxy)phenyl]ethyl]isothiourea methane-sulfonate} inhibits the Na/Ca exchanger more potently than the Na/H exchanger (or the Na/K-ATPase and $Ca^{2+}$-ATPase). Since KB-R7943 has a protective effect against myocardial ischemia/reperfusion injury, stimulation of the Na/Ca exchanger normally must occur immediately after reperfusion begins (Nakamura *et al.*, 1998; Watano and Kimura, 1998). Without the KB-R7943 drug, the intracellular acidosis ($H^+$ overload) produced during ischemia would lead to a marked $H^+$ efflux via the Na/H exchanger and therefore $Na^+$ influx, which, in turn, would cause the Na/Ca exchanger to go into reverse mode operation (i.e. $Ca^{2+}$ influx and $Na^+$ efflux).

## Na/H exchanger

### General

The Na/H exchanger is an important regulator for intracellular pH, cell volume, and transepithelial $Na^+$ transport. It exists in virtually all cells, and it is regulated by a variety of extracellular stimuli, including growth factors, hormones, and mechanical stimuli (e.g. osmotic stress). Five different isoforms of the Na/H exchanger are known. These isoforms differ in tissue localization, sensitivity to inhibitors, and mode of transcriptional and post-transcriptional regulation. This allows the various isoforms to participate in different physiologic processes.

Ischemia results in the accumulation of lactate and other proton donors, thereby causing intracellular (and extracellular) acidification. During reperfusion, when suddenly the extracellular $H^+$ ion concentration is lowered, the Na/H exchanger extrudes protons with concomitant influx of $Na^+$ (elevating $[Na]_i$). The rise in $[Na]_i$ changes the operation of the Na/Ca exchanger to reverse mode ($Ca^{2+}$ influx), resulting in a rise in $[Ca]_i$. Thus, the Na/H exchanger is an important part of a cascade leading from intracellular acidosis to accumulation of $[Na]_i$, followed by $Ca^{2+}$ overload. Therefore, although Na/H exchange represents an important mechanism for pH regulation in the cardiac cell, it may paradoxically mediate tissue damage in the reperfused myocardium. A blockade of this exchanger has been hypothesized to cause stronger intracellular acidification in the course of ischemia, thereby tending to exaggerate ischemic damage. However, acidosis inhibits the $Ca_L$ channels (very quickly and reversibly) (Vogel and Sperelakis, 1977; Irisawa and Sato, 1986), which would diminish $Ca^{2+}$ influx and protect against $Ca^{2+}$ overload.

### Amiloride

Na/H exchange plays an important role not only during reperfusion but also during ischemia and development of post-ischemic cardiac dysfunction. This exchanger induces primary $Na^+$ overload and secondary $Ca^{2+}$ overload. The Na/H exchanger in heart is inhibited by several amiloride analogues: 5-($N$-ethyl-$N$-isopropyl)-amiloride (EIPA), 5-($N,N$-dimethyl)amiloride (DMA), and methylisobutyl amiloride (MIA). When amiloride is administered prior to ischemia, infarct size of the rabbit heart is reduced (Bugge *et al.*, 1996). Therefore, as discussed in the previous section, Na/H exchange inhibitors, like amiloride derivatives, would have a cardioprotective profile in cardiac surgery, especially if added before ischemia is initiated (Myers *et al.*, 1995; Koike *et al.*, 1996; Tani *et al.*, 1996; Docherty *et al.*, 1997).

It is well known that ischemic preconditioning and pH preconditioning (i.e. acidosis) produces cardioprotective effects against cardiac damage by ischemia. The pH preconditioning may involve the inhibition of $Ca_L$ channels, and thereby $Ca^{2+}$ influx and resultant Ca overload, by the residual intracellular acidosis (Vogel and Sperelakis, 1977; Irisawa and Sato, 1986). Amiloride administered during ischemic preconditioning attenuates the cardioprotective effect of ischemic preconditioning. Therefore, the mechanism by which an ischemic preconditioning produces cardioprotection may involve stimulation of the Na/H exchanger (Kaur *et al.*, 1997).

### Cariporide (HOE-642) and HOE-694

The inhibitors of the Na/H exchange system HOE-694 (3-methylsulfonyl-4-piperidinobenzoyl, guanidine hydrochloride) and HOE-642 possess cardioprotective effects in ischemia/reperfusion. Cariporide (4-isopropyl-3-methyl-sulfonylbenzoyl-guanidine methanesulfonate; HOE-642) is a novel Na/H exchanger subtype 1 inhibitor. It has antiarrhythmic effects on ischemia/reperfusion arrhythmias (Aye *et al.*, 1997), but only has a weak suppressing effect on ouabain-induced arrhythmias (Xue *et al.*, 1996). The Na/H exchanger inhibitor may confer protection against arrhythmias during surgery (Mathur and Karmazyn, 1997). HOE-642 also markedly attenuates apoptosis in heart disease (Chakrabarti *et al.*, 1997).

The addition of HOE-694 to cardioplegic solution attenuates the increase of intracellular $Na^+$ during the surgical period (Loh *et al.*, 1996; Choy *et al.*, 1997). Inhibition of the Na/H antiporter with HOE-694 is antiarrhythmic and diminishes myocardial ischemic cell injury by preventing $Na^+$ overload during reperfusion (Sack *et al.*, 1994) (see Table 11.8).

### Palytoxin (PTX)

Palytoxin (PTX) has potent cardiotoxic properties. In embryonic chick ventricular cells under normal ionic conditions, palytoxin produces an intracellular acidification, which is only partially compensated for by the Na/H antiporter. Therefore, this causes an increased rate of $Na^+$ uptake via the Na/H antiporter (ethylisopropylamiloride sensitive). It was proposed that palytoxin acidifies cardiac cells by opening pre-existing $H^+$-conducting pathways in the plasma membrane

*Table 11.8* Summary of some toxins that inhibit the Na/H exchanger of SL

| Name | Action | $IC_{50}$ concentration | Reference |
|---|---|---|---|
| HOE 642(Cariporide) | Inhibition | 1–10 µM | Aye *et al.* (1997) |
| HOE 694 | Inhibition | 1 µM | Choy *et al.* (1997) |
| Amiloride | Inhibition | ~300 µM | Periyasamy (1992) |
| Amiloride analogs | | | |
| HMA | Inhibition | ~30 µM (100% inhibition) | Periyasamy (1992) |
| DMA | Inhibition | 10 µM | Koike *et al.* (1996) |
| MIA | Inhibition | 2 µM | Tani *et al.* (1996) |
| Opioids (U-50,488H) | Inhibition | 100 µM | Periyasamy (1992) |
| Erythrinin B | Inhibition | 1.25 µg ml$^{-1}$ | Kobayashi *et al.* (1997) |

Note

HMA, hexamethylene amiloride; DMA, dimethyl amiloride; MIA, methylisobutyl amiloride; EIPA, ethylisopropyl amiloride (also inhibits, but $IC_{50}$ not given).

(Frelin *et al.*, 1990). Palytoxin also has a pronounced effect in inducing a Na$^+$-selective ion channel that is resistant to TTX (see below).

### Other toxins

Some of the opioids produce inhibition of the cardiac Na/H exchanger in micromolar concentrations. U-50,488H (an opioid) is more potent than amiloride in inhibiting the cardiac Na/H antiporter (Periyasamy, 1992).

Three inhibitors of the Na/H exchange system, erythrinin-B, euchrenone-b10, and 1,3,5-trihydroxy-4-(3-methylbut-2-enyl)xanthen-9-one, were isolated from Indonesian medicinal plants (*Erythrina variegata* and the roots of *Maclura cochinchinensis*). They potently inhibit the Na/H exchanger system of VSM cells (Kobayashi *et al.*, 1997).

Diacetyl monoxime (DAM or BDM) [CH$_3$-CO-(CH$_3$)C=N-OH] produces a phosphatase-like effect (Bauza *et al.*, 1995). It affects the Na/H exchanger indirectly, as evidenced by a reduction in the pH$_i$ recovery rate following ischemia. DAM also has inhibitory action on Ca$_L$ channels (see below) (Sada *et al.*, 1985).

## Summary

In this survey of toxins that affect the cardiovascular system, it was not possible to cover all, or even most, of such agents because of space and time limitations. Instead, we tried to cover representative compounds, with a wide variety of chemical structures, that acted by a variety of mechanisms on the ion channels, ion pumps, and ion exchangers of cardiac muscle and vascular smooth muscle.

Again because of space limitations, the chemical structure of the channels/pumps/ exchangers could not be given, but the reader is referred to a textbook of cell physiology in which these channel structures are given (Sperelakis, 1998a). In addition, it was not possible to provide the chemical structure of the various toxins, but reference is given to articles in which these chemical structures are given and details of the biologic effects are presented. A summary of the various agents and their major actions are presented in a series of tables.

As can be seen from this chapter, a large number of the toxins derived from plants, bacteria, animals, and that are man-made act on the cell membrane of neurons and various types of muscle such as cardiac muscle and vascular smooth muscle. In addition, the primary targets on the cell membrane are the various types of ion channels, but also include the pumps and exchangers. In a few cases, the toxins act on the SR/ER membranes internally, especially on their Ca pump and their Ca-release channels. Ion channels of the sarcolemma particularly can be viewed as being targets of a variety of toxins and therapeutic drugs. In fact, abnormal ion channel structure/function is responsible for a number of diseases, such as myotonic and cystic fibrosis. Some therapeutic drugs, such as many of the antiarrhythmics, act on ion channels, and some of the positive inotropic drugs, such as the cardiac glycosides, act on the ion pumps.

Some toxins that act an the ion channels or pumps can lead indirectly to changes in the ultrastructure of the cells. For example, any toxin that increases $Na^+$ influx (such as BTX, GTX) and producing a higher $[Na]_i$ and $[Ca]_i$ (via the Na/Ca exchanger) can cause Ca overload, with SR swelling, mitochondrial deposits and disruption, and supercontracted myofibrils. In the opposite situation, toxins that act on the SR Ca pump (such as volvatoxin) can cause $[Ca]_i$ to rise, and this would increase $K^+$ conductance of the cell membrane because of the $K_{Ca}$ channels becoming activated. Thus, the cell membrane and SR membrane are effectively interconnected because of special properties of some of the ion channels.

In summary, the major goal of this chapter was to provide the reader with some appreciation of the wide variety of toxins that act on the ion channels of the cardiac sarcolemma to alter their normal function. Some toxins open or stimulate certain types of ion channels, whereas other toxins block the channels. In either case, there are dire consequences for the normal function of the cells. Some plants and animals apparently make use of these toxins as protective mechanisms against predators.

# References

Abbott, G.W., Sesti, F., Splawski, I., Buck, M.E., Lehmann, M.H., Timothy, K.W., Keating, M.T., and Goldstein, S.A.N. 1999. MiRP1 forms IKr potassium channels with HERG and is associated with cardiac arrhythmia. *Cell* 97: 175–187.
Ackerman, M. and Clapham, D. 1993. Cardiac chloride channels. *Trends Cardiovasc Med* 3: 23–28.

Adda, S., Fleischmann, B.K., Freedman, B.D., Yu, M., Hay, D.W.P., and Kotlikoff, M.I. 1996. Expression and function of voltage-dependent potassium channel genes in human airway smooth muscle. *J Biol Chem* 271: 13239–13243.

Agata N., Tanaka H., and Shigenobu K. 1993. Possible action of cyclopiazonic acid on myocardial sarcoplasmic reticulum: inotropic effects on neonatal and adult rat heart. *Br J Pharmacol* 108: 571–572.

Akaike, N. and Sadoshima, J.-I. 1989. Caffeine affects four different ionic currents in the bull-frog sympathetic neuron. *J Physiol* 412: 221–244.

Allen, T.J., Mikala, G., Wu, X., and Dolphin, A.C. 1998. Effects of 2,3-butanedione monoxime (BDM) on calcium channels expressed in *Xenopus oocytes*. *J Physiol* 508: 1–14.

Amédée, T., Benhan, C., Bolton, T., Byrne, N., and Large, W. 1990. Potassium, chloride, and nonselective cation conductances opened by noradrenaline in rabbit ear artery cells. *J Physiol* 423: 551–568.

Ameri, A. 1998. The effects of Aconitum alkaloids on the central nervous system. *Progr Neurobiol* 56: 211–235.

Arai, A., Kodama, I., and Toyama, J. 1996. Roles of Cl⁻ channels and Ca²⁺ mobilization in stretch-induced increase of SA node pacemaker activity. *Am J Physiol* 270: H1726–H1735.

Armstrong, C.M. and Bezanilla, F. 1974. Charge movement associated with the opening and closing of the activation gates of the Na⁺ channels. *J Gen Physiol* 63: 533–552.

Aye, N.N., Xue, Y.X., and Hashimoto, K. 1997. Antiarrhythmic effects of cariporide, a novel Na⁺–H⁺ exchange inhibitor, on reperfusion ventricular arrhythmias in rat hearts. *Eur J Pharmacol* 339: 121–127.

Backs, P.H. and Marban, E. 1993. Background potassium current active during the plateau of the action potential in guinea pig ventricular myocytes. *Circ Res* 72: 890–900.

Baer, M., Best, P.M., and Reuter, H. 1976. Voltage-dependent action of tetrodotoxin in mammalian cardiac muscle. *Nature* 263: 344.

Bahinski, A., Nairn, A., Greengard, P., and Gadsby, D. 1989. Chloride conductance regulated by cyclic AMP-dependent protein kinase in cardiac myocytes. *Nature* 340: 718–721.

Bai, Y.D.H.K. and Pelletier, S.W. 1995. N-oxides of some norditerpenoid alkaloids. *J Nat Prod* 58: 929–933.

Bassani, R.A., Bassani, J.W., and Bers, D.M. 1995. Relaxation in ferret ventricular myocytes: role of the sarcolemmal Ca ATPase. *Pflügers Arch* 430: 573–578.

Bauza, G., Le Moyec, L., and Eugene, M. 1995. pH regulation during ischaemia-reperfusion of isolated rat hearts, and metabolic effects of 2,3-butanedione monoxime. *J Mol Cell Cardiol* 27: 1703–1713.

Bengmann, J.S. and Nechay, B.R. 1982. Maitotoxin inhibits Na⁺ K⁺ ATPase in vitro. *Fed Proc Fed Am Soc Exp Biol* 41: 1562.

Bertrand, P.P. and Galligan, J.J. 1994. Contribution of chloride conductance increase to slow EPSC and tachykinin current in guinea-pig myenteric neurons. *J Physiol* 481: 47–60.

Bialecki, R.A., Kulik, T.J., and Colucci, W.S. 1992. Stretching increases calcium influx and efflux in cultured pulmonary arterial smooth muscle cells. *Am J Physiol* 263: L602–L606.

Bloomquist, J.R. 1993. Toxicology, mode of action and target site-mediated resistance to insecticides acting on chloride channels. *Comp Biochem Physiol C: Comp Pharmacol Toxicol* 106: 301–314.

Blumenthal, K. 1998. Ion channels as targets for toxins. In: *Cell Physiology Source Book*, 2nd edn. Sperelakis, N. (ed.), pp. 547–563. San Diego: Academic Press.

Bontems, F., Roumestand, C., Gilquin, B., Ménez, A., and Toma, F. 1991. Refined structure of charybdotoxin: common motifs in scorpion toxins and insect defensins. *Science* 254: 1521–1523.

Bontems, F., Gilquin, B., Roumestand, C., Ménez, A., and Toma, F. 1992. Analysis of side-chain organization on a refined model of charybdotoxin: structural and functional implications. *Biochemistry* 31: 7756–7764.

Borchard, U., Fox, A.A.L., Greeff, K., and Schlieper, P. 1979. Negative and positive inotropic action of vanadate on atrial and ventricular myocardium. *Nature* 279: 339–341.

Boucek, Jr., R.J., Olson, R.D., Brenner, D.E., Ogunbunmi, E.M., Inui, M., and Fleischer, S. 1987. The major metabolite of doxorubicin is a potent inhibitor of membrane-associated ion pumps. A correlative study of cardiac muscle with isolated membrane fractions. *J Biol Chem* 262: 15851–15856.

Brayden, J.E. 1996. Potassium channels in vascular smooth muscle. *Clin Exp Pharmacol Physiol* 23: 1069–1076.

Brill, D.M. and Wasserstrom, J.A. 1986. Intracellular sodium and the positive inotropic effect of veratridine and cardiac glycoside in sheep Purkinje fibers. *Circ Res* 58: 109–119.

Bugge, E., Munch-Ellingsen, J., and Ytrehus, K. 1996. Reduced infarct size in the rabbit heart in vivo by ethylisopropyl-amiloride. A role for $Na^+/H^+$ exchange. *Basic Res Cardiol* 91: 203–209.

Busch, A.E., Suessbrich, H., Waldegger, S., Sailer, E., Greger, R., Lang, H.J., Lang, F., Gibson, K.J., and Maylie, J.G. 1996. Inhibition of IKs in guinea pig cardiac myocytes and guinea pig IsK channels by the chromanol 293B. *Pflügers Arch* 432: 1094–1096.

Byrne, N. and Large, W. 1988. Membrane ionic mechanisms activated by noradrenaline in cells isolated from the rabbit portal vein. *J Physiol* 404: 557–573.

Cameron, J., Flowers, A.E., and Capra, M.F. 1991. Effects of ciguatoxin on nerve excitability in rats (Part I). *J Neurol Sci* 101: 87–92.

Caterina, M.J., Schumacher, M.A., Tominaga, M., Rosen, T.A., Levine, J.D., and Julius, D. 1997. The capsaicin receptor: a heat-activated ion channel in the pain pathway. *Nature* 389: 816–824.

Catterall, W.A., Trainer, V., and Baden, D.G. 1992. Molecular properties of the sodium channel: a receptor for multiple neurotoxins. *Bull Soc Pathol Exot* 85: 481–485.

Cestele, S., Qu, Y., Rogers, J.C., Rochat, H., Scheuer, T., and Catterall, W.A. 1998. Voltage sensor-trapping: enhanced activation of sodium channels by beta-scorpion toxin bound to the S3–S4 loop in domain II. *Neuron* 21: 919–931.

Chakrabarti, S., Hoque, A.N., and Karmazyn, M. 1997. A rapid ischemia-induced apoptosis in isolated rat hearts and its attenuation by the sodium–hydrogen exchange inhibitor HOE 642 (cariporide). *J Mol Cell Cardiol* 29: 3169–3174.

Chang, G.J., Wu, M.H., Wu, Y.C., and Su, M.J. 1996. Electrophysiological mechanisms for antiarrhythmic efficacy and positive inotropy of liriodenine, a natural aporphine alkaloid from *Fissistigma glaucescens*. *Br J Pharmacol* 118: 1571–1583.

Chapman, R.A., Suleiman, M.S., Rodrigo, G.C., Minezaki, K.K., Chatamra, K.R., Little, C.R., Mistry, D.K., and Allen, T.J.A. 1993. *Intracellular Taurine, Intracellular Sodium and Defense Against Cellular Damage*. Norwell: Kluwer Academic Publishers.

Chicheportiche, R., Balerna, M., Lombet, A., Romey, G., and Lazdunski, M. 1979. Synthesis and mode of action on axonal membranes of photoactivable derivatives of tetrodotoxin. *J Biol Chem* 254: 1552–1557.

Choy, I.O., Schepkin, V.D., Budinger, T.F., Obayashi, D.Y., Young, J.N., and DeCampli, W.M. 1997. Effects of specific sodium/hydrogen exchange inhibitor during cardioplegic arrest. *Ann Thorac Surg* 64: 94–99.

Clark, S., Jordt, S.-F., Jentsch, T., and Mathie, A. 1998. Characterization of the hyperpolarization-activated chloride current in dissociated rat sympathetic neurons. *J Physiol* 506: 665–678.

Cohen, C.J., Bean, B.O., Colatsky, T.J., and Tsein, R.W. 1981. Tetrodotoxin block of sodium channels in rabbit purkinje fibers. *J Gen Physiol* 78: 383–411.

Colatsky, T.J. and Gadsby, D.C. 1980. Is tetrodotoxin block of background sodium channels in canine cardiac Purkinje fibers voltage-dependent? *J Physiol* 306: 20.

Collier, M.L. and Hume, J.R. 1995. Unitary chloride channels activated by protein kinase C in guinea pig ventricular myocytes. *Circ Res* 76: 317–324.

Collier, M.L., Levesque, P.C., Kenyon, J.L., and Hume, J.R. 1996. Unitary Cl⁻ channels activated by cytoplasmic $Ca^{2+}$ in canine ventricular myocytes. *Circ Res* 78: 936–944.

DeBin, J., Maggio, J., and Strichartz, G. 1993. Purification and characterization of chlorotoxin, a chloride channel ligand from the venom of the scorpion. *Am J Physiol* 264: C361–C369.

Dick, G., Bradley, K., Horowitz, B., Hume, J., and Sanders, K. 1998. Functional and molecular identification of a novel chloride conductance in canine colonic smooth muscle. *Am J Physiol* 275: C940–C950.

DiFrancesco, D. 1994. Some properties of the UL-FS 49 block of the hyperpolarization-activated current (i(f)) in sino-atrial node myocytes. *Pflügers Arch* 70.

DiFrancesco, D., Porciatti, F., Janigro, D., Maccaferri, G., Mangoni, M., Tritella, T., Chang, F., and Cohen, I.S. 1991. Block of the cardiac pacemaker current ($I_f$) in the rabbit sino-atrial node and in canine Purkinje fibres by 9-amino-1,2,3,4-tetrahydroacridine. *Pflügers Arch* 417: 611–615.

Diochot, S., Schweitz, H., Béress, L., and Lazdunski, M. 1998. Sea anemone peptides with a specific blocking activity against the fast inactivating potassium channel Kv3.4. *J Biol Chem* 273: 6744–6749.

Diochot, S., Drici, M.D., Moinier, D., Fink, M., and Lazdunski, M. 1999. Effects of phrixotoxins on the Kv4 family of potassium channels and implications for the role of Ito1 in cardiac electrogenesis. *Br J Pharmacol* 126: 251–263.

Docherty, J.C., Yang, L., Pierce, G.N., and Deslauriers, R. 1997. Na⁺–H⁺ exchange inhibition at reperfusion is cardioprotective during myocardial ischemia-reperfusion; ³¹P NMR studies. *Mol Cell Biochem* 176: 257–264.

Doorty, K.B., Bevan, S., Wadsworth, J.D., and Strong, P.N. 1997. A novel small conductance $Ca^{2+}$-activated K⁺ channel blocker from *Oxyuranus scutellatus* taipan venom. Re-evaluation of taicatoxin as a selective $Ca^{2+}$ channel probe. *J Biol Chem* 272: 19925–19930.

Droogmans, G., Callewaert, G., Declerck, I., and Casteels, R. 1991. ATP-induced $Ca^{2+}$ release and Cl⁻ current in cultured smooth muscle cells from pig aorta. *J Physiol* 440: 623–634.

Earm, Y.E., Ho, W.K., So, I., Leem, C.H., and Han, J. 1993. *Effect of Taurine on the Activation of Background Current in Cardiac Myocytes of the Rabbit*. Boston: Kluwer.

Ernst, M.E. and Kelly, M.W. 1998. Mibefradil, a pharmacologically distinct calcium antagonist. *Pharmacotherapy* 18: 463–485.

Ertel, E.A., Warren, V.A., Adams, M.E., Griffin, P.R., Cohen, C.J., and Smith, M.M. 1994. Type III omega-agatoxins: a family of probes for similar binding sites on L- and N-type calcium channels. *Biochemistry* 33: 5098–5108.

Evangeline, D.M., Paul, R.J., and Matlib, M.A. 1993. Role of $Na^+$–$Ca^{2+}$ exchange in the regulation of vascular smooth muscle tension. *Am Physiol Soc*: H1028–H1040.

Fainzibler, M., Kofman, O., Zlotkin, E., and Gordon, D. 1994. A new neurotoxin receptor site on sodium channels is identified by a conotoxin that affects sodium channel inactivation in molluscs and acts as an antagonist in rat brain. *J Biol Chem* 269: 2574–2580.

Fainzibler, M., Lodder, J., Kits, K.S., Kofman, O., Vinnitsky, I., VanRietschoten, J., Zlotkin, E., and Gordon, D. 1995. A new conotoxin affecting sodium current inactivation interacts with the δ-conotoxin receptor site. *J Biol Chem* 270: 1123–1129.

Fassold, E., Slade, A.M., Lin, J.Y., and Nayler, W.G. 1976. An effect of the cardiotoxic protein volvatoxin A on the function and structure of heart muscle cells. *J Mol Cell Cardiol* 8: 501.

Fermini, B., Jurkiewicz, N.K., Jow, B., Guinosso, Jr., P.J., Baskin, E.P., Lynch, Jr., J.J., and Salata, J.J. 1995. Use-dependent effects of the class III antiarrhythmic agent NE-10064 (azimilide) on cardiac repolarization: block of delayed rectifier potassium and L-type calcium currents. *J Cardiovasc Pharmacol* 26: 259–271.

Forbes M.S. and Sperelakis, N. 1972. ($Na^+$,$K^+$)-ATPase activity in tubular systems of mouse cardiac and skeletal muscles. *Z Zellforsch MiLrosk Anat* 134: 1–11.

Frelin, C., Vigne, P., and Breittmayer, J.P. 1990. Palytoxin acidifies chick cardiac cells and activates the $Na^+$/$H^+$ antiporter. *FEBS Lett* 264: 63–66.

Fuchs, S., Gertz, E.W., and Briggs, F.N. 1968. The effect of quinidine on calcium accumulation by isolated sarcoplasmic reticulum of skeletal and cardiac muscle. *J Gen Physiol* 52: 955.

Galvez, A., Gimenez-Gallego, G., Reuben, J.P., Roy-Contancin, L., Feigenbaum, P., Kaczorowski, G.J., and Garcia, M.L. 1990. Purification and characterization of a unique, potent, peptidyl probe for the high conductance calcium-activated potassium channel from venom of the scorpion *Buthus tamulus*. *J Biol Chem* 265: 11083–11090.

Gannier, F., White, E., Lacampagne, A., Garnier, D., and Le Guennec, J.Y. 1994. Streptomycin reverses a large stretch induced increases in $[Ca^{2+}]_i$ in isolated guinea pig ventricular myocytes. *Cardiovasc Res* 28: 1193–1198.

Garcia, M.L., Garcia-Calvo, M., Hidalgo, P., Lee, A., and MacKinnon, R. 1994. Purification and characterization of three inhibitors of voltage-dependent $K^+$ channels from *Leiurus quinquestriatus* var. hebraeus venom. *Biochemistry* 33: 6834–6839.

Garcia, M.L., Hanner, M., Koch, R., Schmalhofer, W., Slaughter, R.S., and Kaczorowski, G.J. 1997. Pharmacology of potassium channels. *Adv Pharmacol* 39: 425–471.

Gasparini, S. and DiFrancesco, D. 1997. Action of the hyperpolarization-activated current (Ih) blocker ZD 7288 in hippocampal CA1 neurons. *Pflügers Arch* 435: 99–106.

Gatto, C., Hale, C.C., Xu, W., and Milanick, M.A. 1995. Eosin, a potent inhibitor of the plasma membrane Ca pump, does not inhibit the cardiac Na–Ca exchanger. *Biochemistry* 34: 965–972.

Gerstheimer, F., Muhleisen, M., Nehring, D., and Kreye, V. 1987. A chloride–bicarbonate exchanging anion carrier in vascular smooth muscle of the rabbit. *Pflügers Arch* 409: 60–66.

Goethals, M., Raes, A., and van Bogaert, P.P. 1993. Use-dependent block of the pacemaker current $I_f$ in rabbit sinoatrial node cells by zatebradine (UL-FS 49). On the mode of action of sinus node inhibitors. *Circulation* 88: 2389–2401.

Gray, D.F., Mihailidou, A.S., Hansen, P.S., Buhagiar, K.A., Bewick, N.L., Rasmussen, H.H., and Whalley, D.W. 1998. Amiodarone inhibits the Na$^+$–K$^+$ pump in rabbit cardiac myocytes after acute and chronic treatment. *J Pharmacol Exp Ther* 284: 75–82.

Gray, M., Plant, S., and Argent, B. 1993. cAMP-regulated whole cell chloride currents in pancreatic duct cells. *Am J Physiol* 264: C591–C602.

Gusovsky, F., Padgett, W.L., Creveling, C.R., and Daly, J.W. 1992. Interaction of pumiliotoxin B with an "alkaloid-binding domain" on the voltage-dependent sodium channel. *Mol Pharmacol* 42: 1104–1108.

Gutser, U.T., Friese, J., Heubach, J.F., Matthiesen, T., Selve, N., Wilffert, B., and Gleitz, J. 1998. Mode of antinociceptive and toxic action of alkaloids of *Aconitum* spec. *Naunyn-Schmiedebergs Arch Pharmacol* 357: 39–48.

Gyori, J., Fejtl, M., Carpenter, D.O., and Salanki, J. 1994. Effect of HgCl$_2$ on acetylcholine, carbachol, and glutamate currents of Aplysia neurons. *Cell Mol Neurobiol* 14: 653–664.

Hagiwara, N., Masuda, H., Shoda, M., and Irisawa, H. 1992. Stretch-activated anion currents of rabbit cardiac myocytes. *J Physiol* 456: 285–302.

Hansen, D.E., Borganelli, M., Stacy, Jr., G.P., and Taylor, L.K. 1991. Dose-dependent inhibition of stretch-induced arrhythmias by gadolinium in isolated canine ventricles. Evidence for a unique mode of antiarrhythmic action. *Circ Res* 69: 820–831.

Harvey, R. and Hume, J. 1989. Autonomic regulation of a chloride current in heart. *Science* 244: 983–985.

Harvey, R.D. 1993. Effects of stilbenedisulfonic acid derivatives on the cAMP-regulated chloride current in cardiac myocytes. *Pflügers Arch* 422: 436–442.

Harvey, R.D., Clark, C.D., and Hume, J.R. 1990. Chloride current in mammalian cardiac myocytes. Novel mechanism for autonomic regulation of action potential duration and resting membrane potential. *J Gen Physiol* 95: 1077–1102.

Hisada, T., Singer, J.J., and Walsh, Jr., J.V. 1993. Aluminofluoride activates hyperpolarization- and stretch-activated cationic channels in single smooth muscle cells. *Pflügers Arch* 422: 397–400.

Hobai, I.A. 1996. Correlated biochemical modifications of plasma lipoproteins in coronary heart disease: an accelerating pathologic factor. *Rom J Intern Med* 34(1–2): 55–64.

Hobai, I.A., Bates, J.A., Howarth, F.C., and Levi, A.J. 1997a. Inhibition by external Cd$^{2+}$ of Na/Ca exchange and L-type Ca channel in rabbit ventricular myocytes. *Am J Physiol* 272: H2164–H2172.

Hobai, I.A., Khananshvili, D., and Levi, A.J. 1997b. The peptide "FRCRCFa", dialysed intracellularly, inhibits the Na/Ca exchange in rabbit ventricular myocytes with high affinity. *Pflügers Arch* 433: 455–463.

Hoffmann, E. and Dunham, P. 1995. Membrane mechanisms and intracellular signaling in cell volume regulation. *Int Rev Cytol* 161: 173–262.

Hogg, R.C., Wang, Q., and Large, W.A. 1994. Effects of Cl channel blockers on Ca-activated chloride and potassium currents in smooth muscle cells from rabbit portal vein. *Br J Pharmacol* 111: 1333–1341.

Hogg, R.C., Lewis, R.J., and Adams, D.J. 1998. Ciguatoxin (CTX-1) modulates single tetrodotoxin-sensitive sodium channels in rat parasympathetic neurons. *Neurosci Lett* 252: 103–106.

Holevinsky, K.O., Fan, Z., Frame, M., Makielski, J.C., Groppi, V., and Nelson, D.J. ATP-sensitive K$^+$ channel opener acts as a potent Cl$^-$ channel inhibitor in vascular smooth muscle cells. 1994. *J Membr Biol* 137: 59–70.

Hoyer, J., Kohler, R., and Distler, A. 1997. Mechanosensitive cation channels in aortic endothelium of normotensive and hypertensive rats. *Hypertension* 30: 112–119.

Hu, H. and Sachs, F. 1996. Mechanically activated currents in chick heart cells. *J Membr Biol* 154: 205–216.

Huang, L.Y., Yatani, A., and Brown, A.M. 1987. The properties of batrachotoxin-modified cardiac Na channels, including state-dependent block by tetrodotoxin. *J Gen Physiol* 90: 341–360.

Huang, Y., Quayle, J.M., Worley, J.F., Standen, N.B., and Nelson, M.T. 1989. External cadmium and internal calcium block of single calcium channels in smooth muscle cells from rabbit mesenteric artery. *Biophys J* 56: 1023–1028.

Hwang, T.-C., Horie, M., Dousmanis, A., and Gadsby, D. 1992. Regulation of PK-A activated Cl conductance in guinea pig ventricular myocytes: whole-cell studies. *J Gen Physiol* 100: 69a.

Irisawa, H. and Sato, R. 1986. Intra- and extracellular action of proton on the calcium current of isolated guinea pig ventricular cells. *Circ Res* 59: 348–355.

Ishii, T.M., Silvia, C., Hirschberg, B., Bond, C.T., Adelman, J.P., and Maylie J. 1997. A human intermediate conductance calcium-activated potassium channel. *Proc Natl Acad Sci USA* 94: 11651–11656.

Janigro, D., Martenson, M.E., and Baumann, T.K. 1997. Preferential inhibition of Ih in rat trigeminal ganglion neurons by an organic blocker. *J Membr Biol* 160: 101–109.

Joiner, W.J., Wang, L.Y., Tang, M.D., and Kaczmarek, L.K. 1997. hSk4, a member of a novel subfamily of calcium-activated potassium channels. *Proc Natl Acad Sci USA* 94: 11013–11018.

Josephson, I.R. and Sperelakis, N. 1990. Fast activation of cardiac $Ca^{2+}$ channel gating charge by the dihydropyridine agonist, BAY K 8644. *Biophys J* 58: 1307–1311.

Jung, F., Selvaraj, S., and Gargus, J.J. 1992. Blockers of platelet-derived growth factor-activated nonselective cation channel inhibit cell proliferation. *Am J Physiol* 262: C1464–C1470.

Kääb, S., Dixon, J., Duc, J., Ashen, D., Näbauer, M., Beuckelmann, D.J., Steinbeck, G., McKinnon, D., and Tomaselli, G.F. 1998. Molecular basis of transient outward potassium current downregulation in human heart failure. A decrease in Kv4.3 mRNA correlates with a reduction in current density. *Circulation* 98: 1383–1393.

Kaneda, M., Fukui, K., and Doi, K. 1994. Activation of chloride current by P2-purinoceptors in rat ventricular myocytes. *Br J Pharmacol* 111: 1355–1360.

Karhu, S., Perttula, S., Weckstrom, M., Kivisto, T., and Sellin, L.C. 1995. Salicylaldoxime blocks $K^+$ and $Ca^{2+}$ currents in rat cardiac myocytes. *Eur J Pharmacol* 279: 7–13.

Kaur, H., Parikh, V., Sharma, A., and Singh, M. 1997. Effect of amiloride A $Na^+/H^+$ exchange inhibitor on cardioprotective effect of ischaemic preconditioning: possible involvement of resident cardiac mast cells. *Pharmacol Res* 36: 95–102.

Kerrison, J. and Freschi, J.E. 1992. The effects of gamma-aminobutyric acid on voltage-clamped motoneurons of the lobster cardiac ganglion. *Comp Biochem Physiol C: Comp Pharmacol Toxicol* 101: 227–233.

Khan, S.A., Higdon, N.R., Hester, J.B., and Meisheri, K.D. 1997. Pharmacological characterization of novel cyanoguanidines as vascular KATP channel blockers. *J Pharmacol Exp Ther* 283: 1207–1213.

Kim, D., Fujita, A., Horio, Y., and Kurachi, Y. 1998. Cloning and functional expression of a novel cardiac two-pore background $K^+$ channel (cTBAK-1). *Circ Res* 82: 513–518.

Kimura, J., Miyamae, S., and Noma, A. 1987. Identification of sodium–calcium exchange current in single ventricular cells of guinea-pig. *J Physiol* 384: 199–222.

Kini, R.M., Caldwell, R.A., Wu, Q.Y., Baumgarten, C.M., Feher, J.J., and Evans, H.J. 1998. Flanking proline residues identify the L-type $Ca^{2+}$ channel binding site of calciseptine and FS2. *Biochemistry* 37: 9058–9063.

Kito, M., Maehara, M., and Watanabe, K. 1996. Mechanisms of T-type calcium channel blockade by zonisamide. *Seizure* 5: 115–119.

Klöckner, U. and Isenberg, G. 1991. Endothelin depolarizes myocytes from porcine coronary and human mesenteric arteries through a Ca-activated chloride current. *Pflügers Arch* 418: 168–175.

Kobayashi, M., Mahmud, T., Yoshioka, N., Shibuya, H., and Kitagawa, I. 1997. Indonesian medicinal plants. XXI. Inhibitors of $Na^+/H^+$ exchanger from the bark of *Erythrina variegata* and the roots of *Maclura cochinchinensis*. *Chem Pharm Bull* 45: 1615–1619.

Kobrin, I., Bieska, G., Charlon, V., Lindberg, E., and Pordy, R. 1998. Anti-anginal and anti-ischemic effects of mibefradil, a new T-type calcium channel antagonist. *Cardiology* 89: 23–32.

Köhler, M., Hirschberg, B., Bond, C.T., Kinzie, J.M., Marrion, N.V., Maylie, J., and Adelman, J.P. 1996. Small-conductance, calcium-activated potassium channels from mammalian brain. *Science* 273: 1709–1714.

Kohlhardt, M., Frobe, U., and Herzig, J.W. 1987. Removal of inactivation and blockade of cardiac $Na^+$ channels by DPI 201-106: different voltage-dependencies of the drug actions. *Naunyn-Schmiedebergs Arch Pharmacol* 335: 183–188.

Koike, A., Akita, T., Hotta, Y., Takeya, K., Kodama, I., Murase, M., Abe, T., and Toyama, J. 1996. Protective effects of dimethyl amiloride against postischemic myocardial dysfunction in rabbit hearts: phosphorus 31-nuclear magnetic resonance measurements of intracellular pH and cellular energy. *J Thorac Cardiovasc Surg* 112: 765–775.

Korbmacher, C., Volk, T., Segal, A.S., Boulpaep, E.L., and Fromter, E. 1995. A calcium-activated and nucleotide-sensitive nonselective cation channel in M-1 mouse cortical collecting duct cells. *J Membr Biol* 146: 29–45.

Krafte, D.S., Volberg, W.A., Dillon, K., and Ezrin, A.M. 1991. Expression of cardiac Na channels with appropriate physiological and pharmacological properties in *Xenopus* oocytes. *Proc Natl Acad Sci USA* 88: 4071–4074.

Lambert, P., Kuroda, H., Chino, N., Watanabe, T.X., Kimura, T., and Sakakibara, S. 1990. Solution synthesis of charybdotoxin (ChTX), a $K^+$ channel blocker. *Biochem Biophys Res Commun* 170: 684–690.

Lawrence, J.C. and Catterall, W.A. 1981. Tetrodotoxin-insensitive sodium channels. Binding of polypeptide neurotoxins in primary cultures of rat muscle cells. *J Biol Chem* 256: 6223–6229.

Lee, C.Y. 1972. Chemistry and pharmacology of polypeptide toxins in snake venom. *Am Rev Pharmacol* 12: 265–286.

Legrand, A.M., Galonnier, M., and Bagnis, R. 1982. Studies on the mode of action of ciguateric toxins. *Toxicon* 20: 311–315.

Legros, C. and Martin-Eauclaire, M.F. 1997. Scorpion toxins. *C R Seances Soc Biol Filiales* 191: 345–380.

Levesque, P.C. and Hume, J.R. 1995. $ATP_o$ but not $cAMP_i$ activates a chloride conductance in mouse ventricular myocytes. *Cardiovasc Res* 29: 336–343.

Levesque, P.C., Clark, C.D., Zakarov, S.I., Rosenshtraukh, L.V., and Hume, J.R. 1993. Anion and cation modulation of the guinea-pig ventricular action potential during β-adrenoceptor stimulation. *Pflügers Arch* 424: 54–62.

Lewis, R.J. 1992. Ciguatoxins are potent ichthyotoxins. *Toxicon* 30: 207–211.

Lin, J.Y., Jeng, T.W., Chen, C.C., Shi, G.Y., and Tung, T.C. 1973. Isolation of a new cardiotoxic protein from the edible mushroom. *Nature* 246: 524–525.

Lippens, G., Najib, J., Wodak, S., and Tartar, A. 1995. NMR sequential assignments and solution structure of chlorotoxin, a small scorpion toxin that blocks chloride channels. *Biochemistry* 34: 13–21.

Little, M.J., Zappia, C., Gilles, N., Connor, M., Tyler, M.I., Martin-Eauclaire, M.F., Gordon, D., and Nicholson, G.M. 1998. delta-Atracotoxins from Australian funnel-web spiders compete with scorpion alpha-toxin binding but differentially modulate alkaloid toxin activation of voltage-gated sodium channels. *J Biol Chem* 273: 27076–27083.

Loh, S.H., Sun, B., and Vaughan-Jones, R.D. 1996. Effect of Hoe 694, a novel Na$^+$–H$^+$ exchange inhibitor, on intracellular pH regulation in the guinea-pig ventricular myocyte. *Br J Pharmacol* 118: 1905–1912.

Lombet, A., Renaud, J.F., and Chicheportiche, M. 1981. A cardiac tetrodotoxin binding component: biochemical identification, characterization, and properties. *Biochemistry* 20: 1279–1285.

Lombet, A., Bidard, J.N., and Lazdunski, M. 1987. Ciguatoxin and brevetoxins share a common receptor site on the neuronal voltage-dependent Na$^+$ channel. *FEBS Lett* 219: 355–359.

Lu, Z. and MacKinnon, R. 1997. Purification, characterization, and synthesis of an inward-rectifier K$^+$ channel inhibitor from scorpion venom. *Biochemistry* 36: 6936–6940.

McDonald, T.V., Yu, Z., Ming, Z., Palma, E., Meyers, M.B., Wang, K.-W., Goldstein, S.A.N., and Fishman, G.I. 1997. A minK–HERG complex regulates the cardiac potassium current IKr. *Nature* 388: 289–292.

McMahon, E. and Jones, A. 1988. Altered chloride transport in arteries from aldosterone-salt hypertensive rats. *J Hypertension* 6: 593–599.

McManus, O.B., Helms, L.M.H., Pallanck, L., Ganetzky, B., Swanson, R., and Leonard, R.J. 1995. Functional role of the β-subunit of high conductance calcium-activated potassium channels. *Neuron* 14: 645–650.

Martinez, M., Salvador, C., Farias, J., Vaca, L., and Escobar, L. 1999. Modulation of a calcium-activated chloride current by Maitotoxin. *Toxicon* 37: 359–370.

Mathur, S. and Karmazyn, M. 1997. Interaction between anesthetics and the sodium–hydrogen exchange inhibitor HOE 642 (cariporide) in ischemic and reperfused rat hearts. *Anesthesiology* 87: 1460–1469.

Matsuoka, T., Nishizaki, T., and Nomura, T. 1997. The voltage-dependent non-selective cation channel sensitive to the L-type calcium channel blocker efonidipine regulates Ca$^{2+}$ influx in brain vascular smooth muscle cells. *Biochem Biophys Res Commun* 240: 484–487.

Matsuura, H. and Ehara, T. 1992. Activation of chloride current by purinergic stimulation in guinea pig heart cells. *Circ Res* 70: 851–855.

Morales, J.A., Ram, J.L., Song, J., and Brown, R.A. 1997. Acetaldehyde inhibits current through voltage-dependent calcium channels. *Toxicol Appl Pharmacol* 143: 70–74.

Myers, M.L., Mathur, S., Li, G.H., and Karmazyn, M. 1995. Sodium–hydrogen exchange inhibitors improve postischemic recovery of function in the perfused rabbit heart. *Cardiovasc Res* 29: 209–214.

Nakajima, T., Kitazawa, T., Hamada, E., Hazama, H., Omata, M., and Kurachi, Y. 1995. 17beta-Estradiol inhibits the voltage-dependent L-type Ca$^{2+}$ currents in aortic smooth muscle cells. *Eur J Pharmacol* 294: 625–635.

Nakamura, A., Harada, K., Sugimoto, H., Nakajima, F., and Nishimura, N. 1998. Effects of KB-R7943, a novel $Na^+/Ca^{2+}$ exchange inhibitor, on myocardial ischemia/reperfusion injury. *Folia Pharmacol Jpn* 111: 105–115.

Narahashi, T. 1974. Chemicals as tools in the study of excitable membranes. *Physiol Rev* 54: 813–889.

Narahashi, T. 1986. Toxins that modulate the sodium channel gating mechanism. *Ann NY Acad Sci* 479: 133–151.

Narahashi, T. 1996. Neuronal ion channels as the target sites of insecticides. *Pharmacol Toxicol* 79: 1–14.

Narahashi, T., Moore, J.W., and Scott, W.R. 1964. Tetrodotoxin blockage of sodium conductance increase in lobster giant axon. *J Gen Physiol* 47: 965.

Nayler, W.G., Sullivan, A.T., Dunnett, J., Slade, A.M., and Trethewie, E.R. 1976. The effect of a cardiotoxic component of the venom of the Indian cobra (*Naja nigricollis*) on the subcellular structure and function of heart muscle. *J Mol Cell Cardiol* 8: 341–360.

Nelson, M.T. and Quayle, J.M. 1995. Physiological roles and properties of potassium channels in arterial smooth muscle. *Am J Physiol* 268: C799–C822.

Nicholson, G.M., Little, M.J., Tyler, M., and Narahashi, T. 1996. Selective alteration of sodium channel gating by Australian funnel-web spider toxins. *Toxicon* 34: 1443–1453.

Nilius, B. 1998. Ion channels in nonexcitable cells. In: *Cell Physiology Source Book*, 2nd edn. Sperelakis, N. (ed.), pp. 436–455. San Diego: Academic Press.

Nilius, B., Sehrer, J., and Droogmans, G. 1994. Permeation properties and modulation of volume-activated $Cl^-$-currents in human endothelial cells. *Br J Pharmacol* 112: 1049–1056.

Nilius, B., Eggermon, J., Voets, T., and Droogmans, G. 1996. Volume-activated $Cl^-$ channels. *Gen Pharmacol* 27: 1131–1140.

Nilius, B., Prenen, J., Szücs, G., Wei, L., Tanzi, F., Voets, T., and Droogmans, G. 1997. Calcium-activated chloride channels in bovine pulmonary artery endothelial cells. *J Physiol* 498: 381–396.

Norris, T.M., Moya, E., Blagbrough, I.S., and Adams, M.E. 1996. Block of high-threshold calcium channels by the synthetic polyamines sFTX-3.3 and FTX-3.3. *Mol Pharmacol* 50: 939–946.

Ohya, Y., Adachi, N., Nakamura, Y., Setoguchi, M., Abe, I., and Fujishima, M. 1998. Stretch-activated channels in arterial smooth muscle of genetic hypertensive rats. *Hypertension* 31: 254–258.

Oren, D.A., Froy, O., Amit, E., Kleinberger-Doron, N., Gurevitz, M., and Shaanan, B. 1998. An excitatory scorpion toxin with a distinctive feature: an additional alpha helix at the C terminus and its implications for interaction with insect sodium channels. *Structure* 6: 1095–1103.

Pankucsi, C., Banyasz, T., Magyar, J., Gyonos, I., Kovacs, A., Varro, A., Szenasi, G., and Nanasi, P.P. 1997. Electrophysiological effects of EGIS-7229, a new antiarrhythmic agent, in isolated mammalian and human cardiac tissues. *Naunyn-Schmiedebergs Arch Pharmacol* 355: 398–405.

Patkar, S.A., Rasmussen, U., and Diamant, B. 1979. On the mechanism of histamine release induced by thapsigargin from *Thapsia garganica* L. *Agents Actions* 9: 53–57.

Periyasamy, S.M. 1992. Inhibition of cardiac sarcolemmal $Na^+/H^+$ antiporter by opioids. *Can J Physiol Pharmacol* 70: 1048–1056.

Popp, R., Englert, H.C., Lang, H.J., and Gogelein, H. 1993. Inhibitors of nonselective cation channels in cells of the blood–brain barrier. *Exs* 66: 213–218.

Poronnik, P., Cook, D.I., Allen, D.G., and Young, J.A. 1991. Diphenylamine-2-carboxylate (DPC) reduces calcium influx in a mouse mandibular cell line (ST885). *Cell Calcium* 12: 441–447.

Poronnik, P., Ward, M.C., and Cook, D.I. 1992. Intracellular $Ca^{2+}$ release by flufenamic acid and other blockers of the non-selective cation channel. *FEBS Lett* 296: 245–248.

Possani, L.D., Martin, B.M., Yatani, A., Mochca-Morales, J., Zamudio, F.Z., Gurrola, G.B., and Brown, A.M. 1992. Isolation and physiological characterization of taicatoxin, a complex toxin with specific effects on calcium channels. *Toxicon* 30: 1343–1364.

Proks, P. and Ashcroft, F.M. 1997. Phentolamine block of KATP channels is mediated by Kir6.2. *Proc Natl Acad Sci USA* 94: 11716–11720.

Ray, D.E., Sutharsan, S., and Forshaw, P.J. 1997. Actions of pyrethroid insecticides on voltage-gated chloride channels in neuroblastoma cells. *Neurotoxicology* 18: 755–760.

Renaud, J.F. and Lazdunski, M. 1988. Action of natural toxins on cardiac ionic channels. In: *Physiology and Pathophysiology of the Heart*, 1st edn. Sperelakis, N. (ed.), pp. 551–572. Boston: Kluwer Academic Press.

Renaud, J.F., Kazazoglou, T., Lombet, A., Chicheportiche, R., Jaimovich, E., Romey, G., and Lazdunski, M. 1983. The $Na^+$ channel in mammalian cardiac cells. Two kinds of tetrodotoxin receptors in rat heart membranes. *J Biol Chem* 258: 8799–8805.

Richards, N.W. and Dawson, D.C. 1993. Selective block of specific $K^+$-conducting channels by diphenylamine-2-carboxylate in turtle colon epithelial cells. *J Physiol* 462: 715–734.

Robineau, P., Leclercq, Y., Gerbi, A., Berrebi-Bertrand, I., and Lelievre, L.G. 1991. An organophosphorus compound, VX, selectively inhibits the rat cardiac $Na^+$, $K^+$-ATPase alpha 1 isoform. Biochemical basis of the cardiotoxicity of VX. *FEBS Lett* 281: 145–148.

Roden, D.M. and George, J.A.L. 1997. Structure and function of cardiac sodium and potassium channels. *Am J Physiol* 273: H511–H525.

Rodgers, R.L., Chou, H.N., Temma, K., Akera, T., and Shimizu, Y. 1984. Positive inotropic and toxic effects of brevetoxin-B on rat and guinea pig heart. *Toxicol Appl Pharmacol* 76: 296–305.

Rudy, B. 1988. Diversity and ubiquity of K channels. *Neuroscience* 25: 729–749.

Ruknudin, A., Sachs, F., and Bustamante, J.O. 1993. Stretch-activated ion channels in tissue-cultured chick heart. *Am J Physiol* 264: H960–H972.

Sack, S., Mohri, M., Schwarz, E.R., Arras, M., Schaper, J., Ballagi-Pordany, G., Scholz, W., Lang, H.J., Scholkens, B.A., and Schaper, W. 1994. Effects of a new $Na^+/H^+$ antiporter inhibitor on postischemic reperfusion in pig heart. *J Cardiovasc Pharmacol* 23: 72–78.

Sada, H., Sada, S., and Sperelakis, N. 1985. Effects of diacetyl monoxine (DAM) on slow and fast action potentials of young and old embryonic chick hearts and rabbit hearts. *Eur J Pharmacol* 112: 145–152.

Salanki, J., Gyori, J., and Carpenter, D.O. 1994. Action of lead on glutamate-activated chloride currents in *Helix pomatia* L. neurons. *Cell Mol Neurobiol* 14: 755–768.

Sanguinetti, M.C., and Jurkiewicz, N.K. 1990. Two components of cardiac delayed rectifier $K^+$ current. Differential sensitivity to block by class III antiarrhythmic agents. *J Gen Physiol* 96: 195–215.

Sanguinetti, M.C., Johnson, J.H., Hammerland, L.G., Kelbaugh, P.R., Volkmann, R.A., Saccomano, N.A., and Mueller, A.L. 1997 Heteropodatoxins: peptides isolated from spider venom that block Kv4.2 potassium channels. *Mol Pharmacol* 51: 491–498.

Sanna, E., Motzo, C., Usala, M., Pau, D., Cagetti, E., and Biggio, G. 1998. Functional changes in rat nigral $GABA_A$ receptors induced by degeneration of the striatonigral GABAergic pathway: an electrophysiological study of receptors incorporated into *Xenopus* oocytes. *J Neurochem* 70: 2539–2544.

Satoh, H. and Sperelakis, N. 1998. Review of some actions of taurine on ion channels of cardiac muscle cells and others. *Gen Pharmacol* 30: 451–463.

Sauviat, M.P. 1997. Effect of neurotoxins on the electrical activity and contraction of the heart muscle. *C R Seances Soc Biol Filiales* 191: 451–471.

Schreibmayer, W. and Jeglitsch, G. 1992. The sodium channel activator Brevetoxin-3 uncovers a multiplicity of different open states of the cardiac sodium channel. *Biochim Biophys Acta* 1104: 233–242.

Schwartz, A., Lindenmayer, G.E., and Allen, J.C. 1975. The sodium–potassium adenosine triphosphatase: pharmacological, physiological and biochemical aspects. *Pharmacol Rev* 27: 3–134.

Schweitz, H., Heurteaux, C., Bois, P., Moinier, D., Romey, G., and Lazdunski, M. 1994. Calcicludine, a venom peptide of the Kunitz-type protease inhibitor family, is a potent blocker of high-threshold $Ca^{2+}$ channels with a high affinity for L-type channels in cerebellar granule neurons. *Proc Natl Acad Sci USA* 91: 878–882.

Schweitz, H., Bruhn, T., Guillemare, T., Moinier, D., Lancelin, J.M., Béress, L., and Lazdunski, M. 1995. Two different classes of sea anemone toxins for voltage-sensitive $K^+$ channels. *J Biol Chem* 270: 25121–25126.

Scott, R.H., Sutton, K.G., Griffin, A., Stapleton, S.R., and Currie, K.P. 1995. Aspects of calcium-activated chloride currents: a neuronal perspective. *Pharm Ther* 66: 535–565.

Seitz, U. and Ameri, A. 1998. Different effects on [³H]noradrenaline uptake of the Aconitum alkaloids aconitine, 3-acetylaconitine, lappaconitine, and N-desacetyllappaconitine in rat hippocampus. *Biochem Pharmacol* 55: 883–888.

Sheppard, D. and Welsh, M. 1992. Effect of ATP-sensitive $K^+$ channel regulators on cystic fibrosis transmembrane conductance regulator chloride currents. *J Gen Physiol* 100: 573–592.

Shier, W.T. and DuBourdieu, D.J. 1992. Sodium- and calcium-dependent steps in the mechanism of neonatal rat cardiac myocyte killing by ionophores. I. The sodium-carrying ionophore, monensin. *Toxicol Appl Pharmacol* 116: 38–46.

Soejima, M. and Kokubun, S. 1988. Single anion-selective channel and its ion selectivity in the vascular smooth muscle cells. *Pflügers Arch* 411: 304–311.

Sorota, S. 1992. Swelling-induced chloride-sensitive current in canine atrial cells revealed by whole-cell patch-clamp method. *Circ Res* 70: 679–687.

Sorota, S. 1994. Pharmacologic properties of the swelling-induced chloride current of dog atrial myocytes. *J Cardiovasc Electrophysiol* 5: 1006–1016.

Sperelakis, N. 1967. *Electrophysiology of Cultured Chick Heart Cells*. Tokyo: Bunkodo Co.

Sperelakis, N. 1992. Chemical agent actions on ion channels and electrophysiology of the heart. In: *Cardiovascular Toxicology*, 2nd edn. Acosta, D. (ed.), pp. 283–337. New York: Raven Press.

Sperelakis, N. 1995. Origin of resting membrane potentials. In: *Cell Physiology Source Book*. Sperelakis, N. (ed.), pp. 67–90. San Diego: Academic Press.

Sperelakis, N. 1998a. *Cell Physiology Source Book*. San Diego: Academic Press.

Sperelakis, N. 1998b. Regulation of ion channels by phosphorylation. In: *Cell Physiology Source Book*, 2nd edn. Sperelakis, N. (ed.), pp. 499–509. San Diego: Academic Press.

Sperelakis, N. 1998c. Origin of resting membrane potentials. In: *Cell Physiology Source Book*, 2nd edn. Sperelakis, N. (ed.), pp. 178–201. San Diego: Academic Press.

Sperelakis, N., Katsube, Y., and Kusaka, M. 1996. *Some Actions of Taurine on Ionic Currents of Myocardial Cells and Myometrial Cells*. New York: Raven Press.

Stacy, Jr., G.P., Jobe, R.L., Taylor, L.K., and Hansen, D.E. 1992. Stretch-induced depolarizations as a trigger of arrhythmias in isolated canine left ventricles. *Am J Physiol* 263: H613–H621.

Strange, K. and Jackson, P. 1995. Swelling-activated organic osmolyte efflux: A new role for anion channels. *Kidney Int* 48: 994–1003.

Suleymanian, M.A., Clemo, H.F., Cohen, N.M., and Baumgarten, C.M. 1995. Stretch-activated channel blockers modulate cell volume in cardiac ventricular myocytes. *J Mol Cell Cardiol* 27: 721–728.

Sullivan, M.J., Sharma, R.V., Wachtel, R.E., Chapleau, M.W., Waite, L.J., Bhalla, R.C., and Abboud, F.M. 1997. Non-voltage-gated $Ca^{2+}$ influx through mechanosensitive ion channels in aortic baroreceptor neurons. *Circ Res* 80: 861–867.

Sunami, A., Sasano, T., Matsunaga, A., Fan, Z., Swanobori, T., and Hiraoka, M. 1993. Properties of veratridine-modified single $Na^+$ channels in guinea pig ventricular myocytes. *Am J Physiol* 264: H454–H463.

Suzuki, M., Murata, M., Ikeda, M., Miyoshi, T., and Imai, M. 1998. Primary structure and functional expression of a novel non-selective cation channel. *Biochem Biophys Res Commun* 242: 191–196.

Swartz, K.J. and MacKinnon, R. 1995. An inhibitor of the Kv2.1 potassium channel isolated from the venom of a Chilean tarantula. *Neuron* 15: 941–949.

Swartz, K.J. and MacKinnon, R. 1997. Mapping the receptor site for Hanatoxin, a gating modifier of voltage-dependent $K^+$ channels. *Neuron* 18: 675–682.

Szück, G., Buyse, G., Eggermont, J., Droogmans, G., and Nilius, B. 1996. Characterisation of volume-activated chloride currents in endothelial cells from bovine pulmonary artery. *J Membr Biol* 149: 189–197.

Tang, C.M., Presser, F., and Morad, M. 1988. Amiloride selectively blocks the low threshold (T) calcium channel. *Science* 240: 213–215.

Tani, M., Shinmura, K., Hasegawa, H., and Nakamura, Y. 1996. Effect of methylisobutyl amiloride on $[Na^+]_i$, reperfusion arrhythmias, and function in ischemic rat hearts. *J Cardiovasc Pharmacol* 27: 794–801.

Tatsukawa, Y., Kiyosue, T., and Arita, M. 1997. Mechanical stretch increases intracellular calcium concentration in cultured ventricular cells from neonatal rats. *Heart and Vessels* 12: 128–135.

Tazieff-Depierre, F., Czajka, M., and Lowagie, C. 1969. Action pharmacologique des fractions pures de venin de Naja nigricollis et liberation de calcium dans les muscles stries. *CR Acad Sci Ser D* 268: 2511.

Thastrup, O. 1990. Role of $Ca^{2+}$-ATPases in regulation of cellular $Ca^{2+}$ signalling, as studied with the selective microsomal $Ca^{2+}$-ATPase inhibitor, thapsigargin. *Agents Actions* 29: 8–15.

Tominaga, M., Horie, M., and Okada, Y. 1994. Additional similarity of cardiac cAMP-activated $Cl^-$ channels to CFTR $Cl^-$ channels. *Jpn J Physiol* 44: S215–S218.

Tseng, G. 1999. Molecular structure of cardiac Ito channels: Kv4.2, Kv4.3, and other possibilities? *Cardiovasc Res* 41: 16–18.

Tseng, G.N. 1992. Cell swelling increases membrane conductance of canine cardiac cells: evidence for a volume-sensitive Cl channel. *Am J Physiol* 262: C1056–C1068.

Tucker, S.J., Gribble, F.M., Zhao, C., Trapp, S., and Ashcroft, F.M. 1997. Truncation of Kir6.2 produces ATP-sensitive K$^+$ channels in the absence of the sulfonylurea receptor. *Nature* 387: 179–183.

Tytgat, J., Vereecke, J., and Carmeliet, E. 1988. Differential effects of verapamil and flunarizine on cardiac L-type and T-type Ca channels. *Naunyn-Schmiedebergs Arch Pharmacol* 337: 690–692.

Ueda, K., Komine, J., Matsuo, M., Seino, S., and Amachi, T. 1999. Cooperative binding of ATP and MgADP in the sulfonylurea receptor is modulated by glibenclamide. *Proc Natl Acad Sci USA* 96: 1268–1272.

Valverde, M., Hardy, S., and Sepulveda, F. 1995. Chloride channels: a state of flux. *FASEB J* 9: 509–515.

Vandenberg, J.I., Yoshida, A., Kirk, K., and Powell, T. 1994. Swelling-activated and isoprenaline-activated chloride currents in guinea pig cardiac myocytes have distinct electrophysiology and pharmacology. *J Gen Physiol* 104: 997–1017.

Van Bogaert, P.P. and Goethals, M. 1987. Pharmacological influence of specific bradycardic agents on the pacemaker current of sheep cardiac Purkinje fibres. A comparison between three different molecules. *Eur Heart J* 42: 35–42.

Vengralik, C., DeBoos, A., Singh, A., Schultz, B., Frizzell, R., and Bridges, R. 1994. Sulfonylureas cause open channel blockade of CFTR. *Biophys J* 66: A421.

Vogel, S. and Sperelakis, N. 1977. Blockade of myocardial slow inward current at low pH. *Am J Physiol* 233: C99-C103.

Walsh, K. 1994. Agents which block heart Cl$^-$ channels also inhibit Ca$^{2+}$ current regulation. *Biophys J* 66: A239.

Walsh, K.B. and Long, K.J. 1994. Properties of a protein kinase C-activated chloride current in guinea pig ventricular myocytes. *Circ Res* 74: 121–129.

Walsh, K.B. and Wang, C. 1996. Effect of chloride channel blockers on the cardiac CFTR chloride and L-type calcium currents. *Cardiovasc Res* 32: 391–399.

Wang, D.J., Mao, H.Y., and Lei, M. 1993. Rotundium in the treatment of atrial fibrillation. *Chung Kuo Chung Hsi i Chieh Ho Tsa Chih* 13: 455–457.

Wang, Y. and Rosenberg, R.L. 1991. Ethaverine, a derivative of papaverine, inhibits cardiac L-type calcium channels. *Mol Pharmacol* 40: 750–755.

Wang, Z., Fermini, B., and Nattel, S. 1993. Sustained depolarization-induced outward current in human atrial myocytes. Evidence for a novel delayed rectifier K$^+$ current similar to Kv1.5 cloned channel currents. *Circ Res* 73: 1061–1076.

Wang, Z., Feng, J., Shi, H., Pond, A., Nerbonne, J.M., and Nattel, S. 1999. Potential molecular basis of different physiological properties of the transient outward K$^+$ current in rabbit and human atrial myocytes. *Circ Res* 84: 551–561.

Warashina, A., Ogura, T., and Fujita, S. 1988. Binding properties of sea anemone toxins to sodium channels in the crayfish giant axon. *Comp Biochem Physiol C: Comp Pharmacol Toxicol* 90: 351–359.

Watano, T. and Kimura, J. 1998. Calcium-dependent inhibition of the sodium–calcium exchange current by KB-R7943. *Can J Cardiol* 14: 259–262.

White, R., Elton, T., Shoemaker, R., and Brock, T. 1995. Calcium-sensitive chloride channels in vascular smooth muscle cells. *Exp Biol Med* 208: 255–262.

Wu, G. and Hamil, O. 1993. NPPB block of Ca$^{2+}$-activated Cl$^-$ currents in *Xenopus* oocytes. *Pflügers Arch* 420: 227–229.

Xu, W., Denison, H., Hale, C.C., Gatto, C., and Milanick, M.A. 1997. Identification of critical positive charges in XIP, the Na/Ca exchange inhibitory peptide. *Arch Biochem Biophys* 341: 273–279.

Xue, Y.X., Aye, N.N., and Hashimoto, K. 1996. Antiarrhythmic effects of HOE642, a novel $Na^+-H^+$ exchange inhibitor, on ventricular arrhythmias in animal hearts. *Eur J Pharmacol* 317: 309–316.

Yakehiro, M., Yamamoto, S., Baba, N., Nakajima, S., Iwasa, J., and Seyama, I. 1993. Structure–activity relationship for D-ring derivatives of grayanotoxin in the squid giant axon. *J Pharmacol Exp Ther* 265: 1328–1332.

Yakehiro, M., Seyama, I., and Narahashi, T. 1997. Kinetics of grayanotoxin evoked modification of sodium channels in squid giant axons. *Pflügers Arch* 433: 403–412.

Yamamoto, Y. and Suzuki, H. 1996. Two types of stretch-activated channel activities in guinea-pig gastric smooth muscle cells. *Jpn J Physiol* 46: 337–345.

Yamazaki, J. and Hume, J.R. 1997. Inhibitory effects of glibenclamide on cystic fibrosis transmembrane regulator, swelling-activated, and $Ca^{2+}$-activated Cl⁻ channels in mammalian cardiac myocytes. *Circ Res* 81: 101–109.

Yokoshiki, H., Sunagawa, M., Seki, T., and Sperelakis, N. 1998. ATP-sensitive $K^+$ channels in pancreatic, cardiac, and vascular smooth muscle cells. *Am J Physiol* 274: C25–C37.

Yokoshiki, H., Sunagawa, M., Seki, T., and Sperelakis, N. 1999. Antisense oligodeoxynucleotides of sulfonylurea receptors inhibit ATP-sensitive $K^+$ channels in cultured neonatal rat ventricular cells. *Pflügers Arch* 437: 400–408.

Young, R.C., McLaren, M., and Ramsdell, J.S. 1995. Maitotoxin increases voltage independent chloride and sodium currents in GH4C1 rat pituitary cells. *Nat Toxins* 3: 419–427.

Yu, M., Zhang, L., Rishi, A.K., Khadeer, M., Inesi, G., and Hussain, A. 1998. Specific substitutions at amino acid 256 of the sarcoplasmic/endoplasmic reticulum $Ca^{2+}$ transport ATPase mediate resistance to thapsigargin in thapsigargin-resistant hamster cells. *J Biol Chem* 273: 3542–3546.

Zhang, J., Rasmusson, R.L., Hall, S.K., and Lieberman, M. 1993. A chloride current associated with swelling of cultured chick heart cells. *J Physiol* 472: 801–820.

Zygmunt, A.C. and Gibbons, W.R. 1991. Calcium-activated chloride current in rabbit ventricular myocytes. *Circ Res* 68: 424–437.

# 12

# CARDIOTOXICITY OF ANTHRACYCLINES AND OTHER ANTINEOPLASTIC AGENTS

*Jane Pruemer*

*University of Cincinnati College of Pharmacy,*
*Department of Pharmacy Services, The University Hospital,*
*Cincinnati, OH, USA*

The treatment of malignant disease with antineoplastic agents has become more widespread with the availability of additional active drugs and treatment regimens. Adjuvant treatment programs attempting to eradicate microscopic disease are commonplace for breast, colon, osteosarcoma, and testicular tumors, and investigational in a number of other solid tumors. Neoadjuvant chemotherapy programs preceding definitive local treatment are now used in the therapy of locally advanced breast cancer, osteosarcomas, head and neck tumors, and, in some cases, non-small-cell lung cancer. Patients with advanced testicular tumors, small-cell lung cancer, lymphomas, myeloma, and leukemias can experience prolonged survival and, in some cases, are cured with chemotherapy as the primary treatment. Many patients with metastatic and/or advanced disease will receive successful palliative treatment with antineoplastics. The gains of these treatment programs are not without risks of complications because of the toxic nature of the agents used. Late abnormalities of left ventricular performance have been reported in survivors of childhood cancers (Hancock *et al.*, 1993; Lipshultz *et al.*, 1995; Sorensen *et al.*, 1997; Nysom *et al.*, 1998). Late cardiotoxicity has been observed in bone marrow transplant patients who received anthracyclines (Lele *et al.*, 1996). Cardiac failure and dysrhythmias have occurred from 6 to 19 years after anthracycline therapy in some patients (Steinherz *et al.*, 1995). This chapter is a review of the cardiotoxic effects of the commonly used anthracyclines, a discussion of possible mechanisms of action and prevention, as well as additional discussion of other antineoplastics with cardiotoxic effects.

## Anthracyclines

### *Doxorubicin and daunorubicin*

The anthracyclines doxorubicin and daunorubicin are among the most widely used antineoplastics, with established response rates in leukemias as well as in a variety of solid tumors (Blum *et al.*, 1974; Young *et al.*, 1981). Daunorubicin has the more limited spectrum of activity, primarily being used in acute leukemias. Three distinct types of anthracycline-induced cardiotoxicity have been described. First, acute or subacute injury can occur immediately after treatment. This rare form of cardiotoxicity may cause transient arrhythmias (Lenaz and Page, 1976; Steinberg *et al.*, 1987), a pericarditis–myocarditis syndrome, or acute failure of the left ventricle (Ferrans, 1978). Second, anthracyclines can induce chronic cardiotoxicity that results in cardiomyopathy. This is a more common form of damage and is clinically the most important (Von Hoff *et al.*, 1977; Bristow *et al.*, 1978b; Friedman *et al.*, 1978). Finally, late-onset ventricular dysfunction (Haq *et al.*, 1985; Schwartz *et al.*, 1987; Steinherz *et al.*, 1991) and arrhythmias (Lipshultz *et al.*, 1991; Yeung *et al.*, 1991; Larsen *et al.*, 1992) that manifest years to decades after anthracycline treatment has been completed are increasingly being recognized.

Electrocardiographic changes noted in association with the administration of the anthracyclines include ST–T wave changes, sinus tachycardia, ventricular and atrial ectopy, atrial tachyarrhythmia, and low voltage QRS complex (Minow *et al.*, 1975; Von Hoff *et al.*, 1977; Praga *et al.*, 1979). The most common electrocardiogram (EKG) finding noted in studies using continuous electrographic recording devices is ventricular ectopy (Freiss *et al.*, 1985; Steinberg *et al.*, 1987). In general, EKG changes are reversible and of little clinical consequence; however, cardiac arrest, presumably due to a dysrhythmia, has been reported (Wortman *et al.*, 1979).

The more serious toxicity of the anthracyclines and their dose-limiting effect is a dose-dependent cardiomyopathy. The overall incidence of cardiomyopathy has ranged from 0.4 to 10 percent, with an associated mortality rate of 28–61 percent (Halazun *et al.*, 1974; LaFrak *et al.*, 1975; Minow *et al.*, 1975; Von Hoff *et al.*, 1979). Based on a number of studies, the onset of symptoms of congestive heart failure (CHF) following the last dose of anthracycline ranged from 2 days to 10.3 years (Von Hoff *et al.*, 1979; Freter *et al.*, 1986; Lipshultz *et al.*, 1991). One study (Minow *et al.*, 1975) reported a shorter median time (25 days) to CHF in fatal cases than in non-fatal cases (56 days).

Risk factors for the development of anthracycline cardiomyopathy have been identified. For both doxorubicin and daunorubicin, a dose–response relationship exists between the total dose of anthracycline and the development of CHF. Initial studies reporting doxorubicin cardiotoxicity identified a dose of 600 mg m$^{-2}$ as the cardiotoxic threshold above which CHF was more likely to occur (Bonadonna *et al.*, 1975; Cortes *et al.*, 1975). In large retrospective reviews of over 4000 patients, Von Hoff and colleagues identified an increasing probability of developing CHF as the dose of the anthracycline was increased. The cumulative probability of developing CHF with doxorubicin was 3 percent at 400 mg m$^{-2}$ and 7 percent at 550 mg m$^{-2}$. The greatest increase in the slope of the curve was noted at the 550 mg m$^{-2}$ total dose level (Von Hoff *et al.*, 1979) (Figure 12.1). For daunorubicin, the incidence of CHF at 600 mg m$^{-2}$ was 1.5 percent, with an increase to 12 percent

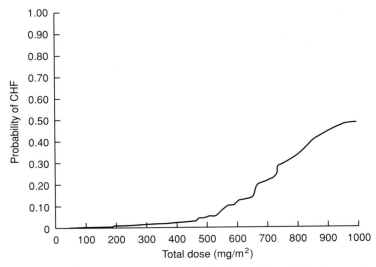

*Figure 12.1* Cumulative probability of developing doxorubicin-induced congestive heart failure (CHF) versus total cumulative dose of doxorubicin in 3941 patients receiving doxorubicin. Reproduced with permission from Von Hoff *et al.* (1979).

at a total dose of 1000 mg m$^{-2}$ (Von Hoff *et al.*, 1977). More recently, a study of escalating doses of doxorubicin in patients with advanced breast cancer noted significant decreases in left ventricular function by radionuclide multigated blood pool scans (MUGA) at a mean dose of 459 mg m$^{-2}$ (SD + 165 mg m$^{-2}$) (Jones *et al.*, 1987). These data continue to support an approximate dose of 550 mg m$^{-2}$ as a threshold for increased risk for the development of cardiotoxicity, as identified by Von Hoff and colleagues.

The schedule of doxorubicin administration has been shown to influence the incidence of both drug-induced non-cardiac as well as cardiac toxicity. Multiple studies have shown that weekly administration or prolonged infusions of doxorubicin decrease the incidence of drug-induced cardiomyopathy without sacrificing efficacy (Weiss *et al.*, 1976; Chlebowski *et al.*, 1979; Legha *et al.*, 1982; Lum *et al.*, 1985; Gundersen *et al.*, 1986). Other risk factors frequently mentioned for the development of anthracycline-induced CHF include advanced age of the patient (Bristow *et al.*, 1978a; Von Hoff *et al.*, 1979), pre-existing cardiac disease (Cortes *et al.*, 1975; Minow *et al.*, 1975), prior mediastinal radiation (Cortes *et al.*, 1975; Merrill *et al.*, 1975; Minow *et al.*, 1975), and concomitant administration of other cytotoxic agents (Kushner *et al.*, 1975; Minow *et al.*, 1975; Smith *et al.*, 1977; Buzdar *et al.*, 1978; Praga *et al.*, 1979; Watts, 1991).

Prospective evaluation of cardiac function during treatment with anthracyclines has become standard practice. Non-invasive methods in use include serial EKGs for change in QRS voltage (Minow *et al.*, 1977), rest and exercise radionuclide angiography for measurement of left ventricular ejection fraction (Singer *et al.*, 1978; Alexander *et al.*, 1979; Palmeri *et al.*, 1986), exercise and Doppler echocardiographic analysis of left ventricular function (Bloom *et al.*, 1978; Marchandise *et al.*, 1989; Weesner *et al.*, 1991), and QRS–Korotkoff interval (Greco, 1978). The gold standard for measurement of cardiac damage due to anthracyclines is endomyocardial biopsy with the designated pathologic changes, rated 1–3, correlating with the degree of toxicity. A pathologic score of 0 denotes no changes; 1 denotes early myofibrillar drop out and/or swelling of the sarcoplasmic reticulum; 2 reveals progressive myofibrillar drop out with cytoplasmic vacuolization, or both; 3 reveals diffuse myocyte damage with marked cellular changes in mitochondria, nuclei, and sarcoplasmic reticulum, and cell necrosis (Billingham *et al.*, 1977). Despite some evidence of lack of correlation between cardiac biopsy scores and radionuclide measurement of left ventricular ejection fraction, of the non-invasive methods radionuclide angiography appears to be the most practical and reliable method of serial assessment of cardiac function (Marshall *et al.*, 1978; Ewer *et al.*, 1984). Recommendations for discontinuation of anthracycline therapy include ejection fractions (EFs) less than 45 percent at rest, failure to increase the EF with exercise, or greater than 10 percent decrease from a normal pretreatment level (Piver *et al.*, 1985; Steinberg and Wasserman, 1985; Palmeri *et al.*, 1986).

The actual mechanism of anthracycline cardiotoxicity remains elusive. No single theory adequately explains or integrates our current understanding of the clinical, biochemical, and molecular effects of these agents on cardiac structure and function. Similarly, the cytotoxicity of the anthracyclines has undergone extensive scrutiny over the years. A variety of biochemical effects are known, including inhibition of nucleic acid metabolism as a result of intercalation with DNA, chelation of transition metal ions, participation in oxidation–reduction reactions, and binding to cell membranes (Pigram *et al.*, 1972; Murphree *et al.*, 1976; Sinha, 1980). Unfortunately, the precise mechanism of the cytotoxic action of anthracyclines has yet to be defined. There is emerging evidence, however, that the cytotoxic/anti-tumor effect may be related to the activation of topoisomerase II-mediated DNA cleavage rather than the DNA intercalation itself (Tewey *et al.*, 1984).

The ultrastructural changes seen with anthracycline therapy are well documented and reproducible in a variety of laboratory animals as well as in humans (Janke, 1974; Meyers *et al.*, 1977; Billingham, 1979; Singal *et al.*, 1985). As mentioned earlier, these changes reveal several cellular abnormalities linking myofibrillar loss and cytoplasmic vacuolization due to swelling of the sarcotubular system, structural abnormalities in the mitochondria with deposits of electron-dense bodies, and increased numbers of lysosomes (Olson *et al.*, 1974; Ferrans, 1978).

Multiple researchers have attempted to explain the ultrastructural changes seen in myocardial cells after treatment with anthracyclines in terms of a unifying theory of action. There are several leading hypotheses of anthracycline cardiotoxicity. These include (1) free radical formation with subsequent membrane damage and interference with energy metabolism; (2) interference with calcium metabolism; (3) the effect of histamine and other catecholamines; and (4) toxicity due to a cardiotoxic metabolite.

Free radical formation by doxorubicin and the resulting cardiac DNA and membrane damage have been extensively studied and considered critical in the evolution of anthracycline-induced cardiotoxicity (Meyers *et al.*, 1977; Doroshow, 1983; Rajagopalan *et al.*, 1988). The quinone-containing anthracyclines (doxorubicin, daunorubicin, epirubicin) were first noted to produce free radicals in the mid-1970s. Under aerobic conditions such as those in the myocardium, the quinone can be reduced to a free radical (semiquinone) by several electron-donating enzyme systems, such as NADPH and cytochrome P450 reductase and NADH dehydrogenase. The semiquinone free radicals subsequently react with molecular oxygen to form superoxide, hydrogen peroxide, and hydroxyl radicals and, in turn, result in lipid peroxidation of cell membranes with continued generation of additional free radicals. Interaction with and damage to the cell membrane then influences cell permeability and function. The generation of these free radicals with accumulation of lipid peroxides is well documented (Meyers *et al.*, 1977; Singal and Pierce, 1986). In addition, it is clear that free radical formation occurs at a variety of sites including the cytosol, mitochondria, and sarcoplasmic reticulum and possibly explains the ultrastructural lesions commonly seen (Doroshow, 1988). Free radicals also impair sequestration of calcium by the sarcoplasmic reticulum and ultimately may result in decreased calcium stores, resulting in impaired contractility and relaxation of cardiac muscle (Abramson and Salama, 1988; Olson and Muslin, 1990). Increased calcium influx and myocardial calcium content have also been described in treatment with doxorubicin (Olson *et al.*, 1974; Azuma *et al.*, 1981). Free radicals may also be generated by non-enzymatic reactions of iron with doxorubicin with similar consequences. Although little free iron is present within the myocardium, there is evidence that doxorubicin can abstract iron from ferritin (Zweier *et al.*, 1986).

Interference with calcium metabolism may be a direct result of effects on cellular membranes rather than on the inciting event in anthracycline-induced cardiotoxicity. Early on, it was thought that increased levels of intracellular calcium were responsible for mitochondria dysfunction, with resultant depletion of high-energy phosphate stores and contractile dysfunction. The electron-dense bodies seen in mitochondria were found to contain calcium (Singal *et al.*, 1983). Accumulation of calcium was well documented *in vivo* in mitochondria in a variety of organs in the rabbit treated with chronic administration of doxorubicin (Olson *et al.*, 1974; Revis and Marusic, 1979). Recent data, however, point more toward an initial deficiency of intracellular calcium and its resultant effects on calcium flux and muscle contraction (Jensen, 1986). Studies with combinations of calcium channel-blocking drugs thought to prevent calcium accumulation with anthracycline treatment have provided conflicting data regarding their influence on cardiotoxic effects (Suzuki *et al.*, 1979; Rabkin, 1983; Maisch *et al.*, 1985).

Another theory of anthracycline cardiotoxicity revolves around the involvement of histamine and other vasoactive substances as causative agents. Support for this theory comes from experiments examining histopathologic lesions produced in rabbits after histamine infusions, which were found to be similar to doxorubicin-induced lesions (Bristow *et al.*, 1983). These same authors were able to show that histamine release was stimulated *in vitro* by doxorubicin. Additional studies by others have supported these findings as well as documented prevention of histamine release with the use of inhibitors such as theophylline and disodium cromoglycate and with the free radical scavenger *N*-acetylcysteine, which was also found to inhibit the release of histamine (Klugman *et al.*, 1986). Klugman and colleagues also noted the absence of typical histopathologic cardiac lesions in the animals treated with the inhibitors.

The possibility of a metabolite of doxorubicin as the offending cardiotoxic agent has also been previously suggested (Del Tacca *et al.*, 1985; Boucek *et al.*, 1987; Olson *et al.*, 1988). Olson and colleagues compared the *in vitro* cardiotoxic effects of doxorubicin and doxorubicinol, the carbon-13 alcohol metabolite of doxorubicin. In their study, doxorubicinol was found to be a more potent inhibitor of contractile function, of membrane-associated ion pumps, and greatly decreased calcium loading within the sarcoplasmic reticulum vesicles. In addition, the authors noted intracardiac conversion of doxorubicin to doxorubicinol, further supporting previous evidence of accumulation in cardiac tissue in a time-dependent fashion (Peters *et al.*, 1981; Del Tacca *et al.*, 1985). Of interest, these authors found that doxorubicin maintained greater cytotoxicity in three pancreatic adenocarcinoma cell lines over the metabolite, suggesting separation of cytotoxic and cardiotoxic effects.

## Cardioprotectants

Perhaps one of the more enlightening aspects providing some insight into mechanisms of cardiotoxicity has been the various agents tested to prevent cardiac toxicity. These agents include coenzyme Q (Cortes, 1978), *N*-acetylcysteine (NAC) (Doroshow *et al.*, 1981), prenylamine (Milei *et al.*, 1987), and the bispiperazinedione ICRF-187 (Speyer *et al.*, 1992), which is now known as dexrazoxane and is FDA approved for the prevention of anthracylcine-induced cardiotoxicity. Inhibition of coenzyme Q ($CoQ_{10}$), a mitochondrial enzyme involved in oxidative phosphorylation, results in cardiac lesions in the rat similar to those seen with doxorubicin cardiotoxicity (Combs *et al.*, 1976). Investigators described the prevention of experimental cardiotoxicity by doxorubicin with the addition of $CoQ_{10}$ (ubiquinone) in the isolated rabbit heart model (Bertazzoli *et al.*, 1975a). These same investigators administered ubiquinone to rabbits and were able to demonstrate prevention of doxorubicin cardiotoxicity *in vivo* (Bertazzoli *et al.*, 1975b). More recently, $CoQ_{10}$ has been studied for its therapeutic effect in dilated cardiomyopathy, with evidence of efficacy (Langsjoen *et al.*, 1990).

Prenylamine is a calcium channel-blocking agent that has undergone investigation in Argentina. After obtaining laboratory evidence of cardioprotection in animals, investigators proceeded with a small randomized trial in patients (Milei *et al.*, 1987, 1988). Cardiotoxicity as evidenced by congestive cardiomyopathy and supraventricular dysrhythmia was seen in the untreated patients. There were no cardiac events in the group treated with prenylamine. As mentioned earlier, other studies have not revealed a benefit with the use of other calcium channel blockers.

N-Acetylcysteine (NAC) is a sulfhydryl compound shown in mice to confer cardiac protection from doxorubicin treatment theoretically through increased sulfhydryl content in the heart (Doroshow *et al.*, 1981). However, when a randomized trial with the oral form was conducted in cancer patients, treatment with NAC did not confer significant cardioprotection (Myers *et al.*, 1983).

Of all these agents, only dexrazoxane has been studied in a randomized, prospective fashion and has shown consistent evidence of modulating cardiotoxicity due to anthracyclines (Speyer *et al.*, 1992).

### Dexrazoxane (Zinecard$^{TM}$)

Dexrazoxane, previously known as ICRF-187, is an iron-chelating agent whose chelating properties were first noted during phase I testing of the compound as an antineoplastic agent (Von Hoff *et al.*, 1981). Anthracycline cardiotoxicity is thought to be prevented by the binding of dexrazoxane to ferrous ions at intracellular sites that would normally complex with doxorubicin. It is the iron–doxorubicin complex that is thought to be responsible for the generation of free radicals, with the subsequent cascade of events leading to cardiac damage (Meyers *et al.*, 1977; Hasinoff, 1990).

Dexrazoxane was studied extensively in women with advanced breast cancer receiving doxorubicin as well as epirubicin therapy (Speyer *et al.*, 1992; Venturi *et al.*, 1996; Swain *et al.*, 1997). Dexrazoxane has a significant cardioprotectant effect, as measured by non-invasive testing and clinical CHF when given with doxorubicin, but has been implicated in causing a lower response rate than doxorubicin alone (Swain *et al.*, 1997). For this reason, many clinicians are reluctant to utilize this agent in patients who are responding to anthracycline therapy. The FDA has approved the agent for use in women with metastatic breast cancer who have previously received a total of 300 mg m$^{-2}$ of doxorubicin and who are continuing to respond to therapy. It is not approved for use in the adjuvant treatment of breast cancer. Dexrazoxane has also been studied in the prevention of cardiotoxicity associated with epirubicin (Lopez *et al.*, 1998).

In summary, there are several theories of the mechanism of anthracycline cardiotoxicity without an all-encompassing theory to explain the myriad properties and effects of this class of antineoplastic agent. Further investigation and elucidation are required and are ongoing. Dexrazoxane continues to show promise as a clinically useful agent in the prevention of doxorubicin cardiotoxicity.

### Liposomal doxorubicin and liposomal daunorubicin

More recently, doxorubicin has been administered to patients in a liposome-encapsulated form with a suggestion of less cardiac toxicity, as determined by radionuclide ejection fraction and, in a few patients, Billingham score on endomyocardial biopsy (Balazsovits *et al.*, 1989; Treat *et al.*, 1990). Liposomal doxorubicin has been studied extensively in the treatment of acquired immune deficiency syndrome (AIDS)-associated Kaposi's sarcoma (Wagner *et al.*, 1994; Harrison *et al.*, 1995), as well as in the treatment of refractory ovarian cancer. Liposomal daunorubicin is approved for the treatment of human immunodeficiency virus (HIV)-associated Kaposi's sarcoma with similar potential for cardiac effects.

### Anthracycline analogs

Over 1000 anthracycline derivatives have been synthesized with the hope of retaining therapeutic efficacy with less toxicity of both myelosuppression and cardiotoxicity (Weiss *et al.*, 1986a). Studies of correlations between structure and activity demonstrate that changes at the 4' position of the amino sugar moiety affect toxicity and indicate that cardiotoxicity can be separated from therapeutic effect (Casazza, 1979). Only compounds with cytotoxicity that preclinically is at least equal to doxorubicin are then tested further to ascertain their toxicity profile. Determining whether these analogs are beneficial and less toxic than doxorubicin continues to be an active area of investigation. The following briefly reviews the cardiotoxicity seen with several of the compounds in clinical use or undergoing clinical evaluation (Figure 12.2).

### Esorubicin (4'-deoxydoxorubicin)

Esorubicin is an anthracycline analog synthesized by the removal of the hydroxyl group from the 4' carbon of the sugar moiety of the parent compound doxorubicin. Recent follow-up of 136 patients treated with esorubicin on one of two Cancer and Leukemia Group B phase II protocols has been reported (Ringenberg *et al.*, 1990). Serial MUGA scans were obtained in thirty-six of forty-four patients who received more than four cycles of therapy. Decreases in left ventricular ejection fraction of more than 5 percent were noted at doses of 240 mg m$^{-2}$ and of more than 10 percent at doses of 480 mg m$^{-2}$. Overall, cardiotoxicity was observed in eleven patients (8 percent) without previous anthracycline or history of cardiovascular disease. The cardiotoxicity described included overt congestive heart failure asymptomatic decreases in left ventricular ejection fraction, sinus tachycardia, and one myocardial infarction.

### 4'-Epidoxorubicin

Epirubicin is a stereoisomer of doxorubicin with a different configuration of the hydroxyl group in the 4' position of the sugar moiety. Cardiotoxicity similar in scope to that reported for doxorubicin has been reported with epirubicin. In two studies of patients with advanced breast cancer without prior treatment with an anthracycline, congestive heart failure was reported in four patients who received

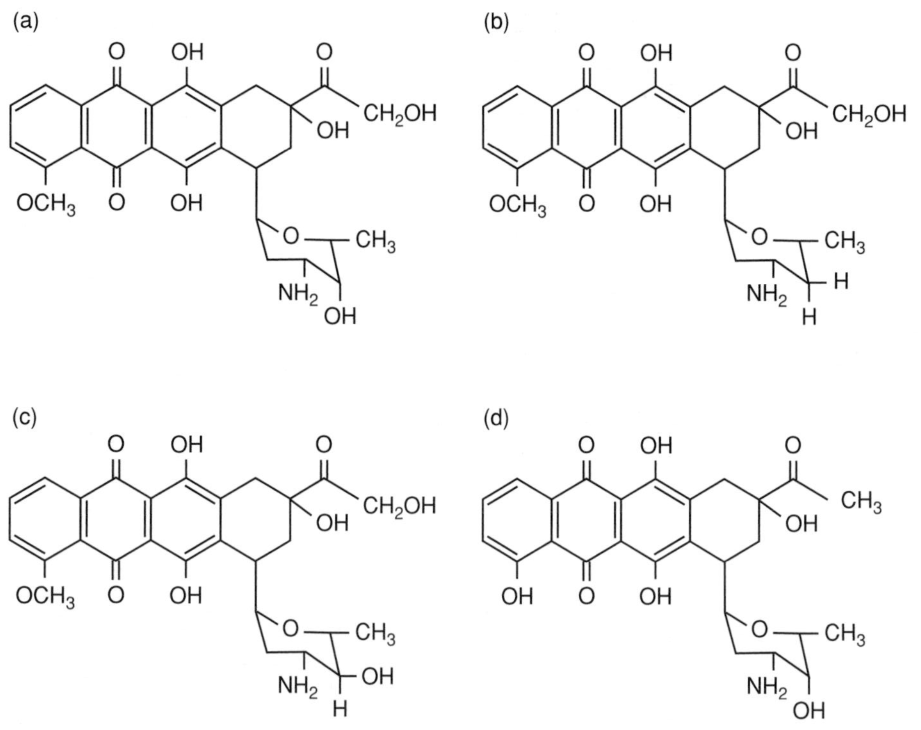

*Figure 12.2* Anthracyclines. (a) Doxorubicin. (b) Epirubicin. (c) Esorubicin. (d) Idarubicin.

cumulative doses of epirubicin greater that 1000 mg m$^{-2}$ (Jain *et al.*, 1985) and in one patient who received a total dose of 797 mg m$^{-2}$ (Havsteen *et al.*, 1989). There have been several studies reported that have included endomyocardial biopsies as part of the evaluation documenting cardiotoxicity due to epirubicin (Dardir *et al.*, 1989; Macchiarini *et al.*, 1990; Nielsen *et al.*, 1990). In all these studies, the type and severity of histologic abnormalities were similar to those seen with doxorubicin and correlated with increasing doses of epirubicin. Dardir and colleagues noted a statistically significant correlation ($P = 0.0006$) between the total dose of epirubicin and pathologic changes quantified by the use of the Billingham scale (Myers *et al.*, 1983). In one study, doses smaller than 500 mg m$^{-2}$ were not associated with cardiotoxicity. However, at doses of 500–1000 mg m$^{-2}$, 2 percent of the patients developed congestive heart failure, with an increase to 35 percent of the patients developing congestive heart failure at cumulative doses greater than 1000 mg m$^{-2}$ (Von Hoff *et al.*, 1981).

Nair and colleagues evaluated the efficacy and toxicity of epirubicin and doxorubicin in 211 patients with non-Hodgkin's lymphoma. In their study, the maximum dose of epirubicin was 480 mg m$^{-2}$ (75 mg m$^{-2}$ per dose) and that of doxorubicin was 300 mg m$^{-2}$ (50 mg m$^{-2}$ per dose). The MUGA scan indicated a similar reduction in the global EF, peak ejection, and peak flow rates in the two arms. Thus, epirubicin was found to have the same cardiotoxicity at the subclinical level as doxorubicin (Nair *et al.*, 1998). This was supported by a retrospective analysis of epirubicin cardiotoxicity in 469 patients with metastatic breast cancer (Ryberg *et al.*, 1998). This analysis confirmed a significantly increasing risk of CHF in patients who receive cumulative doses greater than 950 mg m$^{-2}$ of epirubicin.

### Idarubicin (4-demethoxydaunorubicin)

Idarubicin differs from the parent compound doxorubicin in substitution of the C-4 methoxyl group with a hydrogen atom. During phase I testing with the agents, the significant cardiotoxicity described was limited to patients who had received previous treatment with anthracyclines. Therefore, postulating a direct cause and effect was not possible (Berman *et al.*, 1983; Daghestani *et al.*, 1985; Tan *et al.*, 1987). The cardiotoxicity described ranged from asymptomatic EKG changes to overt congestive heart failure requiring therapy and discontinuation of the idarubicin. In phase II studies, decreases in left ventricular ejection fraction without clinical signs of cardiac failure were seen infrequently and were limited to patients who had received prior anthracyclines (Kris *et al.*, 1985; Martoni *et al.*, 1985; Chisesi *et al.*, 1988; Gillies *et al.*, 1988; Villani *et al.*, 1989). In these studies, cumulative doses of 800 mg m$^{-2}$ orally and 169 mg m$^{-2}$ intravenously were tolerated without signs of clinical congestive heart failure.

Anderlini and colleagues performed a retrospective review of idarubicin cardiotoxicity in patients with acute myeloid leukemia or myelodysplasia. They analyzed a group of 127 patients who had received idarubicin-based induction and post-remission or salvage therapy and who achieved a complete remission. They determined the probability of idarubicin-related cardiomyopathy was 5 percent at a cumulative idarubicin dose of 150–290 mg m$^{-2}$ and that cardiomyopathy was uncommon with cumulative doses greater than this (Anderlini *et al.*, 1995).

## *Mitoxantrone (Novantrone$^{TM}$)*

Mitoxantrone, a substituted anthraquinone, was developed in an attempt to achieve similar anti-tumor activity to the anthracyclines but with less toxicity. Despite modifications, mitoxantrone has been reported to have cardiac effects, although on a lesser scale than the anthracyclines. Described cardiac toxicity includes decreases in left ventricular ejection fraction (LVEF) and congestive heart failure (Shenkenberg and Von Hoff, 1986). Dysrhythmias have been noted infrequently (Gams and Wesler, 1984). In a large series including a randomized study comparing cyclophosphamide, doxorubicin, and 5-fluorouracil with cyclophosphamide, mitoxantrone, and 5-fluorouracil in patients with metastatic breast cancer, the incidence of congestive heart failure was less than 2 percent (Berman *et al.*, 1983; Clark *et al.*, 1984; Bennett *et al.*, 1988). The majority of patients experiencing congestive heart failure have received more than 120 mg m$^{-2}$ of mitoxantrone, but similar toxicity has been reported at lower doses in patients both with and without prior exposure to an anthracycline (Coleman *et al.*, 1982; Schell *et al.*, 1982; Daghestani *et al.*, 1985). Treatment of CHF related to mitoxantrone therapy usually responds to management with digoxin, diuretics, and discontinuation of mitoxantrone, with the possibility of eventual return to a baseline cardiac status (Martoni *et al.*, 1985). A small number of endomyocardial biopsies have been carried out and revealed changes consistent with anthracycline-induced cardiomyopathy (Aapro *et al.*, 1983; Unverferth *et al.*, 1984). Predisposing factors to mitoxantrone cardiotoxicity include prior anthracycline therapy, mediastinal irradiation, and prior cardiovascular disease; prior anthracycline therapy is the most important factor (Crossley, 1984). In patients previously treated with anthracyclines, the incidence of CHF is negligible up to doses of 100 mg m$^{-2}$. In patients without previous treatment with anthracyclines, doses up to 160 mg m$^{-2}$ appear to be tolerated without significant cardiotoxicity (Posner *et al.*, 1985). Careful monitoring of cardiac ejection fraction at cumulative doses greater than 100 mg m$^{-2}$ is recommended, especially in those at risk for development of cardiac toxicity. Toxicology studies performed in beagle dogs did not reveal clinical manifestations of CHF or EKG changes (Henderson *et al.*, 1982). Abnormalities on endomyocardial biopsies in dogs were limited to dilatation of the sarcoplasmic reticulum (Sparano *et al.*, 1982). In one study, mitoxantrone was shown to be an antioxidant inhibiting both basal and drug-induced peroxidation of lipids (Kharasch and Novak, 1982). It follows that as lipid peroxidation is important in the development of cardiotoxicity of anthracyclines and anthracycline-like drugs mitoxantrone theoretically has the potential for causing less cardiotoxicity. To date, this has also been shown to be the case clinically.

# Other anti-tumor agents

## Cyclophosphamide

Severe hemorrhagic cardiac necrosis has been reported in the transplant setting at doses of 120–240 mg kg$^{-1}$ given over 1–4 days (O'Connell and Berenbaum, 1974; Applebaum et al., 1976; Goldberg et al., 1986). The presenting symptoms are tachycardia and refractory congestive heart failure. EKG changes reveal sinus tachycardia, low-voltage QRS complex, ST segment elevation, and non-specific ST–T wave changes. Left ventricular systolic function, as assessed by echocardiographic fractional shortening, has been shown to be significantly decreased from baseline in patients with and without clinical symptoms of heart failure (Gottdiener et al., 1981). Significant increases in lactate dehydrogenase (LDH) and creatine phosphokinase (CPK) suggesting myocardial damage are seen in approximately one-half of the patients. Symptoms of cardiac necrosis may not become evident until 2 weeks after dosing, but are rapidly fatal when present (Slavin et al., 1975). Pathologic findings at autopsy include dilated heart, patchy transmural hemorrhages, focal areas of fibrinous pericarditis and myocardial necrosis, and interstitial lesions consisting of hemorrhage, edema, and fibrin deposition (Crossley, 1984; Unverferth et al., 1984). There are emerging data that the intracellular thiol glutathione may play a role in the protection against cardiac injury caused by cyclophosphamide (Friedman et al., 1990).

There is some evidence that cyclophosphamide in combination with other agents, particularly carmustine (BCNU), 6-thioguanine, cytosine arabinoside, and total body irradiation, may be more cardiotoxic than cyclophosphamide alone (Trigg et al., 1987). In one study, four of fifteen patients died of acute myopericarditis using the combination of BCNU, cyclophosphamide, 6-thioguanine, and cytosine arabinoside (Coleman et al., 1982). Another study reported a 9 percent incidence of fatal cardiomyopathy and/or pericarditis with this same combination or high-dose cyclophosphamide and total body irradiation (Cazin et al., 1986). An additional 22 percent of patients experienced non-fatal congestive heart failure. The majority of patients in each of these studies had received prior anthracyclines, possibly compounding their risk of developing cardiotoxicity from these regimens.

A more recent study has evaluated the cardiotoxicity of cyclophosphamide in a twice-daily higher dose compared with a lower daily dose schedule (Braverman et al., 1991). Left ventricular ejection fractions did not change significantly in either group; however, four of the five patients who developed clinical cardiotoxicity (four pericarditis and one congestive heart failure) were in the higher dose group. The conclusion of the authors was that the twice-daily dosing schedule, although not completely without cardiotoxicity, resulted in less ventricular dysfunction. As more experience is gained in bone marrow transplantation, it will be important to identify regimens and dosing schedules that allow for efficacy without excessive toxicity.

## Cisplatin

Cisplatin, a bifunctional alkylating agent with a broad spectrum of activity, is associated with rare reports of cardiotoxicity. Cisplatin-induced bradycardia (Schlaeffer *et al.*, 1983) and paroxysmal supraventricular tachycardia have also been reported (Hashimi *et al.*, 1984; Fassio *et al.*, 1986). Ischemic vascular events with myocardial infarctions in young patients with and without mediastinal radiation who were treated with cisplatin-based combination chemotherapy are among the most serious toxicities reported with the agent (Doll *et al.*, 1986; Talcott and Herman, 1987). Coronary artery spasm was documented in one patient at cardiac catheterization in the absence of atherosclerotic disease. Two cases of severe coronary artery atherosclerosis and one case of fibrous intimal proliferation in young males with testicular cancer after cisplatin-based chemotherapy have been documented (Edwards *et al.*, 1979; Bodensteiner, 1981). None of the patients was considered to have had significant risk factors for coronary artery disease; only one patient had received thoracic irradiation.

## 5-Fluorouracil (5-FU)

The reported incidence of cardiac side-effects with 5-fluorouracil (5-FU), a widely used antimetabolite, is low at approximately 1.6 percent (La Bianca *et al.*, 1982). However, with high-dose continuous infusion 5-FU, the incidence has been reported to be as high as 7.6 percent (de Forni *et al.*, 1992). Angina with ischemic EKG changes is the most frequent cardiac toxicity noted. The first reports of chest pain associated with ischemic EKG changes in patients receiving 5-FU occurred in 1975. All three patients failed to have subsequent evidence of a myocardial infarction; EKG abnormalities resolved with discontinuation of the drug (Dent and McCall, 1975). Ischemic EKG changes, left ventricular dysfunction, and hypotension with dyspnea associated with infusions of 5-FU alone and in combination with cisplatin have been reported previously (Jakubowski and Kemeny, 1988; Rezkalla *et al.*, 1989). Severe but reversible heart failure with global hypokinesis and cardiogenic shock has been reported in association with continuous infusions of 5-FU (Chaudary *et al.*, 1988; McKendall *et al.*, 1988; Martin *et al.*, 1989). Extensive cardiac evaluations have been performed in a small number of these patients without documentation of significant coronary artery disease or clear evidence of vasospasm (Slavin *et al.*, 1975; Collins and Weiden, 1987; Freeman and Constanza, 1988; Ensley *et al.*, 1989; Trigg *et al.*, 1987; Friedman *et al.*, 1990). The episodes of severe heart failure and cardiogenic shock resolved with aggressive support following discontinuation of the 5-FU infusion in most reported cases. Conflicting evidence exists regarding the efficacy of nitrates and/or calcium channel-blocking agents in preventing anginal episodes, which suggests that mechanisms other than coronary vasospasm may be involved in the cardiac effects of 5-fluorouracil (Kleiman *et al.*, 1987; Patel *et al.*, 1987; Oleksowicz and Bruckner, 1988). Myocardial infarctions have been reported in a small number of patients as well as deaths in patients refractory to supportive therapy (La Bianca *et al.*, 1982; Cazin *et al.*, 1986; Trigg *et al.*, 1987; Braverman *et al.*, 1991).

The mechanism by which 5-FU causes cardiotoxicity is unknown. Possible etiologies include vasospasm, a direct cardiotoxic effect either from 5-FU or one of its metabolites, or some other metabolic derangement leading to either an increase in metabolic demands or a decrease in the available energy to meet those demands. Comparisons have been made to the "stunned myocardium," a syndrome of reversible post-ischemic ventricular dysfunction (Braunwald and Kloner, 1982). Few animal data exist to support any particular theory at the present time. There is laboratory evidence of persistent radioactivity in the myocardium of mice injected with $^{14}$C-labeled 5-FU 96 h after injection, suggesting delayed metabolism in the heart (Liss and Chadwick, 1974). In addition, both the pharmacokinetics and the toxicity profiles of oral, bolus intravenous, and prolonged intravenous administration of 5-FU are known to differ. Lower but sustained plasma levels and less myelosuppression and greater mucositis are noted with the prolonged infusion (Fraile *et al.*, 1980). These differences may ultimately provide insight into the mechanism of 5-FU cardiotoxicity.

Today, 5-FU is often combined with leucovorin (folinic acid) in an effort to improve its anti-tumor effect. Grandi and colleagues have reported a non-invasive evaluation of the cardiotoxicity of this combination in patients with colorectal cancer. They evaluated blood pressure, EKG, and two-dimensional and digitized M-mode echocardiograms before and after several doses and cycles of the combination. They concluded that 5-FU and low-dose folinic acid treatment induced a decrease in LV systolic function and an impairment of diastolic function, which developed without symptoms, were transient and reversible (Grandi *et al.*, 1997).

### Cytosine arabinoside (Ara-C)

Cytarabine, a nucleoside analog effective in treating acute leukemia, rarely causes cardiotoxicity. There are, however, case reports of a cardiac dysrhythmia (Willemze *et al.*, 1982) and acute pericarditis (Vaickus and Letendre, 1984) encountered during high-dose therapy. At the time of the pericarditis, the patient was in complete clinical remission from acute lymphocytic leukemia. Pericardial fluid analysis was negative for tumor or an infectious agent. No evidence of myocardial damage either clinically or by laboratory studies was noted during the episode of pericarditis.

### Paclitaxel (Taxol$^{TM}$)

Paclitaxel, a taxane derived from the Pacific yew tree, has become a major agent in the treatment of breast cancer, ovarian cancer, and non-small-cell lung cancer. In the early clinical development of paclitaxel, the drug was recognized to have a unique toxicity profile. In addition to the more routine side-effects observed with antineoplastic agents (bone marrow suppression, alopecia, etc.), hypersensitivity reactions were observed. Patients were also found to develop cardiac arrhythmia, particularly bradycardia, and episodes of sudden cardiac death were reported (Kris *et al.*, 1986; Rowinsky *et al.*, 1991; Rowinsky and Donehower, 1995; Shek *et al.*, 1996).

In a retrospective review of gynecologic cancer patients treated with paclitaxel with or without a platinum agent, Markman and colleagues found fifteen patients who had major cardiac risk factors before therapy. These risk factors included pre-existing congestive heart failure, severe coronary artery disease, angina, and patients who were being treated for rhythm disturbances with agents such as β-blockers. There was no deterioration in cardiac function observed in these patients subsequent to paclitaxel therapy (Markman *et al.*, 1998). It is now recognized that much of the initial concern for the cardiac effects of paclitaxel were related to severe hypersensitivity reactions, and that with appropriate premedication patients are unlikely to experience these dysrhythmias.

In the doxorubicin plus paclitaxel trials of Gianni *et al.* (1995) and Gehl *et al.* (1996), an alarming incidence of cardiac dysfunction and clinical congestive heart failure (about 20 percent) was observed. However, in the randomized phase II trial of Sledge *et al.* (1997), there was no increased incidence of cardiac toxicity in the group of patients receiving doxorubicin plus paclitaxel compared with the group receiving doxorubicin alone. It should be noted that the combination of doxorubicin plus paclitaxel used by Sledge *et al.* (1997) differed from that used by both Gianni *et al.* (1995) and Gehl *et al.* (1996) with regard to dose, duration of administration, interval between administration of doxorubicin and paclitaxel, and dose of doxorubicin. Subsequently, Gianni *et al.* (1997) studied the pharmacokinetic interference between paclitaxel and doxorubicin which results in non-linear doxorubicin plasma disposition and increased concentrations of doxorubicin and its metabolite doxorubicinol. Therefore, it is believed that the exposure of the patients to higher concentrations of doxorubicin could be responsible for the increased cardiotoxicity when given with paclitaxel.

### Amsacrine (AMSA)

This drug is an acridine orange derivative with documented activity in acute leukemia and lymphoma. Reported cardiac toxicity with this agent has included dysrhythmias (Von Hoff *et al.*, 1980; McLaughlin *et al.*, 1983; Dhaliwal *et al.*, 1986), ventricular dysfunction (Steinherz *et al.*, 1982), and acute myocardial necrosis (Lindpainter *et al.*, 1986), although the last occurred after administration of multiple drugs and in the setting of progressive disease. Significant QT prolongation may be the initial effect resulting in increased vulnerability to ventricular dysrhythmias, as noted by some authors (Weiss *et al.*, 1983; Shinar and Hasin, 1984). The presence of hypokalemia may compound the risk of developing a dysrhythmia (Fraile *et al.*, 1980; Schlaeffer *et al.*, 1983; Weiss *et al.*, 1986b). One study of heavily pretreated patients concluded that an anthracycline dose greater than 400 mg m$^{-2}$ and administration of more than 200 mg m$^{-2}$ of AMSA over 48 h were related to an increased risk of cardiac effects associated with the AMSA therapy (Weiss *et al.*, 1986a). Four of the six patients who developed clinical congestive heart failure in that study were in this high-risk group. To date, a cumulative dose effect and its relationship to cardiotoxicity have not been demonstrated for this agent (Weiss *et al.*, 1986a).

Studies in rabbits at high doses and in dogs using toxic doses of high, lethal, and supralethal doses of AMSA revealed marked effects of atrioventricular and intraventricular conduction systems (D'Alessandro *et al.*, 1983). First- and second-degree AV block, prolongation of QRS and QT intervals, ventricular premature contractions, atrial flutter, and ventricular tachycardia were among the noted effects.

## Biologics

### *Interferon*

The incidence of cardiovascular toxicity associated with interferon therapy has been in the range of 5–12 percent (Kirkwood and Ernstoff, 1984). Increasing dose, increasing age, and a prior history of cardiovascular disease appear to be risk factors for the development of cardiotoxicity with the interferons (Spiegel, 1987).

The most frequently reported cardiac toxicities are primarily hypotension and tachycardia and may be related to the febrile reaction commonly seen rather than a direct cardiotoxic effect (Quesada *et al.*, 1986). Non-fatal dysrhythmias, predominantly supraventricular tachyarrhythmias, have been described in patients receiving interferon therapy (Martino *et al.*, 1987). Early clinical trials in France were temporarily halted because of four deaths from myocardial infarctions in patients treated with interferon (Dickson, 1982). Myocardial infarctions in patients with and without prior cardiac histories have been reported previously (Sarna *et al.*, 1983; Foon *et al.*, 1984; Grunberg *et al.*, 1985; Martino *et al.*, 1987). Infrequent reports of congestive heart failure with short-term and prolonged administration of interferons have been described by Cooper *et al.* (1986), Martino *et al.* (1987), Brown *et al.* (1987), and Deyton *et al.* (1989). The report of three patients with Kaposi's sarcoma and HIV-positive status suggests a possible synergism between interferon and HIV. Post-mortem findings in one case revealed four-chamber enlargement without evidence of coronary artery disease, fibrosis, or amyloid or inflammatory infiltrates, suggesting a drug-related etiology of the cardiomyopathy (Cohen *et al.*, 1988).

Although the reports of cardiovascular toxicities with interferon treatment overall are infrequent, older patients and those with a history of previous cardiac events may be at increased risk for the development of cardiac toxicity from interferons.

## *Interleukin-2 (IL-2)/lymphokine-activated killer cells (LAK)*

Significant cardiotoxicity with interleukin-2 alone and in combination with lymphokine-activated killer cells has been documented by all centers involved in these investigations. The incidence of hypotension requiring pharmacologic support with vasopressors was 65 percent in 317 patients treated at the National Cancer Institute (NCI) (Lee *et al.*, 1989). Dysrhythmias, primarily supraventricular tachyarrhythmias, occurred in 9.7 percent of courses. Angina or ischemic changes were noted in 2.6 percent of patients and myocardial infarction in 1.5 percent. Hemodynamic changes seen in patients receiving IL-2/LAK therapy consisted of a decrease in mean arterial pressure and systemic vascular resistance with an increase in heart rate and cardiac index (Gaynor *et al.*, 1988). Cardiac dysfunction with significantly decreased stroke index and left ventricular stroke work associated with a reduction in left ventricular ejection fraction was also noted in the NCI study. Complete heart block has been documented in one patient (Vaitkus *et al.*, 1990). Severe myocarditis with lymphocytic and eosinophilic infiltrates with areas of myocardial necrosis on autopsy have been documented in one patient on high-dose IL-2 therapy (Samlowski *et al.*, 1989). The hemodynamic changes seen are consistent with those seen in early septic shock (Ognibene *et al.*, 1988). The etiology of the hypotension is thought to be due to an increase in vascular permeability (capillary leak phenomenon) leading to both a decrease in intravascular volume and a reduction in systemic vascular resistance (Foon *et al.*, 1984; Nora *et al.*, 1989). The actual mechanism by which this high-output/low-resistance state occurs is currently unknown. Leading possibilities include a direct effect of IL-2 or an indirect effect mediated by another cytokine or substance released by IL-2. Investigational studies with IL-2 in various schedules and doses are ongoing.

## Summary

Cardiotoxicity primarily due to treatment with anthracyclines continues to provide a fertile area of research for scientists and physicians. Further research is required to unravel the precise mechanism of anthracycline cardiotoxicity. The search for a less cardiotoxic but equivalent cytotoxic anthracycline analog continues to be an active focus of preclinical and clinical research. With the increasing use of antineoplastics in the treatment of malignant disease, there has been increased recognition of varied cardiac effects with multiple agents. Undoubtedly, this body of knowledge will continue to grow and result in additional research questions over the coming years.

## References

Aapro MS, Alberts DS, Woolfenden JM, Mackel C. 1983. Prospective study of left ventricular function using radionuclide scans in patients receiving mitoxantrone. *Invest New Drugs* 1: 341–347.

Abramson JJ, Salama G. 1988. Sulfhydryl oxidation and calcium release from sarcoplasmic reticulum. *Mol Cell Biochem* 82: 81–84.

Alexander J, Dainiak N, Berger HJ, *et al*. 1979. Serial assessment of doxorubicin cardiotoxicity with quantitative radionuclide angiocardiography. *N Engl J Med* 300: 278–283.

Anderlini P, Benjamin RS, Wong FC, *et al*. 1995. Idarubicin cardiotoxicity: a retrospective study in acute myeloid leukemia and myelodysplasia. *J Clin Oncol* 13: 2827–2834.

Applebaum FR, Strauchen JA, Graw Jr., GR, *et al*. 1976. Acute lethal carditis caused by high dose combination chemotherapy. *Lancet* 1: 58–62.

Azuma J, Sperelakis N, Hasegawa H, *et al*. 1981. Adriamycin cardiotoxicity: possible pathogenic mechanisms. *J Mol Cell Cardiol* 13: 381–397.

Balazsovits JAE, Mayer LD, Bally MB, *et al*. 1989. Analysis of the effect of liposome encapsulation on the vesicant properties, acute and cardiac toxicities, and antitumor efficacy of doxorubicin. *Cancer Chemother Pharmacol* 23: 81–86.

Bennett JM, Muss HD, Doroshow JH, *et al*. 1988. A randomized multicenter trial comparing mitoxantrone, cyclophosphamide, and fluorouracil in the therapy of metastatic breast carcinoma. *J Clin Oncol* 6: 1611–1620.

Berman E, Wittes RE, Leyland-Jones B, *et al*. 1983. Phase I and clinical pharmacology studies of intravenous and oral administration of 4-demethoxydaunorubicin in patients with advanced cancer. *Cancer Res* 43: 6096–6101.

Bertazzoli C, Sala L, Tosano MG. 1975a. Antagonistic action of ubiquinone on experimental cardiotoxicity of adriamycin in isolated rabbit heart. *Int Res Commun Sys Med Sci* 3: 367.

Bertazzoli C, Sala L, Socia E, Ghione M. 1975b. Experimental adriamycin cardiotoxicity prevented by ubiquinone *in vivo*. *Int Res Commun Sys Med Sci* 3: 468.

Billingham ME. 1979. Some recent advances in cardiac pathology. *Hum Pathol* 10: 367–386.

Billingham ME, Bristow MR, Glatstein E, *et al*. 1977. Adriamycin cardiotoxicity: endomyocardial biopsy evidence of enhancement by irradiation. *Am J Surg Pathol* 1: 17–23.

Bloom KR, Bini RM, Williams CM, *et al*. 1978. Echocardiography in adriamycin cardiotoxicity. *Cancer* 41: 1265–1269.

Blum RH, Carter SK. 1974. Adriamycin: a new anticancer drug with significant clinical activity. *Ann Intern Med* 80: 249–259.

Bodensteiner DC. 1981. Fatal coronary artery fibrosis after treatment with bleomycin, vincristine, and cisplatinum. *South Med J* 74: 898–899.

Bonadonna G, Beretta B, Tancini G, *et al*. 1975. Adriamycin (NSC-123127) studies at the Instituto Nazionale Tumori, Milan. *Cancer Chemother Rep* 6: 231–245.

Boucek RJ, Olson RD, Brenner DE, *et al*. 1987. The major metabolite of doxorubicin is a potent inhibitor of membrane-associated ion pumps: a correlative study of cardiac muscle with isolated membrane fractions. *J Biol Chem* 262: 15851–15856.

Braunwald E, Kloner RA. 1982. The stunned myocardium: prolonged postischemic ventricular dysfunction. *Circulation* 66: 1146–1149.

Braverman AC, Antin JH, Plappert MT, *et al*. 1991. Cyclophosphamide cardiotoxicity in bone marrow transplantation: a prospective evaluation of new dosing regimens. *J Clin Oncol* 9: 1215–1223.

Bristow MR, Mason JW, Billingham ME, Daniels JR. 1978a. Doxorubicin cardiomyopathy: evaluation by phonocardiography, endomyocardial biopsy, and cardiac catheterization. *Ann Intern Med* 88: 168–175.

Bristow MR, Billingham ME, Mason JW, Daniels JR. 1978b. Clinical spectrum of anthracycline antibiotic cardiotoxicity. *Cancer Treat Rep* 62: 873–879.

Bristow MR, Kantrowitz NE, Harrison WD, *et al.* 1983. Mediation of subacute anthracycline cardiotoxicity in rabbits by cardiac histamine release. *J Cardiovasc Pharmacol* 5: 913.

Brown TD, Koeller J, Beougher K, *et al.* 1987. A phase I clinical trial of recombinant DNA gamma interferon. *J Clin Oncol* 1987; 5: 790–798.

Buzdar AV, Legha SS, Tashima CK, *et al.* 1978. Adriamycin and mitomycin-C: possible synergistic cardiotoxicity. *Cancer Treat Rep* 62: 1005–1008.

Casazza AM. 1979. Experimental evaluation of anthracycline analogs. *Cancer Treat Rep* 63: 835–844.

Cazin B, Gorin NC, Laporte JP, *et al.* 1986. Cardiac complications after bone marrow transplantation. *Cancer* 57: 2061–2069.

Chaudary S, Song SYT, Jaski BE. 1988. Profound yet reversible heart failure secondary to 5-fluorouracil. *Am J Med* 85: 454–456.

Chisesi T, Capnist G, De Dominicis E, Dini E. 1988. A phase II study of idarubicin (4-demethoxydaunorubicin) in advanced myeloma. *Eur J Cancer Clin Oncol* 24: 681–684.

Chlebowski R, Pugh R, Paroly W, *et al.* 1979. Adriamycin on a weekly schedule: clinically effective with low incidence of cardiotoxicity. *Clin Res* 27: 53A.

Clark GM, Tokaz KL, Von Hoff DD, *et al.* 1984. Cardiotoxicity in patients treated with mitoxantrone on Southwest Oncology Group phase II protocols. *Cancer Treat Symp* 3: 25–30.

Cohen MC, Huberman MS, Nesto RW. 1988. Recombinant alpha$_2$ interferon-related cardiomyopathy. *Am J Med* 85: 549–551.

Coleman RE, Maisey MN, Khight RK, Rubens TD. 1982. Mitoxantrone in advanced breast cancer – a phase II study with special attention to cardiotoxicity. *Eur J Cancer Clin Oncol* 20: 771–776.

Collins C, Weiden PL. 1987. Cardiotoxicity of 5-fluorouracil. *Cancer Treat Rep* 71: 733–736.

Combs AB, Kishi T, Poter TH, Folkers K. 1976. Models for clinical disease. I. Biochemical cardiotoxicity of coenzyme Q$_{10}$ inhibitor in rats. *Res Commun Chem Pathol Pharmacol* 13: 333–339.

Cooper MR, Fefer A, Thompson J, *et al.* 1986. Alpha$_2$ interferon/melphalan/prednisone in previously untreated patients with multiple myeloma: a phase I–II trial. *Cancer Treat Rep* 70: 473–476.

Cortes EP. 1978. Adriamycin cardiotoxicity: early detection by systolic time interval and possible prevention by coenzyme Q10. *Cancer Treat Rep* 62: 887.

Cortes EP, Lutman G, Wanka J, *et al.* 1975. Adriamycin (NSC-123127) cardiotoxicity: a clinicopathologic correlation. *Cancer Chemother Rep* 6: 215–225.

Crossley RJ. 1984. Clinical safety and tolerance of mitoxantrone. *Semin Oncol* 11 (3 Suppl. 1): 54–58.

Daghestani AN, Arlin ZA, Leyland-Jones B, *et al.* 1985. Phase I and II clinical and pharmacological study of 4-demethoxydaunorubicin (idarubicin) in adult patients with acute leukemia. *Cancer Res* 45: 1408–1412.

D'Alessandro N, Gebbia N, Crescimanno M, *et al.* 1983. Effects of amsacrine (m-AMSA), a new aminoacridine antitumor drug, on the rabbit heart. *Cancer Treat Rep* 67: 467–474.

Dardir MD, Ferrans VJ, Mikhael YS, *et al*. 1989. Cardiac morphologic and functional changes induced by epirubicin chemotherapy. *J Clin Oncol* 7: 947–958.

de Forni M, Malet-Martino MC, Jaillais P, *et al*. 1992. Cardiotoxicity of high-dose continuous infusion fluorouracil: a prospective clinical study. *J Clin Oncol* 10: 1795–1801.

Del Tacca M, Danesi R, Ducci M, *et al*. 1985. Might adriamycinol contribute to adriamycin-induced cardiotoxicity? *Pharmacol Res Commun* 17: 1073–1084.

Dent RG, McCall I. 1975. 5-Fluorouracil and angina. *Lancet* 1: 347–348.

Deyton LR, Walker RE, Kovacs JA, *et al*. 1989. Reversible cardiac dysfunction associated with interferon alpha therapy in AIDS patients with Kaposi's sarcoma. *N Engl J Med* 321: 1246–1249.

Dhaliwal HS, Shannon MS, Barnett MJ, *et al*. 1986. Treatment of acute leukemia with m-AMSA in combination with cytosine arabinoside. *Cancer Chemother Pharmacol* 18: 59–62.

Dickson D. 1982. Death halts interferon trials in France. *Science* 218: 772.

Doll DC, List AF, Greco FA, *et al*. 1986. Acute vascular ischemic events after cisplatin-based combination chemotherapy for germ-cell tumors of the testis. *Ann Intern Med* 105: 48–51.

Doroshow JH. 1983. Effect of anthracycline antibiotics on oxygen radical formation in rat heart. *Cancer Res* 43: 460–472.

Doroshow JH. 1988. Role of reactive oxygen production in doxorubicin cardiac toxicity. In *Organ Directed Toxicities of Anticancer Drugs*. Hacker MP, Lazo JS, Tritton TR (eds), pp. 31–40. The Hague: Martinus Nijhoff.

Doroshow JH, Locker GY, Ifrim I, Myers CE. 1981. Prevention of doxorubicin cardiotoxicity in the mouse by *N*-acetylcysteine. *J Clin Invest* 68: 1053–1064.

Edwards BS, Lane M, Smith FE. 1979. Long-term treatment with cis-dichloro-diamineplatinum(II)-vinblastine-bleomycin: possible association with severe coronary artery disease. *Cancer Treat Rep* 63: 551–552.

Ensley JF, Patel B, Kloner R, *et al*. 1989. The clinical syndrome of 5-fluorouracil cardiotoxicity. *Invest New Drugs* 7: 101–109.

Ewer MS, Ali MK, Mackay B, *et al*. 1984. A comparison of cardiac biopsy grades and ejection fraction estimations in patients receiving adriamycin. *J Clin Oncol* 2: 112–117.

Fassio T, Canobbio L, Gasparini G, Villani F. 1986. Paroxysmal supraventricular tachycardia during treatment with cisplatin and etoposide combination. *Oncology* 43: 219–220.

Ferrans VJ. 1978. Overview of cardiac pathology in relation to anthracycline cardiotoxicity. *Cancer Treat Rep* 62: 955–961.

Foon KA, Sherwin SA, Abrams PG, *et al*. 1984. Treatment of advanced non-Hodgkin's lymphoma with recombinant leukocyte interferon in human malignancy. *N Engl J Med* 311: 1148–1152.

Fraile RJ, Baker LH, Buroker TR, *et al*. 1980. Pharmacokinetics of 5-fluorouracil administered orally, by rapid intravenous and by slow infusion. *Cancer Res* 20: 2223–2228.

Freeman NJ, Costanza ME. 1988. 5-Fluorouracil-associated cardiotoxicity. *Cancer* 61: 36–45.

Freiss GG, Boyd JF, Geer MR, Carcia JC. 1985. Effects of first-dose doxorubicin on cardiac rhythm as evaluated by continuous 24-hour monitoring. *Cancer* 56: 2762–2764.

Freter CE, Lee TC, Billingham ME, *et al.* 1986. Doxorubicin cardiac toxicity manifesting seven years after treatment. *Am J Med* 80: 483–485.

Friedman MA, Bozdech MJ, Billingham ME, Rider AK. 1978. Doxorubicin cardiotoxicity. Serial endomyocardial biopsies and systolic time intervals. *J Am Med Assoc* 240: 1603–1606.

Friedman HS, Colvin OM, Aisaka K, *et al.* 1990. Glutathione protects cardiac and skeletal muscle from cyclophosphamide-induced toxicity. *Cancer Res* 50: 2455–2462.

Gams RA, Wesler MJ. 1984. Mitoxantrone cardiotoxicity: results from Southeastern Cancer Study Group. *Cancer Treat Symp* 3: 31–33.

Gaynor ER, Vitek L, Sticklin L, *et al.* 1988. The hemodynamic effects of treatment with interleukin-2 and lymphokine-activated killer cells. *Ann Intern Med* 109: 953–958.

Gehl J, Boesgaard M, Paaske T, *et al.* 1996. Combined doxorubicin and paclitaxel in advanced breast cancer: effective and cardiotoxic. *Ann Oncol* 7: 687–693.

Gianni L, Munzone E, Capri G, *et al.* 1995. Paclitaxel by 3-hour infusion in combination with bolus doxorubicin in women with untreated metastatic breast cancer: high antitumor efficacy and cardiac effects in a dose-finding and sequence-finding study. *J Clin Oncol* 13: 2688–2699.

Gianni L, Vigano L, Locatelli A, *et al.* 1997. Human pharmacokinetic characterization and in vitro study of the interaction between doxorubicin and paclitaxel in patients with breast cancer. *J Clin Oncol* 15: 1906–1915.

Gillies H, Liang R, Rogers H, *et al.* 1988. Phase II trial of idarubicin in patients with advanced lymphoma. *Cancer Chemother Pharmacol* 21: 261–264.

Goldberg MA, Antin JH, Guinan EC, Rappeport JM. 1986. Cyclophosphamide cardiotoxicity: an analysis of dosing as a risk factor. *Blood* 68: 1114–1118.

Gottdiener JS, Applebaum FR, Ferrans VJ, *et al.* 1981. Cardiotoxicity associated with high-dose cyclophosphamide therapy. *Arch Intern Med* 141: 758–763.

Grandi AM, Pinotti G, Morandi E, *et al.* 1997. Noninvasive evaluation of cardiotoxicity of 5-fluorouracil and low doses of folinic acid: a one-year follow-up study. *Ann Oncol.* 8: 705–708.

Greco FA. 1978. Subclinical adriamycin cardiotoxicity: detection by timing the arterial sounds. *Cancer Treat Rep* 62: 901–905.

Grunberg SM, Kempf RA, Itri LM, *et al.* 1985. Phase II study of recombinant alpha interferon in the treatment of advanced non-small cell lung carcinoma. *Cancer Treat Rep* 70: 1031–1032.

Gundersen S, Kvinnsland S, Klepp O, *et al.* 1986. Weekly adriamycin versus VAC in advanced breast cancer. A randomized trial. *Eur J Cancer Clin Oncol* 22: 1431–1434.

Halazun JF, Wagner HR, Gaeta JF, Sinks LF. 1974. Daunorubicin cardiac toxicity in children with acute lymphocytic leukemia. *Cancer* 33: 545–554.

Hancock SL, Donaldson SS, Hoppe RT. 1993. Cardiac disease following treatment of Hodgkin's disease in children and adolescents. *J Clin Oncol* 11: 1208–1215.

Haq MM, Legha SS, Choksi J, *et al.* 1985. Doxorubicin-induced congestive heart failure in adults. *Cancer* 56: 1361–1365.

Harrison M, Tomlinson D, Stewart S. 1995. Liposomal-entrapped doxorubicin: an active agent in AIDS-related Kaposi's sarcoma. *J Clin Oncol* 13: 914–920.

Hashimi LA, Khalyl MF, Salem PA. 1984. Supraventricular tachycardia: a probable complication of platinum treatment. *Oncology* 41: 174–175.

Hasinoff BB. 1990. The interaction of the cardioprotective agent ICRF-187 ((+)-1,2-bis(3,5-dioxopiperazinyl-1-yl)propane): its hydrolysis product (ICRF-198); and other chelating agents with the Fe(III) and Cu(II) complexes of adriamycin. *Agents Actions* 29: 374–381.

Havsteen H, Brynjolf I, Svahn T, *et al.* 1989. Prospective evaluation of chronic cardiotoxicity due to high-dose epirubicin of combination chemotherapy with cyclophosphamide, methotrexate, and 5-fluorouracil. *Cancer Chemother Pharmacol* 23: 101–104.

Henderson BM, Dougherty WJ, James VC, *et al.* 1982. Safety assessment of a new anticancer compound, mitoxantrone, in beagle dogs: comparison with doxorubicin. I. Clinical observations. *Cancer Treat Rep* 66: 1139–1143.

Jain KK, Casper ES, Geller NL, *et al.* 1985. A prospective randomized comparison of epirubicin and doxorubicin in patients with advanced breast cancer. *J Clin Oncol* 3: 818–826.

Jakubowski AA, Kemeny N. 1988. Hypotension as a manifestation of cardiotoxicity in three patients receiving cisplatin and 5-fluorouracil. *Cancer* 62: 266–269.

Janke RA. 1974. An anthracycline antibiotic-induced cardiomyopathy in rabbits. *Lab Invest* 30: 292–303.

Jensen RA. 1986. Doxorubicin cardiotoxicity: contractile changes after long term treatment in the rat. *J Pharmacol Exp Ther* 236: 197–203.

Jones RB, Holland JF, Bhardwaj S, *et al.* 1987. A phase I–II study of intensive-dose adriamycin for advanced breast cancer. *J Clin Oncol* 5: 172–177.

Kharasch ED, Novak RF. 1982. Inhibition of adriamycin-stimulated microsomal lipid peroxidation by mitoxantrone and ametantrone, two new anthracenedione antineoplastic agents. *Biochem Biophys Res Commun* 108: 1346–1352.

Kirkwood JM, Ernstoff MS. 1984. Interferons in the treatment of human cancer. *J Clin Oncol* 2: 336–352.

Kleiman NS, Lehane DE, Geyer CE, *et al.* 1987. Prinzmetal's angina during 5-fluorouracil chemotherapy. *Am J Med* 82: 566–568.

Klugman FB, Decorti G, Candussio L, *et al.* 1986. Inhibitors of adriamycin-induced histamine release *in vitro* limit adriamycin cardiotoxicity *in vivo*. *Br J Cancer* 54: 743–748.

Kris MG, Gralla RJ, Kelsen DP, *et al.* 1985. Phase II trial of oral 4-demethoxydaunorubicin in patients with non-small cell lung cancer. *Am J Clin Oncol* 8: 377–379.

Kris MG, O'Connell JP, Gralla RJ, *et al.* 1986. Phase I trial of Taxol given as a 3-hour infusion every 21 days. *Cancer Treat Rep* 70: 605–607.

Kushner JP, Hansen VL, Hammar SP. 1975. Cardiomyopathy after widely separated courses of adriamycin exacerbated by actinomycin-D and mithramycin. *Cancer* 36: 1577–1584.

La Bianca R, Berretta G, Clerici M, *et al.* 1982. Cardiac toxicity of 5-fluorouracil: a study of 1083 patients. *Tumori* 68: 505–510.

LaFrak EA, Pitha J, Rosenheim S, *et al.* 1975. Adriamycin (NSC 123127) cardiomyopathy. *Cancer Chemother Rep* 6: 203–208.

Langsjoen PH, Langsjoen PH, Folkers K. 1990. A six-year clinical study of therapy of cardiomyopathy with coenzyme $Q_{10}$. *Int J Tissue React* 12: 169–171.

Larsen RL, Jakacki RI, Vetter VL, *et al.* 1992. Electrocardiographic changes and arrhythmias after cancer therapy in children and young adults. *Am J Cardiol* 70: 73–77.

Lee RE, Lotze MT, Skibber JM, *et al.* 1989. Cardiorespiratory effects of immunotherapy with interleukin-2. *J Clin Oncol* 7: 7–20.

Legha SS, Benjamin RS, Mackay B, *et al.* 1982. Reduction of doxorubicin cardiotoxicity by prolonged continuous intravenous infusion. *Ann Intern Med* 96: 133–139.

Lele SS, Durrant STS, Atherton JJ, *et al.* 1996. Demonstration of late cardiotoxicity following bone marrow transplantation by assessment of exercise diastolic filling characteristics. *Bone Marrow Transplant* 17: 1113–1118.

Lenaz L, Page JA. 1976. Cardiotoxicity of adriamycin and related anthracyclines. *Cancer Treat Rev* 3: 111–120.

Lindpainter K, Lindpainter LS, Wentworth M, Burns CP. 1986. Acute myocardial necrosis during administration of amsacrine. *Cancer* 57: 1284–1286.

Lipshultz SE, Colan SD, Gelber RD, *et al.* 1991. Late cardiac effects of doxorubicin therapy for acute lymphoblastic leukemia in childhood. *N Engl J Med* 324: 808–815.

Lipshultz SE, Lipsitz SR, Mone SM, *et al.* 1995. Female sex and higher drug dose as risk factors for late cardiotoxic effects of doxorubicin therapy for childhood cancer. *N Engl J Med* 332: 1738–1743.

Liss RH, Chadwick M. 1974. Correlation of 5-fluorouracil (NSC-19893) distribution in rodents with toxicity and chemotherapy in man. *Cancer Chemother Rep* 58: 777–786.

Lopez M, Vici P, Di Lauro L, *et al.* 1998. Randomized prospective clinical trial of high-dose epirubicin and dexrazoxane in patients with advanced breast cancer and soft tissue sarcomas. *J Clin Oncol* 16: 86–92.

Lum BL, Svec JM, Torti FM. 1985. Doxorubicin: alteration of dose scheduling as a means of reducing cardiotoxicity. *Drug Intell Clin Pharm* 19: 259–264.

Macchiarini P, Danesi R, Mariotti R, *et al.* 1990. Phase II study of high-dose epirubicin in untreated patients with small-cell lung cancer. *Am J Clin Oncol* 13: 302–307.

McKendall GR, Shurman A, Anamur M, Most AS. 1988. Toxic cardiogenic shock associated with infusion of 5-fluorouracil. *Am Heart J* 118: 184–186.

McLaughlin P, Salvador PG, Cabanillas F, Legha SS. 1983. Ventricular fibrillation following AMSA. *Cancer* 52: 557–558.

Maisch B, Gregor O, Zuess M, Kocksiek K. 1985. Acute effect of calcium channel blockers on adriamycin exposed adult cardiocytes. *Basic Res Cardiol* 80: 626–635.

Marchandise B, Schroeder E, Boslv A, *et al.* 1989. Early detection of doxorubicin cardiotoxicity: interest of Doppler echocardiographic analysis of the left ventricular filling dynamics. *Am Heart J* 118: 92–98.

Markman M, Kennedy A, Webster K, *et al.* 1998. Paclitaxel administration to gynecologic cancer patients with major risk factors. *J Clin Oncol* 16: 3483–3485.

Marshall RC, Berger HJ, Reduto LA, *et al.* 1978. Variability in sequential measures of left ventricular performance assessed with radionuclide angiocardiography. *Am J Cardiol* 41: 531–536.

Martin M, Diaz-Rubio E, Furio V, *et al.* 1989. Lethal cardiac toxicity after cisplatin and 5-fluoruracil chemotherapy. *Am J Clin Oncol* 12: 229–234.

Martino S, Ratanatharathorn V, Karanes C, *et al.* 1987. Reversible arrhythmias observed in patients treated with recombinant alpha$_2$ interferon. *J Cancer Res Clin Oncol* 113: 376–378.

Martoni A, Pacciarini MA, Pannuti F. 1985. Activity of 4-demethoxydaunorubicin by the oral route in advanced breast cancer. *Eur J Cancer Clin Oncol* 21: 803–806.

Merrill J, Greco FA, Zimbler H, *et al.* 1975. Adriamycin and radiation: synergistic cardiotoxicity. *Ann Intern Med* 82: 122–123.

Meyers CE, McGuire WP, Liss RH, *et al.* 1977. Adriamycin: the role of lipid peroxidation in cardiac toxicity and tumor response. *Science* 197: 165–167.

Milei J, Marantz A, Ale J, *et al.* 1987. Prevention of adriamycin-induced cardiotoxicity by prenylamine: a pilot double blind study. *Cancer Drug Deliv* 4: 129–136.

Milei J, Vazquez A, Boveris A, *et al.* 1988. The role of prenylamine in the prevention of adriamycin-induced cardiotoxicity. A review of experimental and clinical findings. *J Int Med Res* 16: 19–30.

Minow RA, Benjamin RS, Gottlieb JA. 1975. Adriamycin (NSC-123127) cardiomyopathy – an overview with determination of risk factors. *Cancer Chemother Rep* 6: 195–201.

Minow RA, Benjamin RS, Leo ET, Gottlieb JA. 1977. Adriamycin cardiomyopathy – risk factors. *Cancer* 39: 1397–1402.

Murphree SA, Cunningham LS, Hwang KM, *et al.* 1976. Effects of adriamycin on surface properties of sarcoma 180 ascites cells. *Biochem Pharmacol* 25: 1227–1231.

Myers CE, Bonow R, Palmeri S, *et al.* 1983. A randomized controlled trial assessing the prevention of doxorubicin cardiomyopathy by *N*-acetylcysteine. *Semin Oncol* 10 (1 Suppl. 1): 53–55.

Nair R, Ramakrishnan G, Nair NN, *et al.* 1998. A randomized comparison of the efficacy and toxicity of epirubicin and doxorubicin in the treatment of patients with non-Hodgkin's lymphoma. *Cancer* 82: 2282–2288.

Nielsen D, Jensen NB, Dombernowsky O, *et al.* 1990. Epirubicin cardiotoxicity: a study of 135 patients with advanced breast cancer. *J Clin Oncol* 8: 1806–1810.

Nora R, Abrams JS, Tait NS, *et al.* 1989. Myocardiac toxic effects during recombinant interleukin-2 therapy. *J Natl Cancer Inst* 81: 59–63.

Nysom K, Holm K, Lipsitz SR, *et al.* 1998. Relationship between cumulative anthracycline dose and late cardiotoxicity in childhood acute lymphoblastic leukemia. *J Clin Oncol* 16: 545–550.

O'Connell TX, Berenbaum MC. 1974. Cardiac and pulmonary effects of high doses of cyclophosphamide and isophosphamide. *Cancer Res* 34: 1586–1591.

Ognibene FP, Rosenberg SA, Lotze M, *et al.* 1988. Interleukin-2 administration causes reversible hemodynamic changes and left ventricular dysfunction similar to those seen in septic shock. *Chest* 94: 750–754.

Oleksowicz L, Bruckner HW. 1988. Prophylaxis of 5-fluorouracil induces coronary vasospasm with calcium channel blockers. *Am J Med* 85: 750–751.

Olson HM, Young DM, Prieur DJ, *et al.* 1974. Electrolyte and morphologic alterations of myocardium in adriamycin-treated rabbits. *Am J Pathol* 77: 439–454.

Olson RD, Mushlin PS. 1990. Doxorubicin cardiotoxicity: analysis of prevailing hypotheses. *FASEB J* 4: 3076–3086.

Olson RD, Mushlin PS, Brenner DE, *et al.* 1988. Doxorubicin cardiotoxicity may be due to its metabolite, doxorubicinol. *Proc Natl Acad Sci USA* 85: 3585–3589.

Palmeri ST, Bonow RO, Myers CE, *et al.* 1986. Prospective evaluation of doxorubicin cardiotoxicity by rest and exercise radionuclide angiography. *Am J Cardiol* 58: 607–613.

Patel B, Kloner RA, Ensley J, *et al.* 1987. 5-Fluorouracil cardiotoxicity: left ventricular dysfunction and effect of coronary vasodilators. *Am J Med Sci* 294: 238–243.

Peters JH, Gordon GR, Kashiwase D, Acton EM. 1981. Tissue distribution of doxorubicin and doxorubicinol in rats receiving multiple doses of doxorubicin. *Cancer Chemother Pharmacol* 7: 65–70.

Pigram WJ, Fuller W, Amilton LDH. 1972. Stereochemistry of intercalation: interaction of daunomycin with DNA. *Nature* 235: 17–19.

Piver MS, Marchetti DL, Parthasarathy KL, *et al.* 1985. Doxorubicin hydrochloride (adriamycin) cardiotoxicity evaluated by sequential radionuclide angiocardiography. *Cancer* 56: 76–80.

Posner LE, Dukart G, Goldberg J, *et al.* 1985. Mitoxantrone: an overview of safety and toxicity. *Invest New Drugs* 3: 123–132.

Praga C, Beretta G, Vigo PL, *et al.* 1979. Adriamycin cardiotoxicity: a survey of 1273 patients. *Cancer Treat Rep* 63: 827–834.

Quesada JR, Talpaz M, Rios A, *et al.* 1986. Clinical toxicity of interferons in cancer patients: a review. *J Clin Oncol* 4: 234–243.

Rabkin SW. 1983. Interaction of external calcium concentrations and verapamil on the effects of doxorubicin (adriamycin) in the isolated heart preparation. *J Cardiovasc Pharmacol* 5: 848–855.

Rajagopalan S, Politi PM, Sinha BK, Myers CE. 1988. Adriamycin-induced free radical formation in the perfused rat heart: implications for cardiotoxicity. *Cancer Res* 48: 4766–4769.

Revis N, Marusic N. 1979. Effects of doxorubicin and its aglycone metabolite on calcium sequestration by rabbit heart, liver, and kidney mitochondria. *Life Sci* 25: 1055–1064.

Rezkalla S, Kloner RA, Enslev J, *et al.* 1989. Continuous ambulatory ECG monitoring during fluorouracil therapy: a prospective study. *J Clin Oncol* 7: 509–514.

Ringenberg QS, Propert KJ, Muss HB, *et al.* 1990. Clinical cardiotoxicity of esorubicin (4′-deoxydoxorubicin, DxDx): prospective studies with serial gated heart scans and reports of selected cases. *Invest New Drugs* 8: 221–226.

Rowinsky EK, Donehower RC. 1995. Paclitaxel (Taxol). *N Engl J Med* 332: 1004–1014.

Rowinsky EK, McGuire WP, Guarnieri T, *et al.* 1991. Cardiac disturbances during the administration of Taxol. *J Clin Oncol* 9: 1704–1712.

Ryberg M, Nielsen D, Skovsgaard T, *et al.* 1998. Epirubicin cardiotoxicity: an analysis of 469 patients with metastatic breast cancer. *J Clin Oncol* 16: 3502–3508.

Samlowski WE, Ward JH, Craven CM, Freedman RA. 1989. Severe myocarditis following high-dose interleukin-2 administration. *Arch Pathol Lab Med* 113: 838–841.

Sarna G, Figlin R, Callaghan M. 1983. Alpha (human leukocyte)-interferon as treatment for non-small cell carcinoma of the lung: a phase II trial. *J Biol Response Mod* 2: 343–347.

Schell FC, Yap H-Y, Blumenschein G, *et al.* 1982. Potential cardiotoxicity with mitoxantrone. *Cancer Treat Rep* 66: 1641–1643.

Schlaeffer F, Tovi F, Leiberman A. 1983. Cisplatin-induced bradycardia. *Drug Intell Clin Pharm* 17: 899–901.

Schwartz RG, McKenzie WB, Alexander J, *et al.* 1987. Congestive heart failure and left ventricular dysfunction complicating doxorubicin therapy. Seven-year experience using serial radionuclide angiocardiography. *Am J Med* 82: 1109–1118.

Shek TW, Luk ISC, Ma L, Cheung KL. 1996. Paclitaxel-induced cardiotoxicity: an ultrastructural study. *Arch Pathol Lab Med* 120: 89–91.

Shenkenberg TD, Von Hoff DD. 1986. Mitoxantrone: a new anticancer drug with significant clinical activity. *Ann Intern Med* 105: 67–81.

Shinar E, Hasin Y. 1984. Acute electrocardiographic changes induced by amsacrine. *Cancer Treat Rep* 68: 1169–1172.

Singal PK, Pierce GN. 1986. Adriamycin stimulates low-affinity $Ca^{2+}$ binding and lipid peroxidation but depresses myocardial function. *Am J Physiol* 250: H419–H425.

Singal PK, Forbes MS, Sperelakis N. 1983. Occurrence of intramitochondrial $Ca^{2+}$ granules in a hypertrophied heart exposed to adriamycin. *Can J Physiol Pharmacol* 62: 1239–1244.

Singal PK, Segstro RJ, Singh RP, Kutryk MJ. 1985. Changes in lysosomal morphology and enzyme activities during the development of adriamycin-induced cardiomyopathy. *Can J Cardiol* 1: 139–147.

Singer JW, Narahara KA, Ritchie JL, *et al.* 1978. Time and dose-dependent changes in ejection fraction determined by radionuclide angiography after anthracycline therapy. *Cancer Treat Rep* 62: 945.

Sinha BK. 1980. Binding specificity of chemically and enzymatically activated anthracycline anticancer agents to nucleic acids. *Chem Biol Interact* 30: 67–77.

Slavin RE, Millan JC, Mullins CM. 1975. Pathology of high dose intermittent cyclophosphamide therapy. *Hum Pathol* 6: 693–709.

Sledge GW, Neuberg D, Ingle J, *et al.* 1997. Phase II trial of doxorubicin vs. paclitaxel vs. doxorubicin + paclitaxel as first-line therapy for metastatic breast cancer: an intergroup trial. *Proc Am Soc Clin Oncol* 16: 1a.

Smith PJ, Ekert H, Waters KD, Matthews RN. 1977. High incidence of cardiomyopathy in children treated with adriamycin and DTIC in combination chemotherapy. *Cancer Treat Rep* 61: 1736–1738.

Sorensen K, Levitt G, Bull C, *et al.* 1997. Anthracycline dose in childhood acute lymphoblastic leukemia: issues of early survival versus late cardiotoxicity. *J Clin Oncol* 15: 61–68.

Sparano BM, Gordon G, Hall C, *et al.* 1982. Safety assessment of a new anticancer compound, mitoxantrone, in beagle dogs: comparison with doxorubicin. II. Histologic and ultrastructural pathology. *Cancer Treat Rep* 66: 1145–1158.

Speyer JL, Green MD, Jacquotte AZ, *et al.* 1992. ICRF-187 permits longer treatment with doxorubicin in women with breast cancer. *J Clin Oncol* 10: 117–127.

Spiegel RJ. 1987. The alpha interferons: clinical overview. *Semin Oncol* 14: 1–12.

Steinberg JS, Wasserman AG. 1985. Radionuclide ventriculography for evaluation and prevention of doxorubicin cardiotoxicity. *Clin Ther* 7: 660–667.

Steinberg JS, Cohen AJ, Wasserman AG, *et al.* 1987. Acute arrhythmogenicity of doxorubicin administration. *Cancer* 60: 1213–1218.

Steinherz LJ, Steinherz PG, Mangiacasale D, *et al.* 1982. Cardiac abnormalities after AMSA administration. *Cancer Treat Rep* 66: 483–488.

Steinherz LJ, Steinherz PG, Tan CT, *et al.* 1991. Cardiac toxicity 4 to 20 years after completing anthracycline therapy. *J Am Med Assoc* 266: 1672–1677.

Steinherz LJ, Steinherz PG, Tan CT. 1995. Cardiac failure and dysrhythmias 6–19 years after anthracycline therapy: a series of 15 patients. *Med Pediatr Oncol* 24: 352–361.

Suzuki T, Kanda H, Kawai Y, *et al.* 1979. Cardiotoxicity of anthracycline antineoplastic drugs – clinicopathological and experimental studies. *Jpn Circ J* 43: 1000–1008.

Swain SM, Whaley FS, Gerber MC, *et al.* 1997. Cardioprotection with dexrazoxane for doxorubicin-containing therapy in advanced breast cancer. *J Clin Oncol* 15: 1318–1332.

Talcott JA, Herman TS. 1987. Acute ischemic vascular events and cisplatin. *Ann Intern Med* 107: 121–122.

Tan CTC, Hancock C, Steinherz P, *et al*. 1987. Phase I clinical pharmacological study of 4-demethoxydaunorubicin (idarubicin) in children with advanced cancer. *Cancer Res* 47: 2990–2995.

Tewey KM, Chen GI, Nelson EM, Lui LF. 1984. Intercalative antitumor drugs interfere with the breakage-reunion of mammalian DNA topoisomerase II. *J Biol Chem* 259: 9182–9187.

Treat J, Greenspan A, Forst D, *et al*. 1990. Anti-tumor activity of liposome-encapsulated doxorubicin in advanced breast cancer: Phase II study. *J Natl Cancer Inst* 82: 1706–1710.

Trigg ME, Finlay JL, Bozdech M, Gilnbert E. 1987. Fatal cardiac toxicity in bone marrow transplant patients receiving cytosine arabinoside, cyclophosphamide, and total body irradiation. *Cancer* 59: 38–42.

Unverferth DV, Bashore TM, Magrien RD, *et al*. 1984. Histologic and function characteristics of human heart after mitoxantrone therapy. *Cancer Treat Symp* 3: 47–53.

Vaickus L, Letendre L. 1984. Pericarditis induced by high-dose cytarabine therapy. *Arch Intern Med* 144: 1868–1869.

Vaitkus PT, Grossman D, Fox KR, *et al*. 1990. Complete heart block due to interleukin-2 therapy. *Am Heart J* 119: 978–980.

Venturi M, Michelotti A, Del Mastro L, *et al*. 1996. Multicenter randomized controlled clinical trial to evaluate cardioprotection of dexrazoxane versus no cardioprotection in women receiving epirubicin chemotherapy for advanced breast cancer. *J Clin Oncol* 14: 3112–3120.

Villani F, Galimberti M, Comazzi R, Crippa F. 1989. Evaluation of cardiac toxicity of idarubicin (4-demethoxydaunorubicin). *Eur J Cancer Clin Oncol* 25: 13–18.

Von Hoff DD, Rozenoweig M, Layard M, *et al*. 1977. Daunomycin-induced cardiotoxicity in children and adults. A review of 110 cases. *Am J Med* 62: 200–208.

Von Hoff DD, Layard MW, Basa P, *et al*. 1979. Risk factors for doxorubicin-induced congestive heart failure. *Ann Intern Med* 91: 710–717.

Von Hoff DD, Elson D, Polk G, Coltman C. 1980. Acute ventricular fibrillation and death during infusion of 4′(9-acridinylamino)methanesulfon-*m*-anisidide (AMSA). *Cancer Treat Rep* 64: 356–358.

Von Hoff DD, Howser D, Lewis B, *et al*. 1981. Phase I study of ICRF-187 using a daily for 3 days schedule. *Cancer Treat Rep* 65: 249–252.

Wagner D, Kern WV, Kern P. 1994. Liposomal doxorubicin in AIDS-related Kaposi's sarcoma: long-term experience. *Clin Invest* 72: 417–423.

Watts RG. 1991. Severe and fatal anthracycline cardiotoxicity at cumulative doses below 400 mg/m$^2$: evidence for enhanced toxicity with multiagent chemotherapy. *Am J Hematol* 36: 217–218.

Weesner KM, Bledsoe M, Chauvenet A, Wofford M. 1991. Exercise echocardiography in the detection of anthracycline cardiotoxicity. *Cancer* 68: 435–438.

Weiss AJ, Metter GE, Fletcher WS, *et al*. 1976. Studies on adriamycin using a weekly regimen demonstrating its clinical effectiveness and lack of cardiac toxicity. *Cancer Chemother Rep* 60: 813–822.

Weiss RB, Moquin D, Adams JD, *et al*. 1983. Electrocardiogram abnormalities iduced by amsacrine. *Cancer Chemother Pharmacol* 10: 133–134.

Weiss RB, Grillo-Lopez AJ, Marsoni S, *et al*. 1986a. Amsacrine-associated cardiotoxicity: an analysis of 82 cases. *J Clin Oncol* 4: 918–928.

Weiss RB, Sarosy G, Clagett-Carr K, *et al.* 1986b. Anthracycline analogs: the past, present, and future. *Cancer Chemother Pharmacol* 18: 185–197.

Willemze R, Zwaan FE, Colpin G, *et al.* 1982. High dose cytosine arabinoside in the management of refractory acute leukemia. *Scand J Haematol* 29: 141–146.

Wortman JE, Lucas JS. Schuster E, *et al.* 1979. Sudden death during doxorubicin administration. *Cancer* 44: 1588–1591.

Yeung ST, Yoong C, Spink J, *et al.* 1991. Functional myocardial impairment in children treated with anthracyclines for cancer. *Lancet* 337: 816–818.

Young RC, Ozols RF, Myers CE. 1981. The anthracycline antineoplastic drugs. *N Engl J Med* 305: 139–153.

Zweier JL, Gianni L, Muindi J, Myers CE. 1986. Differences in $O_2$ reduction by the iron complexes of adriamycin and daunomycin: the importance of side chain hydroxyl group. *Biochim Biophys Acta* 884: 326–336.

# 13

# PASSIVE SMOKING CAUSES HEART DISEASE

*Stanton A. Glantz and William W. Parmley*

*Division of Cardiology, Department of Medicine,
Cardiovascular Research Institute, University of California,
San Francisco, CA, USA*

Although most of the discussion of the health effects of passive smoking on non-smokers has concentrated on lung cancer (US Environmental Protection Agency, 1992), heart disease is a much more important end-point (Wells, 1988, 1994, 1998; Glantz and Parmley, 1991, 1995; Office of Environmental Health Hazard Assessment, 1997). Whereas passive smoking-induced lung cancer accounts for about 3000 deaths per year, passive smoking-induced heart disease accounts for up to 62 000 deaths annually (Office of Environmental Health Hazard Assessment, 1997), with about an equal number of non-fatal events (Glantz and Parmley, 1991, 1995; Wells, 1994, 1998). Epidemiologic studies of the effects of passive smoking on both fatal and non-fatal end-points associated with heart disease reveal about a 30 percent increase in risk (Law *et al.*, 1997), and the American Heart Association has formally concluded that passive smoking is an important risk factor for heart disease in both adults (Taylor *et al.*, 1992) and children (Gidding *et al.*, 1994). The primary issue related to passive smoking and heart disease has been the size of this effect compared with the effect of active smoking on smokers. Active smoking, which involves a dose of the toxins in second-hand smoke that is at least two orders of magnitude greater than a non-smoker receives, only about doubles the risk of heart disease. Thus, the effect of second-hand smoke seems large for the dose, assuming a linear dose–response relationship. There are, however, a wide variety of clinical and experimental studies which demonstrate that the effects of second-hand smoke on the cardiovascular system occur at low doses in non-smokers, with the effects being about one-third of that observed in active smokers. These effects are manifest through effects on platelets and vascular function, among other end-points. The dose–response relationship between second-hand smoke exposure and heart disease is probably not linear; it is superlinear.

# Effects of second-hand smoke on oxygen delivery, processing, and exercise

Passive smoking reduces the blood's ability to deliver oxygen to the myocardium. The carbon monoxide in second-hand smoke competes with oxygen for binding sites on red blood cells and displaces the oxygen (USPHS, 1983; USDHHS, 1986; Moskowitz et al., 1990; Leone et al., 1991; US Environmental Protection Agency, 1992). Children of smoking parents have elevated levels of 2,3-diphosphoglycerate (DPG), a compound that appears in red blood cells in an effort to modify how they handle oxygen to compensate for chronic oxygen deprivation (Moskowitz et al., 1990, 1993; Pomrehn et al., 1990; Feldman et al., 1991; Gidding et al., 1994). While the reduction in oxygen-carrying capacity of blood due to increased carboxyhemoglobin is small compared with smokers, it can have important physiologic implications because the body normally extracts more than 90 percent of the oxygen from the blood during exercise (Lamb, 1984). People with existing heart disease showed increasing electrocardiographic evidence of ischemia (Allred et al., 1989; Dwyer and Turino, 1989) and experienced more arrhythmias (Sheps et al., 1990) as carboxyhemoglobin increased, even at low levels.

In addition to reducing the blood's ability to deliver oxygen to the heart, there is direct evidence from animal studies that passive smoking reduces the ability of the heart muscle to convert oxygen into the "energy molecule" adenosine triphosphate (ATP). The mitochondrial enzymes that facilitate this process do not work as efficiently in rabbits exposed to second-hand smoke. Cytochrome oxidase exhibited a 25 percent reduction in its activity after a single 30-min exposure to second-hand smoke, and the activity continued to drop with prolonged exposure (Gvozdjak et al., 1987). After 8 weeks of 30 min per day exposure, its activity was cut in half. Thus, not only does second-hand smoke reduce the ability of the blood to deliver oxygen to the myocardium but it also reduces the ability of the myocardium to use effectively the oxygen it does get (Gvozdjakova et al., 1992).

Passive smoking also significantly increased the amount of lactate in venous blood, which indicates that during passive smoking the heart switches to a greater reliance on anaerobic metabolism (McMurray et al., 1985). People with coronary heart disease cannot exercise as long or reach as high a level of exercise after breathing second-hand smoke than when breathing clean air (Aronow, 1978; Khaifen and Klochkov, 1987; Leone et al., 1991) and they are more likely to develop arrhythmias with exercise (Leone et al., 1992). Experiments on healthy young adults exposed to second-hand smoke show higher resting heart rates, higher blood carboxyhemoglobin, a significant reduction in the amount of oxygen absorbed during exercise, and a shorter time to exhaustion when running on a treadmill. Exposure to second-hand smoke also increased perceived level of exertion during exercise, the maximum heart rate, carbon dioxide output, and the time to recover resting heart rate at the end of exercise, to the point that normal healthy individuals took as long as people with heart disease to recover their resting heart rate following exercise (McMurray et al., 1985; Leone et al., 1991).

## Platelets

Second-hand cigarette smoke activates blood platelets, which increases the likelihood of formation of a thrombus and can damage the lining of the coronary arteries and facilitate the development of atherosclerotic lesions (Pittilo *et al.*, 1982; Sinzinger and Kefalides, 1982; Burghuber *et al.*, 1986; Davis *et al.*, 1989; Sinzinger and Virgolini, 1989; Steinberg *et al.*, 1989). Large platelets and mean platelet volume are independent risk factors for recurrent or more serious myocardial infarction (Martin *et al.*, 1991). Increased platelet activity is associated with increased relative risk for ischemic heart disease (Elwood *et al.*, 1991); the increases in platelet activity observed in passive smokers would be expected to have acute effects, increasing the risk by 34 percent (Law *et al.*, 1997), which is approximately that observed in the epidemiologic studies.

In one experiment, non-smokers and smokers were asked to smoke two cigarettes (Figure 13.1) (Burghuber *et al.*, 1986). The smokers' platelets, which were "stickier" than the non-smokers' platelets at the beginning of the experiment, did not significantly change activity in response to the two cigarettes. Most likely, the smokers' platelets were maximally activated because of the chronic exposure to the toxins in cigarette smoke, so the addition of the relatively small (compared with what a smoker receives on an ongoing basis) amount of toxins in two cigarettes had no additional effects. In contrast, smoking just two cigarettes significantly increased non-smokers' platelet activity, to the point that it was not significantly different from that of the habitual smoker. This situation demonstrates that the responses of non-smokers and smokers to the toxins in the cigarette smoke are often very different.

More important, Burghuber *et al.* (1986) measured platelet activity in smokers and non-smokers before and after they had been sitting in a room for 20 min where cigarettes had been smoked just before the experimental subjects entered (Figure 13.1). Again, there was no significant change in the platelet activity among the smokers, but there was a significant increase in platelet stickiness among the non-smokers, to the point that their platelet activation was not discernibly different

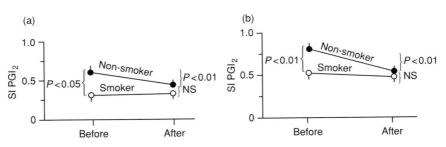

*Figure 13.1* Effect of active (a) and passive (b) smoking on platelet aggregation in smokers and non-smokers. The sensitivity index, $SI_{PGI2}$, is defined as the inverse of the concentration of prostaglandin $I_2$ necessary to inhibit ADP-induced platelet aggregation by 50 percent. Lower values of $SI_{PGI2}$ indicate greater platelet aggregation. Reprinted from Glantz and Parmley (1991) with the permission of the American Heart Association.

from the smokers. These data, together with other human experiments (Davis *et al.*, 1985a,b, 1986, 1987, 1989), indicate that non-smokers are much more sensitive to second-hand smoke than smokers and that very low levels of second-hand smoke exposure can have a major impact on non-smokers' platelet activity (Table 13.1). It also appears that the process saturates at low doses: once the non-smoker has been exposed to even a low dose of second-hand smoke, the platelets are maximally activated, similar to that of a habitual smoker. These data also indicate that dose-based extrapolations from smokers to non-smokers using "cigarette equivalents" will grossly underestimate the risks to non-smokers of breathing second-hand smoke.

Animal data support this conclusion. In our studies of the effects of passive smoking on heart disease, we have found that bleeding time (another measure of platelet activity) is significantly shortened (meaning more activated platelets) in both rabbits (Zhu *et al.*, 1993; Sun *et al.*, 1994) and rats (Zhu *et al.*, 1994) exposed at even the lowest doses of second-hand smoke; there were no additional effects at higher doses.

At a biochemical level, studies of cigarette smoke extract on the effects of platelet activity suggest that the toxins in the cigarette smoke increase platelet-activating factor by interfering with the activity of the plasma enzyme platelet-activating factor acetylhydrolase (PAF-AH) (Miyaura *et al.*, 1992). PAF-AH

*Table 13.1* Effects of passive and active smoking on platelet aggregation and endothelial cell damage

| | Platelet aggregate ratio | | | Endothelial cell count | | | |
|---|---|---|---|---|---|---|---|
| | Before | After | Change | Before | After | Change | n |
| Passive smoking (non-smoker) | 0.87 | 0.78 | −0.09 | 2.8 | 3.7 | 0.9 | 10 |
| Tobacco (non-smoker) vs. | 0.80 | 0.65 | −0.15 | 2.3 | 4.8 | 2.5 | 20 |
| Non-tobacco cigarette (non-smoker) | 0.81 | 0.78 | −0.03 | 2.5 | 3.0 | 0.5 | |
| Inhale cigarette (smoker) vs. | 0.81 | 0.68 | −0.13 | 4.0 | 5.4 | 1.4 | 24 |
| Not inhale cigarette (non-smoker) | 0.82 | 0.73 | −0.09 | 3.3 | 4.7 | 1.4 | 22 |
| Smoke (smoker) vs. | 0.85 | 0.70 | −0.15 | 4.4 | 6.4 | 2.0 | 17 |
| Snuff (smoker) | 0.82 | 0.76 | −0.06 | 3.9 | 4.7 | 0.8 | |

Note
All studies are paired and reflect significant differences ($P < 0.005$). Platelet aggregate ratio is the ratio of platelet count of platelet-rich plasma, prepared immediately after venipuncture with a solution containing edetic acid and formaldehyde, to that of platelet-rich plasma prepared in the same manner except for the absence of formaldehyde. A decrease in the platelet aggregate ratio reflects an increased formation of platelet aggregates. Endothelial cell count is mean number of anuclear cell carcasses in 0.9-μl chambers. Sources: Davis *et al.* (1985a,b, 1986, 1987, 1989, 1990) and Davis (1990). Table reprinted with permission of the American Heart Association from Glantz and Parmley (1991).

reduces platelet activity by neutralizing platelet activating factor. Because toxins in the cigarette smoke appear to reduce the effectiveness of PAF-AH in neutralizing platelet activating factor, these toxins may contribute to an increase in platelet activity. Nicotine does not appear to be the only active agent in tobacco smoke, but rather some other as yet undefined element in the smoke also contributes to these effects on the platelets (Davis *et al.*, 1985b; Miyaura *et al.*, 1992). This biochemical result is reinforced by clinical studies which find that smokers treated with nicotine patches show fewer changes in platelet activity than continuing smokers despite having similar nicotine levels (Benowitz *et al.*, 1993).

## Endothelial function

Arteries have a one-cell-thick lining known as the vascular endothelium. The endothelium plays an important role in controlling the ability of arteries to dilate and constrict (and so regulate blood flow). In addition, damage to the vascular endothelium facilitates development of atherosclerosis. There is good evidence, in both animals (Hutchinson *et al.*, 1995; Zhu and Parmley, 1995; Hutchison *et al.*, 1997a, 1998) and humans (Sumida *et al.*, 1998), that second-hand smoke interferes with endothelium-dependent vasodilation. Moreover, it is possible to block these effects by increasing the amount of L-arginine, an amino acid that is a precursor for nitric oxide, which mediates endothelium-dependent vasodilation (Hutchinson *et al.*, 1996; Hutchison *et al.*, 1997b, 1999). This result indicates that second-hand smoke specifically interferes with the production of nitric oxide production. Consistent with other experimental results which indicate that non-smokers are very sensitive to the effects of second-hand smoke, exposure to second-hand smoke causes increases in constriction of coronary arteries in human non-smokers that are nearly as large as the changes observed in smokers (Sumida *et al.*, 1998).

Although not clearly related to changes in endothelial function, experiments in humans show that acute exposure to second-hand smoke reduces the distensibility of the aorta (Stefanadis *et al.*, 1998). The distensibilty of the aorta in non-smokers exposed to second-hand smoke for 5 min was 21 percent compared with 27 percent in the active smoking group (and no change in sham-exposed patients). As with the other acute effects of second-hand smoke on the vasculature, the effects of second-hand smoke were of similar magnitude to that of active smoking, further buttressing the plausibility of the relatively large risks of heart disease associated with second-hand smoke compared with active smoking.

## Atherosclerosis

In addition to the short-term toxicity of cigarette smoke, there are long-term permanent effects. In particular, smoking contributes to the development of atherosclerosis. In addition to their role in acute thrombus formation, platelets are also important in the development of atherosclerosis (Ross, 1986; Steinberg *et al.*, 1989). Once there is damage to the arterial endothelium, either through mechanical or chemical factors, platelets interact with or adhere to the subendothelial connective tissue and initiate a sequence that leads to the formation of an atherosclerotic plaque. When platelets interact with or adhere to subendocardial connective tissue, they are stimulated to release their granule contents. Endothelial cells normally prevent platelet adherence because of the non-thrombogenic character of their surface and because of their capacity to form antithrombotic substances such as prostacyclin. Once the endothelial cells have been damaged, the platelets can stick to them and release mitogens such as platelet-derived growth factor, which encourages migration and proliferation of smooth muscle cells in the region of the endothelial injury. If platelet aggregation is increased because of exposure to second-hand smoke, the chances of platelets building up at that endothelial injury site will be increased.

Experiments in humans have indicated that even short-term exposure to second-hand smoke – like active smoking (Prerovsky and Hladovec, 1979) – significantly increases the appearance of anuclear endothelial cell carcasses in the blood of people exposed to second-hand smoke (or other tobacco products) constituents (Davis *et al.*, 1989). The appearance of these cell carcasses indicates damage to the endothelium, which is the initiating step in the atherosclerotic process. The appearance of endothelial cells after passive smoking in non-smokers is almost as great as in primary smoking in non-smokers.

Passive smoking both among adolescents whose parents smoke and among adults working in places where smoking is permitted exhibit lower levels of high-density lipoprotein (HDL) than children breathing clean air (Moskowitz *et al.*, 1990; Feldman *et al.*, 1991). Similar results have been reported in adults who work in smoky environments (White and Froeb, 1991). This effect on cholesterol and on the ratio of HDL to total cholesterol also increases the risk of developing atherosclerosis. Adults breathing second-hand smoke for only 5.5 h exhibit compromised antioxidant biochemical defenses and increased accumulation of low-density lipoprotein (LDL) cholesterol in macrophages (Valkonen and Kuusi, 1998).

Many atherosclerotic plaques in humans either are monoclonal (meaning they arose from a single cell) or possess a predominantly monoclonal component, which indicates that the smooth muscle cells of each plaque have a predominant cell type. Several animal studies (Albert *et al.*, 1977; Penn *et al.*, 1981, 1986, 1992, 1994, 1996; Majesky *et al.*, 1983; Revis *et al.*, 1984; Penn and Snyder, 1993, 1994, 1996a,b) demonstrated that polycyclic aromatic hydrocarbons (PAHs), in particular 7,12-dimethylbenz(a,h)anthracene (DMBA), 1,3-butadiene, and benzo(a)pyrene (BAP), accelerate the development of atherosclerosis. BAP is an important constituent of second-hand smoke. The PAHs appear to bind preferentially to both the LDL and HDL subfragments of cholesterol, which may facilitate incorporation of the carcinogenic compounds into the cells lining the coronary arteries and hence contribute to both cell injury and the hyperplasia in the atherosclerotic process.

Humans exposed to second-hand smoke at work exhibit increased production of 8-hydroxy-2'-deoxyguanosine, an indicator of DNA damage that has been linked to increased risk of cancer and heart disease (Howard *et al.*, 1998).

In addition to this biochemical evidence demonstrating the effects of specific components in second-hand smoke on the development of atherosclerotic lesions at a cellular and molecular level, animal experiments have demonstrated that short-term exposure to environmental tobacco smoke significantly speeds the atherosclerotic process. Zhu *et al.* (1993) exposed two groups of rabbits on a high-cholesterol diet to 10 weeks of second-hand smoke from Marlboro cigarettes. The animals were exposed to the second-hand smoke for 6 h per day for 5 days per week for just 10 weeks. One group (high dose) was exposed to smoke at levels that would be observed in a smoky bar and the other group (low dose) was exposed to levels about half as high. A third group of rabbits on a high-cholesterol diet was exposed to clean air. The high-dose group was exposed to pollution levels similar to those observed in a medium-sized car with the windows rolled up and four cigarettes per hour being smoked (Ott *et al.*, 1992). With just 10 weeks of exposure (a total of 300 h), the fraction of pulmonary artery and aorta covered with lipid deposits nearly doubled compared with the rabbits exposed to clean air (Figure 13.2). This is short-term exposure, even for a rabbit.

This effect appears to be directly caused by elements in the cigarette smoke itself rather than by a reaction to the second-hand smoke, which might have increased circulating catecholamines. (Increased levels of circulating catecholamines is one of the mechanisms by which cigarette smoking increases the risk of heart disease in active smokers.) Sun *et al.* (1994) exposed rabbits in an experiment similar to that described above to second-hand smoke but gave half of the rabbits the beta-blocking drug metropolol. As expected, the animals receiving metropolol developed fewer lipid deposits than those who were receiving a placebo (saline), but this effect was independent of whether the rabbits were breathing second-hand smoke. Therefore, the second-hand smoke effects on the development of atherosclerotic-type lesions in the arteries were not mediated by the increased levels of catecholamines.

One criticism that tobacco industry consultants have raised is that this rabbit model of atherosclerosis requires the rabbits to be on a high-cholesterol diet (Wu, 1993). This experimental model of atherosclerosis, which has been used since 1908, requires the rabbits to have a high-cholesterol diet in order to develop any lesions within a reasonable length of time (Zhu *et al.*, 1993). More important, Penn and Snyder (1993) and Penn *et al.* (1994) showed similar increases in plaque development in young cockerels (between 6 and 22 weeks old) who were exposed to second-hand smoke for 6 h per day for 5 days per week for 12 weeks. The cockerels were exposed to lower levels of second-hand smoke than the rabbits and were eating a normal, low-cholesterol, diet. Although there was no difference in the plaque incidence between the cockerels breathing second-hand smoke and the cockerels breathing clean air, there was a significant dose-dependent acceleration in the growth of these plaques associated with passive smoking.

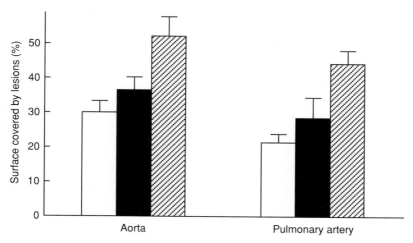

*Figure 13.2* Passive smoking increases lipid deposits in arteries of rabbits in a dose-dependent manner. Bars are for control (clean air), low-dose, and high-dose second-hand smoke exposures. Reproduced with permission of the American College of Cardiology from Zhu *et al.* (1993).

The carcinogens in smoke appear to be acting as a promoter to facilitate the development of plaques rather than to initiate them. In addition, it is unlikely that these effects are due to the carbon monoxide in the smoke because other experiments in which chickens were exposed to high doses of carbon monoxide did not produce similar effects (Penn *et al.*, 1992). In contrast, exposure to second-hand smoke for a relatively brief time (corresponding to about 0.4 percent of their life span) significantly accelerated the development of plaques. The fact that it is possible to induce atherosclerotic-like changes in two different species of experimental animals with only a few weeks' exposure to second-hand smoke similar to that experienced by people in normal day-to-day life is an important finding linking the epidemiologic and biochemical evidence that passive smoking causes heart disease. The experimental studies on rabbits and cockerels, which do not suffer from the potential confounding variables in epidemiologic studies, bridge this gap by showing that it is possible to induce atherosclerosis in experimental animals with second-hand smoke. Finally, there are also data in humans showing that passive smokers have significantly thicker carotid artery walls than people who were never exposed to passive or active smoking, with a dose–response relationship (Howard *et al.*, 1994). Moreover, He *et al.* (1996) observed that the number of stenotic (blocked or narrowed) coronary arteries observed in patients during coronary angiography was related to the amount of second-hand smoke to which they had been exposed. These results are consistent with what one would expect from the animal experiments. The causal link between passive smoking and atherosclerosis is complete.

## Free radicals in second-hand smoke and ischemic damage

Free radicals are highly reactive oxygen products (Church and Pryor, 1985; Ferrari *et al.*, 1991) which are extremely destructive to the heart muscle cell membrane as well as other processes within the cell. Passive smoking worsens the outcome of an ischemic event in the heart through the activity of free radicals during reperfusion injury. Animal studies indicate that low exposures to nicotine or other cigarette smoke constituents significantly worsens reperfusion injury.

The nicotine of just one cigarette doubled the reperfusion injury in dogs (Przyklenk, 1994). This is so low a dose of nicotine that it had no effect on heart rate, blood pressure, regional myocardial shortening, or other hemodynamic measures of cardiac function commonly affected by nicotine in active and passive smokers (Benowitz, 1991). In a dog, after an ischemic episode in which the left anterior descending coronary artery was litigated for 15 min, the regional shortening during reperfusion was reduced by 50 percent of the preischemic values. When the dog was exposed to the nicotine from just a single cigarette, the muscle shortened by 25 percent of control values. When the dog was given a free radical scavenger with the nicotine, this effect was obliterated. Thus, exposure to a very low dose of nicotine doubled the impact of the reperfusion injury.

The effects of free radicals induced by passive smoking have been explored at the cellular level (van Jaarsveld *et al.*, 1992a,b). Rats who were exposed to second-hand smoke from two cigarettes per day for 2 months exhibited severely damaged mitochondrial function during reperfusion injury, such that the ability of cardiac mitochondrial cells to convert oxygen into ATP was much more compromised during reperfusion injury among rats exposed to these low doses of second-hand smoke than among control rats. This is another way in which the toxins in second-hand smoke interfere with myocardial energy metabolism.

There is also some evidence that smokers are less sensitive to free radical damage from cigarette smoke than non-smokers because of changes in the levels of enzymes that control free radicals (McCusker and Hoidal, 1990). When hamsters were exposed to second-hand smoke from six cigarettes per day for 8 weeks, the activity of antioxidant enzymes in their lungs nearly doubled. Similar changes were found in the lungs of smokers compared with non-smokers. This is another piece of evidence that the effects of passive cigarette smoking on smokers and non-smokers may be different. Chronic exposure to cigarette smoke appears to increase the free radical scavenging systems in smokers, a benefit that non-smokers would not have when breathing someone else's smoke.

In addition, passive smoking by humans sensitizes lung neutrophils (Anderson *et al.*, 1991). As with platelets, neutrophils are an important element of the body's defenses against infection and damage. Inappropriately activated neutrophils, however, release oxidants, and these elements can play a role in tissue damage in passive smokers. In a group of passive smokers exposed to just 3 h of sidestream smoke, there were significant increases in the circulating leukocyte counts and stimulated neutrophil migration. (This study deals with neutrophils in the lungs, but it is reasonable to assume that the neutrophils exhibit similar effects throughout the body as they are transported by the blood.) Like the other responses, the responses to exposure to second-hand smoke were greater in non-smokers than in smokers, again suggesting that the biochemistry of second-hand smoke in passive smokers is different from that in active smokers, with the passive smokers being more sensitive to the toxins in second-hand smoke.

## Myocardial infarction

There are also direct animal data to show that second-hand smoke promotes more tissue damage following myocardial infarction. Dogs exposed to second-hand smoke for 1 h daily for 10 days and then subjected to blockage of a coronary artery developed myocardial infarctions that were twice as large as those of control dogs that breathed clean air (Prentice *et al.*, 1989). This effect was not due to elevated circulating levels of nicotine or carboxyhemoglobin, because the infarcts were created the day after the last day of second-hand smoke exposure. Zhu *et al.* (1994) conducted an experiment in rats, similar to the rabbit experiment discussed above, to investigate the effects of second-hand smoke exposure on infarct size. Rats were exposed to second-hand smoke for 6 h per day for 3 days, 3 weeks, or 6 weeks and were then subjected to a left coronary artery occlusion for 35 min, followed by reperfusion. There was a dose-dependent increase in infarct size, with the longest exposure (180 h total second-hand smoke exposure) yielding infarcts that were nearly twice as large as those in the control group that breathed clean air (Figure 13.3). It was also possible to block this effect by feeding the animals L-arginine, the amino acid which is a precursor for nitric oxide (Zhu *et al.*, 1996). This result suggests that the fact that second-hand smoke interferes with the vascular endothelium helps to mediate the effects of second-hand smoke on myocardial infarction. There is no evidence of a threshold effect.

Although smokers seem to be less sensitive to effects of passive smoking than non-smokers, it is important to recognize that even low doses of cigarette smoke can have important effects for smokers. For patients with coronary artery disease, smoking one cigarette significantly increases the coronary vascular resistance (Quillen *et al.*, 1993). Thus, at a time when demands for oxygen and blood supply to the heart are increasing (Fenton and Dobson, 1985; Benowitz, 1991), even a single cigarette can dramatically reduce the ability of smokers' coronaries to transmit blood. In addition, in habitual smokers, smoking a single cigarette causes an increase in the stiffness of coronary arterial walls, and this increased stiffness may be related to the rupturing of the atherosclerotic plaque, which can be an important element in myocardial infarction (Kool *et al.*, 1993). It is likely that low doses of cigarette smoke will have similar effects in passive smokers.

## Epidemiologic studies

Several investigators have reviewed the epidemiologic studies of passive smoking and heart disease (Wells, 1988, 1994, 1998; Glantz and Parmley, 1991, 1995;

411

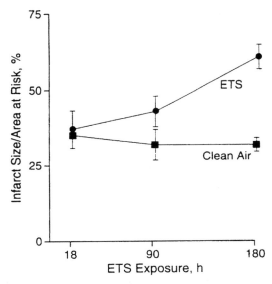

*Figure 13.3* Passive smoking increases infarct size in rats subjected to a 35-min occlusion of the left coronary artery in a dose-dependent manner. There is no evidence of a threshold effect. Data from Zhu *et al.* (1994), used with permission of the American Heart Association.

Law *et al.*, 1997; Office of Environmental Health Hazard Assessment, 1997). There are now adequate epidemiologic data to conclude that passive smoking causes both fatal and non-fatal cardiac events.

Wells (1994) summarized twelve studies (counting end-points for men and women separately, even if they were reported in the same paper) that examined heart disease mortality associated with passive smoking: seven of non-smoking women married to men who smoke (Garland *et al.*, 1985; Butler, 1988, 1990; Helsing *et al.*, 1988; Hole *et al.*, 1989; Jackson, 1989; Sandler *et al.*, 1989; Hirayama, 1990; Humble *et al.*, 1990) and five of non-smoking men married to women who smoke (Svendsen *et al.*, 1987; Butler, 1988, 1990; Helsing *et al.*, 1988; Hole *et al.*, 1989; Jackson, 1989; Sandler *et al.*, 1989). [Two other studies, published as abstracts (Hunt *et al.*, 1986; Palmer *et al.*, 1988), showed increased risk, but Wells excluded them from his formal analysis because they were never published in full. The fact that the only known unpublished data on passive smoking and heart disease are positive is evidence against the claim (Rennie, 1993, 1994; Bero *et al.*, 1994) that there is a publication bias against negative studies on second-hand smoke.] Of these twelve studies, eleven show an elevation in risk of death from heart disease for non-smokers married to smokers, after controlling for other risk factors for ischemic heart disease (e.g. diet, weight, and age). The probability of observing eleven of twelve studies with an increased risk by chance if passive smoking did not affect the risk of heart disease death is only 0.003, or about 3 in 1000. In addition, eight of these studies show a positive dose–response relationship.

These results are consistent with the conclusion that passive smoking increases the risk of heart disease death.

The problem in interpreting any epidemiologic study is that the results depend not only on the true effect of the toxic agent being studied (in this case, environmental tobacco smoke) but also on the specific individuals who happen to be selected in the random sample obtained for the study. This uncertainty is commonly quantified using a confidence interval, which provides a range within which the true relative risk is likely to lie. The 95 percent confidence interval covers the range in which one can be 95 percent confident that the true relative risk lies. While the question of statistical significance deals with whether or not the confidence interval includes 1.0, the fact is that we can be 95 percent confident that the true relative risk lies somewhere in the confidence interval. It is equally likely that the true risk could be at the upper end of the interval as at the lower end, a fact that the tobacco industry rarely notes. In other words, the risk of heart disease from second-hand smoke could be substantially larger than estimated based on the point estimates or lower bounds of the confidence intervals, even if the lower bound is below 1.0. If the 95 percent confidence interval excludes 1.0, one can conclude with 95 percent confidence that passive smoking changes the risk of dying of heart disease. Note that this is a two-tailed test, in which one considers not only the possibility that passive smoking increases the risk of heart disease but also that passive smoking reduces the risk of heart disease, i.e. breathing second-hand smoke would be protective of coronary artery disease. As no one – not even the tobacco industry – has asserted that passive smoking is good for people's health, a two-tailed test seems overly conservative. It is probably more appropriate to use a one-tailed test which tests the question of whether or not passive smoking increases the risk of heart disease. In this case, it would be more appropriate to see whether or not the two-tailed 90 percent confidence interval includes 1.0, because the lower bound of the two-tailed 90 percent confidence interval is exactly equal to the lower bound for the one-tailed 95 percent confidence interval. By examining the confidence intervals, we can conclude that three of the studies, taken individually, each provides strong enough evidence to be 95 percent certain that passive smoking changes the risk of dying of heart disease. Moreover, we can be 97.5 percent confident that it increases the risk of dying from heart disease. The probability of obtaining three such positive tests by chance is $(1-0.975)^3 = 0.00002$, or about 2 in 100 000. These three positive studies alone provide adequate evidence to conclude that secondhand tobacco smoke exposure increases the risk of death from heart disease.

This situation leaves us with the question of how to interpret the remaining nine studies, which did not reach statistical significance. There are two reasons that a test may not reach statistical significance. The first reason would be that the toxin being investigated, in this case secondhand smoke, in fact did not affect the risk of death. In this case, failure to reach statistical significance would be a true negative, meaning that the statistical test did not detect an effect because none existed. Unfortunately, however, there is a second reason that a test may not reach statistical significance: the sample size was too small. The sensitivity of any statistical test – its power – increases with the size of the study. Just as it is traditionally considered desirable to be able to reach statistical significance on a positive conclusion with 95 percent confidence, it is considered desirable to reach an 80 percent power before confidently reaching a negative conclusion from a statistical analysis. Unfortunately, because of small sample sizes, none of the studies of passive smoking and heart disease reach this level of power. Indeed, most of the studies have power below 10 percent (to detect a 20 percent increase in risk associated with passive smoking) (Glantz and Parmley, 1991). This low power makes it unreliable to reach a negative conclusion based on many of these studies, taken one at a time.

The solution to this problem is to treat all of the studies together as one large study, which increases the effective sample size and raises the power of the analysis. As a result of this increased power, we can be more confident in both positive and negative conclusions. Wells (1994) pooled the results from all twelve studies using the same approach that the US Environmental Protection Agency (1992) did to evaluate passive smoking and lung cancer. This procedure demonstrated that the relative risk for dying of heart disease was 1.2 (with a 95 percent confidence interval extending from 1.1 to 1.4). Therefore, we can be more than 95 percent confident that passive smoking affects the risk of dying from heart disease and more than 97.5 percent confident that passive smoking increases the risk of death from heart disease.

Applying this risk on a population basis yields an estimated 62 000 heart disease deaths in 1985 (Wells, 1994), compared with only 3000 from lung cancer (US Environmental Protection Agency, 1992). Because of declines in smoking and increases in smoke-free environments, Wells (1994) estimates that this toll has fallen to 47 000 in 1994.

When Wells (1994) limited his analysis to just the best five of the studies for heart disease deaths, he obtained a higher adjusted relative risk for passive smoking and heart disease mortality of 1.7 (with a 95 percent confidence interval extending from 1.3 to 2.3). The fact that excluding the lower quality studies increased the pooled relative risk estimate is a very interesting point because it indicates that the better the quality of the study – defined as controlling for other factors which contribute to heart disease – the higher the risk attributed to second-hand smoke. The tobacco industry and its consultants (Barnes and Bero, 1998) often criticize studies for failing to account for confounding variables on the grounds that failure to account for confounders artificially inflates the observed relative risk and makes it appear that ETS is more dangerous than it really is. The actual situation is just the opposite.

Law et al. (1997) conducted a similar analysis of nineteen studies (Garland et al., 1985; Lee et al., 1986; Svendsen et al., 1987; He et al., 1989, 1994; Hole et al., 1989; Sandler et al., 1989; Hirayama, 1990; Humble et al., 1990; Dobson et al., 1991; LaVecchia et al., 1993; Muscat and Wynder, 1995; Tunstall-Pedoe et al., 1995; Ciruzzi et al., 1996; Steenland et al., 1996; Kawachi et al.,

1997) of the risk of ischemic heart disease in never-smokers whose spouses currently smoked. They found an overall relative risk of 1.30 (95 percent confidence interval 1.18 to 1.38) due to passive smoking (Figure 13.4). Moreover, they demonstrated that this effect was unlikely to be the result of confounding with other variables. They also showed that this risk was consistent with the observed increase in risk of heart disease in active smokers who smoked one cigarette per day, providing epidemiologic evidence to support the existence of a superlinear dose–response curve.

In addition to the epidemiologic studies that used death as an end-point, there are also thirteen studies (considering men and women separately) that examined non-fatal cardiac disease, such as a non-fatal myocardial infarction, presence of angina, or malignant electrocardiographic changes (Svendsen *et al.*, 1987; He *et al.*, 1989, 1994; Hole *et al.*, 1989; Jackson, 1989; Lee, 1989; Dobson *et al.*, 1991; LaVecchia *et al.*, 1993; Ciruzzi *et al.*, 1998). Eleven of these studies show an elevation in risk. The probability of observing eleven positive studies out of thirteen if there was no effect of passive smoking on non-fatal cardiac events is only 0.01. A formal analysis (A. J. Wells, personal communication) to pool the first eleven of these studies yields a relative risk for non-fatal coronary events associated with exposure to second-hand smoke of 1.3 (with a 95 percent confidence interval of 1.1 to 1.6). Three of these studies show a dose–response relationship, with

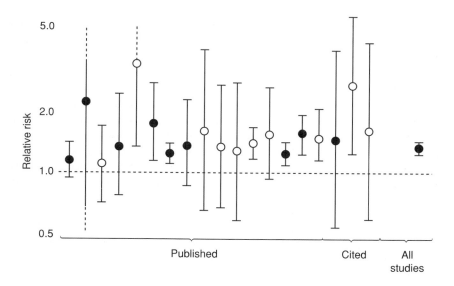

*Figure 13.4* Relative risk estimates (with 95 percent confidence intervals), adjusted for age and sex, from nine prospective studies (solid circles) and ten case–control studies (open circles) comparing ischemic heart disease in lifelong non-smokers whose spouse currently smokes with those whose spouse never smoked. Reproduced with permission of the *British Medical Journal* from Law *et al.* (1997).

higher exposures of second-hand smoke associated with larger increases in risk. Wells (1998) also demonstrated similar increases in risk for second-hand smoke exposure in the workplace. The fact that passive smoking increases the risk of non-fatal coronary events as well as fatal coronary events is consistent with what we know about the physiology and biochemistry of how passive smoking affects the heart.

Some of these studies used marriage to a current smoker as the measure of exposure to secondhand smoke, whereas others used marriage to an ever-smoker (even if the spouse was currently a non-smoker) as the measure of exposure to secondhand smoke. Given the fact that the effects of smoking (and, presumably, passive smoking) on the heart decline quickly (USDHHS, 1990; Lightwood and Glantz, 1997) when exposure ends, the design of these studies is often biased against detecting an effect of secondhand smoke on heart disease. In addition, the facts that the observed risks are of similar magnitude across studies carried out in many countries and that controlling for a variety of the other risk factors for heart disease strengthen the confidence one can have in reaching a conclusion that passive smoking causes heart disease.

The only difference between a fatal and non-fatal coronary event is the severity of the event, i.e. whether or not the insult to the heart is so large that the cardiovascular system's natural adaptive defenses can compensate for it. If the cardiovascular system can compensate, or the individual reaches medical care quickly enough, the coronary event will not be fatal. Thus, the presence of an effect of passive smoking on both fatal and non-fatal coronary events is additional important evidence supporting the fact that passive smoking causes heart disease.

## Conclusion

The ability of the heart and vascular system to adapt to changing conditions is very important when considering the health effects of environmental tobacco smoke, particularly when one compares the effects of secondhand smoke in non-smokers and smokers. People who smoke cigarettes are chronically and continually adversely affecting their cardiovascular system (USPHS, 1983), which adapts to compensate for all the deleterious effects of smoking. Non-smokers, however, do not have the "benefit" of this adaptation, so the effects of passive smoking on non-smokers are much greater than on smokers. This difference probably arises for two reasons. First, non-smokers' hearts and vascular systems have not attempted to adapt to the chemicals in the second-hand smoke. Second, it appears that the cardiovascular system is extremely sensitive to many of the chemicals in second-hand smoke and that smokers may have achieved the maximum response possible to at least some of the toxins in the smoke; so, the small additional exposures associated with passive smoking have little or no effect on habitual smokers because the additional dose of these toxins is so tiny compared with what the smoker normally receives.

These two facts make it imperative to consider the effects of environmental tobacco smoke on the cardiovascular system of passive smokers separately from the effects on active smokers. The qualitative differences between the effects of secondhand smoke on smokers and non-smokers explains the high relative risks associated with passive smoking compared with active smoking, even though passive smokers absorb much smaller doses of the toxins in cigarette smoke than do smokers (Wu-Williams and Samet, 1990). In particular, the practice – often advocated by the tobacco industry when considering second-hand smoke – of thinking about "cigarette equivalents" or dose-based extrapolations from smokers to non-smokers will lead to gross underestimations of the risks of passive smoking to the cardiovascular system. The tobacco industry is fond of saying that even a heavily exposed passive smoker only breathes in the equivalent of about of one cigarette per day. Leaving aside the philosophical question of whether anyone ought to be required to breathe one cigarette a day under any circumstances, the smoke from one cigarette is enough to produce substantial effects on the cardiovascular system.

Using different methodologies, several investigators have estimated the population burden associated with passive smoking and heart disease, yielding estimates of 30 000–62 000 deaths annually in the USA (Wells, 1988, 1994, 1998; Glantz and Parmley, 1991; Steenland, 1992; Office of Environmental Health Hazard Assessment, 1997) with about three times as many non-fatal cardiovascular events. This is a tremendous public health impact and one that warrants strong action, commensurate with that devoted to other smaller health problems such as illegal drugs and AIDS (Glantz, 1994), to protect workers, children, and the general public. The simplest and most cost-effective control measure is to mandate smoke-free workplaces, schools, and public places (Stillman *et al.*, 1990; Siegel, 1993; Woodruff *et al.*, 1993; Pierce *et al.*, 1994a,b; Glantz, 1997).

## Acknowledgment

This chapter is an updated version of two earlier papers by the authors (Glantz and Parmley, 1991, 1995). This material is used with permission of the American Heart Association and American Medical Association.

## References

Albert, R.E., Vanderlaan, M., Burns, F.J., and Nishizumi, M. 1977. Effect of carcinogens on chicken atherosclerosis. *Cancer Res* 37: 2232–2235.

Allred, E.N., Bleecker, E.R., Chaitman, B.R., Dahms, T.E., Gottlieb, S.O., Hackney, J.D., Pagano, M., Selvester, R.H., Walden, S.M., and Warren, J. 1989. Short-term effects of carbon monoxide exposure on the exercise performance of subjects with coronary artery disease. *N Engl J Med* 321: 1426–1432.

Anderson, R., Theron, A.J., Richards, G.A., Myer, M.S., and van Rensburg, A.J. 1991. Passive smoking by humans sensitizes circulating neutrophils. *Am Rev Respir Dis* 144: 570–574.

Aronow, W. 1978. Effect of passive smoking on angina pectoris. *N Engl J Med* 299: 21–24.

Barnes, D.E. and Bero, L.A. 1998. Why review articles on the health effects of passive smoking reach different conclusions. *J Am Med Assoc* 279: 1566–70.

Benowitz, N.L. 1991. Nicotine and coronary heart disease. *Trends Cardiovasc Med* 1: 315–321.

Benowitz, N.L., Fitzgerald, G.A., Wilson, M., and Zhang, Q. 1993. Nicotine effects on eicosanoid formation and hemostatic function: Comparison of transdermal nicotine and cigarette smoking. *J Am Coll Cardiol* 22: 1159–1167.

Bero, L.A., Glantz, S.A., and Rennie, D. 1994. Publication bias and public health policy on environmental tobacco smoke. *J Am Med Assoc* 272: 133–136.

Burghuber, O., Punzengruber, C., Sinzinger, H., Haber, P., and Silberbauer, K. 1986. Platelet sensitivity to prostacyclin in smokers and non-smokers. *Chest* 90: 34–38.

Butler, T.L. 1988. *The Relationship of Passive Smoking to Various Health Outcomes Among Seventh Day Adventists in California.* University of California, Los Angeles.

Butler, T. 1990. The relationship of passive smoking to various health outcomes among Seventh-Day Adventists in California. In *Proceedings of the Seventh World Conference on Tobacco and Health*, 1–5 April 1990, Perth, Australia, p. 316.

Church, D.F. and Pryor, W.A. 1985. Free-radical chemistry of cigarette smoke and its toxicological implications. *Environ Health Persp* 64: 111–126.

Ciruzzi, M., Esteban, O., Rozlosnik, J., Montagna, H., Caccavo, A., and De La Cruz, J. 1996. Passive smoking and the risk of acute myocardial infarction. *Eur Heart J* 17 (Suppl.): 309.

Ciruzzi, M., Pramparo, P., Esteban, O., Rozlosnik, J., Tartagilone, J., Abecasis, B., Cesar, J., De Rosa, J., Paterno, C., and Schargrodsky, H. 1998. Case–control study of passive smoking at home and risk of acute myocardial infarction. *J Am Coll Cardiol* 31: 797–803.

Davis, J. 1990. Some acute effects of smoking on endothelial cells and platelets. In *Tobacco Smoking and Atherosclerosis: Pathogenesis and Cellular Mechanisms.* Diana, J. (ed.), pp. 107–119. Plenum Press, New York.

Davis, J., Shelton, L., Hartman, C., Eigenberg, D., and Ruttinger, H. 1986. Smoking-induced changes in endothelium and platelets are not affected by hydroxyethylrutosides. *Br J Exp Pathol* 67: 765–771.

Davis, J., Shelton, L., Watanabe, I., and Arnold, J. 1989. Passive smoking affects endothelium and platelets. *Arch Intern Med* 149: 386–389.

Davis, J., Shelton, L., and Zucker, M. 1990. A comparison of some acute effects of smoking and smokeless tobacco on platelets and endothelium. *J Vasc Med Biol* 2: 289–293.

Davis, J.W., Hartman, C.R., Lewis, Jr., H.D., Shelton, L., Eigenberg, D.A., Hassanein, K.M., Hignite, C.E., and Ruttinger, H.A. 1985a. Cigarette smoking-induced enhancement of platelet function: Lack of prevention by aspirin in men with coronary artery disease. *J Lab Clin Med* 105: 479–483.

Davis, J.W., Shelton, L., Eigenberg, D.A., Hignite, C.E., and Watanabe, I.S. 1985b. Effects of tobacco and non-tobacco cigarette smoking on endothelium and platelets. *Clin Pharmacol Ther* 37: 529–533.

Davis, J.W., Shelton, L., Eigenberg, D.A., and Hignite, C.E. 1987. Lack of effect of aspirin on cigarette smoke-induced increase in circulating endothelial cells. *Haemostasis* 7: 66–69.

Dobson, A.J., Alexander, H.M., Heller, R.F., and Lloyd, D.M. 1991. Passive smoking and the risk of heart attack or coronary death. *Med J. Aust* 154: 793–797.

Dwyer, E.M.J. and Turino, G.M. 1989. Carbon monoxide and cardiovascular disease. *N Engl J Med* 21: 1474–1475.

Elwood, P.S.R., Sharp, D., Beswick, A., O'Brien, J., and Yarnell, J. 1991. Ischemic heart disease and platelet aggregation: The Caerphilly collaborative heart disease study. *Circulation* 83: 38–44.

Feldman, J., Shenker, I.R., Etzel, R.A., Spierto, F.W., Lilienfeld, D.E., Nussbaum, M., and Jacobson, M.S. 1991. Passive smoking alters lipid profiles in adolescents. *Pediatrics* 88: 259–264.

Fenton, R.A. and Dobson, J.G.J. 1985. Nicotine increases heart adenosine release, oxygen consumption, and contractility. *Am J Physiol (Heart)* 249: H463–H469.

Ferrari, R., Ceconi, C., Curello, S., Cargnoni, A., Alfieri, O., Pardini, A., Marzollo, P., and Visioli, O. 1991. Oxygen free radicals and myocardial damage: Protective role of thiol-containing agents. *Am J Med* 91 (Suppl. 3C): 95S–105S.

Garland, C., Barrett-Connor, E., Suarez, L., Criqui, M., and Wingard, D. 1985. Effects of passive smoking on ischemic heart disease mortality of nonsmokers. *Am J Epidemiol* 121: 645–650.

Gidding, S.S., Morgan, W., Perry, C., Isabel-Jones, J., Bricker, J.T., Kavey, R.W., Bricker, J.T., Daniels, S.R., Deckelbaum, R., Fisher, E., Marx, G.R., Teske, D., Wilmore, J., Wall, M., and Schydlower, M. 1994. Active and passive tobacco exposure: a serious pediatric health problem: A statement from the Committee on Atherosclerosis and Hypertension in Children, Council on Cardiovascular Disease in the Young, American Heart Association. *Circulation* 90: 2582–2590.

Glantz, S.A. 1994. Actual causes of death in the United States (letter). *J Am Med Assoc* 271: 660.

Glantz, S.A. 1997. Back to basics: Getting smoke free workplaces back on track (editorial). *Tobacco Control* 6: 164–166.

Glantz, S.A. and Parmley, W. 1995. Passive smoking and heart disease: Mechanisms and risk. *J Am Med Assoc* 273: 1047–1053.

Glantz, S.A. and Parmley, W.W. 1991. Passive smoking and heart disease: Epidemiology, physiology, and biochemistry. *Circulation* 83: 1–12.

Gvozdjak, J., Gvozdjakova, A., Kucharska, J. and Bada, V. 1987. The effect of smoking on myocardial metabolism. *Czech Med* 10: 47–53.

Gvozdjakova, A., Kucharska, J., and Gvozdjak, J. 1992. Effect of smoking on the oxidative processes of cardiomyocytes. *Cardiology* 81: 81–84.

He, Y., Li, L.-S., Wan, Z.-H., Li, L.-S., Zheng, X.-L., and Gru, L.-L. 1989. Women's passive smoking and coronary heart disease. *Chung-Hua-Yu-Fang-I-Hsueh-Tsa-Chin* 23: 19–22.

He, Y., Lam, T.H., Li, T.S., Li, L.S., Du, R.Y., Jia, G.L., Huang, J.Y., and Zheng, J.S. 1994. Passive smoking at work as a risk factor for coronary heart disease in Chinese women who have never smoked. *Br Med J* 308: 380–384.

He, Y., Lam, T., Li, L.S., Li, L., Du, R., Jia, G., Huang, J., and Zheng, J. 1996. The number of stenotic coronary arteries is associated with the amount of passive smoking exposure. *Atherosclerosis* 127: 229–238.

Helsing, K., Sandler, D.G.C., and Chee, E. 1988. Heart disease mortality in nonsmokers living with smokers. *Am J Epidemiol* 127: 915–922.

Hirayama, T. 1990. Passive smoking. *NZ Med J* 103: 54.

Hole, D.J., Gillis, C.R., Chopra, C., and Hawthorne, V.M. 1989. Passive smoking and cardiorespiratory health in a general population in the west of Scotland. *Br Med J* 299: 423–427.

Howard, D., Ota, R., Briggs, L., Hampton, M., and Pritscos, C. 1998. Environmental tobacco smoke in the workplace induces oxidative stress in employees, including increased production of 8-hydroxy-2'-deoxyguanosine. *Cancer Epidemiol Biomarkers Prev* 7: 141–146.

Howard, G., Burke, G.L., Szklo, M., Tell, G., Eckfeldt, J., Evans, G., and Heiss, G. 1994. Active and passive smoking are associated with increased carotid artery wall thickness: The Atherosclerosis Risk in Communities Study. *Arch Intern Med* 154: 1277–1282.

Humble, C., Croft, J., Gerber, A.M.C., Hames, C., and Tyroler, H. 1990. Passive smoking and twenty year cardiovascular disease mortality among nonsmoking wives in Evans County, Georgia. *Am J Public Health* 80: 599–601.

Hunt, S.C., Martin, M.J., and Williams, R.R. 1986. *Passive Smoking by Nonsmoking Wives is Associated with an Increased Incidence of Heart Disease.* American Public Health Association, Las Vegas.

Hutchinson, S., Sievers, R., Zhu, B.-Q., Sun, Y.-P., Sudhir, K., Deedwania, P., Parmley, W., and Chaterjee, K. 1995. Physiological concentrations of testosterone impair endothelium-dependent vasodilation in hypercholesterolemic rabbits exposed to tobacco smoke. *Circulation* 92: I-68.

Hutchinson, S., Ibarra, M., Chou, T., Sievers, R., Chaterjee, K., Glantz, S., Deedwania, P., and Parmley, W. 1996. L-arginine restores normal endothelium-mediated relaxation in hypercholesterolemic rabbits exposed to environmental tobacco smoke. *J Am Coll Cardiol* 27 (Suppl.): 39A.

Hutchison, S., Sudhir, K., Chou, T., Sievers, R., Zhu, B., Sun, Y., Deedwania, P., Glantz, S., Parmely, W., and Chatterjee, K. 1997a. Testosterone worsens endothelial dysfunction associated with hypercholesterolemia and environmental tobacco smoke exposure in male rabbit aorta. *J Am Coll Cardiol* 29: 800–807.

Hutchison, S., Reitz, M., Sudhir, K., Sievers, R., Zhu, B., Sun, Y., Chou, T., Deedwania, P., Chatterjee, K., Glantz, S., and Parmley, W. 1997b. Chronic dietary L-arginine prevents endothelial dysfunction secondary to environmental tobacco smoke in normocholesterolemic rabbits. *Hypertension* 29: 1186–1191.

Hutchison, S., Glantz, S., Zhu, B.-Q., Sun, Y.P., Chou, T., Chaterjee, K., Deedwania, P., Parmley, W., and Sudhir, K. 1998. In-utero and neonatal exposure to secondhand smoke causes vascular dysfunction in newborn rats. *J Am Coll Cardiol* 32: 1463–1467.

Hutchison, S., Sudhir, K., Sievers, R., Zhu, B., Sun, Y., Chou, T., Chatterjee, K., Deedwania, P., Cooke, J., Glantz, S., and Parmley, W. 1999. Beneficial effects of chronic L-arginine supplementation on atherogenesis, endothelium-mediated relaxation, and nitric oxide production in hypercholesterolemic rabbits exposed to second hand smoke. *Hypertension* 34: 44–50.

van Jaarsveld, H., Kuyl, J.M., and Alberts, D.W. 1992a. Antioxidant vitamin supplementation of smoke-exposed rats partially protects against myocardial ischaemic/reperfusion injury. *Free Radical Res Commun* 17: 263–269.

van Jaarsveld, H., Kuyl, J.M., and Alberts, D.W. 1992b. Exposure of rats to low concentration of cigarette smoke increases myocardial sensitivity to ischaemia/reperfusion. *Basic Res Cardiol* 87: 393–399.

Jackson, R.T. 1989. *The Auckland Heart Study.* University of Auckland, Auckland, New Zealand.

Kawachi, I., Colditz, G., Speizer, F., Manson, J., Stampfer, M., Willett, W., and Hennekens, C. 1997. A prospective study of passive smoking and coronary heart disease. *Circulation* 95: 2374–2379.

Khaifen, E.S. and Klochkov, V.A. 1987. Effect of passive smoking on physical tolerance of ischemia heart disease patients. *Ter Arkh* 59: 112–115.

Kool, M.J.F., Hoeks, A.P.G., Boudier, H.A.J.S., Reneman, R.S., and Van Bortel, L.M.A.B. 1993. Acute and chronic effects of smoking on arterial wall properties in habitual smokers. *J Am Coll Cardiol* 22: 1881–1886.

Lamb, D. 1984. *Physiology of Exercise: Responses and Adaptation*. Macmillan Publishing, New York.

LaVecchia, C., D'Avanzo, B., Franzosi, M.G., and Tognoni, G. 1993. Passive smoking and the risk of acute myocardial infarction. *Lancet* 341: 505–506.

Law, M., Morris, J., and Wald, N. 1997. Environmental tobacco smoke exposure and ischaemic heart disease: An evaluation of the evidence. *Br Med J* 315: 973–980.

Lee, P. 1989. Deaths from lung cancer and ischaemic heart disease due to passive smoking in New Zealand. *NZ Med J* 102: 448.

Lee, P., Chamberlain, J., and Alderson, M. 1986. Relationship of passive smoking to risk of lung cancer and other smoking-associated diseases. *Br J Cancer* 54: 97–105.

Leone, A., Mori, L., Bertanelli, F., Fabiano, P., and Filippelli, M. 1991. Indoor passive smoking: Its effect on cardiac performance. *Int J Cardiol* 33: 247–252.

Leone, A., Bertanelli, F., Mori, L., Fabiato, P., and Bertanelli, G. 1992. Ventricular arrhythmias by passive smoke in patients with pre-existing myocardial infarction. *Am J Cardiol* 19: 256A.

Lightwood, J.M. and Glantz, S.A. 1997. Short-term economic and health benefits of smoking cessation: myocardial infarction and stroke. *Circulation* 96: 1089–1096.

McCusker, K. and Hoidal, J. 1990. Selective increase of antioxidant enzyme activity in the alveolar macrophages from cigarette smokers and smoke-exposed hamsters. *Am Rev Respir Dis* 141: 678–682.

McMurray, R.G., Hicks, L.L., and Thompson, D.L. 1985. The effects of passive inhalation of cigarette smoke on exercise performance. *Eur J Appl Physiol* 54: 196–200.

Majesky, M., Yang, H., and Benditt, E. 1983. Carcinogenesis and atherogenesis: Differences in monoxygenase inducibility and bioactivation of benzo(a)pyrene in aortic and hepatic tissues of atherosclerosis-susceptible versus resistant pigeons. *Carcinogenesis* 4: 647–652.

Martin, J.F., Bath, P.M., and Burr, M.L. 1991. Influence of platelet size on outcome after myocardial infarction. *Lancet* 338: 1409–1411.

Miyaura, S., Eguchi, H., and Johnson, J.M. 1992. Effect of a cigarette smoke extract on the metabolism of the proinflammatory autacoid, platelet-activating factor. *Circ Res* 70: 341–347.

Moskowitz, W., Mosteller, M., Schieken, R., Bossano, R., Hewitt, J., Bodurtha, J., and Segrest, J. 1990. Lipoprotein and oxygen transport alterations in passive smoking preadolescent children: The MCV Irwin study. *Circulation* 81: 586–592.

Moskowitz, W.B., Mosteller, M., Hewitt, J.K., Eaves, L.J., Nance, W.E., and Schieken, R.M. 1993. Univariate genetic analysis of oxygen transport regulation in children: The Medical College of Virginia twin study. *Pediatr Res* 33: 645–648.

Muscat, J. and Wynder, E. 1995. Exposure to environmental tobacco smoke and risk of heart attack. *Int J Epidemiol* 24: 715–719.

Office of Environmental Health Hazard Assessment. 1997. *Health Effects of Exposure to Environmental Tobacco Smoke.* California Environmental Protection Agency, Sacramento, CA.

Ott, W., Landan, L., and Switzer, P. 1992. A time series model for cigarette smoking activity patterns: Model validation for carbon monoxide and respirable particles in a chamber and an automobile. *J Exposure Anal Environ Epidemiol* 2 (Suppl. 2): 175–200.

Palmer, J., Rosenberg, L., and Shapiro, S. 1988. Passive smoking and myocardial infarction. *CVD Epidemiol Newsletter* 43: 29.

Penn, A. and Snyder, C.A. 1993. Inhalation of sidestream cigarette smoke accelerates development of arteriosclerotic plaques. *Circulation* 88 (Part 1): 1820–1825.

Penn, A. and Snyder, C. 1994. Sidestream cigarette smoke; reply. *Circulation* 89: 2943–2944.

Penn, A. and Snyder, C. 1996a. 1,3 Butadiene, a vapor phase component of environmental tobacco smoke, accelerates atherosclerotic plaque development. *Circulation* 93: 552–557.

Penn, A. and Snyder, C. 1996b. Butadiene inhalation accelerates arteriosclerotic plaque development in cockerels. *Toxicology* 113: 351–354.

Penn, A., Batastini, G., Soloman, J., Burns, F., and Albert, R. 1981. Dose-dependent size increases of aortic lesions following chronic exposure to 7.12-dimethybenz(a)-anthracene. *Cancer Res* 41: 588–592.

Penn, A., Garte, S., Warren, L., Nesta, D., and Mindich, B. 1986. Transforming gene is human atherosclerotic plaque DNA. *Proc Natl Acad Sci USA* 83: 7951–7955.

Penn, A., Currie, J., and Snyder, C.A. 1992. Inhalation of carbon monoxide does not accelerate arteriosclerosis in cockerels. *Eur J Pharmacol* 228: 155–164.

Penn, A., Chen, L.C., and Snyder, C.A. 1994. Inhalation of steady-state sidestream smoke from one cigarette promotes atherosclerotic plaque development. *Circulation* 90: 1363–1367.

Penn, A., Keller, K., Snyder, C., Nadas, A., and Chen, L. 1996. The tar fraction of cigarette smoke does not promote arteriosclerotic plaque development. *Environ Health Perspect* 104: 1108–1113.

Pierce, J.P., Evans, N., Farkas, A.J., Cavin, S.W., Berry, C., Kramer, M., Kealey, S., Rosbrook, B., Choi, W., and Kaplan, R.M. 1994a. *Tobacco Use in California: An Evaluation of the Tobacco Control Program, 1989–1993.* University of California, San Diego.

Pierce, J.P., Shanks, T.G., Pertschuk, M., Gilpin, E., Shopland, D., Johnson, M., and Bal, D. 1994b. Do smoking ordinances protect non-smokers from environmental tobacco smoke at work? *Tobacco Control* 3: 15–20.

Pittilo, R.M., Mackie, I.J., Rowles, P.M., Machine, S.J., and Woolf, N. 1982. Effects of cigarette smoking on the ultrastructure of rat thoracic aorta and its ability to produce prostacyclin. *Thromb Haemost* 48: 173–176.

Pomrehn, P., Hollarbush, J., Clarke, W., and Lauer, R. 1990. Children's HDL-chol: The effects of tobacco, smoking, smokeless, and parental smoking. *Circulation* 81: 726.

Prentice, R.C., Carroll, R., Scanlon, P.J., and Thomas, J.X.J. 1989. Recent exposure to cigarette smoke increases myocardial infarct size. *J Am Coll Cardiol* 13: 124A.

Prerovsky, I. and Hladovec, J. 1979. Suppression of the desquamating effect of smoking on the human endothelium by hydroxyethylrutosides. *Blood Vessels* 16: 239–240.

Przyklenk, K. 1994. Nicotine exacerbates postischemic contractile dysfunction of "stunned" myocardium in the canine model: Possible role of free radicals. *Circulation* 89: 1272–1281.

Quillen, J.E., Rossen, J.D., Oskarsson, H.J., Minor, R.L.J., Lopez, A.G., and Winniford, M.D. 1993. Acute effect of cigarette smoking on the coronary circulation: Constriction of epicardial and resistance vessels. *J Am Coll Cardiol* 22: 642–647.

Rennie, D. 1993. Smoke and letters. *J Am Med Assoc* 270: 1742–1743.

Rennie, D. 1994. Smoke and letters. *J Am Med Assoc* 271: 1575.

Revis, N., Bull, R., Laurie, D., and Schiller, C. 1984. The effectiveness of chemical carcinogens to induce atherosclerosis in the white carneau pigeon. *Toxicology* 32: 215–227.

Ross, R. 1986. The pathology of atherosclerosis: An Update. *N Engl J Med* 314: 488–500.

Sandler, D.P., Comstock, G.W., Helsing, K.J., and Shore, D.L. 1989. Deaths from all causes in nonsmokers who lived with smokers. *Am J Public Health* 79: 163–7.

Sheps, D.S., Herbst, M.C., Hinderliter, A.L., Adams, K.F., Ekelund, L.G., O'Neil, J.J., Goldstein, G.M., Bromberg, P.A., Dalton, J.L., Ballenger, M.N., *et al.* 1990. Production of arrhythmias by elevated carboxyhemoglobin in patients with coronary artery disease. *Ann Intern Med* 113: 343–351.

Siegel, M. 1993. Involuntary smoking in the restaurant workplace: A review of employee exposure and health effects. *J Am Med Assoc* 270: 490–493.

Sinzinger, H. and Kefalides, A. 1982. Passive smoking severely decreases platelet sensitivity to antiaggregatory prostaglandins. *Lancet* 2: 392–393.

Sinzinger, H. and Virgolini, I. 1989. Are passive smokers at greater risk of thrombosis? *Wien Klin Wochenschr* 20: 694–698.

Steenland, K. 1992. Passive smoking and the risk of heart disease. *J Am Med Assoc* 267: 94–99.

Steenland, K., Thun, M., Lally, C., and Heath, C.J. 1996. Environmental tobacco smoke and coronary heart disease in the American Cancer Society CPS-II cohort. *Circulation* 94: 622–628.

Stefanadis, C., Vlachopoulos, C., Tsiamis, E., Diamantopoulos, L., Toutouzas, K., Giatrakos, N., Vaina, S., Tsekoura, D., and Toutouzas, P. 1998. Unfavorable effects of passive smoking on aortic function in men. *Ann Intern Med* 128: 426–34.

Steinberg, D., Parthasarathy, S., Carew, T.E., Khoo, J.C., and Witztum, J.L. 1989. Beyond cholesterol: modifications of low-density lipoprotein that increase its atherogenicity. *N Engl J Med* 320: 915–924.

Stillman, F., Becker, D., Swank, R., Hantual, D., Moses, H., Glantz, S., and Waranch, H. 1990. Ending smoking at the Johns Hopkins Medical Institutions: An evaluation of smoking prevalence and indoor pollution. *J Am Med Assoc* 264: 1565–1569.

Sumida, H., Watanabe, H., Kugiyama, K., Ohgushi, M., Matsumura, T., and Yasue, H. 1998. Does passive smoking impair endothelium-dependent coronary artery dilation in women? *J Am Coll Cardiol* 31: 811–5.

Sun, Y.-P., Zhu, B.-Q., Sievers, R.E., Glantz, S.A., and Parmley, W.W. 1994. Metoprolol does not attenuate atherosclerosis in lipid-fed rabbits exposed to environmental tobacco smoke. *Circulation* 89: 2260–2265.

Svendsen, K.H., Kuller, L.H., Martin, M.J., and Ockene, J.K. 1987. Effects of passive smoking in the Multiple Risk Factor Intervention Trial. *Am J Epidemiol* 126: 783–795.

Taylor, A.E., Johnson, D.C., and Kazemi, H. 1992. Environmental tobacco smoke and cardiovascular disease: A position paper from the Council on Cardiopulmonary and Critical Care, American Heart Association. *Circulation* 86: 1–4.

Tunstall-Pedoe, H., Brown, C.A., Woodward, M., and Tavendale, R. 1995. Passive smoking by self report and serum cotinine and the prevalence of respiratory and coronary heart disease in the Scottish heart health study. *J Epidemiol Community Health* 49: 139–43.

USDHHS. 1986. *The Health Consequences of Involuntary Smoking. A Report of the Surgeon General*. US Department of Health and Human Services, Public Health Service, Centers for Disease Control, Washington, DC.

USDHHS. 1990. *The Health Benefits of Smoking Cessation: A Report of the Surgeon General, 1990*. US Department of Health and Human Services, Public Health Service, Centers for Disease Control, Center for Chronic disease Prevention and Health Promotion, Office on Smoking and Health, Washington, DC.

US Environmental Protection Agency. 1992. *Respiratory Health Effects of Passive Smoking: Lung Cancer and Other Disorders*. US Environmental Protection Agency, Washington, DC.

USPHS. 1983. *The Health Consequences of Smoking: Cardiovascular Disease. A Report of the Surgeon General*. USPHS, Washington, DC.

Valkonen, M. and Kuusi, T. 1998. Passive smoking induces atherogenic changes in low-density lipoprotein. *Circulation* 97: 2012–2016.

Wells, A.J. 1988. An estimate of adult mortality in the United States from passive smoking. *Environ Int* 14: 249–265.

Wells, A.J. 1994. Passive smoking as a cause of heart disease. *J Am Coll Cardiol* 24: 546–554.

Wells, A.J. 1998. Heart disease from passive smoking in the workplace. *J Am Coll Cardiol* 31: 1–9.

White, J.R. and Froeb, H.F. 1991. Serum lipoproteins in nonsmokers chronically exposed to tobacco smoke in the workplace. In *Proceedings of the 8th World Conference on Tobacco or Health*, 30 March to 3 April, 1992. Buenos Aires, Argentina.

Woodruff, T., Rosebrook, B., Pierce, J., and Glantz, S. 1993. Lower levels of cigarette consumption found in smoke-free workplaces in California. *Arch Intern Med* 153: 1485–1493.

Wu, J.M. 1993. Increased experimental atherosclerosis in cholesterol-fed rabbits exposed to passive smoke: Taking issue with study design and methods of analysis. *J Am Coll Cardiol* 22: 1751–1752.

Wu-Williams, A. and Samet, J. 1990. Environmental tobacco smoke: Exposure–response relationships in epidemiologic studies. *Risk Analysis* 10: 39–48.

Zhu, B., Sun, Y., Sievers, R.E., Shuman, J.L., Glantz, S.A., Chatterjee, K., Parmley, W.W., and Wolfe, C.L. 1996. L-arginine decreases infarct size in rats exposed to environmental tobacco smoke. *Am Heart J* 132: 91–100.

Zhu, B.Q. and Parmley, W.W. 1995. Hemodynamic and vascular effects of active and passive smoking. *Am Heart J* 130: 1270–1275.

Zhu, B.-Q., Sun, Y.-P., Sievers, R., Isenberg, R., Glantz, S.A., and Parlmey, W.W. 1993. Passive smoking increases experimental atherosclerosis in cholesterol-fed rabbits. *J Am Coll Cardiol* 21: 225–232.

Zhu, B.-Q., Sun, Y.-P., Sievers, R.E., Glantz, S.A., Parmley, W.W., and Wolfe, C.L. 1994. Exposure to environmental tobacco smoke increases myocardial infarct size in rats. *Circulation* 889: 1282–1290.

# 14

# CARDIOVASCULAR EFFECTS OF STEROIDAL AGENTS

*Russell B. Melchert,\* Richard H. Kennedy,\**
*and Daniel Acosta, Jr.†*

*\*Department of Pharmaceutical Sciences,*
*University of Arkansas for Medical Sciences, College of Pharmacy,*
*Little Rock, AR, USA; and †University of Cincinnati,*
*College of Pharmacy, Cincinnati, OH, USA*

## Introduction

### Overview

The steroidal agents are a group of compounds with remarkable diversity in target tissues and actions. Steroidal agents include androgens, estrogens, progestins, glucocorticoids, mineralocorticoids, cholesterol, bile acids, and cardiac glycosides. Receptors for steroids are found throughout the cardiovascular system of nearly every species examined. Not surprisingly, the cardiovascular system is the target of many steroid actions through either indirect effects or direct effects mediated by direct interaction of the steroids with vascular or cardiac cells. In addition, continued identification of non-genomic mechanisms of steroid action raise questions as to the diversity of cardiovascular tissues that may be susceptible to steroid-mediated effects. Similarly, increased awareness and identification of environmental or novel synthetic compounds acting through steroid receptors underscores the importance of understanding the cardiovascular effects of steroidal agents, especially with regard to toxicologic implications. Finally, the extensive hepatic metabolism of these agents coupled with the great diversity in target tissues leaves the steroids susceptible to a wide variety of drug, chemical, or physiologic interactions. This chapter is not intended to undermine the importance of steroid function in other classic target tissues; rather, the focus of this chapter will be on the known effects of steroidal agents on the vasculature and the heart, with special emphasis on identification of future areas for steroid research. Where possible, emphasis will be placed on human studies providing mechanistic information regarding the cardiovascular effects of steroidal agents. However, contributions from animal experiments have made a tremendous impact on defining the mechanisms of action of steroidal agents on the cardiovascular system, and these studies are included where necessary and where possible.

## *Review of steroidal agents*

Steroidal agents include both naturally occurring and synthetic derivatives of compounds structurally based on the cyclopentanoperhydrophenanthrene ring illustrated in Table 14.1. For a thorough review of the chemical structures of steroidal agents, see Brueggemeier *et al.* (1995). This group of compounds includes classic sex-steroid hormones (androgens, estrogens, progestins), mineralo-corticoids, glucocorticoids, cholesterol and bile acids, and the cardiotonic steroids known as cardiac glycosides. All of these classes of steroidal agents may influence cardiovascular function through either systemic neurohumoral effects or direct interactions with myocardial and vascular tissue.

## *Androgens and anabolic steroids*

Androgens and synthetic derivatives of androgens are more appropriately known as androgenic anabolic steroids (AASs). The AASs are divided into two structural classes: (1) non-alkylated AASs (e.g. testosterone and ester derivatives of testosterone, 19-nortestosterone or nandrolone, and ester derivatives of nandrolone, boldenone, dehydroepiandrosterone, and androstenedione); and (2) 17α-alkylated AASs (e.g. fluoxymesterone, methandrostenolone, methenolone, methyl-testosterone, oxandrolone, oxymetholone, and stanozolol) (Kopera, 1985; Melchert and Welder, 1995). The essential difference between these two classes of AASs is the ability of the 17α-alkylated compounds to resist first-pass metabolism by the liver and to reach significant blood concentrations following oral administration (Barbosa *et al.*, 1971; Rahwan, 1988). Incidentally, the structural modification to improve oral bioavailability has resulted in AASs that are associated with increased frequency of hepatotoxicity (Haupt and Rovere, 1984). Whether this structural modification results in significant differences in the cardiovascular effects of AASs is not entirely known, but some literature suggests that there is, in fact, a clear structure–activity relationship for effects of AASs on lipid metabolism, as discussed below.

Historically, the AASs have been used clinically to treat anemia, breast cancer, hereditary angioneurotic edema, endometriosis, and osteoporosis (Council on Scientific Affairs, 1988, 1990; Rahwan, 1988). Because improved treatments for those conditions have been developed, the most appropriate clinical use of AASs is currently replacement therapy for hypogonadal males. Many of the AASs have been removed from the US market (e.g. methandrostenolone). Nonetheless, AASs continue to be used illicitly in attempts to improve athletic performance or physical appearance (Yesalis *et al.*, 1997). Importantly, self-administration of AASs for these illicit purposes often follows regimens which incorporate doses of AASs that are 10–200 times the normal therapeutic doses of these agents (Narducci *et al.*, 1990). Therefore, when discussing the adverse cardiovascular effects of AASs, it is critical to include observations from individuals using these high-dose regimens.

*Table 14.1* The steroid nucleus and classification of steroidal agents

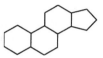

*The steroid nucleus: cyclopentanoperhydrophenanthrene ring*

I Androgens and anabolic steroids
  A Non-alkylated AASs
    Androstenedione
    Boldenone
    Dehydroepiandrosterone
    Dihydrotestosterone
    Nandrolone (19-
      nortestosterone)
    Testosterone (and ester
      formulations)
  B 17α-Alkylated AASs
    Danazol
    Fluoxymesterone
    Methandrostenolone
    Methenolone
    Methyltestosterone
    Oxandrolone
    Oxymetholone
    Stanozolol

II Estrogens
  A Endogenous estrogens
    17β-Estradiol
    Estrone
    Estriol
  B Synthetic estrogens
    Diethylstilbestrol (non-steroidal)
    Equilin
    17β-Estradiol (ester
      formulations)
    Ethinyl estradiol
    Mestranol
    Quinestrol

III Progestins
  A Progesterone-like progestins
    Hydroxyprogesterone
    Medroxyprogesterone
    Progesterone
  B 19-Nortestosterone-like
      progestins
    Desogestrel
    Norethindrone
    Norethynodrel
    Norgestimate
    Norgestrel

IV Mineralocorticoids
  Aldosterone

V Glucocorticoids
  A Endogenous glucocorticoids
    Corticosterone
    Cortisone
    Hydrocortisone (cortisol)
  B Synthetic glucocorticoids
    Alclometasone
    Amcinonide
    Beclomethasone
    Betamethasone
    Clobetasol
    Desonide
    Desoximetasone
    Dexamethasone
    Diflorasone
    Fludrocortisone
    Flunisolide
    Fluocinolone
    Fluocinonide
    Fluorometholone
    Flurandrenolide
    Halcinonide
    Medrysone
    Methylprednisolone
    Mometasone
    Paramethasone
    Prednisolone
    Prednisone
    Triamcinolone

VI Cholesterol and bile acids
  Cholesterol
  Cholic acid
  Chenodeoxycholic acid
  Deoxycholic acid
  Lithocholic acid
  Ursodeoxycholic acid

VII Cardiac glycosides
  Digoxin
  Digitoxin
  Ouabain

## Estrogens

Estrogen, 17β-estradiol, estrone, and estriol are the primary naturally occurring estrogens in animals and humans. Synthetic derivatives of estrogen include esterified versions (e.g. estradiol valerate and estradiol cypionate) and ethinyl estradiol, mestranol, quinestrol, and equilin (Williams and Stancel, 1995). In addition, synthetic non-steroidal estrogens have been made, including diethylstilbestrol, and many other synthetic chemicals have estrogenic activity such as the pesticides DDT [dichlorodiphenyltrichloroethane; 1,1,1-trichloro-2,2-bis(p-chlorophenyl)ethane] and methoxychlor, the plasticizer bisphenol A, and other industrial chemicals such as polychlorinated biphenyls (Williams and Stancel, 1995; Cummings, 1997). Recent attention has focused on the naturally occurring environmental estrogens or phytoestrogens (found in soy-based foods) such as flavones and isoflavones (e.g. genistein) and coumestan derivatives (Santell *et al.*, 1997; Sheehan, 1998). Together, the synthetic chemicals and naturally occurring substances that serve as estrogen receptor agonists fall into the general classification of endocrine disrupters. Thus, discussion of the cardiovascular effects of estrogenic compounds applies to a wide variety of steroidal and non-steroidal agents that are either naturally occurring or man-made.

Estrogens, and synthetic derivatives of estradiol, have been used for 40 years as oral contraceptive drugs or as hormone replacement therapy for ovariectomized or post-menopausal women to reduce the occurrence of osteoporosis, and, more recently, to reduce risk of cardiovascular disease in post-menopausal women. Despite the many years of clinical use, a clear understanding of the cardiovascular effects of exogenous estrogens has been slow to develop. Initial reports were based on high-dose estrogen administration for oral contraception; however, current practice involves a dramatic reduction in total estrogen doses for oral contraception compared with doses used immediately after introduction of these agents in 1960 (Williams and Stancel, 1995; Sidney *et al.*, 1998). Ironically, discussion of the cardiovascular effects of estrogens must include observations from individuals using lower dose regimens of estrogens, which is in direct opposition to examining cardiovascular effects of high-dose androgens.

## Progestins

The primary progestational hormone synthesized and secreted by the ovaries and adrenal glands is progesterone. Like the androgens, progestins can be grouped into two major chemical classes: (1) compounds with high first-pass metabolism by the liver that must be administered by injection (e.g. hydroxyprogesterone caproate and progesterone); and (2) compounds with an ethinyl group at the 17 position or methyl group at the 6 position, which reduces first-pass metabolism and allows oral administration (e.g. desogestrel, medroxyprogesterone, norethindrone, norethynodrel, norgestrel, and norgestimate) (Williams and Stancel, 1995). Importantly, however, these compounds may also be grouped according to structural similarity to either progesterone (hydroxyprogesterone and medroxyprogesterone) or 19-nortestosterone (desogestrel, norethindrone, norethynodrel, norgestimate, and norgestrel). This classification is clinically important as those compounds with structural similarity to 19-nortestosterone retain significant androgenic activity (Hirvonen *et al.*, 1981; Williams and Stancel, 1995).

The primary clinical uses of progestins are for contraception or hormone replacement therapy, and, for such purposes, progestins are more frequently combined with estrogens than used alone (Sorensen *et al.*, 1998). Antagonists of the progesterone receptor (e.g. mifepristone or RU486) have been developed and used as abortifacient agents.

### Mineralocorticoids

Aldosterone is the primary mineralocorticoid, and it is synthesized and secreted by the adrenal glands. Mineralocorticoids are not used for therapeutic purposes, but steroidal agents with mineralocorticoid activity have a profound impact on the cardiovascular system (Christ and Wehling, 1998). The mineralocorticoid receptor may have at least limited affinity for many steroidal agents, including androgens, estrogens, progestins, and glucocorticoids. Therefore, cardiovascular effects associated with mineralocorticoid activity must be considered for many steroidal agents. Structural modifications of mineralocorticoids have produced some therapeutically useful agents which act as antagonists of mineralocorticoid receptors (e.g. spironolactone).

### Glucocorticoids

Cortisol, or hydrocortisone, and corticosterone are the predominant glucocorticoids synthesized and secreted by the adrenal glands. In addition to hydrocortisone, there are presently over twenty different synthetic glucocorticoids used clinically in the USA. Among the numerous glucocorticoids are alclometasone, amcinonide, beclomethasone, betamethasone, clobetasol, desonide, desoximetasone, dexamethasone, diflorasone, fludrocortisone, flunisolide, fluocinolone, fluocinonide, fluorometholone, flurandrenolide, halcinonide, medrysone, methylprednisolone, mometasone, paramethasone, prednisolone, prednisone, and triamcinolone (Schimmer and Parker, 1995). Many of these drugs are used topically, but several are used systemically for the treatment of various inflammatory conditions. In addition, glucocorticoids are most often used in regimens of short duration (1 week or less); however, a significant population of patients with chronic inflammatory conditions exists throughout the world, and many of these patients undergo long-term glucocorticoid therapy. The glucocorticoids have long been known to exert significant effects on cardiovascular function (Page and McCubbin, 1954). Moreover, cardiovascular morbidity and mortality is increased in patients with Cushing's syndrome (Ross and Linch, 1982). Therefore, a clear understanding of the mechanisms responsible for the adverse cardiovascular effects of glucocorticoids is needed.

## Cholesterol and bile acids

Cholesterol and bile acids are steroidal agents, and, as with the aforementioned steroidal agents, the bile acids are synthesized from cholesterol. The cardiovascular effects of cholesterol will not be included in this chapter because of numerous previous reviews; however, the effects of other steroidal agents on lipoprotein–cholesterol metabolism will be considered here. The primary bile acids in the body are cholic acid, chenodeoxycholic acid, deoxycholic acid, lithocholic acid, and ursodeoxycholic acid (Brunton, 1995). These agents are rarely used therapeutically, with the exception of ursodeoxycholic acid, which receives occasional use for dissolution of gallstones (Brunton, 1995). Because the bile acids are primarily found in the intestinal tract and are largely confined to this region via enterohepatic recirculation, potential cardiovascular effects of these agents will not be considered in this chapter.

## Cardiac glycosides

The cardiac glycosides also represent a group of steroidal agents with profound effects on the cardiovascular system. Indeed, these steroidal agents were likely the first identified to have direct actions upon myocardial tissue. Other than to point out that cardiac glycosides share in common with the agents listed above the cyclopentanoperhydrophenanthrene ring, this chapter will not review the cardiovascular effects of these drugs. For a more complete review of the cardiovascular toxicities of cardiac glycosides, see the Chapter 11 and the review by Kennedy and Seifen (1991).

## Mechanisms of steroid action

### The genomic mechanism

The central dogma for the mechanism of steroid action is now well over 30 years old. Classic models for steroid action are based upon intracellular protein receptors specific for androgens, estrogens, progestins, mineralocorticoids, glucocorticoids, and ligands for other members of the steroid superfamily of receptors (e.g. thyroid hormone, retinoic acid, vitamin D, and peroxisome proliferator-activated receptors). It is now understood that many of these receptors, including those activated by estrogen, glucocorticoid, retinoic acid, and peroxisome proliferator, and very likely others, exist in multiple isoforms, thus giving rise to multiple subtypes of steroid receptors. Furthermore, several proteins closely related to receptors of the steroid superfamily (orphan receptors) have been discovered for which ligands have not yet been identified. In the unoccupied state, steroid receptors are frequently found associated with heat shock proteins (e.g. the 90-kDa heat shock protein), and steroid binding results in dissociation of the receptor from the heat shock protein (Carson-Jurica et al., 1990; Wahli and Martinez, 1991; Veldscholte et al., 1992).

Through what now may be called a "genomic" mechanism, steroids first diffuse across the plasma membrane, then bind and form a complex with steroid receptors located either in the cytosol or in the nucleus. The ligand–steroid receptor complex translocates to the nucleus (if cytosolic), binds to one or more steroid response elements, and either up- or down-regulates gene transcription (Carson-Jurica *et al.*, 1990; Christ and Wehling, 1998). Of note, several steroid receptors, including estrogen, progesterone, and glucocorticoid receptors, function through receptor–ligand complex homodimerization before or during interactions with their respective response elements (O'Malley, 1991), while other steroid receptors (e.g. retinoic acid and peroxisome proliferator-activated receptors) are known to form heterodimers before or during interaction with DNA (Jain *et al.*, 1998).

This general genomic mechanism has withstood the tests of time and experimentation and adequately explains most of the effects of steroids on gene transcription. Of course, a long held exception to the genomic model has been the mechanism of action of cardiac glycosides which involves inhibition of Na/K-ATPase. Moreover, the question of how steroidal agents regulate proliferation, metabolism, biosynthesis, and/or secretion has been difficult to answer with explanations imparted solely by the genomic mechanism (Farnsworth, 1990).

## Non-genomic mechanisms

More recently, however, evidence of "non-genomic" mechanisms of steroid action has surfaced, generating questions as to the primary mode of action of steroidal agents (reviewed in Wehling, 1995), and many of these non-genomic mechanisms may be receptor mediated. Examples of non-genomic mechanisms of steroid action are found in a variety of tissues. For example, Koenig and colleagues (1989) demonstrated that nanomolar concentrations of testosterone induce rapid increases in ornithine decarboxylase activity and polyamine concentrations and induce acute stimulation of calcium fluxes and calcium-mediated membrane transport systems in rat ventricular myocytes exposed for less than 1 min. The authors suggested that the effects were consistent with androgen receptor-mediated events (Koenig *et al.*, 1989). However, questions arise as to whether androgen receptor-mediated alterations in gene transcription could have accounted for the aforementioned effects of testosterone because of the swift nature of the responses. The authors hypothesized that testosterone effects on ornithine decarboxylase were, at least in part, mediated by post-translational modification of the enzyme by androgen receptor-mediated phosphorylation or dephosphorylation (Koenig *et al.*, 1989). Therefore, it is possible that testosterone exerts at least some of its effects on rat ventricular myocytes by androgen receptor-mediated non-genomic mechanisms.

Additional support for androgens acting via non-genomic mechanisms comes from studies of prostate cells. Farnsworth (1990) demonstrated that androgens bind to Na/K-ATPase in prostatic plasma membranes and can activate the ATPase to regulate metabolic activity. In addition, evidence strongly suggests the coexistence of non-DNA-binding androgen receptors in endoplasmic reticulum (microsomal fractions) of rat ventral prostate tissue that was not simply due to contamination of the fractions (Steinsapir and Muldoon, 1991). Therefore, it is reasonable to speculate that androgens may also affect cardiac myocyte function through interactions with Na/K-ATPase or other enzyme targets in a non-genomic, receptor- or non-receptor-mediated fashion.

Further support for non-genomic modes of steroid action comes from research into mechanisms of estrogen action. Using MCF-7 (Michigan Cancer Foundation) breast cancer cells, Migliaccio *et al.* (1996) demonstrated that estradiol, coupled to the estrogen receptor, elicited tyrosine kinase activation of the p21ras signaling pathway, resulting in activation of extracellular signal-regulated kinases (ERK 1/2, part of the mitogen-activated protein kinase family) and culminating in stimulation of MCF-7 cell growth. Furthermore, estradiol has been shown to enhance cardiac fibroblast proliferation through non-genomic mechanisms. Lee and Eghbali-Webb (1998) found that estrogen stimulated cardiac fibroblast DNA synthesis through activation of ERK 1/2, and these effects were blocked by the estrogen receptor antagonist tamoxifen or by the mitogen-activated protein kinase inhibitor PD98059. Although dogma associates steroid receptors with the nucleus, a subpopulation of estrogen receptors similar to the classic intracytosolic/nuclear receptors have been localized to the plasma membrane in rat pituitary tumor cells (Pappas *et al.*, 1995). Therefore, evidence suggests that at least part of the mechanism of action of estrogens involves binding to membrane-associated estrogen receptors and stimulation of mitogen-activated protein kinase pathways. Given the similarities of the steroid superfamily of receptors, it is reasonable to speculate that other steroidal agents also act through membrane-localized steroid receptors.

In summary, the literature suggests that steroidal agents act in part by steroid receptor-mediated alterations in gene transcription (i.e. genomic mechanisms) and in part by steroid receptor- or non-receptor-mediated non-genomic mechanisms, many of which likely involve growth or death signaling pathways such as the mitogen-activated protein kinases. Whether this dual mechanism for steroid action exists in the tissues composing the cardiovascular system remains to be determined. Table 14.2 provides a summary of the general characteristics of genomic and non-genomic mechanisms of steroid action.

## Vascular effects of steroidal agents

### *Indirect effects of steroidal agents on the vasculature: lipid metabolism*

The causative relationship between hypercholesterolemia and atherosclerosis is no longer regarded as a controversial theory as the mechanisms responsible for low-density lipoprotein (LDL) cholesterol-induced atherosclerosis are increasingly understood. The major atherogenic carriers of cholesterol are LDL and β-very-low-density lipoprotein (β-VLDL), yet high-density lipoprotein (HDL) is almost

*Table 14.2* Characteristics of steroid mechanisms of action

| Genomic mechanisms | Non-genomic mechanisms |
| --- | --- |
| 1 Receptor-mediated | 1 Receptor- or non-receptor-mediated |
| 2 Slowly developing (> 1–2 h) | 2 Rapidly developing (< 1–2 h) |
| 3 Interaction with steroid response element | 3 No direct interaction with steroid response element |
| 4 Altered gene transcription | 4 No effect on gene transcription or indirect and delayed effects on gene transcription |
| 5 Response inhibited by actinomycin D | 5 Immediate response unaffected by actinomycin D |
| 6 Response inhibited by cycloheximide | 6 Immediate response unaffected by cycloheximide |

universally regarded as non-atherogenic if not antiatherogenic (Grundy, 1990; Steinberg and Witztum, 1990). Furthermore, evidence suggests that LDL cholesterol initiates atherosclerotic plaque development when it is oxidized to a form that initiates injury and inflammation (Steinberg and Witztum, 1990). Conclusions regarding atherogenic lipoproteins were reached following years of clinical research into risk factors for atherosclerosis and observations of patients with familial hypercholesterolemia. Based upon these conclusions, current clinical practice includes monitoring serum LDL and HDL cholesterol and attempting to decrease elevated LDL cholesterol while increasing depressed HDL cholesterol.

### Endogenous sex steroids and risk of coronary artery disease

Endogenous androgens, estrogens, and progestins have long received attention as possible mediators of sex differences in the risk of coronary artery disease. Now well accepted is the approximate twofold increased risk of coronary artery disease in men compared with premenopausal women (Kalin and Zumoff, 1990). The clinical literature from which numerous inconclusive and/or disparate results have been obtained is extensive (reviewed in Kalin and Zumoff, 1990). Thus, the purpose of the following review is not to revisit the entire clinical literature with regard to mortality rates and risk of coronary artery disease as they relate to levels of endogenous sex steroids. Rather, the purpose is to consider the effects of exogenous androgens, estrogens, and progestins on lipid metabolism, as these data likely have significant pharmacologic and toxicologic relevance with regard to the increasing identification of heretofore unknown androgenic, estrogenic, and progestogenic compounds to which humans are exposed. It is, nonetheless, worthwhile to consider some of the conclusions reached by Kalin and Zumoff (1990) regarding endogenous levels of androgens, estrogens, and progestins. First, although both are normal prior to myocardial infarction, endogenous estradiol levels are elevated and testosterone levels are decreased for up to 1 year in men who survive myocardial infarction. Second, progesterone is normal before but is elevated for short periods (less than 1 year) after myocardial infarction, and this alteration may be stress related. Third, pregnancy (high levels of endogenous estrogens and progestins) appears to provide protection against coronary artery disease. Fourth, men with cirrhosis of the liver have high endogenous estrogen levels and low endogenous testosterone levels, and this appears to be associated with a decreased risk of coronary artery disease. Finally, fifth, women with elevated endogenous testosterone appear to have an increased risk of coronary artery disease. In summary, these clinical studies support the hypothesis that estrogens provide protection from coronary artery disease, whereas androgens may increase the risk of coronary artery disease. The observed effects of exogenous androgens, estrogens, and progestins on lipid metabolism also support this hypothesis.

### Androgens and anabolic steroids

The anabolic androgenic steroids (AASs) have long been known to alter lipid metabolism in humans and animals, and the effects of AASs on lipid metabolism have been reviewed previously (Glazer, 1991; Rockhold, 1993; Melchert and Welder, 1995; Sullivan *et al.*, 1998). Net effects of AASs on lipid metabolism are generally observed to include significant elevations in LDL cholesterol and significant reductions in HDL cholesterol. However, as discussed below, effects of individual AASs on lipid metabolism may vary significantly, and a structure–activity relationship appears to explain, at least partially, this variability.

While alterations in lipid metabolism that include significantly elevated LDL and reduced HDL have long been associated with atherosclerosis, and the AASs are known to affect lipid metabolism in such a manner, experimental evidence supporting the hypothesis that AASs promote atherosclerosis is lacking (Glazer, 1991). Nonetheless, potential causes for differences in death rates from coronary artery disease have included androgen-induced alterations in lipid metabolism (Kalin and Zumoff, 1990), and a suggestion has been made to include women with signs of androgen excess as being at a greater risk of coronary artery disease (Wild *et al.*, 1990). Also of note, the reduction of serum HDL induced by AASs in humans is of greater magnitude than alterations produced by any other pharmacologic agent or non-pharmacologic factor, including smoking and obesity (Glazer, 1991). Therefore, understanding the mechanisms responsible for AAS-induced reductions in serum HDL is of utmost importance.

The exact mechanisms for AAS-induced alterations in lipid metabolism are largely unknown; however, the genomic mechanisms could largely account for these effects. In support of this theory, evidence suggests that AASs up-regulate or induce hepatic triglyceride lipase (HTGL), which catabolizes HDL, yet AASs have little effect on lipoprotein lipase, which liberates fatty acids from triglycerides and converts very-low-density lipoproteins (VLDL) and chylomicrons into atherogenic $\beta$-VLDL. For example, subjects given 7.5 mg per day of oxandrolone for 3 weeks had significantly higher activities of post-heparin plasma HTGL activity than control subjects, but no differences in lipoprotein lipase were observed

(Ehnholm *et al.*, 1975). Similarly, subjects given 6 mg per day of stanozolol had significantly increased activity of HTGL but unaltered lipoprotein lipase compared with their pretreatment levels, and the elevated HTGL activity appeared to correlate with reduced serum HDL levels in these subjects (Haffner *et al.*, 1983). Furthermore, increases in HTGL induced by stanozolol were subsequently found to precede decreases in serum HDL (Applebaum-Bowden *et al.*, 1987). Nearly identical results on HDL and HTGL have been reported in men who were self-administering high doses of AASs (Kantor *et al.*, 1985; Lenders *et al.*, 1988). However, these studies were hampered by a general lack of ability to control diet, dose and purity of the AAS, and other factors (Melchert and Welder, 1995).

A structure–activity relationship for the effects of AASs on lipid metabolism appears to exist, and this relationship is most likely unrelated to the relative androgenic potencies of the AASs. In a crossover study in weightlifters given 6 mg per day oral stanozolol or 200 mg per week intramuscular testosterone enanthate for 6 weeks, HDL cholesterol was reduced by 33 percent during stanozolol administration and 9 percent during testosterone administration (Thompson *et al.*, 1989). Stanozolol increased HTGL activity by 123 percent, while testosterone only increased HTGL activity by 25 percent. Interestingly, LDL-cholesterol increased by 29 percent in the stanozolol-treated group, whereas LDL-cholesterol decreased by 16 percent in the testosterone-treated group (Thompson *et al.*, 1989). A subsequent study found similar results (Friedl *et al.*, 1990). Eighteen subjects were divided into three groups and for 12 weeks were given 280 mg per week testosterone enanthate, 280 mg per week testosterone enanthate plus 250 mg testolactone (aromatase inhibitor) orally four times daily, or 20 mg methyl-testosterone orally twice daily (Friedl *et al.*, 1990). Subjects treated with methyltestosterone or testosterone enanthate plus testolactone had significant decreases in HDL cholesterol, whereas subjects treated with testosterone enanthate alone had no significant changes in HDL cholesterol. Reductions in HDL cholesterol were preceded by increases in HTGL in subjects treated with methyltestosterone or testosterone enanthate plus testolactone, but subjects treated with testosterone enanthate alone had no significant changes in HTGL (Friedl *et al.*, 1990). To clarify further the effects of the aromatase inhibitor testolactone, a subsequent study recruited fourteen male weightlifters, and, in a randomized crossover design, administered to them 200 mg per week testosterone enanthate, 250 mg testolactone orally four times daily, or a combination of testosterone enanthate and testolactone (Zmuda *et al.*, 1993). Serum testosterone levels increased during all three treatments; however, serum estradiol was unchanged during treatment with testolactone or testosterone enanthate plus testolactone, and serum estradiol increased by 47 percent when subjects received testosterone enanthate alone. These results strongly suggested that testolactone inhibited testosterone aromatization to estradiol (Zmuda *et al.*, 1993). Although testolactone had minimal effects on lipid metabolism, testosterone decreased HDL cholesterol, and testosterone plus testolactone appeared to decrease further HDL but the changes were not significantly different. There was, however, a significant difference when comparing effects of the regimens on HTGL; testosterone enanthate increased HTGL by 21 percent, whereas testosterone enanthate plus testolactone increased HTGL by 38 percent (Zmuda et al., 1993).

In summary, many clinical studies demonstrate that AASs alter lipid metabolism in humans, and the alterations most frequently include elevated LDL cholesterol and decreased HDL cholesterol. A structure–activity relationship has been established which suggests that 17α-alkylated AASs have a greater effect on lipid metabolism through induction of HTGL and subsequent reduction of plasma HDL cholesterol. When an aromatizable androgen is administered (e.g. testosterone), the effects on HTGL and HDL are not as profound, and evidence suggests that the conversion of testosterone to estradiol may impart a slight protective effect.

### Estrogens and progestins

The effects of estrogens on lipid metabolism are nearly opposite to those of androgens, because estrogens dose dependently increase HDL cholesterol and commonly produce reductions in total and LDL cholesterol (Samsioe, 1998). Higher doses or higher potencies of estrogens produce a different pattern of altered lipid metabolism in which LDL and VLDL may be increased (Samsioe, 1998). In direct contrast to estrogens, the effects of synthetic progestins, particularly those with structural similarity to 19-nortestosterone, on lipid metabolism are nearly identical to those of androgens. These sex hormone-mediated alterations in lipid metabolism may at least partially explain sex differences in coronary artery disease.

From the numerous clinical studies evaluating exogenous estrogens and progestins, Kalin and Zumoff (1990) concluded that (1) post-menopausal estrogen replacement therapy may protect against coronary artery disease; (2) oral contraceptives utilizing high-dose synthetic estrogens likely increase the risk of coronary thrombosis, but not coronary atherosclerosis; and (3) the oral contraceptives utilizing synthetic progestins with androgenic activity may increase the risk of myocardial infarction. A more recent study suggests that the currently used, low-dose estrogen and progestin oral contraceptives do not increase the risk of myocardial infarction (Sidney et al., 1998). In short, the effects of estrogens on lipid metabolism are generally regarded as protective in terms of atherosclerosis, and commonly used combined estrogen and progestin hormone replacement therapy may result in no net beneficial effects because the estrogen effects may be diminished by those of progestins (Hirvonen et al., 1981; Sorenson et al., 1998). For example, in a cross-sectional study of 693 post-menopausal French women over 2 years, twenty-seven received transdermal unopposed (no progestins) estradiol, 165 received transdermal estradiol plus a progestin, and 501 women received no hormone replacement therapy (Bongard et al., 1998). Women receiving hormone replacement therapy had lower serum total cholesterol, triglycerides, apolipoprotein B, and LDL and VLDL cholesterol. However, no significant differences in HDL cholesterol were found, and the results suggested that women administered combined hormone replacement therapy (86 percent of treated women) may have had beneficial effects of estradiol reduced by progestins (Bongard *et al.*, 1998). Interestingly, the effects of estrogens on lipid metabolism may be more profound in those individuals who have hyperlipidemias prior to hormone replacement therapy. For example, in women with normal blood cholesterol levels, estrogen therapy via oral or transdermal administration reduced total and LDL cholesterol by up to 10 percent; whereas in women with hypercholesterolemia estrogen therapy via oral or transdermal administration reduced total and LDL cholesterol levels by up to 20 percent (Samsioe, 1998).

As with androgens, the mechanisms responsible for estrogen- and/or progestin-induced alterations in lipid metabolism are largely unknown; however, the mechanisms involved for estrogens may include steps that are in direct opposition to those observed with androgens. Genomic mechanisms are likely responsible for estrogen- or progestin-induced alterations in lipid metabolism. Estrogens are thought to inhibit HTGL expression or activity, thus promoting HDL levels (Nabulsi *et al.*, 1993; Samsioe, 1998) and working antagonistically to androgens. Conceivably, the estrogen–estrogen receptor complex could act as a regulatory factor that interferes with or reduces HTGL expression. Similar to androgens, estrogens have not been clearly demonstrated to affect lipoprotein lipase (Samsioe, 1998). Because many of the progestins have significant androgenic activity (Hirvonen *et al.*, 1981; Kalin and Zumoff, 1990), it should come as no surprise that at least one mechanism for progestin-induced alterations in lipid metabolism includes up-regulation and/or activation of HTGL (Nabulsi *et al.*, 1993). Furthermore, the human androgen receptor shares 82 percent amino acid homology of the two zinc finger structural motifs and 75 percent and 56 percent amino acid homology of two other important regions (likely hormone binding domains) with that of human progesterone receptors, and the hormone response elements for androgen and progesterone receptors are very similar if not identical (Carson-Jurica, 1990; Distelhorst, 1993).

An additional mechanism regarding potential beneficial effects of estrogens on lipid metabolism deserves mention. That is, experimental evidence suggests that estrogens may serve as antioxidants, thus behaving similarly to $\alpha$-tocopherol. Specifically, estrogen was shown to inhibit the oxidation of LDL induced by copper or by exposure to endothelial cells (White *et al.*, 1997). However, these *in vitro* experiments required extremely high concentrations of estradiol (1.25–2.5 μM). Presumably, the rigorous *in vitro* conditions led to requirements for high estradiol concentrations, and *in vivo* radical production may be much lower than that produced *in vitro* so that conceivably this antioxidant mechanism could function in the intact vasculature (White *et al.*, 1997).

In summary, exogenous estrogens produce alterations in lipid metabolism that are opposite to those elicited by androgens, so total and LDL cholesterol is frequently reduced whereas HDL cholesterol is elevated. Exogenous progestins, in contrast, appear to produce alterations in lipid metabolism that are very similar to those induced by androgens. The primary target leading to sex steroid-altered lipid metabolism appears to be HTGL, and it is likely that sex steroid receptors regulate HTGL expression. Future research into the mechanisms responsible for sex steroid-induced alterations in lipid metabolism should include clear identification of the molecular targets of the receptors and delineation of transcriptional activity of the receptors at the gene encoding HTGL.

### Glucocorticoids

In contrast to androgens, estrogens, and progestins, the effects of glucocorticoids on lipid metabolism are less clear. Even though individuals with Cushing's syndrome frequently have elevated serum levels of all lipids and lipoproteins, including LDL and HDL cholesterol, difficulties have prevented sound conclusions regarding effects of exogenous glucocorticoids on lipid metabolism (Henkin *et al.*, 1992). Nonetheless, treatment with glucocorticoids frequently results in elevated total, LDL, and HDL cholesterol – a lipid profile somewhat different from that induced by androgens, estrogens, and progestins.

Clinical studies evaluating the effects of exogenous glucocorticoid therapy on lipid metabolism have been frequently conducted in heart or kidney transplant recipients; however, not many of these studies have been published. In ninety-two patients who received heart transplants, 52 percent were above the sex- and age-adjusted 75th percentile and 35 percent were above the 90th percentile for total cholesterol, and similar elevations were found in LDL and HDL cholesterol (Becker *et al.*, 1988). Prednisone exposure was the strongest predictor of both total and LDL cholesterol levels independent of other clinical variables (Becker *et al.*, 1988). In 500 renal transplant recipients, hypercholesterolemia occurred in 82 percent of the patients, and there was a strong correlation between prednisone doses and cholesterol levels, which were significantly reduced when prednisone doses were decreased (Vathsala *et al.*, 1989). It is important to note that examination of transplant patients to draw firm conclusions regarding glucocorticoid-induced alterations in lipid metabolism is difficult because of concomitant immuno-suppressant therapy, often with cyclosporine, which may independently alter lipid metabolism. However, some studies in patients with various inflammatory conditions provide some support for the observed glucocorticoid-induced lipid alterations in transplant recipients.

When forty-six female patients with systemic lupus erythematosus (SLE) were compared with thirty matched control subjects, SLE patients receiving prednisone (thirty-two of the forty-six patients) had significantly elevated total and LDL cholesterol compared with SLE patients not receiving prednisone and with control subjects (Ettinger *et al.*, 1987a). In addition, cholesterol levels correlated with daily prednisone dosage in treated patients with SLE (Ettinger *et al.*, 1987a). In contrast, a study involving twenty-three patients with rheumatic disease who received prednisone for 1 month showed that total and HDL cholesterol were significantly increased but LDL cholesterol was unchanged (Ettinger *et al.*, 1987b). Interestingly, women may be more susceptible to glucocorticoid-induced alterations in lipid metabolism. For example, in patients receiving long-term

(> 3 years) glucocorticoid treatment for connective tissue disorders and asthma, women, but not men, had significantly elevated total cholesterol and decreased HDL cholesterol (Jefferys *et al.*, 1980). Overall, available clinical literature suggests that exogenous glucocorticoid therapy frequently results in elevated total, LDL, and HDL cholesterol; however, these changes are inconsistent when comparing the reports. Further studies are required to clarify glucocorticoid effects.

Effects of glucocorticoids on lipid metabolism can surface fairly rapidly. For example, six male and six female subjects given prednisone showed significant increases in total and HDL cholesterol within 48 h after initiation of treatment; LDL cholesterol did not increase significantly (Zimmerman *et al.*, 1984). As with androgens, estrogens, and progestins, mechanisms for glucocorticoid-induced alterations in lipid metabolism are largely unknown. The mechanism could partially be explained by changes in LDL receptor expression (Markell and Friedman, 1989) which are most likely mediated by a genomic mechanism. More detailed information regarding the mechanism(s) could be provided by future animal studies because at least one animal study suggested that glucocorticoids slow the catabolism of LDL cholesterol. Cynomolgus monkeys given prednisone developed increased total cholesterol, including elevated LDL cholesterol and depressed HDL cholesterol, and there was a decrease in the fractional catabolic rate of LDL (Ettinger *et al.*, 1989). Thus, definitive mechanistic studies of glucocorticoid-induced alterations in lipid metabolism are lacking, yet clarification of cellular or molecular mechanisms will be important as new agonists and antagonists of glucocorticoid receptors are identified.

In summary, a major systemic influence of steroidal agents on cardiovascular function is steroid-induced hyperlipidemias. Table 14.3 provides a summary of the potential effects of exogenous steroids on lipoprotein metabolism. Androgens, progestins, and glucocorticoids appear to be the primary steroidal agents that may alter lipid metabolism in such a manner as to favor development of atherosclerosis. The most likely target of these steroidal compounds appears to be hepatic triglyceride lipase. In contrast to androgens, progestins, and glucocorticoids, available evidence suggests that estrogens impart a protective effect against undesirable lipid profiles. If all estrogenic compounds elicit this type of response, then concerns regarding altered lipid metabolism secondary to environmental or industrial chemical estrogens may be unjustified. Nonetheless, as new agonists and antagonists of the steroidal receptors are identified, a clear understanding of the mechanisms responsible for steroid-mediated changes in lipid metabolism will become increasingly important. This importance may be best exemplified by examples listed above in which particular members of a class of steroidal agents (e.g. androgens) display quite different effects on lipid metabolism. Although it is useful to discuss all steroidal agents as classes, a caveat regarding compound-specific differences is in order.

Other indirect hemodynamic actions of steroidal agents, including effects on blood pressure, circulating electrolytes and volume, autonomic function, thrombogenesis, and hematopoiesis will not be discussed in detail in this chapter.

*Table 14.3* Potential effects of exogenous steroids on lipoprotein metabolism

| Steroid class | HTGL | TC | LDL-C | HDL-C |
|---|---|---|---|---|
| Androgens and anabolic steroids | | | | |
|   Non-alkylated | ↑ | ↑ | ↑ | ↓ |
|   17α-Alkylated | ↑↑ | ↑↑ | ↑↑ | ↓↓ |
| Estrogens | ↓ | ↓ | ↓ | ? |
| Progestins | ↑ | ↑ | ↑ | ↓ |
| Mineralocorticoids | – | – | – | – |
| Glucocorticoids | ? | ↑ | ↑ | ↑ or ↓ |

Note
HTGL, hepatic triglyceride lipase; TC, total serum cholesterol; LDL-C, low-density lipoprotein cholesterol; HDL-C, high-density lipoprotein cholesterol. ↑, increased; ↓, decreased; ↑↑, larger increase; ↓↓, larger decrease; –, no significant effect; ?, unknown effects. Supporting references are found throughout the text.

Although these indirect effects may be quite important, either results of numerous human investigations have been inconclusive or only limited information is available regarding effects of steroidal agents. The remainder of the chapter will focus on direct effects of steroidal agents on the vasculature and heart.

### Direct effects of steroidal agents on the vasculature

Increasing evidence suggests that steroidal agents may exert cardiovascular effects through direct actions on smooth muscle and/or endothelial cells lining the vasculature (Christ and Wehling, 1998). However, results are limited in that few human studies have been conducted and confounding factors in these studies, such as hypercholesterolemia and hypertension, are difficult to eliminate. Further evidence for direct steroid-mediated alterations in vascular tone stems largely from whole animal and *in vitro* experiments. Several reports provide experimental results suggesting the presence of steroid receptors in vascular tissue (Table 14.4). Overall, these experiments certainly provide strong support for consideration of the vasculature as a target for direct steroid action. Potential direct effects of exogenous steroids on the vasculature are summarized in Table 14.5.

### Androgens and anabolic steroids

Autoradiographic evidence for the presence of androgen receptors in the vasculature was found when McGill and Sheridan (1981) reported finding specific tritiated dihydrotestosterone binding in vascular smooth muscle and endothelial cells from male and female baboons. These experiments provided the foundation for identification of the vasculature as a target for direct androgen action. Evidence for direct AAS effects on the vasculature comes mostly from animal studies.

*Table 14.4* Evidence for vascular steroid receptors in various species: location, isoforms, and methods used for detection

| | Species | Location | Isoforms | Methods |
|---|---|---|---|---|
| Androgen receptors | Baboon | VSMC, EC | ? | RB |
| Estrogen receptors | Rats, monkeys, humans | VSMC, EC | $\alpha$ and $\beta$ | IB, RNaseP, RT-PCR |
| Progesterone receptors | Rats, rabbits, humans | VSMC | ? | IH, RT-PCR |
| Mineralocorticoid and glucocorticoid receptors | Rats, rabbits, humans | VSMC, EC | Type I and II | RB, SRE |

Note

VSMC, vascular smooth muscle cells; EC, endothelial cells; ?, unknown; SRE, binding or activation of steroid response elements; IB, immunoblotting; IH, immunohistochemistry; RB, radioligand binding; RT-PCR, reverse transcription polymerase chain reaction; RNaseP, ribonuclease protection assay. Supporting references are found throughout the text.

*Table 14.5* Potential direct effects of exogenous steroids on the vasculature

| Steroid class | Types of studies | Endothelium-dependent effects | Endothelium-independent effects | Possible net effects on reactivity |
|---|---|---|---|---|
| Androgens and anabolic steroids | Animal | ↓ NO signaling | ? | Vasoconstriction *in vivo* and vasodilation *in vitro* |
| Estrogens | Human and animal | ↑ NO signaling<br>↑ NOS | ↓ $Ca^{2+}$ influx or ↑ $Ca^{2+}$ efflux | Vasodilation *in vivo* and *in vitro* |
| Progestins | Animal | ↓ NO signaling? | ↓ $Ca^{2+}$ influx | ? |
| Mineralo-corticoids | Human and animal | ? | ↑ $Na^+$ influx<br>↑ $Na^+$ channels<br>↑ $Ca^{2+}$ influx | Vasoconstriction |
| Gluco-corticoids | Human and animal | ↓ NO signaling<br>↓ prostacyclin | ↑ ACE<br>↑ AT receptors<br>↓ $Na^+$ influx<br>↑ $Ca^{2+}$ influx | Vasoconstriction |

Note

NO, nitric oxide signaling; NOS, nitric oxide synthase; ACE, angiotensin-converting enzyme; AT, angiotensin II; ?, unknown effects. Supporting references are found throughout the text.

However, conflicting results preclude conclusion as to whether AASs promote vascular constriction or dilation. First, 1-week treatment of male and female rats with testosterone resulted in increased maximum tension and an increased potency for the vasoconstrictive response to prostaglandin $F_{2\alpha}$ ($PGF_{2\alpha}$) in female, but not in male, aortic rings with intact endothelium (Maddox *et al.*, 1987). This suggested that the female has a greater capacity than the male for AAS-induced changes in vascular smooth muscle contraction (Maddox *et al.*, 1987). Ferrer and colleagues (1994) examined the effects of chronic (4–12 weeks) nandrolone administration in male rabbits on vasodilator responses of isolated aorta. Nandrolone treatment was not associated with any significant changes in blood pressure throughout the treatment period (Ferrer *et al.*, 1994). In thoracic aorta, endothelium-dependent relaxation induced by acetylcholine and the calcium ionophore A23187 was abolished in nandrolone-treated rabbits; however, similar results were not observed in mesenteric and femoral arteries (Ferrer *et al.*, 1994). Furthermore, acetylcholine- or sodium nitroprusside-induced increases in cyclic GMP were abolished by nandrolone treatment, and the authors concluded that nandrolone reduced nitric oxide-mediated relaxation in thoracic aorta by inhibition of guanylate cyclase, whereas endothelial nitric oxide production (surmised from bioassay data) was unaltered (Ferrer *et al.*, 1994).

Further evidence for direct effects of androgens on endothelium-dependent relaxation was obtained by Farhat and colleagues (1995). They administered testosterone to pigs for 2 weeks, then assessed vascular reactivity in segments of left anterior descending coronary artery (LAD). In vessels obtained from male and female pigs, testosterone treatment significantly increased the maximum response of intact vessels to potassium chloride (KCl) and $PGF_{2\alpha}$. Interestingly, endothelial denudation significantly decreased the testosterone effects on vascular responses to KCl and $PGF_{2\alpha}$ in segments obtained from male but not from female pigs, whereas there was no significant sex difference in the response of LAD segments from placebo-treated pigs to KCl and $PGF_{2\alpha}$ (Farhat *et al.*, 1995).

At least one case report stemming from a human study exists in the literature that may confirm the observed effects of AASs on vascular reactivity found in animal models (Green *et al.*, 1993). Seven men were recruited for measurement of forearm blood flow responses to brachial artery infusion of methacholine (MC) and sodium nitroprusside (SNP). The investigators found one man to have vasodilatory responses to MC and SNP that were 71 percent and 51 percent, respectively, lower in the second measurement session than in the first (Green *et al.*, 1993). It was later serendipitously discovered that this individual had been self-administering high-dose testosterone, which he initiated following the first blood flow measurement. The authors concluded that AAS use may induce changes in nitric oxide-mediated vasodilatory responses that appear to lie distal to the endothelium, perhaps in the vascular smooth muscle (Green *et al.*, 1993). This supposition was supported by the observed effects of nandrolone on rabbit aorta discussed previously (Ferrer *et al.*, 1994).

Opposite actions of AASs on vascular reactivity were reported when aortic or coronary artery rings were obtained and acutely exposed to AAS *in vitro*. For example, testosterone elicited an endothelium-independent relaxation of isolated rabbit coronary artery and aortic rings, and coronary artery rings were more sensitive to testosterone-induced relaxation than aortic rings (Yue *et al.*, 1995). Results were similar in preparations isolated from male and non-pregnant female rabbits. Further, testosterone-induced relaxation of coronary artery rings was inhibited by barium chloride, a potassium channel inhibitor. The authors concluded that altered potassium conductance was at least partially involved in the mechanism of testosterone-induced relaxation, but it is important to note that the concentration of testosterone required for relaxation in these experiments was 1 μM or higher (Yue *et al.*, 1995). Similarly, Costarella *et al.* (1996) demonstrated that testosterone produced direct relaxation of rat thoracic aorta when administered to aortic rings *in vitro*. Supraphysiologic concentrations (> 25 μM) of testosterone relaxed phenylephrine-precontracted endothelium-intact aortic rings, and pretreatment of endothelium-denuded rings with 50 μM testosterone reduced the sensitivity to phenylephrine (Costarella *et al.*, 1996). From these experiments, the authors concluded that testosterone has a direct vasodilating effect involving endothelium-dependent and endothelium-independent mechanisms (Costarella *et al.*, 1996).

In summary, the literature suggests that long-term treatment with AASs may promote vasoconstriction through mechanisms involving nitric oxide, perhaps at the level of inhibiting nitric oxide signaling through down-regulation of guanylyl cyclase. However, when AASs are administered in supraphysiologic concentrations to *in vitro* preparations, a net relaxing effect is observed. At this point, it is tempting to speculate that the former effects (chronic administration and vasoconstriction) result from genomic mechanisms of AAS action, whereas the rapid relaxing effects of AAS result from non-genomic mechanisms (Christ and Wehling, 1998); however, confirming data have not been reported. Future studies are required to characterize fully the effects of AAS on vascular reactivity and to identify the mechanisms responsible for the observed effects.

### Estrogens

In contrast to androgens, a considerable amount of work, including human and animal studies, has been completed in attempts to understand the direct effects of estrogens on the vasculature. Impetus for this work stems from epidemiologic data suggesting that the "atheroprotective" effects of estrogens are not entirely explained by beneficial effects on lipid metabolism, and that additional direct effects of estrogens on the vascular wall likely contribute to this phenomenon (Farhat *et al.*, 1996; Christ and Wehling, 1998; Selzman *et al.*, 1998). Functional estrogen receptors have been identified in human vascular smooth muscle cells from mammary artery and saphenous vein (Karas *et al.*, 1994, 1995) and in human endothelial cells isolated from aorta and umbilical vein (Venkov *et al.*, 1996). Recent investigations have demonstrated that both forms of estrogen receptors (classic estrogen receptor α and recently identified β) are expressed in coronary artery and cultured aortic smooth muscle from cynomolgus monkeys (Register and Adams, 1998), and that estrogen receptor β is increased in male rat aortic smooth muscle and endothelial cells as early as 2 days and persists up to 2 weeks following balloon injury (Lindner *et al.*, 1998). These data suggest that estrogen receptor β may participate in vascular remodeling following injury.

Human studies support the hypothesis that estrogens exert beneficial effects on the vasculature. In a human study in the early 1990s, eleven women (mean age 58 ± 8 years) with angina, coronary artery disease, and clinical evidence of estrogen deficiency were recruited, randomly assigned to two groups, 1 mg 17β-estradiol sublingual or placebo, and then subjected to exercise testing on 2 separate days (Rosano *et al.*, 1993). Nitrates other than sublingual nitroglycerine were withdrawn 2 days before the study, whereas calcium channel blockers and β-adrenergic-blocking agents were withdrawn 4 and 5 days, respectively, prior to the study. As for sublingual nitroglycerine, subjects were withdrawn from therapy at least 6 h prior to exercise testing. Interestingly, sublingual estradiol delayed the onset of signs of myocardial ischemia on the electrocardiogram and increased exercise tolerance in a manner similar to that of sublingual nitroglycerin, as demonstrated in other studies (Rosano *et al.*, 1993). These results suggested that estradiol exerts direct coronary vasodilating effects in menopausal women. Subsequent human studies support this observation. For example, flow-mediated, endothelium-dependent brachial artery vasodilation was greater in post-menopausal subjects given 17β-estradiol for 9 weeks than in those given placebo (Lieberman *et al.*, 1994). Similar findings on brachial artery blood flow were reported in a study in which post-menopausal women were given infusions of 17β-estradiol (Gilligan *et al.*, 1994a), suggesting that both long-term and acute administration of estradiol promotes vasodilation. In an investigation using angiography and Doppler analysis of coronary flow velocity, intracoronary infusion of 17β-estradiol prevented epicardial coronary artery constriction induced by acetylcholine and potentiated the vasodilator coronary microvascular response to acetylcholine (Gilligan *et al.*, 1994b). The effect of estradiol on coronary dynamics was similar in women regardless of angiographically apparent left coronary artery atherosclerosis. The authors concluded that physiologic levels of 17β-estradiol acutely potentiated endothelium-dependent vasodilation of both large coronary arteries and coronary microvascular resistance arteries of post-menopausal women (Gilligan *et al.*, 1994b). Interestingly, a subsequent and similar coronary blood flow investigation which included men confirmed previous findings in post-menopausal women but found no evidence that 17β-estradiol modulates acetylcholine-induced coronary artery responses in men (Collins *et al.*, 1995). Overall, these data strongly suggest that estradiol exerts prominent vasodilating effects in the coronary vasculature of post-menopausal women.

*In vitro* and whole animal studies also support the hypothesis that estrogens exert beneficial effects on the vasculature and provide some evidence as to possible mechanisms of action. Given the observed endothelium-dependent effects of estrogens in human studies, numerous whole animal and/or *in vitro* experiments have focused on estrogen modulation of nitric oxide as a potential mechanism. From these studies, sufficient evidence exists to conclude that exogenous estrogens induce nitric oxide synthase and increase nitric oxide release, thus promoting endothelium-dependent vasodilation in a variety of species and vascular beds, and that endogenous estrogens may be responsible for sex differences in vascular responsiveness via nitric oxide-mediated mechanisms (Stallone, 1993; Collins *et al.*, 1994; Weiner *et al.*, 1994; Gorodeski *et al.*, 1995; Sanchez *et al.*, 1996; Node *et al.*, 1997a). Importantly, the observed effects of estrogens on nitric oxide-mediated vasodilation are accompanied by improvements in myocardial function in dogs, as indicated by reductions in myocardial infarct size and occurrence of ischemia- and reperfusion-induced ventricular arrhythmias (Node *et al.*, 1997b).

Alternatively, several studies have demonstrated calcium channel-blocking effects of estrogens in vascular smooth muscle that could account for the observed vasodilation (Collins *et al.*, 1993). These acute exposure studies include electrophysiologic experiments (Zhang *et al.*, 1994; Kitazawa *et al.*, 1997), fluorescent measurements of intracellular calcium (Han *et al.*, 1995), or contraction measurements in response to the calcium channel agonist BayK 8644 (Cohen and Susemichel, 1996). In general, these studies are hampered by the high concentrations (often in excess of 1 $\mu$M) of estrogen required to demonstrate or to suggest calcium channel-blocking effects. It is plausible that non-specific membrane fluidity alterations induced by intercalation of estrogen into the lipid bilayer contributed to the observed effects in these studies (Christ and Wehling, 1998). Nonetheless, sufficient evidence to rule out the possibility of estrogens serving as calcium channel antagonists does not exist, so future studies should be directed at clarifying the effects of estrogens on calcium channels.

Lower concentrations of estrogens (< 400 nM) have been demonstrated to exert antiproliferative effects on rat carotid artery segments (Vargas *et al.*, 1996) and on porcine left anterior descending coronary artery segments (Vargas *et al.*, 1993). Interestingly, preincubation of rat, but not porcine, vascular segments with the partial estrogen receptor agonist tamoxifen inhibited the effects of estradiol. Thus, estrogen receptors could mediate the antiproliferative effects of estrogen on vascular smooth muscle cells, but insufficient data preclude a firm conclusion. Mechanisms for estrogen-induced inhibition of vascular smooth muscle proliferation might also include insulin-like growth factor-I (IGF-I) receptors because estrogen-treated rabbits displayed reduced IGF-I receptor mRNA in their coronary arteries (Lou *et al.*, 1998a). Some precautions regarding experimental models are in order for future studies. For example, in primary rabbit vascular smooth muscle cell cultures, 17$\beta$-estradiol (10 nM) delayed cell cycle re-entry, thus prolonging the quiescent phase prior to rapid proliferation *in vitro*; however, when secondary or tertiary cultures were examined, 17$\beta$-estradiol actually promoted proliferation (Song *et al.*, 1998). This study of rabbit vascular smooth muscle cells is extremely important as future studies must consider the phenotypic state of the cells before examining effects of estrogens.

A final possible mechanism for estrogen's beneficial effects on vasculature involves the potential antioxidant activity of the hormone. As discussed previously, 17β-estradiol was found to inhibit *in vitro* copper-induced oxidation of LDL, but the concentrations required for antioxidant activity were extremely high, in excess of 1 μM (White *et al.*, 1997). Furthermore, estradiol was found to protect DNA from hydroperoxide-induced damage, but again high concentrations (18 μM) of estradiol were required to observe an antioxidant effect (Tang and Subbiah, 1996). Perhaps the most convincing data for antioxidant effects of estradiol are found in a study by Kim and colleagues (1996). Thirty-nine male dogs were given either 100 μg kg$^{-1}$ 17β-estradiol subcutaneously or an equal volume of vehicle for 2 weeks before instigation of ischemia–reperfusion injury. The investigators found a decreased incidence of ventricular arrhythmias in estradiol-treated compared with vehicle-treated dogs, and *n*-pentane in exhaled gas (an index of lipid peroxidation) was lower in estradiol-treated animals (Kim *et al.*, 1996). Moreover, artery segments from estradiol-treated dogs generated less superoxide anion after hypoxia/reoxygenation than those obtained from vehicle-treated dogs (Kim *et al.*, 1996). By considering solely the *in vitro* data currently at hand, concentrations of estrogens required for antioxidant effects are far too high to assume that similar effects occur *in vivo*. However, at least one *in vivo* study suggests that estrogens may indeed act as antioxidants.

In summary, apart from altered lipid metabolism, four mechanisms have been proposed to explain the beneficial vascular effects of estrogens: (1) estrogen-mediated vasodilation through up-regulation of nitric oxide synthase, i.e. endothelium-dependent vasodilation; (2) estrogen-mediated vasodilation through inhibition of L- or T-type calcium channels, i.e. endothelium-independent vasodilation; (3) estrogen modulation of vascular smooth muscle and/or endothelial cell proliferation; and (4) antioxidant effects of estrogen providing protection from endothelial damage. Although further information is required, a logical suggestion would be that up-regulation of nitric oxide synthase could occur through genomic mechanisms and modulation of vascular cell proliferation could be produced by genomic and/or non-genomic mechanisms. Inhibition of calcium channels and antioxidant effects, on the other hand, likely reflect non-genomic and/or non-receptor-mediated events. Whether any or all of these mechanisms are necessary to produce beneficial effects of estrogens on the vasculature is currently unknown.

## *Progestins*

As with androgens, little is known about the direct effects of progestins on the vasculature. Progesterone receptors are most likely expressed throughout the vasculature, including the coronary vasculature; however, evidence for expression of these receptors is limited. Not surprisingly, progesterone receptors are expressed in arterial vessels of the reproductive tract in rabbits and humans, more specifically in uterine arteries (Perrot-Applanat *et al.*, 1988). Perrot-Applanat and colleagues (1995) also found immunocytochemical evidence of progesterone receptor expression in varicose saphenous veins from men, and pre- and post-menopausal women. Progesterone receptors have also been detected in human and rat aortic smooth muscle cells (Lee *et al.*, 1997). The vasculature serves as a target for direct progestin action, and it is plausible that both genomic and non-genomic progesterone receptor-mediated mechanisms could account for progestin actions. In support of the non-genomic mechanism, a full-length cDNA clone for a membrane-bound progesterone receptor has been constructed from porcine vascular smooth muscle cells (Falkenstein *et al.*, 1996).

The effects of progesterone on vascular reactivity are not entirely clear because the limited animal and *in vitro* studies provide some conflicting information. In rabbit coronary artery rings, high concentrations of progesterone ($> 1$ μM) induced significant coronary relaxation in potassium-, $PGF_{2\alpha}$- or BayK 8644-precontracted arteries, and no differences in progesterone-induced relaxation between endothelium-intact and denuded arteries from either male or female rabbits were found (Jiang *et al.*, 1992). The authors concluded that progesterone induced endothelium-independent relaxation by altering calcium influx, but again high concentrations of progesterone were required. Progesterone-induced inhibition of calcium current in smooth muscle was later found using human intestinal cells in electrophysiologic experiments (Bielefeldt *et al.*, 1996). Furthermore, at least one study provided evidence that although estradiol induced nitric oxide synthase activity in tissues from guinea pigs progesterone treatment did not (Weiner *et al.*, 1994). These findings further support an endothelium-independent effect of progesterone on vascular reactivity. Yet, other evidence suggests that, while progesterone minimally alters endothelium-dependent vascular reactivity, it may antagonize estrogen-induced vasodilation. Miller and Vanhoutte (1991) examined ovariectomized dogs treated with estrogen, progesterone, or estrogen plus progesterone. Estrogen-treated dogs had similar coronary vasodilatory responses as described in other studies, but when progesterone was added, the vasodilatory response of estrogen was inhibited (Miller and Vanhoutte, 1991). As with estrogens, studies suggest that progesterone may inhibit arterial smooth muscle proliferation (Lee *et al.*, 1997). Overall, mechanisms and effects of progesterone on vascular reactivity are not understood, and further research is indicated. Furthermore, it is quite possible that the different classes of progestins may have strikingly different effects on the vasculature, where, for example, progestins chemically related to 19-nortestosterone may antagonize the beneficial vasodilation produced by estrogens.

### Glucocorticoids and mineralocorticoids

Adrenal steroids (glucocorticoids and mineralocorticoids) increase blood pressure in humans, and this response is not entirely explained by renal mechanisms such as increased sodium and water retention (Whitworth and Scoggins, 1990). Thus, examination of direct effects of adrenal steroids on the vasculature has been the subject of several investigations. Functional receptors for both glucocorticoids and mineralocorticoids were found in rabbit aorta and femoral and carotid arteries (Kornel *et al.*, 1983, 1984). More recently, evidence for membrane-bound mineralocorticoid receptors was found in membrane preparations from human mononuclear leukocytes (Wehling *et al.*, 1992) and porcine kidney and liver (Christ *et al.*, 1994; Meyer *et al.*, 1995). Despite identification of classic adrenal steroid receptors in vascular cells, whether membrane-bound glucocorticoid or mineralocorticoid receptors are expressed in vascular cells is not known.

Few human and whole animal studies have been conducted to examine direct effects of glucocorticoids or mineralocorticoids on the vasculature; thus, most of the evidence for direct effects was generated with *in vitro* models. Nonetheless, some evidence has been published for possible direct glucocorticoid alterations in vascular reactivity. Six human subjects were placed on a restricted nitrate diet and treated with 80 mg per day cortisol (Kelly *et al.*, 1998). Cortisol significantly increased systolic and mean arterial blood pressure, and there was an associated reduction in plasma nitrate/nitrite after 3, 4, and 5 days of cortisol treatment. The authors concluded that the results supported a role for nitric oxide in cortisol-induced hypertension in humans (Kelly *et al.*, 1998). Indeed, glucocorticoid-induced hypertension may involve endothelium-mediated vasoconstriction and/or reduced vasodilation, but whether reduced nitric oxide production is involved is unknown. For example, direct glucocorticoid-altered vascular reactivity may be produced by inhibition of prostacyclin synthesis. In human endothelial cell cultures, dexamethasone (0.01–100 nM) reduced histamine-, bradykinin-, and calcium ionophore A23187-induced prostaglandin $I_2$ (prostacyclin) and prostaglandin $E_2$ formation within 4 h of exposure (Lewis *et al.*, 1986). Furthermore, a glucocorticoid receptor antagonist (cortisol-21-mesylate) and cycloheximide blocked the effects of dexamethasone on prostaglandin synthesis (Lewis *et al.*, 1986). The hypothesis that glucocorticoid-induced hypertension involves reductions in endothelial prostacyclin production (Axelrod, 1983) is certainly worthwhile, but subsequent data suggest other mechanisms also participate in the hypertensive response.

Additional mechanisms for direct glucocorticoid actions in the vasculature include alterations in the cellular renin–angiotensin system. For example, dexamethasone (100 nM) increased mRNA for angiotensin-converting enzyme (ACE) in rat aortic smooth muscle cell cultures, and ACE activity was also increased in these cells (Fishel *et al.*, 1995). Interestingly, glucocorticoids have also been shown to increase angiotensin II type 1A receptors in vascular smooth muscle cells (Sato *et al.*, 1994a), and this effect was shown to participate in dexamethasone-induced hypertension in rats (Sato *et al.*, 1994b). Furthermore, a glucocorticoid response element for the rat angiotensin II type 1A receptor was later reported (Guo *et al.*, 1995). Overall, glucocorticoids may increase angiotensin II production in vascular smooth muscle and enhance angiotensin II responsiveness by up-regulating angiotensin II receptors.

Glucocorticoids may also affect vascular reactivity by altering electrolyte transport across the vascular smooth muscle cell plasma membrane. For example, in rabbit aortic smooth muscle cell cultures, dexamethasone (100 nM) significantly increased sodium influx within 48 h of exposure (Kornel *et al.*, 1993). This effect was completely blocked by the glucocorticoid antagonist RU486 and significantly reduced by progesterone (Kornel *et al.*, 1993). Actinomycin D and cycloheximide (protein synthesis inhibitors) also blocked the enhanced sodium influx, suggesting a genomic mechanism for dexamethasone (Kornel *et al.*, 1993). Calcium influx may also participate in direct glucocorticoid actions on vascular smooth muscle. When rabbits were given silastic implants containing dexamethasone, blood pressure was elevated compared with sham-treated controls (Kornel *et al.*, 1995). Interestingly, when the treated rabbits' aortas were excised, aortic rings from the dexamethasone-treated animals exhibited calcium influx at a rate twice that of rings from sham-treated animals (Kornel *et al.*, 1995). Thus, glucocorticoids could alter vascular smooth muscle contractions by enhancing sodium and/or calcium influx. The channels or transporters involved have not been elucidated.

Regarding mineralocorticoids, aldosterone rapidly increases vascular resistance in man. Wehling and colleagues (1998) obtained recent evidence for a rapid aldosterone-induced increase in vascular resistance. They recruited seventeen subjects with suspected coronary artery disease, and enrolled them in a double-blind, placebo-controlled, randomized parallel trial. During cardiac catheterization, intravenous administration of 1 mg of aldosterone rapidly (within 10 min) increased systemic vascular resistance and cardiac output compared with placebo (Wehling *et al.*, 1998). Results of this human experiment provide strong evidence for non-genomic direct actions of mineralocorticoids on the vasculature.

Regarding the mechanisms of mineralocorticoid-induced alterations in vascular reactivity, the most likely explanation is that aldosterone mediates electrolyte transport across vascular smooth muscle cell plasma membranes. At least part of this mechanism is similar to that of glucocorticoids. Aldosterone was shown to stimulate sodium influx in vascular smooth muscle cells, and both genomic and non-genomic mechanisms may account for this effect. Support for a genomic mechanism stems from data demonstrating that physiologic concentrations of aldosterone (5 nM) required 7–10 days to increase sodium influx in rabbit aortic smooth muscle cell cultures, and rabbits treated for 4 weeks with 2 mg per day aldosterone had increased sodium channel synthesis in aortic smooth muscle membranes (Kornel and Smoszna-Konaszewska, 1995). In contrast, aldosterone (1 nM) stimulated sodium influx after only 4 min of exposure in rat vascular smooth muscle cells (Christ *et al.*, 1995a). This effect appeared to be mediated by aldosterone stimulation of the Na/H exchanger, and the results suggested a non-genomic mechanism (Christ *et al.*, 1995a).

Other mechanisms may also participate in aldosterone-mediated vascular reactivity. For example, aldosterone stimulates calcium influx in rat aortic vascular smooth muscle cells (Wehling *et al.*, 1995) and in porcine endothelial cells (Schneider *et al.*, 1997). The calcium effect of aldosterone in vascular smooth muscle cells may be mediated by phospholipase C (PLC) as aldosterone was shown to increase inositol 1,4,5-trisphosphate (IP$_3$) levels within 30 s of exposure to rat vascular smooth muscle cells, and inhibitors of PLC blocked this effect (Christ *et al.*, 1995a). Furthermore, the involvement of PLC would be expected to increase diacylglycerol (DAG) and activate protein kinase C (PKC). Indeed, increased levels of DAG were observed in rat vascular smooth muscle cells exposed to 1 nM aldosterone for 30 s, and increased translocation of PKC-$\alpha$ from cytosolic to particulate fractions (indicating activation) was observed within 5 min of aldosterone exposure (Christ *et al.*, 1995b). Whether the observed signaling mechanisms of aldosterone in vascular smooth muscle and/or endothelial cells are mediated by membrane-associated mineralocorticoid receptors is not known.

In summary, glucocorticoids and mineralocorticoids induce hypertension, and at least part of this effect is likely produced by direct glucocorticoid- or mineralocorticoid-induced increases in vascular resistance. Mechanisms for adrenal steroid-induced alterations in vascular reactivity are beginning to be understood. Further research is required to determine whether genomic and/or non-genomic receptor-mediated mechanisms are responsible for increased vascular smooth muscle contractility. Further research is also required to understand the effects of adrenal steroids on endothelial cells and whether glucocorticoids or mineralocorticoids might alter the nitric oxide system.

## Cardiac effects of steroidal agents

### Steroid receptors and steroids in the heart

Steroid receptors are expressed in cardiac tissue. Experimental data providing strong evidence for the expression of steroid receptors in the heart is summarized in Table 14.6. Autoradiographic evidence for androgen receptor expression was found in rat heart muscle over 20 years ago (Krieg *et al.*, 1978). Two years later, McGill *et al.* (1980) reported evidence for androgen receptor expression in atrial and ventricular cardiac myocytes from female rhesus monkeys and baboons. More recently, full-length androgen receptors (A form; 110 kDa) were identified in human fetal heart tissue by immunoblotting, whereas truncated androgen receptors (B form; 87 kDa) were not detectable (Wilson and McPhaul, 1996). Most recently, mRNA transcripts for androgen receptors were detected by reverse transcription polymerase chain reaction (RT-PCR) in cardiac myocytes isolated from male and female adult rats, pooled cardiac myocytes isolated from male and female neonatal rats, and heart tissue obtained from male and female adult rats, male and female adult dogs, male and female neonatal humans, and male and female adult humans (Marsh *et al.*, 1998). Thus, androgen receptors are most likely expressed in the hearts of nearly every mammalian species regardless of age or sex – an "equal opportunity" receptor.

Interestingly, the rat heart accumulates testosterone to levels that are greater than those observed in more classic androgen target tissue. For example, in uncastrated adult male rats, radioimmunoassay revealed cardiac tissue testosterone levels that were fourfold higher than skeletal muscle and twofold higher than

*Table 14.6* Evidence for cardiac steroid receptors in various species: location, isoforms, and methods used for detection

|  | *Species* | *Location* | *Isoforms* | *Methods* |
|---|---|---|---|---|
| Androgen receptors | Rats, dogs, monkeys, baboons, humans | Atria and ventricles | A form | AR, IB, RB, RT-PCR |
| Estrogen receptors | Rats, rabbits | Atria and ventricles | α and β | AR, IH, RNaseP, RT-PCR |
| Progesterone receptors | Rats | ? | ? | IB |
| Mineralocorticoid receptors | Rats, guinea pigs | Atria and ventricles | Type I | AR, RB |
| Glucocorticoid receptors | Rats | Ventricles | Type II | AR, RB |

Note
AR, autoradiography; IB, immunoblotting; IH, immunohistochemistry; RB, radioligand binding; RT-PCR, reverse transcription polymerase chain reaction; RNaseP, ribonuclease protection assay; ?, unknown. Supporting references are found throughout the text.

prostate tissue, possibly because of the low levels of 5α-reductase in the heart (Krieg *et al.*, 1978). Similar findings were reported in humans in which men were found to have higher post-mortem cardiac testosterone concentrations than striated muscle, and the cardiac hormone profile suggested low levels of 5α-reductase activity (Deslypere and Vermeulen, 1986). Clearly, the heart is a target organ for androgens, but the physiologic and/or pathophysiologic roles of cardiac androgen receptors are unknown.

Evidence for cardiac estrogen receptors was obtained shortly before evidence for androgen receptors when Stumpf and colleagues (1977) found tritiated estradiol binding in the nuclei of atrial myocytes by autoradiography. Since then, two forms of the estrogen receptor have been identified (α and β), and both forms appear to be expressed in heart tissue. For example, in adult male rats, estrogen receptor β was found by immunohistochemistry (Saunders *et al.*, 1997), and in hearts from adult male and female mice mRNA transcripts for estrogen receptor α and β were found by ribonuclease protection assay (Couse *et al.*, 1997). In addition, functional estrogen receptors were found in both male and female neonatal rat cardiac myocytes and cardiac fibroblasts, and 17β-estradiol treatment (1 nM for 24 h) increased estrogen receptor α and β and progesterone receptor expression in cardiac myocytes (Grohe *et al.*, 1997). Also of note is the possibility that estrogen receptor expression in the heart changes following injury. For example, estrogen receptor α was up-regulated (as determined by immunohistochemistry and RT-PCR) in cholesterol-fed rabbits that received cardiac aorta transplants (Lou *et al.*, 1998b). Furthermore, androstendione and testosterone were found to stimulate estrogen receptor $\alpha$ and $\beta$ expression and activate an estrogen-responsive reporter plasmid in neonatal rat cardiac myocytes, perhaps through cardiac aromatase conversion of these precursors to estrogen (Grohe *et al.*, 1998). These results provide evidence for androgen- and estrogen-mediated up-regulation of estrogen receptors, and suggest local cardiac production of estrogens. Therefore, it is clear that the heart is also a target organ for estrogens, but the physiologic and/or pathophysiologic roles of cardiac estrogen receptors are not known.

As for other steroid receptors in the heart, less information is available. Progesterone receptors are expressed in the hearts of male and female neonatal rats, and expression of progesterone receptors may be induced by estrogen (Grohe *et al.*, 1997). In atrial and ventricular cytosols from adult male and female rats, radioligand evidence for aldosterone binding to type I mineralocorticoid receptors was found, and, in a manner similar to that of classic aldosterone target tissue, aldosterone and corticosterone had similar binding affinities (1–2 nM) whereas dexamethasone had a much lower affinity (Pearce and Funder, 1987). In these experiments, relative levels of type I mineralocorticoid receptors were higher in atria than in ventricles, and relative levels of type II (classic glucocorticoid) receptors were higher in ventricles than in atria (Pearce and Funder, 1987). Type I mineralocorticoid receptors were also found in guinea pig heart, and cortisol and aldosterone appeared to have equivalent affinity for this receptor (Myles and Funder, 1994). Most interestingly, there is evidence for local cardiac production of both aldosterone and corticosterone. Rat hearts were found to express the terminal synthetic enzymes for aldosterone (aldosterone synthase) and corticosterone (11$\beta$-hydroxylase), aldosterone and corticosterone were found in rat heart tissue, and rat hearts responded to angiotensin II or adrenocorticotrophin by increasing aldosterone or corticosterone synthesis respectively (Silvestre *et al.*, 1998). Importantly, cardiac aldosterone concentrations in these rats were estimated to be 16 nM, which would be approximately seventeenfold higher than aldosterone concentrations in the plasma (Silvestre *et al.*, 1998). Regarding progestins, progesterone may also bind to mineralocorticoid receptors. However, in contrast to other guinea pig tissue such as kidney and colon where progesterone and aldosterone appeared to have equal affinity for mineralocorticoid receptors, progesterone demonstrated 10–100 times less affinity than aldosterone for guinea pig heart mineralocorticoid receptors (Myles and Funder, 1996). Worthy of note is that other members of the steroid receptor superfamily are also found in the heart. For example, autoradiography and immunocytochemistry techniques were used to demonstrate the presence of receptors for 1,25-dihydroxyvitamin $D_3$ in the right atrium of male and female mice (Bidmon *et al.*, 1991). Overall, progesterone, mineralocorticoid, and glucocorticoid receptors appear to be expressed in the heart of a variety of species and agonists for these receptors may exhibit binding to all three types of receptors, thus challenging researchers with complex signaling and control mechanisms. As with androgen and estrogen receptors, whether subpopulations of progesterone, mineralocorticoid, or glucocorticoid receptors are associated with plasma membrane is not known.

In summary, the heart is a target organ for steroidal agents. Table 14.7 summarizes the potential direct effects of exogenous steroids on the heart. At present, however, very few studies have been published that attempt to verify physiologic or pathophysiologic roles for these cardiac steroid receptors. In addition, whether steroid receptors in the heart exist in plasma membrane-bound forms is not known. A wide range of future research thus lies nearly untouched regarding cardiac steroid receptors and mechanisms of action.

### *Androgens and anabolic steroids*

Evidence for a direct pathologic effect of androgens on cardiac tissue was first described by Behrendt and Boffin (1977), at about the same time as evidence for cardiac androgen receptors was reported. Adult female Wistar rats were given weekly intramuscular injections of 1.65 mg kg$^{-1}$ methandrostenolone for 3 weeks. Using transmission electron microscopy, hearts from rats treated with methandrostenolone had swollen and elongated mitochondria, and myofibrils demonstrated either disintegrated, widened and twisted Z-bands or complete dissolution of the sarcomeric units. The authors concluded that methandrostenolone administration induced myocardial lesions that were similar to those observed during early heart failure (Behrendt and Boffin, 1977). These results suggested that *in vivo* administration of AASs may induce myocardial necrosis and/or

*Table 14.7* Potential direct effects of exogenous steroids on the heart

| Steroid class | Cardiac myocytes | Cardiac fibroblasts |
|---|---|---|
| Androgens and anabolic steroids | Hypertrophic growth<br>↑ Ornithine decarboxylase<br>↑ Pyruvate kinase<br>↑ Lactate dehydrogenase<br>Altered ion homeostasis | ↑ Collagen synthesis |
| Estrogens | ↑ L-type Ca$^{2+}$ channels<br>↓ L-type Ca$^{2+}$ current<br>↑ Na$^+$/K$^+$-ATPase<br>Prolonged QT interval | ↑ or ↓ proliferation |
| Mineralocorticoids | Hypertrophic growth with high glucose<br>↑ Cl$^-$/HCO$_3^-$ exchange<br>↑ Na$^+$/H$^+$ antiporter<br>↑ Na$^+$/K$^+$-ATPase | ↑ Collagen synthesis |
| Glucocorticoids | Hypertrophic growth<br>↑ Angiotensinogen<br>↑ AT receptors | ↑ Collagen synthesis |

Note
AT, angiotensin II. Supporting references are found throughout the text.

453

apoptosis. Indeed, *in vitro* studies demonstrated that several AASs induce cell death of cultured neonatal rat cardiac myocytes (Melchert *et al.*, 1992; Welder *et al.*, 1995) or apoptosis of skeletal myocytes (Abu-Shakra *et al.*, 1997); however, the concentrations of AASs required to induce cardiac myocyte death or skeletal myocyte apoptosis were in the micromolar range. Therefore, whether AASs may induce myocardial necrosis and/or apoptosis in humans self-administering enormous doses of AASs is unknown and requires further research.

Increasing evidence suggests that androgens may induce hypertrophic growth of cardiac myocytes through an androgen receptor-mediated mechanism. First, however, it is important to note that men have larger hearts than women, even after correction for body weight and height and despite similar numbers of myocytes (de Simone *et al.*, 1995). However, left ventricular mass is only slightly lower in girls than boys prior to puberty (de Simone *et al.*, 1995). Thus, sex differences in cardiac size may be related to sex steroids, and endogenous testosterone-induced cardiac hypertrophy may indeed be a normal physiologic response. Furthermore, even if endogenous testosterone were found to be responsible for increased cardiac size in men, the clinical significance in terms of adverse cardiovascular outcomes following administration of exogenous androgens would not be clear. The increased cardiac size in men may represent a normal physiologic variation without adverse consequences. For example, in a study of 436 Black patients (163 male, 273 female) with no angiographic evidence of coronary artery disease, 52 percent of the men and 44 percent of the women had left ventricular hypertrophy (LVH), and a twofold greater relative risk of cardiac death was found among women with LVH than men with LVH (Liao *et al.*, 1995). Thus, endogenous androgen-induced cardiac hypertrophy as a sole cause of sex differences in cardiac size has not been proven and its relationship to cardiovascular disease is questionable.

Exogenous androgens, on the other hand, may impart an increased risk of pathologic cardiac hypertrophy in those who self-administer supraphysiologic doses. Several human studies demonstrate increased left ventricular mass in AAS users compared with non-users; however, an important disclaimer to all these studies is the inherent inability to control the specific AAS(s) used, the dose, or the purity. Urhausen *et al.* (1989) used one- and two-dimensional echocardiography and found increased left ventricular posterior wall and septum thickness and increased left ventricular wall thickness to left ventricular internal diameter ratios in twenty-one AAS-using body builders compared with seven non-using control body builders. Importantly, there was an impairment of diastolic function in the body builders using AASs (Urhausen *et al.*, 1989). Similar results were reported by De Piccoli and colleagues (1991) when they found echocardiographic evidence for increased ventricular septal thickness, increased left ventricular mass, increased end-diastolic volume indices, and increased isovolumetric relaxation time in fourteen body builders self-administering AAS compared with fourteen body builders not using AASs and fourteen sedentary individuals. The investigators also found that cardiac structural modifications persisted in individuals who withdrew from AASs for approximately 9 weeks (De Piccoli *et al.*, 1991). Sachtleben *et al.* (1993) reported similar findings regarding altered cardiac structure in AAS-using body builders, but they observed no AAS-associated changes in myocardial shortening fraction. Finally, at least one study similar to those previously discussed found no association between AAS use in weight lifters and left ventricular hypertrophy or clinically detectable systolic or diastolic dysfunction (Thompson *et al.*, 1992). Although some controversy exists, an association between high-dose AAS use and left ventricular hypertrophy in humans is likely given the results of animal experiments.

Animal studies have demonstrated similar anabolic effects of androgens on the heart. First, and as with humans, animal hearts are known to exhibit sexual dimorphism. For example, male A/J mice and Sprague-Dawley, Wistar, and Fischer 344 rats have slightly larger ventricles (not corrected for body weight) than their female counterparts (Koenig *et al.*, 1982; Capasso *et al.*, 1983; Bai *et al.*, 1990; Rosenkranz-Weiss *et al.*, 1994). Orchidectomized rats were found to have reduced heart weight compared with normal, sham-operated control males (Schaible *et al.*, 1984). Koenig and colleagues (1982) found that male mice also had substantially higher specific activities of lysosomal hydrolases and mitochondrial cytochrome *c* oxidase than female mice, and that these sex differences were abolished by orchidectomy. Cardiac contractile properties may also exhibit sexual dimorphism. For example, papillary muscle from male rats exhibited markedly different contractile properties from age-matched female rats in that the time-course of isometric contraction was decreased and the velocity of shortening during isotonic contractions was increased in tissue from males (Capasso *et al.*, 1983). Wang and colleagues (1998) found that cardiac muscle isolated from female rats was more sensitive to extracellular calcium than tissue from age-matched males. Adult female rat hearts had greater steady-state messenger RNA levels for contractile proteins (α- and β-myosin heavy chain and sarcomeric actin) and structural proteins (collagen type I, cytoskeletal actin, and connexin 43) than their age-matched male counterparts (Rosenkranz-Weiss *et al.*, 1994). Clearly, there are sex differences in cardiac structure and function, and these differences may confound studies examining effects of exogenous sex steroids.

As in the human studies, administration of exogenous androgens to animals was found to elicit hypertrophic cardiac growth. Initial studies of the effects of exogenous androgens on cardiac ultrastructural morphology demonstrated that methandrostenolone administration ($1.65$ mg kg$^{-1}$ intramuscularly once weekly) to female rats for 13 weeks resulted in an increase in intermediate-sized filaments in muscle cells of the left ventricle (Behrendt, 1977). Several subsequent studies have demonstrated anabolic effects of androgens on the hearts of castrated animals. For example, testosterone (but not estrogen or progesterone) administration for 5–6 weeks to castrated male rats was found to induce significant right ventricular hypertrophy (Moore *et al.*, 1978). Testosterone administration to orchidectomized mice induced a marked anabolic effect, as demonstrated by increased ventricular wet weight and increases in total protein and RNA while total DNA remained constant (Koenig *et al.*, 1982). Furthermore, testosterone administration partially restored the reduced heart weight of orchidectomized rats (Scheuer *et al.*, 1987) and partially restored the reduced $V_1$ myosin heavy chain isoenzyme levels in orchidectomized rats (Malhotra *et al.*, 1990). Interestingly, short-term (2 week) testosterone administration to rats restored the reduced α-myosin heavy chain levels that were observed in ovariectomized rats (Calovini *et al.*, 1995). Finally, testosterone administration to young male rats (30 days old) also restored castration-induced reductions in cardiac protein synthesis (Kinson *et al.*, 1990).

Hearts from other species also respond to androgens in an anabolic manner. In dogs, administration of methandienone (1.5 mg $kg^{-1}$ per day orally for 6 weeks) resulted in a significantly increased heart weight that was associated with reduced cardiac responses to inotropic load, and the pressure–volume diagram revealed that the left ventricles of treated animals worked on larger ventricular volumes (Ramo, 1987). Interestingly, exogenous testosterone and methyltestosterone increased rainbow trout heart growth to levels that were approximately 1.7 times that of control fish (Davie and Thorarensen, 1997). Overall, androgens appear to increase heart weight by producing increases in RNA and protein synthesis. As to mechanisms involved in this effect, little is known. Recently, however, exposure of neonatal rat cardiac myocyte cultures to dihydrotestosterone and testosterone was found to increase protein synthesis to levels similar to those of angiotensin II, and the effects of dihydrotestosterone and testosterone were blocked by the androgen antagonist cyproterone acetate (Marsh *et al.*, 1998). Although high concentrations (1 μM) of androgens were used in these *in vitro* experiments, the results suggest that androgen-induced cardiac hypertrophy is mediated through androgen receptors, and that cultured cardiac myocytes may be a useful model for determining mechanisms of androgen-induced hypertrophy.

A variety of other effects, including alterations in specific enzyme systems, ion fluxes, and structural matrices, may occur in cardiac myocytes exposed to androgens. For example, Koenig and colleagues (1989) demonstrated that exposure of rat ventricular cubes and acutely isolated ventricular myocytes to testosterone (10 nM) resulted in increased ornithine decarboxylase activity and subsequent polyamine levels and in increased endocytosis, hexose transport, and amino acid transport. All of these testosterone effects were blocked by the specific ornithine decarboxylase inhibitor α-difluoromethylornithine. In castrated male rats, testosterone administration increased the activity of pyruvate kinase (Chainy and Kanungo, 1978). In addition, total levels of lactate dehydrogenase decreased in the hearts of guinea pigs exposed to methandrostenolone in combination with inclined treadmill running (Weicker *et al.*, 1982).

As for androgen-induced alterations in cardiac ion fluxes, testosterone (10 nM) produced rapid (< 30 s) stimulation of calcium influx and efflux in rat ventricular cubes and isolated myocytes (Koenig *et al.*, 1989), suggesting that androgens may exert effects in cardiac myocytes via non-genomic mechanisms. However, an *in vitro* study using neonatal rat cardiac myocyte cultures found no immediate (< 13 min) changes in intracellular calcium concentrations when fura-2-loaded myocytes were exposed to high concentrations (100 μM) of testosterone (Welder *et al.*, 1995). Nonetheless, other investigators have reported androgen-induced changes in cardiac electrical properties and/or ion channels. For example, ovariectomized rabbits receiving dihydrotestosterone had down-regulated mRNA for two cardiac potassium channels, and the QT interval was prolonged in these animals (Drici *et al.*, 1996). As for cardiac structural matrices, Takala *et al.* (1991) reported that methandienone (1.5 mg kg$^{-1}$ per day) in combination with endurance exercise in dogs increased collagen concentration in the right ventricular wall. Furthermore, sialic acid in the glycocalyx (participates in maintaining normal electrical activity) was increased in castrated rats receiving testosterone replacement (Gualea *et al.*, 1995). Overall, a variety of cardiac enzyme systems, cardiac ion fluxes, and cardiac extracellular matrices may be altered by exogenous androgen administration.

In summary, endogenous androgens are likely to be at least partially responsible for sex-related differences in cardiac size and possibly function. Exogenous androgens, particularly in the high doses used for illicit purposes, may induce cardiac hypertrophy. It is logical to speculate that these two effects are mediated by genomic mechanisms. However, a variety of acute effects of androgens on cardiac tissue have been found, and the rapidity of these effects suggest that androgens may alter cardiac function through non-genomic mechanisms. Future research is required to clarify these two signaling pathways of androgens in the heart.

### Estrogens and progestins

Although compelling evidence suggests that androgens are at least partially responsible for sex differences in cardiac size and function, these sex differences could, of course, also be a result of direct effects of estrogens and/or progestins on the heart. Most likely, however, is the possibility that sex differences in cardiac size and function are produced by a combination of exposure to variable concentrations of all sex steroids and to the secondary alterations in hemodynamics produced by the sex steroids. In short, and as with androgens, little is known about the direct effects of estrogens and progestins on the heart.

Currently, there is great interest in studying the potential direct effects of estrogens and progestins on cardiac remodeling. This interest stems largely from the fact that sex differences in cardiovascular mortality are not entirely explained by protective effects of estrogens on lipid metabolism and from identification of estrogen receptors in the heart. To this end, some work with estrogen in cardiac fibroblasts has been reported. Cardiac fibroblasts compose approximately 90 percent of the non-muscle cells of the heart, and these cells are certainly involved in maintaining functional and structural integrity of the heart during development and pathophysiologic conditions (Dubey *et al.*, 1998; Lee and Eghbali-Webb, 1998). Clearly, there are sex-related differences in the rate of cardiac fibroblast proliferation, and 17β-estradiol affects cardiac fibroblast proliferation; however, it is not clear whether 17β-estradiol increases or decreases this proliferative process. For example, cardiac fibroblasts isolated from adult female rats had over threefold higher rates of tritiated thymidine incorporation than cardiac fibroblasts from adult male rats (Rosenkranz-Weiss *et al.*, 1994). This sex difference was even more striking in cells isolated from neonatal rats, as cardiac fibroblasts from female rats had over ninefold higher amounts of tritiated thymidine incorporation than fibroblasts from males (Rosenkranze-Weiss *et al.*, 1994). Subsequently, 17β-estradiol (1 nM; 24-h exposure) was shown to increase proliferation of neonatal cardiac fibroblasts by 10 percent, as indicated by bromodeoxyuridine incorporation, whereas the metabolites of estradiol, estrone and 2-hydroxyestrone (both used at 1 nM for 24 h), were shown to increase cardiac fibroblast proliferation by approximately 30 percent and 50 percent respectively (Grohe *et al.*, 1996). Similarly, 17β-estradiol (10–20 nM; 12-h exposure) was shown to increase proliferation of cardiac fibroblasts isolated from adult female rats, as determined by tritiated thymidine incorporation (Lee and Eghbali-Webb, 1998). 17α-Estradiol (inactive estrogen) had no effect on proliferation, and tamoxifen blocked the 17β-estradiol-induced proliferation (Lee and Eghbali-Webb, 1998). Furthermore, 17β-estradiol rapidly (< 10 min) increased mitogen-activated protein kinase (MAPK) activity in these cells, an effect that was blocked by tamoxifen and the MAPK pathway inhibitor PD98059 (Lee and Eghbali-Webb, 1998). Importantly, PD98059 also blocked 17β-estradiol-induced increases in tritiated thymidine incorporation, suggesting that estrogen-induced proliferation of cardiac fibroblasts was produced by estrogen receptor activation of the MAPK pathway (Lee and Eghbali-Webb, 1998). In contrast, other investigators showed that 17β-estradiol (1 nM) and progesterone (10 nM), but not 17α-estradiol, inhibited fetal calf serum-induced proliferation of cardiac fibroblasts isolated from both male and female adult rats (Dubey *et al.*, 1998). The estrogen metabolite 2-hydroxyestradiol was more potent than 17β-estradiol at inhibiting cardiac fibroblast proliferation in these experiments (Dubey *et al.*, 1998). Importantly, progesterone was shown to enhance the antiproliferative effects of estradiol in these experiments, and the phytoestrogens biochanin A and daidzein also inhibited fetal calf serum-induced cardiac fibroblast proliferation (Dubey *et al.*, 1998). Overall, the data suggest that estrogens and progestins modulate cardiac fibroblast proliferation but results are seemingly contradictory, with some demonstrating an increase and others showing a decrease in proliferation. Further research is definitely needed.

As with androgens, estrogens appear to exert a variety of other direct effects on the heart, and these effects primarily involve alterations in membrane ion pumps or channels. First, there appears to exist endogenous sex hormone-related differences in L-type calcium channel expression. Binding studies with tritiated nitrendipine demonstrated that ovariectomized, spontaneously hypertensive rats had decreased numbers of nitrendipine-binding sites and that replacement of estradiol returned those numbers to nearly control values (Ishii *et al.*, 1988). The authors suggested that estrogens may stimulate L-type calcium channel expression in spontaneously hypertensive rats. Other experiments by these investigators suggested that L-type calcium channel numbers were not affected by testosterone (Ishii *et al.*, 1988). In contrast, cardiac myocytes isolated from male mice deficient in estrogen receptors had increased calcium channel current (Johnson *et al.*, 1997); therefore, the effects of estrogen on calcium channel expression are not clear. Other studies suggest that estradiol may directly interfere with calcium current. High concentrations (micromolar range) of 17β-estradiol inhibited L-type calcium current in male rat ventricular myocytes (Berger *et al.*, 1997), in isolated adult guinea pig ventricular myocytes (Grohe *et al.*, 1996), in isolated adult guinea pig ventricular myocytes exposed to endothelin-1 (Liu *et al.*, 1997), and in isolated rat and human ventricular myocytes (Meyer *et al.*, 1998). Importantly, however, Meyer and colleagues (1998) demonstrated that ventricular L-type calcium current stimulated by isoproterenol was much more susceptible to inhibition by 17β-estradiol, and the inhibitory effect could be seen at 1 nM estradiol. Combined with previous investigations, these results suggest that estrogens may inhibit L-type calcium current *in vivo* at physiologic concentrations.

Other ion channels or pumps may also be affected by estrogens. For example, ovariectomized dogs treated with estradiol had increased Na/K-ATPase activity in cardiac sarcolemmal membranes compared with untreated ovariectomized dogs, and the experiments suggested that estradiol allosterically stimulated potassium activation of the enzyme (Dzurba *et al.*, 1997). The authors suggested that estradiol stimulation of Na/K-ATPase may impart a protective effect against ischemic insult by improving the maintenance of cation homeostasis in cardiac myocytes (Dzurba *et al.*, 1997). Also worthy of note, however, is the possibility that some estrogen-induced alterations in ion homeostasis are deleterious. For example, women have longer QT intervals and increased risk of torsade de pointes ventricular tachycardia after exposure to antiarrhythmic agents such as quinidine (Drici *et al.*, 1996). Prolonged QT intervals (Drici *et al.*, 1996) and extended action potential duration of papillary muscle (Hara *et al.*, 1998) have been observed in ovariectomized rabbits treated with estradiol. These results suggest that estrogens may also modulate potassium current.

In summary, the heart is a target organ for estrogens and progestins; however, little is known about the direct effects of progestins on the heart. Available studies indicate that both cardiac myocytes and fibroblasts may be susceptible to endogenous and exogenous estrogens. Further research is needed to clarify the growth-inhibiting or -enhancing effects of estrogens and progestins on cardiac fibroblasts as these studies may very well reveal important roles of sex steroids in cardiac remodeling. More research is also needed to understand the effects of estrogens and progestins on cardiac ion channels and pumps, especially to determine whether these effects involve altered expression of ion homeostatic proteins or non-genomic or direct interference of the channels and/or pumps by estrogens. Finally, as available data suggest that estrogens may affect cardiac myocytes and fibroblasts by both genomic and non-genomic mechanisms, a wide avenue of research is open to clarifying the mechanisms whereby estrogens and progestins directly affect the heart.

### *Mineralocorticoids and glucocorticoids*

Given the presence of mineralocorticoid and glucocorticoid receptors and local aldosterone and corticosterone synthesis in the heart, there is little doubt that cardiac tissue is a target for mineralocorticoids and glucocorticoids. As with androgens, estrogens, and progestins, however, little is known about the direct effects of mineralocorticoids and glucocorticoids on the heart. Both aldosterone and glucocorticoids appear to stimulate cardiac fibrosis by unknown mechanisms (Young *et al.*, 1994; Robert *et al.*, 1995). In rats subjected to renovascular hypertension in which aldosterone and angiotensin II are increased and in rats receiving a chronic infusion of aldosterone, a significant rise in cardiac interstitial collagen was observed in hypertrophied left ventricles and non-hypertrophied right ventricles (Brilla *et al.*, 1990). These data suggested that angiotensin II and/ or aldosterone regulate collagen accumulation in both ventricles (Brilla *et al.*, 1990). Using adult rat cardiac fibroblast cultures, Brilla and colleagues (1994) found significantly increased collagen synthesis in cultures exposed to 1 nM aldosterone for 24 h. Furthermore, the increase in collagen synthesis was completely blocked by the mineralocorticoid receptor antagonist spironolactone (Brilla *et al.*, 1994). Perhaps surprisingly, hemodynamic actions of aldosterone may not be responsible for the cardiac fibrosis. Robert and colleagues (1994) demonstrated that rats treated with aldosterone and increased salt intake for 2 months developed arterial hypertension, moderate left ventricular hypertrophy, and numerous foci of proliferating non-muscle cells with bilateral fibrosis. The investigators found that left ventricular hypertrophy and increased atrial natriuretic peptide messenger RNA was restricted to the left ventricle; because fibrosis was found in both ventricles, these investigators suggested that fibrosis was independent of hemodynamic factors (Robert *et al.*, 1994). As for glucocorticoids, uninephrectomized rats treated with corticosterone and increased salt intake developed increased cardiac interstitial collagen in both ventricles compared with control animals; however, the effect was modest compared with the increased cardiac interstitial collagen induced in aldosterone-treated animals (Young *et al.*, 1994). Overall, these data suggest that mineralocorticoids, and to a lesser extent glucocorticoids, induce cardiac fibrosis, which is likely mediated by direct effects of these steroidal agents on cardiac fibroblasts.

Other direct cardiac effects of mineralocorticoids and glucocorticoids deserve attention. For example, exposure of neonatal rat cardiac myocyte cultures to aldosterone for 24 h resulted in increased chloride/bicarbonate exchanger for 6 days following exposure and increased sodium/hydrogen antiporter for 9 days following exposure (Korichneva *et al.*, 1995). Furthermore, physiologic concentrations of aldosterone (nanomolar range) induced rapid increases in messenger RNA for Na/K-ATPase in both neonatal and adult rat cardiac myocyte cultures (Ikeda *et al.*, 1991). In the adult cardiac myocyte cultures, the increase in messenger RNA was associated with a significant increase in Na/K-ATPase protein and transport activity (Ikeda *et al.*, 1991). Also in neonatal rat cardiac myocyte cultures, Sato and Funder (1996) observed hypertrophic growth in cells exposed to aldosterone (10 nM) with high glucose (30 mM), but not in cells exposed to aldosterone alone, high glucose alone, or dexamethasone (10 nM) with or without high glucose. As for glucocorticoids, oral dexamethasone administration to neonatal rats produced cardiac hypertrophy, as indicated by increased heart weight to body weight ratios, elevated total cardiac protein content, elevated actin content, and increased total protein to total DNA ratios after 5 and 7 days of treatment (La Mear *et al.*, 1997). Regarding a potential mechanism of this effect, hearts from adult rats pretreated with dexamethasone had increased angiotensinogen messenger RNA (Lindpainter *et al.*, 1990). Furthermore, in rats subjected to unilateral renal artery clips and later given subcutaneous dexamethasone, messenger RNAs for angiotensin II type 1a and 1b receptors were both significantly increased (Della Bruna *et al.*, 1995). Finally, glucocorticoid-induced hypertrophic growth may be short-lived and reversed with continued glucocorticoid administration. Czerwinski and colleagues (1991) found that female rats given hydrocortisone developed peak cardiac enlargement after 7 days of treatment, but the enlargement returned nearly to control levels by 15 days of continued treatment. These results suggest the existence of a compensatory mechanism to counter glucocorticoid-induced hypertrophic growth.

In summary, both mineralocorticoids and glucocorticoids appear to induce cardiac fibrosis and possibly hypertrophic growth. Thus, both cardiac fibroblasts and cardiac myocytes may be targets for mineralocorticoids and glucocorticoids. The presence of both a local cardiac mineralocorticoid and renin–angiotensin system strongly suggests that aldosterone and angiotensin II exert effects directly on cardiac tissue in a manner similar to that observed in the systemic circulation. Whether mineralocorticoids and glucocorticoids induce their direct actions in cardiac tissue through genomic or non-genomic mechanisms or both is currently not known.

## Further considerations regarding steroidal agents and cardiovascular function

Until the actions of single steroidal agents on the cardiovascular system are better understood, it is unlikely that the more common situation of multiple steroids present in the circulation, and thus simultaneous exposure of the heart and vasculature to numerous combinations of steroidal agents, will be fully appreciated. For example, multiple classes of endogenous steroids are present in the circulation at any given moment. Even in the case of exogenous steroid administration, rarely is one steroidal agent administered, as demonstrated by illicit AAS use in which numerous androgens are used concomitantly in high doses and by hormone replacement therapy or oral contraceptives in which estrogens are most frequently co-prescribed with progestins. Furthermore, little is known regarding the effects of multiple steroidal agents on circulating transport proteins, so whether concomitant administration of multiple steroidal agents increases the free fraction of circulating steroid is relatively open to question. Thus, the highly likely steroid–steroid interactions in the cardiovascular system will be difficult to study and to understand, but future research must bear this consideration.

Similarly, an ever-increasing body of literature continues to describe potential drug–exogenous steroid interactions. The most obvious example is that most steroidal agents undergo significant hepatic metabolism. Thus, administration of any other chemical entity that may modify hepatic metabolism most certainly subjects an individual to drug–steroid interactions. In addition, there is emerging information regarding other drug–steroid interactions with significant implications regarding cardiovascular function. As a case in point, cocaine and nandrolone (19-nortestosterone) administered concomitantly to spontaneously hypertensive rats resulted in heart weights that were greater than those in rats that received either agent alone (Tseng et al., 1994). Myocardial inflammatory and fibrotic changes were also more evident in rats treated with nandrolone alone or cocaine plus nandrolone than in rats that received vehicle or cocaine alone (Tseng et al., 1994).

Additionally, future research should also consider the possibility that physiologic adaptations may interact with steroidal agents. In pointing to a specific example, recall that exogenous self-administration of high doses of AASs may increase the risk of cardiac hypertrophy. Many users of illicit AASs are weight trainers and/or body builders, and weight lifters have long been known to exhibit increased left ventricular mass, left ventricular wall thickness, and intraventricular septal wall thickness and decreased left ventricular systolic internal dimensions (Fleck et al., 1989, 1993). Thus, the possibility of interactions between physiologic adaptations to exercise training and exogenous androgens should be considered.

Finally, increasing evidence suggests that cytokines and/or growth factors may interact with steroidal agents. For example, it is now known that interleukin-6 can stimulate the androgen receptor in the absence of androgen (Hobisch et al., 1998). Furthermore, epidermal growth factor may activate estrogen receptors independently of estrogen ligand (Bunone et al., 1996). Thus, any physiologic or pathophysiologic condition that alters cytokine and/or growth factor release may impart interactions with endogenous steroids and/or induce cardiovascular effects similar to steroidal agents, but independent of cognate ligand.

In summary, the above interactions represent several issues that require continued research. In addition, it is highly likely that future research will identify even further confounding interactions with steroidal agents. However, as in any area, the need to understand the mechanisms of action of the sex steroids and their direct effects on organ systems remains a primary goal in this field. Interactions can be best understood once the cellular mechanisms of the individual agents and/or conditions are elucidated.

## Conclusions: cardiovascular toxicology and steroidal agents

In considering the toxicologic implications of the information discussed, it is imperative to first point out that limitations prevent complete discussion of every reported cardiovascular consequence of steroidal agents. Therefore, the chapter focused on the effects of steroidal agents on lipid metabolism and direct actions of steroidal agents on the vasculature and heart. As such, the chapter should teach that any exogenous agent that may interact with steroid receptors and/or endogenous steroid ligands should be considered as a potential disrupter of normal cardiovascular function. Focus of the chapter was narrow in that only the major steroidal agents were discussed. Now, however, it is important to realize that continued research into pharmacologic and toxicologic modulators of steroid receptor signaling is identifying an increasing number of ligands for steroid receptors as well as an increasing number of receptor isoforms. Examples include pharmaceutical interest in non-steroidal agonists and antagonists of steroid receptors and their subtypes and toxicologic interest in endocrine disrupters including naturally occurring and industrial chemicals that serve as agonists and/ or antagonists of steroid receptors. Possibilities for future research into cardiovascular effects of steroidal agents appear to be infinite in number.

## References

Abu-Shakra, S., Alhalabi, M.S., Nachtman, F.C., Schemidt, R.A., and Brusilow, W.S.A. 1997. Anabolic steroids induce injury and apoptosis of differentiated skeletal muscle. *Journal of Neuroscience Research* 47: 186–197.

Applebaum-Bowden, D., Haffner, S.M., and Hazzard, W.R. 1987. The dyslipoproteinemia of anabolic steroid therapy: increase in hepatic triglyceride lipase activity precedes the decrease in high density lipoprotein$_2$ cholesterol. *Metabolism* 36: 949–952.

Axelrod, L. 1983. Inhibition of prostacyclin production mediates permissive effects of glucocorticoids on vascular tone. Perturbations of this mechanism contribute to pathogenesis of Cushing's syndrome and Addison's disease. *Lancet* 1: 904–906.

Bai, S., Campbell, S.E., Moore, J.A., Morales, M.C., and Gerdes, A.M. 1990. Influence of age, growth, and sex on cardiac myocyte size and number in rats. *The Anatomical Record* 226: 207–212.

Barbosa, J., Seal, U.S., and Doe, R.P. 1971. Effects of anabolic steroids on haptoglobulin, orosomucoid, plasminogen, fibrinogen, transferrin, ceruloplasmin, $\alpha_1$-antitrypsin, $\beta$-glucuronidase and total serum protein. *Journal of Clinical Endocrinology* 33: 388–398.

Becker, D.M., Chamberlain, B., Swank, R., Hegewald, M.G., Girardet, R., Baughman, K.L., Kwiterovich, P.O., Pearson, T.A., Ettinger, W.H., and Renlund, D. 1988. Relationship between corticosteroid exposure and plasma lipid levels in heart transplant recipients. *American Journal of Medicine* 85: 632–638.

Behrendt, H. 1977. Effect of anabolic steroids on rat heart muscle cells. *Cell and Tissue Research* 180: 303–315.

Behrendt, H. and Boffin, H. 1977. Myocardial cell lesions caused by an anabolic hormone. *Cell and Tissue Research* 181: 423–426.

Berger, F., Borchard, U., Hafner, D., Putz, I., and Weis, T.M. 1997. Effects of 17β-estradiol on action potentials and ionic currents in male rat ventricular myocytes. *Naunyn-Schmiedeberg's Archives of Pharmacology* 356: 788–796.

Bidmon, H.J., Gutkowska, J., Murakami, R., and Stumpf, W.E. 1991. Vitamin D receptors in heart: effects on atrial natriuretic factor. *Experientia* 47: 958–962.

Bielefeldt, K., Waite, L., Abboud, F.M., and Conklin, J.L. 1996. Nongenomic effects of progesterone on human intestinal smooth muscle cells. *American Journal of Physiology* 271: G370–G376.

Bongard, V., Ferrieres, S., Ruidavets, J.-B., Amouyel, P., Arveiler, D., Bingham, A., and Ducimetiere, P. 1998. Transdermal estrogen replacement therapy and plasma lipids in 693 French women. *Maturitas* 30: 265–272.

Brilla, C.G., Pick, R., Tan, L.B., Janicki, J.S., and Weber, K.T. 1990. Remodeling of the rat right and left ventricles in experimental hypertension. *Circulation Research* 67: 1355–1364.

Brilla, C.G., Zhou, G., Matsubara, L., and Weber, K.T. 1994. Collagen metabolism in cultured adult rat cardiac fibroblasts: response to angiotensin II and aldosterone. *Journal of Molecular and Cellular Cardiology* 26: 809–820.

Brueggemeier, R.W., Miller, D.D., and Witiak, D.T. 1995. Cholesterol, adrenocorticoids, and sex hormones. In *Principles of Medicinal Chemistry*, 4th edn. Foye, W.O., Lemke, T.L., and Williams, D.A. (eds), pp. 444–497. Williams & Wilkins, Baltimore, MD.

Brunton, L.L. 1995. Agents affecting gastrointestinal water flux and motility; emesis and antiemetics; bile acids and pancreatic enzymes. In *Goodman & Gilman's The Pharmacological Basis of Therapeutics*, 9th edn. Hardman, J.G., Limbird, L.E., Molinoff, P.B., Ruddon, R.W., and Gilman, A.G. (eds), pp. 917–936. McGraw-Hill, New York, NY.

Bunone, G., Briand, P.A., Miksicek, R.J., Picard, D. 1996. Activation of the unliganded estrogen receptor by EGF involves the MAP kinase pathway and direct phosphorylation. *EMBO Journal* 15: 2174–2183.

Calovini, T., Haase, H., and Morano, I. 1995. Steroid-hormone regulation of myosin subunit expression in smooth and cardiac muscle. *Journal of Cellular Biochemistry* 59: 69–78.

Capasso, J.M., Remily, R.M., Smith, R.H., and Sonnenblick, E.H. 1983. Sex differences in myocardial contractility in the rat. *Basic Research in Cardiology* 78: 156–171.

Carson-Jurica, M.A., Schrader, W.T., and O'Malley, B.W. 1990. Steroid receptor family: structure and functions. *Endocrine Reviews* 11: 201–220.

Chainy, G.B.N. and Kanungo, M.S. 1978. Effects of estradiol and testosterone on the activity of pyruvate kinase of the cardiac and skeletal muscles of rats as a function of age and sex. *Biochimica et Biophysica Acta* 540: 65–72.

Christ, M. and Wehling, M. 1998. Cardiovascular steroid actions: swift swallows or sluggish snails? *Cardiovascular Research* 40: 34–44.

Christ, M., Sippel, K., Eisen, C., and Wehling, M. 1994. Non-classical receptors for aldosterone in plasma membranes from pig kidneys. *Molecular and Cellular Endocrinology* 99: R31–R34.

Christ, M., Douwes, K., Eisen, C., Bechtner, G, Theisen, K., and Wehling, M. 1995a. Rapid effects of aldosterone on sodium transport in vascular smooth muscle cells. *Hypertension* 25: 117–123.

Christ, M., Meyer, C., Sippel, K., and Wehling, M. 1995b. Rapid aldosterone signaling in vascular smooth muscle cells: involvement of phospholipase C, diacylglycerol, and protein kinase C alpha. *Biochemical and Biophysical Research Communications* 213: 123–129.

Cohen, M.L. and Susemichel, A.D. 1996. Effect of 17β-estradiol and the nonsteroidal benzothiophene, LY117018 on in vitro rat aortic responses to norepinephrine, serotonin, U46619, and BAYK 8644. *Drug Development Research* 37: 97–104.

Collins, P., Rosano, G.M.C., Jiang, C., Lindsay, D., Sarrel, P.M., and Poole-Wilson, P.A. 1993. Cardiovascular protection by oestrogen – a calcium antagonist effect? *The Lancet* 341: 1264–1265.

Collins, P., Shay, J., Jiang, C., and Moss, J. 1994. Nitric oxide accounts for dose-dependent estrogen-mediated coronary relaxation after acute estrogen withdrawal. *Circulation* 90: 1964–1968.

Collins, P., Rosano, G.M.C., Sarrel, P.M., Ulrich, L., Adamopoulos, S., Beale, C.M., McNeill, J.G., and Poole-Wilson, P.A. 1995. 17 Beta-estradiol attenuates acetylcholine-induced coronary arterial constriction in women but not men with coronary artery disease. *Circulation* 92: 24–30.

Costarella, C.E., Stallone, J.N., Rutecki, G.W., and Whittier, F.C. 1996. Testosterone causes direct relaxation of rat thoracic aorta. *Journal of Pharmacology and Experimental Therapeutics* 277: 34–39.

Council on Scientific Affairs. 1988. Drug abuse in athletes. Anabolic steroids and growth hormone. *Journal of the American Medical Association* 259: 1703–1705.

Council on Scientific Affairs. 1990. Medical and nonmedical uses of anabolic-androgenic steroids. *Journal of the American Medical Association* 264: 1923–2927.

Couse, J.F., Lindzey, J., Grandien, K., Gustafsson, J.-A., and Korach, K.S. 1997. Tissue distribution and quantitative analysis of estrogen receptor-α (ERα) and estrogen receptor-β (ERβ) messenger ribonucleic acid in the wild-type and ERα-knockout mouse. *Endocrinology* 138: 4613–4621.

Cummings, A.M. 1997. Methoxychlor as a model for environmental estrogens. *Critical Reviews in Toxicology* 27: 367–379.

Czerwinski, S.M., Kurowski, T.T., McKee, E.E., Zak, R., and Hickson, R.C. 1991. Myosin heavy chain turnover during cardiac mass changes by glucocorticoids. *Journal of Applied Physiology* 70: 300–306.

Davie, P.S. and Thorarensen, H. 1997. Heart growth in rainbow trout in response to exogenous testosterone and 17-α methyltestosterone. *Comparative Biochemistry and Physiology* 117A: 227–230.

Della Bruna, R., Ries, S., Himmelstoss, C., and Kurtz, A. 1995. Expression of cardiac angiotensin II AT1 receptor genes in rat hearts is regulated by steroids but not by angiotensin II. *Journal of Hypertension* 13: 763–769.

De Piccoli, B., Giada, F., Benettin, A., Sartori, F., and Piccolo, E. 1991. Anabolic steroid use in body builders: an echocardiographic study of left ventricular morphology and function. *International Journal of Sports Medicine* 12: 408–412.

Deslypere, J.P. and Vermeulen, A. 1986. Influence of age on steroid concentrations in skin and striated muscle in women and in cardiac muscle and lung tissue in men. *Journal of Clinical Endocrinology and Metabolism* 61: 648–653.

Distelhorst, C.W. 1993. Steroid hormone receptors. *Journal of Laboratory and Clinical Medicine* 122: 241–244.

Drici, M.D., Burklow, T.R., Haridasse, V., Glazer, R.I., and Woosley, R.L. 1996. Sex hormones prolong the QT interval and downregulate potassium channel expression in the rabbit heart. *Circulation* 94: 1471–1474.

Dubey, R.K., Gillespie, D.G., Jackson, E.K., and Keller, P.J. 1998. 17β-Estradiol, its metabolites, and progesterone inhibit cardiac fibroblast growth. *Hypertension* 31: 522–528.

Dzurba, A., Ziegelhoffer, A., Vrbjar, N., Styk, J., and Slezak, J. 1997. Estradiol modulates the sodium pump in the heart sarcolemma. *Molecular and Cellular Biochemistry* 176: 113–118.

Ehnholm, C., Huttunen, J.K., Kinnunen, P.J., Miettinen, T.A., and Nikkila, E.A. 1975. Effect of oxandrolone treatment on the activity of lipoprotein lipase, hepatic lipase and phospholipase $A_1$ of human postheparin plasma. *New England Journal of Medicine* 292: 1314–1317.

Ettinger, W.H., Goldberg, A.P., Applebaum-Bowden, D., and Hazzard, W.R. 1987a. Dyslipoproteinemia in systemic lupus erythematosus. Effect of corticosteroids. *American Journal of Medicine* 83: 503–508.

Ettinger, W.H., Klinefelter, H.F., and Kwiterovitch, P.O. 1987b. Effect of short-term, low-dose corticosteroids on plasma lipoprotein lipids. *Atherosclerosis* 63: 167–172.

Ettinger, W.H., Dysko, R.C., and Clarkson, T.B. 1989. Prednisone increases low density lipoprotein in cynomolgus monkeys fed saturated fat and cholesterol. *Arteriosclerosis* 9: 848–855.

Falkenstein, E., Meyer, C., Eisen, C., Scriba, P.C., and Wehling, M. 1996. Full-length cDNA sequence of a progesterone membrane-binding protein from porcine vascular smooth muscle cells. *Biochemical and Biophysical Research Communications* 229: 86–89.

Farhat, M.Y., Wolfe, R., Vargas, R., Foegh, M.L., and Ramwell, P.W. 1995. Effect of testosterone treatment on vasoconstrictor response of left anterior descending coronary artery in male and female pigs. *Journal of Cardiovascular Pharmacology* 25: 495–500.

Farhat, M.Y., Lavigne, M.C., and Ramwell, P.W. 1996. The vascular protective effects of estrogen. *FASEB Journal* 10: 615–624.

Farnsworth, W.E. 1990. The prostate plasma membrane as an androgen receptor. *Membrane Biochemistry* 9: 141–162.

Ferrer, M., Encabo, A., Marin, J., and Balfagon, G. 1994. Chronic treatment with the anabolic steroid, nandrolone, inhibits vasodilator responses in rabbit aorta. *European Journal of Pharmacology* 252: 233–241.

Fishel, R.S., Eisenberg, S., Shai, S.-Y., Redden, R.A., Bernstein, K.E., and Berk, B.C. 1995. Glucocorticoids induce angiotensin-converting enzyme expression in vascular smooth muscle. *Hypertension* 25: 343–349.

Fleck, S.J., Henke, C., and Wilson, W. 1989. Cardiac MRI of elite junior olympic weight lifters. *International Journal of Sports Medicine* 10: 329–333.

Fleck, S.J., Pattany, P.M., Stone, M.H., Kraemer, W.J., Thrush, J., and Wong, K. 1993. Magnetic resonance imaging determination of left ventricular mass: junior olympic weightlifters. *Medicine and Science in Sports and Exercise* 25: 522–527.

Friedl, K.E., Hannan, C.J., Jones, R.E., and Plymate, S.R. 1990. High-density lipoprotein cholesterol is not decreased if an aromatizable androgen is administered. *Metabolism* 39: 69–74.

Gilligan, D.M., Badar, D.M., Panza, J.A., Quyyumi, A.A., and Cannon, R.O. 1994a. Acute vascular effects of estrogen in postmenopausal women. *Circulation* 90: 786–791.

Gilligan, D.M., Quyyumi, A.A., Cannon, R.O., Johnson, G.B., and Schenke, W.H. 1994b. Effects of physiological levels of estrogen on coronary vasomotor function in postmenopausal women. *Circulation* 89: 2545–2551.

Glazer, G. 1991. Atherogenic effects of anabolic steroids on serum lipid levels. *Archives of Internal Medicine* 151: 1925–1933.

Gorodeski, G.I., Yang, T., Levy, M.N., Goldfarb, J., and Utian, W.H. 1995. Effects of estrogen in vivo on coronary vascular resistance in perfused rabbit hearts. *American Journal of Physiology* 269: R1333–R1338.

Green, D.J., Cable, N.T., Rankin, J.M., Fox, C., and Taylor, R.R. 1993. Anabolic steroids and vascular responses. *Lancet* 342: 863.

Grohe, C., Kahlert, S., Lobbert, K., Meyer, R., Linz, K.W., Karas, R.H., and Vetter, H. 1996. Modulation of hypertensive heart disease by estrogen. *Steroids* 61: 201–204.

Grohe, C., Kahlert, S., Lobbert, K., Stimpel, M., Karas, R.H., Vetter, H., and Neyses, L. 1997. Cardiac myocytes and fibroblasts contain functional estrogen receptors. *FEBS Letters* 416: 107–112.

Grohe, C., Kahlert, S., Lobbert, K., and Vetter, H. 1998. Expression of oestrogen receptor alpha and beta in rat heart: role of local oestrogen synthesis. *Journal of Endocrinology* 156: R1–R7.

Grundy, S.M. 1990. Cholesterol and coronary heart disease. Future directions. *Journal of the American Medical Association* 264: 3053–3059.

Gualea, M.R., D'Antona, G., Ceriani, T., and Minelli, R. 1995. Effects of testosterone on the electrical activity of rat ventricular myocardium. *Medical Science Research* 23: 705–707.

Guo, D.-F., Uno, S., Ishihata, A., Nakamura, N., and Inagami, T. 1995. Identification of a cis-acting glucocorticoid responsive element in the rat angiotensin II type 1A promoter. *Circulation Research* 77: 249–257.

Haffner, S.M., Kushwaha, R.S., Foster, D.M., Applebaum-Bowden, D., and Hazzard, W.R. 1983. Studies on the metabolic mechanism of reduced high density lipoproteins during anabolic steroid therapy. *Metabolism* 32: 413–420.

Han, S.-Z., Haraki, H., Ouchi, Y., Akishita, M., and Hajime, O. 1995. 17 Beta-estradiol inhibits $Ca^{2+}$ influx and $Ca^{2+}$ release induced by thromboxane $A_2$ in porcine coronary artery. *Circulation* 91: 2619–2626.

Hara, M., Danilo, P., and Rosen, M.R. 1998. Effects of gonadal steroids on ventricular repolarization and on the response to E4031. *The Journal of Pharmacology and Experimental Therapeutics* 285: 1068–1072.

Haupt, H.A. and Rovere, G.D. 1984. Anabolic steroids: a review of the literature. *The American Journal of Sports Medicine* 12: 469–484.

Henkin, Y., Como, J.A., and Oberman, A. 1992. Secondary dyslipidemia. Inadvertent effects of drugs in clinical practice. *Journal of the American Medical Association* 267: 961–968.

Hirvonen E., Malkonen, M., and Manninen, V. 1981. Effects of different progestogens on lipoproteins during postmenopausal replacement therapy. *New England Journal of Medicine* 304: 560–563.

Hobisch, A., Eder, I.E., Putz, T., Horninger, W., Bartsch, G., Klocker, H., and Culig, Z. 1998. Interleukin-6 regulates prostate-specific protein expression in prostate carcinoma cells by activation of the androgen receptor. *Cancer Research* 58: 4640–4645.

Ikeda, U., Hyman, R., Smith, T.W., and Medford, R.M. 1991. Aldosterone-mediated regulation of $Na^+$, $K^+$-ATPase gene expression in adult and neonatal rat cardiocytes. *The Journal of Biological Chemistry* 266: 12058–12066.

Ishii, K., Kano, T., and Ando, J. 1988. Sex differences in [$^3$H]nitrendipine binding and effects of sex steroid hormones in rat cardiac and cerebral membranes. *Japanese Journal of Pharmacology* 46: 117–125.

Jain, S., Pulikuri, S., Zhu, Y., Qi, C., Kanwar, Y.S., Yeldandi, A.V., Rao, M.S., and Reddy, J.K. 1998. Differential expression of the peroxisome proliferator-activated receptor γ (PPARγ) and its coactivators steroid receptor coactivator-1 and PPAR-binding protein PBP in the brown fat, urinary bladder, colon, and breast of the mouse. *American Journal of Pathology* 153: 349–354.

Jefferys, D.B., Lessof, M.H., and Mattock, M.B. 1980. Corticosteroid treatment, serum lipids, and coronary artery disease. *Postgraduate Medical Journal* 56: 491–493.

Jiang, C.W., Sarrel, P.M., Lindsay, D.C., Poole-Wilson, P.A., and Collins, P. 1992. Progesterone induces endothelium-independent relaxation of rabbit coronary artery in vitro. *European Journal of Pharmacology* 211: 163–167.

Johnson, B.D., Zheng, W., Korach, K.S., Scheuer, T., Catterall, W.A., and Rubanyi, G.M. 1997. Increased expression of the cardiac L-type calcium channel in estrogen receptor-deficient mice. *Journal of General Physiology* 110: 135–140.

Kalin, M.F. and Zumoff, B. 1990. Sex hormones and coronary disease: a review of the clinical studies. *Steroids* 55: 330–352.

Kantor, M.A., Bianchini, A., Bernier, D., Sady, S.P., and Thompson, P.D. 1985. Androgens reduce $HDL_2$-cholesterol and increase hepatic triglyceride lipase activity. *Medicine and Science in Sports and Exercise* 17: 462–465.

Karas, R.H., Patterson, B.L., and Mendelsohn, M.E. 1994. Human vascular smooth muscle cells contain functional estrogen receptor. *Circulation* 89: 1943–1950.

Karas, R.H., Baur, W.E., van Eickles, M., and Mendelsohn, M.E. 1995. Human vascular smooth muscle cells express an estrogen receptor isoform. *FEBS Letters* 377: 103–108.

Kelly, J.J., Tam, S.H., Williamson, P.M., Lawson, J., and Whitworth, J.A. 1998. The nitric oxide system and cortisol-induced hypertension in humans. *Clinical and Experimental Pharmacology and Physiology* 25: 945–946.

Kennedy, R.H. and Seifen, E. 1991. Cardiac toxicology of digitalis. In *Principles of Cardiac Toxicology*. Baskin, S.I. (ed.), pp. 217–274. CRC Press, Boca Raton, FL.

Kim, Y.D., Chen, B., Beauregard, J., Kouretas, P., Thomas, G., Farhat, M.Y., Myers, A.K., and Lees, D.E. 1996. 17Beta-estradiol prevents dysfunction of canine coronary endothelium and myocardium and reperfusion arrhythmias after brief ischemia/reperfusion. *Circulation* 94: 2901–2908.

Kinson, G.A., Layberry, R.A., and Hebert, B. 1990. Influences of anabolic androgens on cardiac growth and metabolism in the rat. *Canadian Journal of Physiology and Pharmacology* 69: 1698–1704.

Kitazawa, T., Hamada, E., Kitazawa, K., and Gaznabi, A.K.M. 1997. Non-genomic mechanism of 17β-oestradiol-induced inhibition of contraction in mammalian vascular smooth muscle. *Journal of Physiology* 499: 497–511.

Koenig, H., Goldstone, A., and Lu, C.Y. 1982. Testosterone-mediated sexual dimorphism of the rodent heart. Ventricular lysosomes, mitochondria, and cell growth are modulated by androgens. *Circulation Research* 50: 782–787.

Koenig, H., Fan, C.-C., Goldstone, A.D., Lu, C.Y., and Trout, J.J. 1989. Polyamines mediate androgenic stimulation of calcium fluxes and membrane transport in rat heart myocytes. *Circulation Research* 64: 415–426.

Kopera, H. 1985. The history of anabolic steroids and a review of the clinical experience with anabolic steroids. *Acta Endocrinologica* 110 (Suppl. 271): 11–18.

Korichneva, I., Puceat, M., Millanvoye-Van Brussel, E., Geraud, G., and Vassort, G. 1995. Aldosterone modulates both the Na/H antiport and $Cl/HCO_3$ exchanger in cultured neonatal rat cardiac cells. *Journal of Molecular and Cellular Cardiology* 27: 2521–2528.

Kornel, L. and Smoszna-Konaszewska, B. 1995. Aldosterone (ALDO) increases transmembrane influx of Na⁺ in vascular smooth muscle (VSM) cells through increased synthesis of Na⁺ channels. *Steroids* 60: 114–119.

Kornel, L., Kanamarlapudi, N., Ramsay, C., Travers, T., Kamath, S., Taff, D.J., Patel, N., Packer, W., and Raynor, W.J. 1983. Arterial steroid receptors and their putative role in the mechanism of hypertension. *Journal of Steroid Biochemistry* 19: 333–344.

Kornel, L., Kanamarlapudi, N., Ramsay, C., and Taff, D.J. 1984. Studies on arterial mineralocorticoid and glucocorticoid receptors: evidence for the translocation of steroid–cytoplasmic receptor complexes to cell nuclei. *Clinical Physiology and Biochemistry* 2: 14–31.

Kornel, L., Manisundaram, B., and Nelson, W.A. 1993. Glucocorticoids regulate Na⁺ transport in vascular smooth muscle through the glucocorticoid receptor-mediated mechanism. *American Journal of Hypertension* 6: 736–744.

Kornel, L., Prancan, A.V., Kanamarlapudi, N., Hynes, J., and Kuzianik, E. 1995. Study on the mechanisms of glucocorticoid-induced hypertension: glucocorticoids increase transmembrane Ca²⁺ influx in vascular smooth muscle in vivo. *Endocrine Research* 21: 203–210.

Krieg, M., Smith, K., and Bartsch, W. 1978. Demonstration of a specific androgen receptor in rat heart muscle: relationship between binding, metabolism, and tissue levels of androgens. *Endocrinology* 103: 1686–1694.

La Mear, N.S., MacGilvray, S.S., and Myers, T.F. 1997. Dexamethasone-induced myocardial hypertrophy in neonatal rats. *Biology of the Neonate* 72: 175–180.

Lee, H.-W. and Eghbali-Webb, M. 1998. Estrogen enhances proliferative capacity of cardiac fibroblasts by estrogen receptor- and mitogen-activated protein kinase-dependent pathways. *Journal of Molecular and Cellular Cardiology* 30: 1359–1368.

Lee, W.S., Harder, J.A., Yoshizumi, M., Lee, M.E., and Haber, E. 1997. Progesterone inhibits arterial smooth muscle cell proliferation. *Nature Medicine* 3: 1005–1008.

Lenders, J.W.M., Demacker, P.N.M., Vos, J.A., Jansen, P.L.M., Hoitsma, A.J., van't Laar, A., and Thien, T. 1988. Deleterious effects of anabolic steroids on serum lipoproteins, blood pressure, and liver function in amateur body builders. *International Journal of Sports Medicine* 9: 19–23.

Lewis, C.D., Campbell, W.B., and Johnson, A.R. 1986. Inhibition of prostaglandin synthesis by glucocorticoids in human endothelial cells. *Endocrinology* 119: 62–69.

Liao, Y., Cooper, R.S., Mensah, G.A., and McGee, D.L. 1995. Left ventricular hypertrophy has a greater impact on survival in women than in men. *Circulation* 92: 805–810.

Lieberman, E.H., Gerhard, M.D., Uehata, A., Walsh, B.W., Selwyn, A.P., Ganz, P., Yeung, A.C., and Creager, M.A. 1994. Estrogen improves endothelium-dependent, flow-mediated vasodilation in postmenopausal women. *Annals of Internal Medicine* 121: 936–941.

Lindner, V., Kim, S.K., Karas, R.H., Kuiper, G.G.J.M., Gustafsson, J.-A., and Mendelsohn, M.E. 1998. Increased expression of estrogen receptor-β mRNA in male blood vessels after vascular injury. *Circulation Research* 83: 224–229.

Lindpainter, K., Jin, M.W., Niedermaier, N., Wilhelm, M.J., and Ganten, D. 1990. Cardiac angiotensinogen and its local activation in the isolated perfused beating heart. *Circulation Research* 67: 564–573.

Liu, B., Hu, D., Wang, J., and Liu, X.-L. 1997. Effects of 17β-estradiol on early afterdepolarizations and L-type Ca²⁺ currents induced by endothelin-1 in guinea pig papillary muscles and ventricular myocytes. *Methods and Findings in Experimental and Clinical Pharmacology* 19: 19–25.

469

Lou, H., Ramwell, P.W., and Foegh, M.L. 1998a. Estradiol 17-β represses insulin-like growth factor I receptor expression in smooth muscle cells from rabbit cardiac recipients. *Transplantation* 66: 419–426.

Lou, H., Martin, M.B., Stoica, A., Ramwell, P.W., and Foegh, M.L. 1998b. Upregulation of estrogen receptor-α expression in rabbit cardiac allograft. *Circulation Research* 83: 947–951.

McGill, H.C. and Sheridan, P.J. 1981. Nuclear uptake of sex steroid hormones in the cardiovascular system of the baboon. *Circulation Research* 48: 238–244.

McGill, H.C., Anselmo, V.C., Buchanan, J.M., and Sheridan, P.J. 1980. The heart is a target organ for androgen. *Science* 207: 775–777.

Maddox, Y.T., Falcon, J.G., Ridinger, M., Cunard, C.M., and Ramwell, P.W. 1987. Endothelium-dependent gender differences in the response of the rat aorta. *The Journal of Pharmacology and Experimental Therapeutics* 240: 392–395.

Malhotra A., Buttrick, P., and Scheuer, J. 1990. Effects of sex hormones on development of physiological and pathological cardiac hypertrophy in male and female rats. *American Journal of Physiology* 259: H866–H871.

Markell, M.S. and Friedman, E.A. 1989. Hyperlipidemia after organ transplantation. *American Journal of Medicine* 87: 61N–67N.

Marsh, J.D., Lehmann, M.H., Ritchie, R.H., Gwathmey, J.K., Green, G.E., and Schiebinger, R.J. 1998. Androgen receptors mediate hypertrophy in cardiac myocytes. *Circulation* 98: 256–261.

Melchert, R.B. and Welder, A.A. 1995. Cardiovascular effects of androgenic-anabolic steroids. *Medicine and Science in Sports and Exercise* 27: 1252–1262.

Melchert, R.B., Herron, T.J., and Welder, A.A. 1992. The effect of anabolic-androgenic steroids on primary myocardial cell cultures. *Medicine and Science in Sports and Exercise* 24: 206–212.

Meyer, C., Christ, M., and Wehling, M. 1995. Characterization and solubilization of novel aldosterone-binding proteins in porcine liver microsomes. *European Journal of Biochemistry* 229: 736–740.

Meyer, R., Linz, K.W., Surges, R., Meinardus, S., Vees, J., Hoffmann, A., Windholz, O., and Grohe, C. 1998. Rapid modulation of L-type calcium current by acutely applied oestrogens in isolated cardiac myocytes from human, guinea-pig and rat. *Experimental Physiology* 83: 305–321.

Migliaccio, A., Di Domenico, M., Castoria, G., de Falco, A., Bontempo, P., Nola, E., and Auricchio, F. 1996. Tyrosine kinase/p21ras/MAP-kinase pathway activation by estradiol-receptor complex in MCF-7 cells. *EMBO Journal* 15: 1292–1300.

Miller, V.M. and Vanhoutte, P.M. 1991. Progesterone and modulation of endothelium-dependent responses in canine coronary arteries. *American Journal of Physiology* 261: R1022–R1027.

Moore, L.G., McMurtry, I.F., and Reeves, J.T. 1978. Effects of sex hormones on cardiovascular and hematologic responses to chronic hypoxia in rats. *Proceedings of the Society for Experimental Biology and Medicine* 158: 658–662.

Myles, K. and Funder, J.W. 1994. Type I (mineralocorticoid) receptors in the guinea pig. *American Journal of Physiology* 267: E268–E272.

Myles, K. and Funder, J.W. 1996. Progesterone binding to mineralocorticoid receptors: in vitro and in vivo. *American Journal of Physiology* 270: E601–E607.

Nabulsi, A.A., Folsom, A.R., White, A., Patsch, W., Heiss, G., Wu, K.K., Szklo, M., and the Atherosclerosis Risk in Communities Study Investigators. 1993. Association of

470

hormone-replacement therapy with various cardiovascular risk factors in postmenopausal women. *New England Journal of Medicine* 328: 1069–1075.

Narducci, W.A., Wagner, J.C., Hendrickson, T.P., and Jeffrey, T.P. 1990. Anabolic steroids – A review of the clinical toxicology and diagnostic screening. *Clinical Toxicology* 28: 287–310.

Node, K., Kitakaze, M., Kosaka, H., Minamino, T., Sato, H., Kuzuya, T., and Hori, M. 1997a. Roles of NO and $Ca^{2+}$-activated $K^+$ channels in coronary vasodilation induced by 17β-estradiol in ischemic heart failure. *FASEB Journal* 11: 793–799.

Node, K., Kitakaze, M., Kosaka, H., Minamino, T., Funaya, H., and Hori, M. 1997b. Amelioration of ischemia- and reperfusion-induced myocardial injury by 17β-estradiol. Role of nitric oxide and calcium-activated potassium channels. *Circulation* 96: 1953–1963.

O'Malley, B.W. 1991. Steroid hormone receptors as transactivators of gene expression. *Breast Cancer Research and Treatment* 18: 67–71.

Page, I.H. and McCubbin, J.W. 1954. Cardiovascular reactivity. *Circulation Research* 2: 395–408.

Pappas, T.C., Gametchu, B., and Watson, C.S. 1995. Membrane estrogen receptors identified by multiple antibody labeling and impeded-ligand binding. *FASEB Journal* 9: 404–410.

Pearce, P. and Funder, J.W. 1987. High affinity aldosterone binding sites (type I receptors) in rat heart. *Clinical and Experimental Pharmacology and Physiology* 14: 859–866.

Perrot-Applanat, M., Groyer-Picard, M.T., Garcia, E., Lorenzo, F., and Milgrom, E. 1988. Immunocytochemical demonstration of estrogen and progesterone receptors in muscle cells of uterine arteries in rabbits and humans. *Endocrinology* 123: 1511–1519.

Perrot-Applanat, M., Cohen-Solal, K., Milgrom, E., and Finet, M. 1995. Progesterone receptor expression in human saphenous veins. *Circulation* 92: 2975–2983.

Rahwan, R.G. 1988. The pharmacology of androgens and anabolic steroids. *American Journal of Pharmaceutical Education* 52: 167–177.

Ramo, P. 1987. Anabolic steroids alter the haemodynamic responses of the canine left ventricle. *Acta Physiologica Scandinavica* 130: 209–217.

Register, T.C. and Adams, M.R. 1998. Coronary artery and cultured aortic smooth muscle cells express mRNA for both the classical estrogen receptor and the newly described estrogen receptor beta. *Journal of Steroid Biochemistry and Molecular Biology* 64: 187–191.

Robert, V., Van Thiem, N., Cheav, S.L., Mouas, C., Swynghedauw, B., and Delcayre, C. 1994. Increased cardiac types I and III collagen mRNAs in aldosterone-salt hypertension. *Hypertension* 24: 30–36.

Robert, V., Silvestre, J.-S., Charlemagne, D., Sabri, A., Trouve, P., Wassef, M., Swynghedauw, B., and Delcayre, C. 1995. Biological determinants of aldosterone-induced cardiac fibrosis in rats. *Hypertension* 26: 971–978.

Rockhold, R.W. 1993. Cardiovascular toxicity of anabolic steroids. *Annual Reviews of Pharmacology and Toxicology* 33: 497–520.

Rosano, G.M.C., Sarrel, P.M., Poole-Wilson, P.A., and Collins, P. 1993. Beneficial effect of oestrogen on exercise-induced myocardial ischemia in women with coronary artery disease. *Lancet* 342: 133–136.

Rosenkranz-Weiss, P., Tomek, R.J., Mathew, J., and Eghbali, M. 1994. Gender-specific differences in expression of mRNAs for functional and structural proteins in rat ventricular myocardium. *Journal of Molecular and Cellular Cardiology* 26: 261–270.

Ross, E.J. and Linch, D.C. 1982. Cushing's syndrome – killing disease. Discriminatory value of signs and symptoms aiding early diagnosis. *Lancet* 2: 646–649.

Sachtleben, T.R., Berg, K.E., Elias, B.A., Cheatham, J.P., Felix, G.L., and Hofschire, P.J. 1993. The effects of anabolic steroids on myocardial structure and cardiovascular fitness. *Medicine and Science in Sports and Exercise* 25: 1240–1245.

Samsioe, G. 1998. Cardiovascular disease in postmenopausal women. *Maturitas* 30: 11–18.

Sanchez, A., Gomez, M.J., Dorantes, A.L., Rosales, J.L., Pastelin, G., Diaz, V., Posadas, F., and Escalante, B. 1996. The effect of ovariectomy on depressed contractions to phenylephrine and KCl and increased relaxation to acetylcholine in isolated aortic rings of female compared to male rabbits. *British Journal of Pharmacology* 118: 2017–2022.

Santell, R.C., Chang, Y.C., Nair, M.G., and Helferich, W.G. 1997. Dietary genistein exerts estrogenic effects upon the uterus, mammary gland and the hypothalamic/pituitary axis in rats. *Journal of Nutrition* 127: 263–269.

Sato, A. and Funder, J.W. 1996. High glucose stimulates aldosterone-induced hypertrophy via Type I mineralocorticoid receptors in neonatal rat cardiomyocytes. *Endocrinology* 137: 4145–4153.

Sato, A., Suzuki, H., Murakami, M., Nakazato, Y., Iwaita, Y., and Saruta, T. 1994a. Glucocorticoid increases angiotensin II type 1 receptor and its gene expression. *Hypertension* 23: 25–30.

Sato, A., Suzuki, H., Nakazato, Y., Shibata, H., Inagami, T., and Saruta, T. 1994b. Increased expression of vascular angiotensin II type 1A receptor gene in glucocorticoid-induced hypertension. *Journal of Hypertension* 12: 511–516.

Saunders, P.T.K., Maguire, S.M., Gaughan, J., and Millar, M.R. 1997. Expression of oestrogen receptor beta (ERβ) in multiple rat tissues visualised by immuno-histochemistry. *Journal of Endocrinology* 154: R13–R16.

Schaible, T.F., Malhotra A., Ciambrone, G., and Scheuer, J. 1984. The effects of gonadectomy on left ventricular function and cardiac contractile proteins in male and female rats. *Circulation Research* 54: 38–49.

Scheuer, J., Malhotra, A., Schaible, T.F., and Capasso, J. 1987. Effects of gonadectomy and hormonal replacement on rat hearts. *Circulation Research* 61: 12–19.

Schimmer, B.P. and Parker, K.L. 1995. Adrenocorticotropic hormone; adrenocorticol steroids and their synthetic analogs; synthesis and actions of adrenocortical hormones. In *Goodman & Gilman's The Pharmacological Basis of Therapeutics*, 9th edn. Hardman, J.G., Limbird, L.E., Molinoff, P.B., Ruddon, R.W., and Gilman, A.G. (eds), pp. 1459–1485. McGraw-Hill, New York, NY.

Schneider, M., Ulsenheimer, A., Christ, M., and Wehling, M. 1997. Nongenomic effects of aldosterone on intracellular calcium in porcine endothelial cells. *American Journal of Physiology* 272: E616–E620.

Selzman, C.H., Whitehill, T.A., Shames, B.D., Pulido, E.J., Cain, B.C., and Harken, A.H. 1998. The biology of estrogen-mediated repair of cardiovascular injury. *Annals of Thoracic Surgery* 65: 868–874.

Sheehan, D.M. 1998. Herbal medicines, phytoestrogens and toxicity: risk:benefit considerations. *Proceedings of the Society for Experimental Biology and Medicine* 217: 379–385.

Sidney, S., Siscovick, D.S., Petitti, D.B., Schwartz, S.M., Quesenberry, C.P., Psaty, B.M., Raghunathan, T.E., Kelaghan, J., and Koepsell, T.D. 1998. Myocardial infarction and use of low-dose oral contraceptives. A pooled analysis of 2 US studies. *Circulation* 98: 1058–1063.

Silvestre, J.-S., Robert, V., Heymes, C., Aupetit-Faisant, B., Mouas, C., Moalic, J.-M., Swynghedauw, B., and Delcayre, C. 1998. Myocardial production of aldosterone and corticosterone in the rat. *The Journal of Biological Chemistry* 273: 4883–4891.

de Simone, G., Devereux, R.B., Daniels, S.R., and Meyer, R.A. 1995. Gender differences in left ventricular growth. *Hypertension* 26: 979–983.

Song, J., Wan, Y., Rolfe, B.E., Campbell, J.H., and Campbell, G.R. 1998. Effect of estrogen on vascular smooth muscle cells is dependent upon cellular phenotype. *Atherosclerosis* 140: 97–104.

Sorensen, K.E., Dorup, I., Hermann, A.P., and Mosekilde, L. 1998. Combined hormone replacement therapy does not protect women against the age-related decline in endothelium-dependent vasomotor function. *Circulation* 97: 1234–1238.

Stallone, J.N. 1993. Role of endothelium in sexual dimorphism in vasopressin-induced contraction of rat aorta. *American Journal of Physiology* 265: H2073–H2080.

Steinberg, D. and Witztum J.L. 1990. Lipoproteins and atherogenesis. Current concepts. *Journal of the American Medical Association* 264: 3047–3052.

Steinsapir, J. and Muldoon, T.G. 1991. Role of microsomal receptors in steroid hormone action. *Steroids* 56: 66–71.

Stumpf, W.E., Sar, M., and Aumuller, G. 1977. The heart: a target organ for estradiol. *Science* 196: 319–321.

Sullivan, M.L., Martinez, C.M., Gennis, P., and Gallagher, E.J. 1998. The cardiac toxicity of anabolic steroids. *Progress in Cardiovascular Diseases* 41: 1–15.

Takala, T.E.S., Ramo, P., Kiviluoma, K., Vihko, V., Kainulainen, H., and Kettunen, R. 1991. Effects of training and anabolic steroids on collagen synthesis in dog heart. *European Journal of Applied Physiology* 62: 1–6.

Tang, M. and Subbiah, M.T. 1996. Estrogens protect against hydrogen peroxide and arachidonic acid induced DNA damage. *Biochimica et Biophysica Acta* 1299: 155–159.

Thompson, P.D., Cullinane, E.M., Sady, S.P., Chenevert, C., Saritelli, A.L., Sady, M.A., and Herbert, P.N. 1989. Contrasting effects of testosterone and stanozolol on serum lipoprotein levels. *Journal of the American Medical Association* 261: 1165–1168.

Thompson, P.D., Sadaniantz, A., Cullinane, E.M., Bodziony, K.S., Catlin, D.H., Torek-Both, G., and Douglas, P.S. 1992. Left ventricular function is not impaired in weight-lifters who use anabolic steroids. *Journal of the American College of Cardiology* 19: 278–282.

Tseng, Y.T., Rockhold, R.W., Hoskins, B., and Ho, I.K. 1994. Cardiovascular toxicities of nandrolone and cocaine in spontaneously hypertensive rats. *Fundamental and Applied Toxicology* 22: 113–121.

Urhausen, A., Holpes, R., and Kindermann, W. 1989. One- and two-dimensional echocardiography in bodybuilders using anabolic steroids. *European Journal of Applied Physiology* 58: 633–640.

Vargas, R., Wroblewska, B., Rego, A., Hatch, J., and Ramwell, P.W. 1993. Oestradiol inhibits smooth muscle cell proliferation of pig coronary artery. *British Journal of Pharmacology* 109: 612–617.

Vargas, R., Hewes, B., Rego, A., Farhat, M.Y., Suarez, R., and Ramwell, P.W. 1996. Estradiol effect on rate of proliferation of rat carotid segments: effect of gender and tamoxifen. *Journal of Cardiovascular Pharmacology* 27: 495–499.

Vathsala, A., Weinberg, R.B., Schoenberg, L., Grevel, J., Goldstein, R.A., Van Buren, C.T., Lewis, R.M., and Kahan, B.D. 1989. Lipid abnormalities in cyclosporine-prednisone-treated renal transplant recipients. *Transplantation* 48: 37–43.

473

Veldscholte, J., Berrevoets, C.A., Zegers, N.D., van der Kwast, T.H., Grootegoed, J.A., and Mulder, E. 1992. Hormone-induced dissociation of the androgen receptor-heat-shock protein complex: use of a new monoclonal antibody to distinguish transformed from nontransformed receptors. *Biochemistry* 31: 7422–7430.

Venkov, C.D., Rankin, A.B., and Vaughan, D.E. 1996. Identification of authentic estrogen receptor in cultured endothelial cells: a potential mechanism for steroid hormone regulation of endothelial function. *Circulation* 94: 727–733.

Wahli, W. and Martinez, E. 1991. Superfamily of steroid nuclear receptors: positive and negative regulators of gene expression. *FASEB Journal* 5: 2243–2249.

Wang, S.-N., Wyeth, R.P., and Kennedy, R.H. 1998. Effects of gender on the sensitivity of rat cardiac muscle to extracellular calcium. *European Journal of Pharmacology* 361: 73–77.

Wehling, M. 1995. Looking beyond the dogma of genomic steroid action: insights and facts of the 1990s. *Journal of Molecular Medicine* 73: 439–447.

Wehling, M., Christ, M., and Theisen, K. 1992. Membrane receptors for aldosterone: a novel pathway for mineralocorticoid action. *American Journal of Physiology* 263: E974–E979.

Wehling, M., Neylon, C.B., Fullerton, M., Bobik, A., and Funder, J.W. 1995. Nongenomic effects of aldosterone on intracellular $Ca^{2+}$ in vascular smooth muscle cells. *Circulation Research* 76: 973–979.

Wehling, M., Spes, C.H., Win, N., Janson, C.P., Schmidt, B.M., Theisen, K., and Christ, M. 1998. Rapid cardiovascular action of aldosterone in man. *Journal of Clinical Endocrinology and Metabolism* 83: 3517–3522.

Weicker, H., Hagele, H., Repp, B., and Kolb, J. 1982. Influence of training and anabolic steroids on the LDH isozyme pattern of skeletal and heart muscle fibers of guinea pigs. *International Journal of Sports Medicine* 3: 90–96.

Weiner, C.P., Lizasoain, I., Baylis, S.A., Knowles, R.G., Charles, I.G., and Moncada, S. 1994. Induction of calcium-dependent nitric oxide synthase by sex hormones. *Proceedings of the National Academy of Sciences of the United States of America* 91: 5212–5216.

Welder, A.A., Robertson, J.W., Fugate, R.D., and Melchert, R.B. 1995. Anabolic-androgenic steroid-induced toxicity in primary neonatal rat myocardial cell cultures. *Toxicology and Applied Pharmacology* 133: 328–342.

White, C.R., Darley-Usmar, V., and Oparil, S. 1997. Gender and cardiovascular disease. Recent insights. *Trends in Cardiovascular Medicine* 7: 94–100.

Whitworth, J.A. and Scoggins, B.A. 1990. A "hypertensinogenic" class of steroid hormone activity in man? *Clinical and Experimental Pharmacology and Physiology* 17: 163–166.

Wild, R.A., Grubb, B., Hartz, A., Van Nort, J.J., Bachman, W., and Bartholomew, M. 1990. Clinical signs of androgen excess as risk factors for coronary artery disease. *Fertility and Sterility* 54: 255–259.

Williams, C.L. and Stancel, G.M. 1995. Estrogens and progestins. In *Goodman & Gilman's The Pharmacological Basis of Therapeutics*, 9th edn. Hardman, J.G., Limbird, L.E., Molinoff, P.B., Ruddon, R.W. and Gilman, A.G. (eds), pp. 1411–1440. McGraw-Hill, New York, NY.

Wilson, C.M. and McPhaul, M.J. 1996. A and B forms of the androgen receptor are expressed in a variety of human tissues. *Molecular and Cellular Endocrinology* 120: 51–57.

Yesalis, C.E., Barsukiewicz, C.K., Kopstein, A.N., and Bahrke, M.S. 1997. Trends in anabolic-androgenic steroid use among adolescents. *Archives of Pediatric and Adolescent Medicine* 151: 1197–1206.

Young, M., Fullerton, M., Dilley, R., and Funder, J. 1994. Mineralocorticoids, hypertension, and cardiac fibrosis. *The Journal of Clinical Investigation* 93: 2578–2583.

Yue, P., Kanu, C., Beale, C., Poole-Wilson, P.A., and Collins, P. 1995. Testosterone relaxes rabbit coronary arteries and aorta. *Circulation* 91: 1154–1160.

Zhang, F., Ram, J.L., Standley, P.R., and Sowers, J.R. 1994. 17 β-Estradiol attenuates voltage-dependent $Ca^{2+}$ currents in A7r5 vascular smooth muscle cell line. *American Journal of Physiology* 266: C975–C980.

Zimmerman, J., Fainaru, M., and Eisenberg, S. 1984. The effects of prednisone therapy on plasma lipoprotein and apolipoproteins: a prospective study. *Metabolism: Clinical and Experimental* 33: 521–526.

Zmuda, J.M., Fahrenbach, M.C., Younkin, B.T., Bausserman, L.L., Terry, R.B., Catlin, D.H., and Thompson, P.D. 1993. The effect of testosterone aromatization on high-density lipoprotein cholesterol level and postheparin lipolytic activity. *Metabolism* 42: 446–450.

# Part V

# VASCULAR TOXICITY

# 15

# VASCULAR TOXICOLOGY

## A CELLULAR AND MOLECULAR PERSPECTIVE

*Kenneth S. Ramos, J. Kevin Kerzee,*
*Napoleon F. Alejandro, and Kim P. Lu*

*Department of Physiology and Pharmacology, College of*
*Veterinary Medicine, Texas A & M University,*
*College Station, TX, USA*

## Introduction

Epidemiologic and experimental evidence suggests that a direct correlation exists between occupational and environmental exposure to toxic chemicals and cardiovascular morbidity and mortality. This correlation is best exemplified by the recognition that exposure to tobacco smoke constituents is a major contributor to myocardial infarction, sudden cardiac death, arteriosclerotic peripheral vascular disease, and atherosclerotic aneurysm of the aorta. Although progress has been made in the elucidation of mechanisms of vascular toxicity, the slow onset and long latency periods often associated with vasculotoxic insult continue to pose challenges. Evidence continues to accumulate implicating lipoproteins and chemically derived free radicals in the modulation of vascular cell growth and differentiation. Vascular toxins affect any of the vessels that serve as the circuitry for the transport and delivery of oxygen and nutrients to tissues throughout the body and for the removal of waste products of metabolism.

## Structural and functional characteristics of the blood vessel wall

In view of the heterogeneous characteristics of the vascular tree, knowledge of blood vessel structure and function is essential to the elucidation of molecular mechanisms of chemical toxicity. Blood vessels are often classified as elastic or muscular vessels based on their relative composition and abundance of extracellular matrix proteins. In primates, arteries vary in size from 300 μm internal diameter for large elastic vessels, such as the aorta and the carotid, to 30 μm for peripheral vessels, such as muscular arterioles. Veins are similar to their arterial counterparts, but often are thinner and are of larger diameter than arteries. Arterioles, capillaries, post-capillary venules, and venules constitute the microcirculation. In contrast to large blood vessels, which are distinct anatomical entities, microvessels are considered a part of the tissue in which they reside.

Mammalian blood vessels of large and medium-sized diameter are organized into three morphologically distinct layers (for a comprehensive review, see Rhodin, 1980). The innermost layer, referred to as the tunica intima, consists of a single layer of endothelial cells which rests on a loose layer of connective tissue formed by a thin basal lamina and a subendothelial layer. Luminal endothelial cells are flat and elongated with their long axis parallel to the blood flow. These cells act as a semipermeable barrier between the blood and underlying components of the vessel wall. The subendothelial layer is formed by connective tissue bundles and elastic fibrils in which a few cells of smooth muscle origin may occasionally be oriented parallel to the long axis of the vessel. The subendothelial layer is only seen in large elastic arteries such as the human aorta. The medial layer, or tunica media, is composed of elastin and collagen interwoven between multiple layers of smooth muscle cells. The media is separated from the outermost layer, the tunica adventitia, by a poorly defined external lamina. In the majority of vascular beds, smooth muscle cells dominate the media, but may also be present in the intima of some arteries and veins, as well as the adventitia of veins. The adventitial layer consists of a loose layer of fibroblasts, collagen, elastin, and glycosamino-glycans.

With the exception of capillaries, the walls of smaller vessels also have three distinct layers which share many of the features described for larger vessels. However, in vessels of smaller diameter, the media is less elastic and consists of one to three layers of smooth muscle cells. An interesting feature of these vessels is the presence of myoendothelial junctions. Although the exact role of these structures is unknown, they may serve to enhance the stability of the vessel wall and to facilitate molecular transport and intercellular communication. A recent review suggests that myoendothelial junctions are selective and communicate mainly in one direction, from endothelial cells to smooth muscle cells, to regulate cell–cell communication via secondary messengers (Little *et al.*, 1995). As described for muscular arteries, venules are structurally similar to their arteriole counterparts. Because muscular venules are larger than arterioles, a large fraction of blood is contained in these capacitance vessels. Capillaries are endothelial tubes measuring 4–8 μm in diameter which rest on a thin basal lamina to which pericytes are often attached. When one capillary converges with another, the vessel formed is referred to as a post-capillary venule. The capillary and the pericytic venule are the principal sites of exchange between the blood and tissues.

It has become increasingly apparent that the responses of smooth muscle cells are influenced by their relative location along the vascular tree. These distinctions are illustrated by phenotypic differences in growth characteristics and matrix-producing capabilities (Frid *et al.*, 1997).

## Vascular cell biology

In humans, the development of the blood circulation (i.e. vasculogenesis) begins at 4 weeks of gestation, when simple diffusion of nutrients is no longer sufficient to support growth (Hudlicka, 1980). Developing vessels are formed by cells of mesenchymal origin which become angioblasts, and in turn differentiate into blood cells or endothelial cells. Endothelial cells form capillaries which give rise to larger vessels by the apposition of pericytes and/or fibroblasts that ultimately differentiate into vascular smooth muscle cells. For many years, vascular endothelial cells were considered passive participants in the transport of blood. It is now recognized that endothelial cells play integral roles in the regulation of hemostasis, vascular tone, and angiogenesis. Endothelial cells are also involved in the regulation of macromolecular transport across the vessel wall, attachment and recruitment of inflammatory cells, synthesis of connective tissue proteins, and generation of reactive oxygen species (Jaffe, 1985; King and Johnson, 1985; Friedl et al., 1989). Endothelial cells release von Willebrand factor by 48 h after a single dose of γ-radiation, leading to enhanced platelet adhesion to the endothelial extracellular matrix. This event is important in radiation-induced vascular damage because binding of von Willebrand factor to platelet surface receptor GPIb initiates formation of the thrombotic plug, which ultimately results in vascular occlusion and microthrombus formation (Verheij et al., 1994). Endothelial cells can also be a target of *Rickettsia rickettsii* infection. During infection, coagulation pathway initiator tissue factor mRNA is increased transcriptionally, possibly through activation of the transcription factor NF-κB (Shi et al., 1998). Activated platelets adherent to subendothelial connective tissue release platelet-derived growth factor-BB (PDGF-BB). PDGF-BB is a major chemotactic factor of vascular smooth muscle cells (vSMCs). Inhibition of PDGF-BB and PDGF receptor-β by antisense oligonucleotides suppresses neointimal formation (Sirois et al., 1997).

Under normal conditions, medial smooth muscle cells are found primarily in a quiescent state of growth specialized for muscle contraction (Campbell and Campbell, 1985; Gordon and Schwartz, 1987). Smooth muscle cell responses to contractile agonists are mediated by receptors located on the plasma membrane. Activation of these receptors by endogenous transmitters, hormones, or xenobiotics is associated with changes in ionic conductance that ultimately activate the contractile apparatus. Membrane channels, sarcolemmal pumps, energy-dependent sequestration of calcium by intracellular organelles, and a number of calcium-binding proteins participate in the maintenance of ionic transport. In addition to their central role in the regulation of vasomotor tone, smooth muscle cells participate in the synthesis of extracellular matrix proteins during arterial repair, the metabolism and/or secretion of bioactive substances, the regulation of monocyte function, and the generation of reactive oxygen species (Campbell and Campbell, 1985; Gordon and Schwartz, 1987). Fibroblasts within the adventitial layer secrete some of the collagen and glycosaminoglycans needed to lend structural support to the vessel wall (Sappino et al., 1990). By using direct gene transfer techniques, it has been shown that fibroblast growth factor (FGF) induces intimal hyperplasia in the arterial wall as well as new capillary formation from adjacent luminal endothelial cells (Nabel *et al.*, 1993).

Under the influence of various stimuli, smooth muscle cells lose their ability to contract and shift toward a phenotypic state characterized by enhanced synthetic and proliferative activity. Cells in the synthetic state are distinguished from contractile counterparts by their ability to migrate, proliferate, and secrete extracellular matrix components. Phenotypic modulation of smooth muscle cells occurs during various physiologic processes, such as fetal and post-natal development, regeneration and repair of blood vessels, and myometrial development during pregnancy (Campbell and Chamley-Campbell, 1981). Modulation of smooth muscle cell phenotype from a contractile to a synthetic state is also observed during atherogenesis. In its early stages, atherosclerosis is characterized by focal intimal thickenings of smooth muscle cells that migrate to the intima and proliferate in an uncontrolled fashion (McGill, 1988). Macrophages, extracellular matrix components, and intra- and extracellular lipids accumulate as the lesion advances. The proliferation of smooth muscle cells and accumulation of extracellular matrix components within the lesion contribute to occlusion of the vessel lumen.

PDGF plays a central role in the modulation of this vascular smooth muscle cell proliferation, migration, and contraction (Hughes *et al.*, 1996). Transcriptional activation of the growth-related proto-oncogene c-*Ha-ras* via redox mechanisms is associated with proliferation of vSMCs (Gran *et al.*, 1996). The protein product of *ras* is a guanosine triphosphate (GTP)-binding protein, p21[ras]. Neurofibromin, the protein product of the *nf1* gene, which causes neurofibromatosis-1, accelerates the GTPase activity of p21[ras] in proliferating vSMCs (Ahlgren-Beckendorf *et al.*, 1993). High levels of glucose may also regulate some expression in aortic smooth muscle cells (Delmolino and Castellot, 1997). Proliferation of vSMCs can be inhibited by heparin following binding to cell-surface receptors. Among the genes involved in this early response is the early response gene *sgk* (serum and glucocorticoid-regulated kinase) (Nishio *et al.*, 1994). Recently, nitric oxide has been shown to inhibit proliferation and migration of vSMCs during atherosclerotic lesion development. This effect involves activation of guanylate cyclase and cyclic GMP-dependent protein kinase (Sarkar *et al.*, 1996; Boerth *et al.*, 1997). In addition, vascular smooth muscle cell mitogenesis can also be inhibited by estrogen and progesterone, in agreement with the suggestion that these hormones afford protective effects in the development of cardiovascular disease (Morey *et al.*, 1997). The genetic basis for transition of vSMCs to proliferative phenotypes may involve activation of mobile genetic elements, retrotransposons, as described recently by this laboratory (Lu and Ramos, 1998).

A popular theory of atherosclerosis, as proposed originally by Russell Ross (Ross and Glomset, 1976) and later modified (Ross, 1986, 1993), states that atherosclerotic lesions develop as a result of chronic cycles of vascular injury and repair. Consistent with this hypothesis, mechanical or toxic injury to the endothelium has been associated with initiation of the atherogenic response (Peng *et al.*, 1985; Miano *et al.*, 1990; Nishida *et al.*, 1990). As part of the repair process, smooth muscle cell mitogens and chemotactic agents are released from one or more of the cell types involved in the disease process, including endothelial cells, smooth muscle cells, macrophages, and fibroblasts. An alternate hypothesis is the monoclonal theory of atherogenesis as proposed by Benditt (1974) and recently updated by Murry *et al.* (1997). Based on the monotypism of glucose-6-phosphate dehydrogenase, these investigators proposed that smooth muscle cells within the atherosclerotic plaque are the progeny of a single smooth muscle cell. As such, the atherosclerotic process would resemble benign neoplastic growth of smooth muscle tumors (leiomyomas). Upon exposure to a toxic or viral agent, smooth muscle cells may exist in a genetically altered state which gives rise to lesions upon exposure to chemotactic/growth-promoting factors. Alternatively, mutations could induce constitutive production of growth factors within smooth muscle cells themselves, resulting in autocrine stimulation of growth. DNA isolated from human atherosclerotic plaques is capable of transforming NIH3T3 cells and producing tumors in nude mice (Penn *et al.*, 1986). In recent years, the formation of oxidized low-density lipoprotein (oxLDL) within the intima and the removal of oxLDL by macrophage scavenger receptors have been implicated in the development of atherosclerotic disease (Kroon, 1997). A potent mediator of this oxidation is believed to be the oxidant peroxynitrite ($ONOO^-$), which is the product of the reaction of superoxide ($O_2^-$) and nitric oxide ($NO^-$) (Roger White *et al.*, 1994).

Hypertension is typically characterized by a net increase in peripheral vascular resistance. Such increases in vascular resistance may involve increased levels of circulating vasoconstrictors, such as angiotensin II or catecholamines. However, local regulation by metabolic, myogenic, or angiogenic mechanisms may also be involved in the pressor response (Granger *et al.*, 1988). Increased vascular resistance has been associated with an overall increase in wall thickness and smooth muscle mass (Owens and Schwartz, 1982). These changes appear to be due, at least in part, to hypertrophy of smooth muscle cells. Studies have shown that programmed cell death can be detected in human atherosclerosis and restenosis (Isner *et al.*, 1995) and during vascular wall remodeling in hypertension (Hamet *et al.*, 1996). A sustained elevation in blood pressure has also been associated with destruction of capillaries at the tissue level. In recent years, the recognition that local degradation of the basement membrane in parent vessels leads to new capillary growth, and that such alterations may be related to toxic insult, has served as a stimulus for intense study in the area of angiogenesis. The angiogenic process involves the formation of blood vessels *in situ* secondary to migration, proliferation, and differentiation of vascular cells. Thus, angiogenesis is a critical process in organogenesis and wound repair, as well as during the pathogenesis of cancer and atherosclerosis.

# Principles of vasculotoxic specificity

A wide spectrum of chemicals, including natural products, drugs, and anthropogenic chemicals, have been recognized as potential vascular toxins. Angiotoxicity may be expressed at the mechanical, metabolic, epigenetic, or genetic level. As a general rule, vascular toxicity *in vivo* involves interactions of multiple cellular elements (Table 15.1). Alterations in the expression of cytoskeletal proteins, second messenger molecules, or growth factors from any of these cell types may result in vascular toxicity. Endothelial cells represent the first cellular barrier to the movement of bloodborne toxins from the lumen of the vessel to deeper regions of the wall. This strategic location makes them particularly susceptible to toxic insult, a feature which may be targeted for selective toxicity in angiogenesis-dependent disorders. Toxic chemicals which reach the subendothelial space as a protoxin or as a metabolically active substance produced by endothelial cells may cause injury to medial smooth muscle cells and/or

*Table 15.1* Cell types implicated in the vasculotoxic response

| Cell type | Function |
|---|---|
| Endothelial cells | First barrier to bloodborne toxins; synthesis and release of endothelium-derived relaxing factor; synthesis of pro- and antiaggregatory factors; attachment and recruitment of inflammatory cells; synthesis of connective tissue proteins; generation of oxygen-derived free radicals and other radical moieties |
| Smooth muscle cells | Maintenance of vasomotor tone; synthesis of extracellular matrix proteins including collagen and elastin; synthesis of prostaglandins and other biologically active lipids; regulation of monocyte function; formation of free radicals |
| Fibroblasts | Synthesis of extracellular matrix proteins including collagens, structural support to the vessel wall |
| Monocytes/ macrophages | Scavenger potential; synthesis of macrophage-derived growth factor; generation of reactive oxygen species; lymphocyte activation, progenitor of foam cells |
| Platelets | Synthesis of proaggregatory substances and smooth muscle mitogens such as platelet-derived growth factor |
| Lymphocytes | Release of activated oxygen species; cellular immunity; production of immunoglobulins |

adventitial fibroblasts. Adventitial and medial cells within large elastic arteries, such as the human aorta, may also be reached via the vasa vasorum, the intrinsic blood supply to the vessel wall. These toxic exposures may result in covalent interactions with cellular macromolecules, such as protein and DNA. In addition, the vasculotoxic response may be dependent upon the influence of (1) extracellular matrix proteins which actively interact with vascular cells to modulate biologic behavior, (2) coagulation factors which dictate the extent of hemostatic involvement, (3) hormones and growth factors which regulate proliferative/ differentiation programs, and (4) plasma lipoproteins, some of which modulate cellular metabolism. Acute vascular injury may be associated with local inflammatory reactions that sometimes compromise end-organ function. Chronic vasculotoxic insult involves repeated cycles of injury and repair which often lead to irreversible changes of blood vessel structure and function. Such alterations may promote the pathologic progression of disorders such as atherosclerosis, hypertension, peripheral vascular disease, and vascular aneurysm.

The most prevalent cellular mechanisms of vascular toxicity are listed in Table 15.2. These mechanisms include (1) selective alterations of vascular reactivity, (2) vessel-specific bioactivation of protoxicants, (3) erratic chemical detoxification, and (4) preferential accumulation of the active toxin within vascular cells. As illustrated in Figure 15.1, multiple mechanisms may operate simultaneously for a given toxic agent. Vascular reactivity, as it relates to the intrinsic ability of blood vessels to respond to biologically active substances, can be regulated at multiple levels, including changes in signal transduction from the surface to the interior of the cell and/or modulation of contractile protein structure and function. As described for other organ systems, non-toxic chemicals can be converted by vascular enzymes to highly reactive species capable of causing injury to both intra- and extracellular targets. Enzyme systems present in vascular cells which

*Table 15.2* Putative mechanisms of vasculotoxic insult

| Mechanism | Prototype toxins |
|---|---|
| Alterations of vascular reactivity | Metals, catecholamines, carbon monoxide, nicotine, T-2 toxin |
| Vessel-specific bioactivation | Allylamine, polycyclic aromatic hydrocarbons, catecholamine, homocysteine, carbon disulfide |
| Erratic detoxification | Allylamine, dinitrotoluene, hydrazinobenzoic acid, metals |
| Preferential accumulation | Allylamine, polycyclic aromatic hydrocarbons, TCDD |
| Altered signal transduction | Allylamine, vitamin D, oxidized lipoproteins |

Note
TCDD, tetrachlorodibenzo-*p*-dioxin.

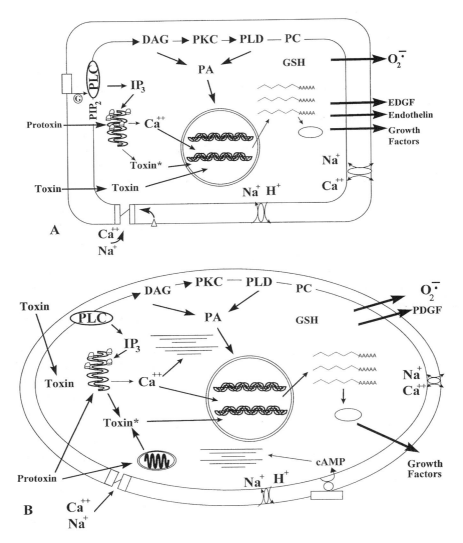

*Figure 15.1* Selected cellular and molecular targets of vasculotoxic insult in endothelial (A) and smooth muscle cells (B). Alterations of vascular reactivity are often mediated by changes in the distribution of ions across the membrane of vascular endothelial and/or smooth muscle cells. Alternatively, toxicant interference with signal transduction mechanisms at the receptor or second messenger level or structural/ functional changes of contractile proteins may also interfere with vascular function. Enzyme systems capable of converting inactive chemicals to reactive forms that cause cell injury have also been identified. Deficient antioxidant capacity in vascular cells has also been suspected as a contributor to enhanced susceptibility to toxic injury. As in other organ systems, accumulation of toxicants within vascular cells has also been implicated in several vascular toxicities. DAG, diacylglycerol; GSH, glutathione; PA, phosphatidic acid; PC, phosphatidylcholine; $PIP_2$, phosphatidylinositol-4,5-biphosphate; PKC, phosphokinase C; PLD, phospholipase D; PLC, phospholipase C; $IP_3$, inositol triphosphate.

have been implicated in the bioactivation of vascular toxins include amine oxidases, cytochrome P450 monooxygenases, and prostaglandin synthetase. These enzymes play important roles in the regulation of vascular function under physiologic conditions. For instance, copper-containing amine oxidases are widespread enzymes which catalyze the oxidative removal of biogenic amines from blood plasma, the cross-linking of collagen and elastin in connective tissue, and the regulation of intracellular spermine and spermidine levels (Janes *et al.*, 1990). The existence of several cytochrome P450 metabolites of arachidonic acid involved in the regulation of vascular tone and sodium pump activity has also been recognized (Escalante *et al.*, 1990). A complex of microsomal enzymes, collectively referred to as prostaglandin synthetase, catalyze the formation of biologically active lipids, including prostacyclin and thromboxane $A_2$. Prostacyclin, the major arachidonic acid metabolite in blood vessels, is a strong vasodilator and endogenous inhibitor of platelet aggregation, whereas thromboxane $A_2$, the major arachidonic acid metabolite in platelets, is a potent vasoconstrictor and promoter of platelet aggregation. Evidence continues to accumulate suggesting that vascular-specific activation of protoxins is a significant contributor to vasculotoxic insult. Cytochrome P450 monooxygenases in both endothelial cells and vSMCs can activate protoxins to toxins, as shown recently for human cells (Zhao *et al.*, 1998). However, the bioactivation of vascular toxins need not be confined to vascular tissue. Angiotoxic chemicals may be bioactivated by other metabolically active organs such as liver and lung. In such instances, migration of activated species from the site of activation to the blood vessel is likely involved. Lipophilic metabolites may be transported and delivered to the vessel wall by association with plasma lipoproteins (Ferrario *et al.*, 1985). Vascular toxicity may also be due to deficiencies in the capacity of target cells to detoxify the active toxin. Key components of the endogenous antioxidant defense system operative in vascular cells include the glutathione/glutathione reductase/glutathione peroxidase system, superoxide dismutase, and catalase. At low oxidant levels, glutathione is believed to be critical for cellular redox balance, whereas catalase is a major detoxifying enzyme at higher oxidant levels. Our laboratory has shown that alterations in cellular redox status in vSMCs is associated with transcriptional deregulation of c-*Ha-ras* (Kerzee and Ramos, 1999). The relevance of this observation lies in the important signaling disturbance that follows *ras* gene activation. Significant differences in the antioxidant capacity of vascular cells relative to other cell types have been documented. For instance, vascular endothelial cells are more sensitive to oxidative stress than fibroblasts (Bishop *et al.*, 1985), whereas vSMCs appear to be fairly resistant to peroxide-induced injury relative to hepatocytes (Ramos and Thurlow, 1993). Limited information is presently available regarding the cellular bases for the differential response of vascular and non-vascular cells, but the response is species-specific since rat cells are clearly more resistant to peroxide injury than murine counterparts. The contractile properties of vSMCs and the role of reactive oxygen species in intracellular signaling may account for the differential response to cellular oxidants. Finally, vascular toxicity may be due to selective accumulation of chemicals within the vascular wall. For example, benzo(a)pyrene, a prototypical polycyclic aromatic hydrocarbon, preferentially accumulates in the endoplasmic reticulum and the mitochondria of target cells (Barhoumi *et al.*, 1999). Although the mechanisms responsible for preferential accumulation of toxins within the vessel wall are not yet known, receptor-mediated internalization of low-density lipoproteins and chemical properties of the toxins in question may be critical in this process.

Ultimately, the consequences of vasculotoxic insult are dictated by the interplay between vascular and non-vascular cells, as well as intracellular signaling molecules and non-cellular factors such as extracellular matrix proteins, coagulation factors, hormones, immune complexes, and plasma lipoproteins. This concept is exemplified by the lymphocytic and platelet involvement in various forms of toxic injury. Furthermore, the toxic response can be modulated by mechanical and hemodynamic factors such as arterial pressure, shear stress, and blood viscosity. An additional consideration is that kinetic and pharmacodynamic differences among different animal species, as well as age and sex, may also alter the toxicologic profile of a given toxicant.

## Selected vascular toxins

### *Allylamine*

Allylamine (3-aminopropene) is an unsaturated aliphatic amine utilized as a precursor in the vulcanization of rubber and the synthesis of pharmaceuticals (Sutton, 1963). In addition, several allylamine compounds have been developed as antifungal agents for human and veterinary use (Ryder, 1988). Allylamine is more toxic than other unsaturated primary amines of higher molecular weight (Beard and Noe, 1981). Exposure to allylamine by a variety of routes in multiple animal species is associated with selective cardiovascular toxicity (Hine *et al.*, 1960; Guzman *et al.*, 1961; Lalich *et al.*, 1972; Boor *et al.*, 1979). The specificity of the toxic response may be related to its ability to accumulate in elastic and muscular arteries upon administration *in vivo* (Boor, 1985). Gross lesions are evident in the myocardium, aorta, and coronary arteries of animals exposed to allylamine. Subacute and chronic administration is associated with the development of atherosclerotic-like lesions characterized by smooth muscle cell proliferation and fibrosis.

Boor and colleagues first proposed that allylamine toxicity results from bioactivation of the parent compound to a toxic aldehyde, acrolein (for a review, see Boor *et al.*, 1990). Vascular-specific bioactivation of allylamine to acrolein and hydrogen peroxide by semicarbazide-sensitive amine oxidase is considered a prerequisite for the manifestation of toxicity (Ramos *et al.*, 1988; Boor *et al.*, 1990). Semicarbazide-sensitive amine oxidase (SSAO) is a copper-containing amine oxidase found in cardiovascular tissue in higher concentrations than in any other tissue (Buffoni, 1983; Lyles, 1996). Inhibition of this enzyme protects vascular cells from allylamine cytotoxicity. SSAO is most abundant in smooth muscle cells, both vascular and non-vascular, as well as adipocytes, chondrocytes, and odontoblasts. As such, allylamine preferentially injures smooth muscle cells relative to other cell types within the vascular wall. The selectivity of allylamine toxicity has been attributed to accumulation and preferential toxification, but other mechanisms including deficient detoxification may also contribute to the specificity of the toxic response. Glutathione-S-transferase 8–8 and γ-glutamylcysteine synthetase activity are up-regulated in vSMCs exposed to allylamine (Misra et al., 1995). The mechanism by which allylamine modulates glutathione levels in multiple organs is not yet clear. Past work has shown that the enzymatic activity responsible for the metabolic conversion of allylamine to acrolein in aortic tissue is localized in the mitochondrial and microsomal fractions (Grossman et al., 1990). These observations are in agreement with studies by others showing that allylamine, or its metabolites, are sequestered in close proximity to endoplasmic reticulum and mitochondria (Hysmith and Boor, 1985).

Acrolein is an extremely reactive aldehyde which disrupts the thiol balance of vascular cells (Ramos and Cox, 1987). Although a large number of compounds react with acrolein under physiologic conditions, the main reaction products result from nucleophilic addition at the terminal ethylenic carbon. As such, toxicity most likely results from the reaction of acrolein with critical cellular sulfhydryls. Hydrogen peroxide and ammonia formed during the deamination process may contribute to allylamine-induced vascular injury. However, acute cytotoxicity studies have shown that vascular cells are relatively resistant to hydrogen peroxide. The absence of overt cytotoxicity does not rule out the possibility that hydrogen peroxide ($H_2O_2$) enhances cellular proliferation, especially at low concentrations, and additional work to define its contribution to the overall cytotoxic injury is warranted (Ramos et al., 1988). Acrolein can also be converted via NADPH-dependent microsomal enzymes to glycidaldehyde and acrylic acid (Patel et al., 1983). Acrolein itself is a ubiquitous toxic chemical found in engine exhaust and cigarette smoke, as well as in cooked foods. Acrolein is formed endogenously upon oxidation of allylamine and as a by-product of lipid peroxidation in biologic systems (Uchida et al., 1998). A limited number of studies have been conducted to examine the direct vascular toxicity of this aldehyde. Within the context of allylamine cytotoxicity, these studies are important as the toxicologic profile of acrolein may not replicate that of the parent compound. Exogenous acrolein results in extensive injury to the plasmalemma before critical subcellular targets are compromised. In contrast, intracellular formation of acrolein allows simultaneous interaction of the aldehyde with multiple subcellular targets. In particular, acrolein can interfere with oxidative phosphorylation processes in the myocardium, resulting in loss of cellular ATP (Ghilarducci and Tjeerdema, 1995). Using Dahl hypertension-resistant and -sensitive rat strains, Kutzman et al. (1984) demonstrated that exposure to acrolein for 62 days is more toxic to hypertension-sensitive animals than hypertension-resistant counterparts. Since differences between these strains are not usually manifested in the absence of hypertensive stimuli, the mechanisms responsible for increased susceptibility to acrolein toxicity remain unclear. It is possible that the underlying mechanism is a function of the aldehyde's ability to alter cellular redox status and interfere with cellular signaling. In response to allylamine exposure, vasoconstriction has been related to competitive interactions between endogenous amines for SSAO, resulting in an overall increase in catecholamine production. The indirect sympathomimetic activity of aldehydes including acrolein, acetaldehyde, and formaldehyde may contribute to the enhanced sensitivity of hypertension-prone animals (Beckner *et al.*, 1974).

Because the expression of vasculotoxic insult is often a multifactorial phenomenon characterized by long latency periods, an *in vivo/in vitro* regimen has been used in our laboratory to evaluate the toxicity of allylamine (Cox and Ramos, 1990; Cox *et al.*, 1990). Upon completion of defined dosing regimens *in vivo*, aortic smooth muscle cells are isolated and established in primary or secondary culture. This culture system has been used to evaluate the impact of repeated cycles of injury and repair *in vivo* upon smooth muscle cell phenotypes. Smooth muscle cells from rats exposed subchronically to allylamine grow more rapidly in primary culture than cells isolated from control animals (Cox and Ramos, 1990). When seeded on a glass surface, control cells are elongated and spindle shaped, whereas allylamine cells are more broad and round. In contrast to cells from control animals, smooth muscle cells isolated from allylamine-treated animals do not respond to contractile challenge *in vitro*. Allylamine cells are characterized by numerous ribosomes and rough endoplasmic reticulum. These features are consistent with their enhanced ability to synthesize DNA and collagen relative to cells from control animals. Similar increases in collagenous proteins have been reported by Awasthi and Boor (1998). Subsequent studies showed that allylamine modulates both precursors and products of phosphoinositide metabolism in vSMCs (Cox *et al.*, 1990). These actions appear to be mediated by enhanced phospholipase C-mediated turnover of membrane phospholipids. Manipulation of phospho-inositide metabolism upon exposure to dibutyryl cAMP modulates the phenotypic expression of allylamine cells, as judged by changes in morphology, DNA synthesis, and inositol phosphate production (Cox *et al.*, 1990). Although an intriguing association between cAMP levels and the phenotypic state of vSMCs has been established, the role of cAMP as a regulatory factor in phosphoinositide metabolism and phenotypic modulation is not yet clear. It is likely that integrin-mediated signaling may regulate these intracellular processes through interactions with an allylamine-induced, thrombin-generated cleavage product of osteopontin in vascular smooth muscle cells, with $\alpha_v$-coupled integrins (Parrish and Ramos, 1997).

### *Carbon monoxide*

Carbon monoxide induces vascular injury in laboratory animals at concentrations to which humans may be exposed from environmental sources such as automobile exhaust, tobacco smoke, and fossil fuels (Astrup *et al.*, 1966). Because most sources of carbon monoxide represent a complex mixture of chemicals, attempts to distinguish the direct effects of carbon monoxide from those of other chemicals such as sulfur oxides, nitrogen oxides, aldehydes, and hydrocarbons have been difficult. Short-term exposure to carbon monoxide is associated with direct damage to vascular endothelial (Levene *et al.*, 1985) and smooth muscle cells (Paule *et al.*, 1976). Injury to endothelial cells increases intimal permeability and allows the interaction of blood constituents with underlying components of the vascular wall. This response may account, at least in part, for the ability of carbon monoxide to induce atherosclerotic lesions in several animal species. Although carbon monoxide enhances total arterial deposition of cholesterol in animals fed a lipid-rich diet (Astrup *et al.*, 1967), its vascular effects appear to be independent of serum cholesterol levels. Carbon monoxide potentiates cellular growth and suppresses collagen synthesis of cultured porcine endothelial cells, but inhibits cellular growth and causes no changes in the collagen synthesis of bovine endothelial cells (Levene *et al.*, 1985). The mechanisms responsible for species differences have not been defined, but may account for conflicting reports in the literature. Smooth muscle cells exposed to carbon monoxide *in vitro* exhibit partial loss of myofilaments and proliferation of intracellular organelles (Paule *et al.*, 1976). A relative increase in the number of pinocytic vesicles at and below the cell surface and an increase in the number of lysosomes have also been observed. These alterations resemble those observed when smooth muscle cells are grown under hypoxic conditions (Paule *et al.*, 1976). Hypoxia can also lead to increased cell mitogens, such as platelet-derived growth factor-B, endothelin-1, and vascular endothelial growth factor in endothelial cells (Morita and Kourembanas, 1995). Furthermore, hypoxia suppresses nitric oxide synthase, thereby decreasing cellular levels of nitric oxide. Vascular smooth muscle cells respond to hypoxia by increasing heme oxygenase, an enzyme that metabolizes heme to carbon monoxide and biliverdin. Carbon monoxide in turn suppresses endothelin-1 and platelet-derived growth factor-B (Kourembanas *et al.*, 1997).

The toxic effects of carbon monoxide have been attributed to its reversible interaction with hemoglobin. The formation of carboxyhemoglobin *in vivo* is favored because binding of carbon monoxide to hemoglobin is more co-operative than that of oxygen. As a result of this interaction, carboxyhemoglobin decreases the oxygen-carrying capacity of blood and shifts the oxyhemoglobin saturation curve to the left. These actions make it more difficult to unload oxygen and eventually cause functional anemia because of reduced oxygen availability. Evidence has also been presented that carbon monoxide exerts toxic effects independent of those associated with carboxyhemoglobin formation. Elevated partial pressures of carbon monoxide in the tissues may lead to the interaction of carbon monoxide with cellular proteins such as myoglobin and cytochrome *c* oxidase (Cobarn and Mayers, 1971; Young and Caughey, 1990). These metalloproteins contain iron and/or copper centers that form metal–ligand complexes with carbon monoxide in competition with molecular oxygen.

Carbon monoxide elicits a direct vasodilatory response of the coronary circulation (McFaul and McGrath, 1987; Vedernikov *et al.*, 1989; Graser *et al.*, 1990). This response is not mediated by hypoxia, nor by interference with adrenergic, adenosine, or prostaglandin receptors (McFaul and McGrath, 1987). Lin and McGrath (1988) showed that carbon monoxide directly relaxes the rat thoracic aorta. This relaxation is independent of the endothelium and does not appear to be agonist specific. Because norepinephrine-induced contractions are inhibited to a greater extent than those induced by potassium, these investigators suggested that carbon monoxide preferentially inhibits contractions initiated by calcium release from intracellular stores. In subsequent experiments, the relaxation of vascular smooth muscle induced by carbon monoxide has been linked to activation of guanylate cyclase in a manner analogous to that of nitric oxide (Brune and Ullrich, 1987; Durante *et al.*, 1997). Carbon monoxide produced in vSMCs under hypoxic conditions can modify guanylate cyclase levels in endothelial and smooth muscle cells (Morita *et al.*, 1997). Furthermore, carbon monoxide increases nitric oxide release from human platelets and bovine endothelial cells (Thom and Ishirpoulos, 1997). This response is independent of nitric oxide synthase, and appears to involve inhibition of nitric oxide sequestration in the tissue. These observations are consistent with studies showing that carbon monoxide increases cGMP levels in cultured aortic smooth muscle cells (Ramos *et al.*, 1989). A role for hypoxia in carbon monoxide-induced alterations of vascular tone should not be dismissed, given that cyanide, a well-known inhibitor of mitochondrial respiration and inducer of cytotoxic hypoxia, modulates aortic contractility (Robinson *et al.*, 1985).

## *Catecholamines*

Endogenous sympathomimetic amines including epinephrine, norepinephrine, and dopamine exert prominent physiologic effects mediated by receptors on the surface of target cells. Acute exposure to toxic concentrations of catecholamines is associated with cardiovascular and hemodynamic changes, some of which are mediated by alterations in peripheral vascular resistance. That catecholamines modulate progression of arterial disease is consistent with the observed enhancement of vascular reactivity to infused norepinephrine in essential hypertension (Grimm *et al.*, 1980). Repeated exposure to catecholamines induces atherosclerotic lesions in several animal species (Helin *et al.*, 1970; Kukreja *et al.*, 1981; Bauch *et al.*, 1987). The atherosclerotic effect of catecholamines is related to their ability to induce endothelial cell injury and modulate the proliferation of vascular cells. The proliferative disturbances induced by catecholamines are partly mediated via $\alpha$-receptors since prasozin, an $\alpha$-receptor antagonist, effectively prevents the toxic response (Nakaki *et al.*, 1989). Stimulation of $\alpha_1$-adrenergic receptors results in activation of protein kinase C and mitogen-activated protein kinase leading to up-regulation of c-*fos*, c-*jun*, and c-*myc* mRNAs (Yu *et al.*, 1996) and stimulation of DNA synthesis in the vessel wall (DeBlois *et al.*, 1996). Other studies have suggested that tyrosine kinase and phosphatidylinositol-3-kinase mediate the gene induction response (Hu *et al.*, 1996). Therefore, $\alpha_1$ stimulation may contribute to vascular remodeling in atherogenesis (DeBlois *et al.*, 1996). However, Pettersson *et al.* (1990) have shown that potentiation of the atherosclerotic process by sympathetic activation can be inhibited by β-adrenergic receptor blockade. Thus, the relative contribution of adrenergic receptor subtypes to changes in proliferation of vascular cells are not clear. The observation that both parent compounds and metabolites may be involved in the toxic response further complicates interpretation of these data (Bauch *et al.*, 1987). Sholley and co-workers (1976) demonstrated that catecholamines inhibit endothelial migration and repopulation of small denuded areas *in vitro*. In this manner, catecholamines may interfere with repair of blood vessels *in vivo*. Smooth muscle cells exposed to atherosclerotic risk factors, such as diabetes, hypertension, and balloon injury are more susceptible to the effects of catecholamines (Grunwald *et al.*, 1982; Grunwald and Haudenschild, 1984). Hyperinsulinemia has also been linked to cardiovascular disease. For example, insulin and insulin-like growth factor-1 up-regulate $\alpha_1$-D receptors, but not $\alpha_1$-B receptors, a pattern suggestive of differential $\alpha_1$-receptor functions (Yu *et al.*, 1996). This suggestion is consistent with reports by Xin and co-workers (1997) that norepinephrine-induced smooth muscle cell growth is mediated by $\alpha_1$-D receptors via a mitogen-activated protein kinase pathway. Thus, formation of arteriosclerotic lesions in certain forms of hypertension may be initiated and/or supported by high levels of circulating catecholamines. The atherogenic effect of catecholamines may also be related to their ability to induce contraction of vSMCs. A link may exist between vasoconstrictor and mitogenic mechanisms in vSMCs (Berk *et al.*, 1985, 1986). The ability of vasoconstrictor agents to modulate the proliferation of smooth muscle cells may be related to modulation of oncogene expression. Angiotensin II, a powerful vasoconstrictor, increases the expression of various oncogenes including c-*fos* and c-*jun* (Naftilan *et al.*, 1990) as well as $\alpha_1$-D and B receptors (Hu *et al.*, 1995). Furthermore, angiotensin-converting enzyme inhibitors "reverse" remodeling of the vessel wall after injury (reviewed in Chrysant, 1998).

Oxidative by-products of catecholamines have been implicated in their cardiac toxicity (Dhalla *et al.*, 1978; Ramos, 1990). The oxidation of catecholamines generates adrenochrome-like products that undergo spontaneous or enzyme-catalyzed oxidation to form oxygen-derived free radicals. Although a similar correlation has not been established for vascular cells, recent studies have demonstrated that 6-hydroxydopa, an oxidative by-product of catecholamines, is present at the active site of serum amine oxidase (Janes *et al.*, 1990). These observations raise the possibility that oxidative by-products of catecholamines formed under physiologic conditions selectively modulate vascular function. In fact, superoxide anions selectively attenuate the contractile responses to catecholamines (Wolin and Belloni, 1985). The vascular effects of oxygen-derived radicals have been reviewed by Rubanyi (1988). Free radicals *in vivo* can be generated secondary to anoxic/reoxygenation injury (McCord, 1985), metabolism of xenobiotics (Machlin and Bendich, 1987), neutrophil/monocyte-mediated inflammation (Babior *et al.*, 1976), and oxidative modification of low-density lipoproteins (Heinecke, 1987). Superoxide anions inactivate endothelium-derived relaxing factor, whereas hydrogen peroxide and hydroxyl radicals cause direct vasodilation and stimulate the synthesis and release of relaxation factors. Oxygen radicals are considered important mediators of vascular damage in acute arterial hypertension and experimental brain injury (Kontos *et al.*, 1981; Wei *et al.*, 1981, 1985). Hiebert and Liu (1990) have suggested that toxic oxygen metabolites can damage endothelial cells and play an important role in the progression of atherosclerotic lesions. Free radicals generated from the xanthine/xanthine oxidase reaction increase the transfer of albumin across a barrier of endothelial cells *in vitro* (Shasby *et al.*, 1985). Rosenblum and Bryan (1987) have presented evidence that hydroxyl radicals mediate the endothelium-dependent relaxation of brain microvessels. It has been suggested that calcium mobilization and activation of protein kinase C play significant roles in the generation and release of superoxide by endothelial cells (Matsubara and Ziff, 1986). This release of superoxide may modulate vascular cell functions. Activated endothelial cells produce and secrete proteases in association with vessel penetration into surrounding connective tissue in response to angiogenic stimuli (Gross *et al.*, 1983).

### *Dinitrotoluene*

Dinitrotoluene is a nitroaromatic chemical used as a precursor in the synthesis of polyurethane foams, coatings, elastomers, and explosives. The manufacture of dinitrotoluene generates a technical grade mixture which consists of 75.8 percent 2,4-dinitrotoluene, 19.5 percent 2,6-dinitrotoluene, and 4.7 percent other isomers. Several chronic toxicity studies in laboratory animals have shown that 2,4- and/ or 2,6-dinitrotoluene cause cancers of the liver, gall bladder, and kidney, as well as benign tumors of the connective tissues (Ellis *et al.*, 1978; Chemical Industry Institute of Toxicology, 1982; Leonard *et al.*, 1987). In humans, however, retrospective mortality studies in workers exposed daily to dinitrotoluene showed that dinitrotoluenes cause circulatory disorders of atherosclerotic etiology (Levine *et al.*, 1986; Levine, 1987). As in other instances of chronic occupational illness, increased mortality from cardiovascular disorders upon exposure to dinitrotoluenes has been related to duration and intensity of exposure.

Studies in this laboratory established that repeated *in vivo* exposure of rats to 2,4- or 2,6-dinitrotoluene is associated with dysplasia and rearrangement of aortic smooth muscle cells (Ramos *et al.*, 1991). Marked inhibition of DNA synthesis occurred in medial smooth muscle cells isolated from dinitrotoluene-treated animals. The ability of dinitrotoluenes to modulate DNA synthesis in aortic smooth muscle cells was not due to direct genotoxic or cytotoxic effects (Ramos *et al.*, 1990). Dinitrotoluenes are metabolized in the liver to dinitrobenzylalcohol, which is then conjugated to form a glucoronide excreted in bile or urine. This conjugate is thought to be hydrolyzed by intestinal microflora and subsequently reduced to a toxic metabolite, or the precursor of a toxic metabolite (Long and Rickert, 1982; Mirsalis *et al.*, 1982). Dent *et al.* (1981) showed that rat cecal microflora convert dinitrotoluene to nitrosonitrotoluenes, aminonitrotoluenes, and diaminotoluenes. *In vitro* exposure of rat aortic smooth muscle cells to 2,4- or 2,6-diaminotoluene modulates DNA synthesis in a manner which resembles that observed upon dinitrotoluene treatment *in vivo* (Ramos *et al.*, 1991). Interestingly, diaminotoluene retards the progression of smooth muscle cells through the $G_1$ phase of the cell cycle (Ramos *et al.*, unpublished observations). This response resembles that observed upon exposure of smooth muscle cells to other chemical carcinogens (Sadhu *et al.*, 1991). However, diaminotoluene has not been detected in metabolism studies upon *in vivo* exposure to dinitrotoluene (Mirsalis *et al.*, 1982). Because both dinitrotoluene and diaminotoluene must be activated to elicit toxic effects, metabolic intermediates common to both agents may actually be responsible for the vascular toxicity of dinitrotoluene.

The modulation of DNA synthesis in rat aortic smooth muscle cells by dinitrotoluene may be related to its ability to promote the atherosclerotic process in humans. Interestingly, in rats pretreated with Aroclor 1254, a complex mixture of PAHs and chlorinated hydrocarbons, the genotoxicity of dinitrotoluene was potentiated possibly through alteration of nitroreductase activity, reduced pH, and/ or changes in the microfloral population (Chadwick *et al.*, 1993). However, additional studies are required to evaluate species differences in response to atherogenic insult as the rat is relatively resistant to both spontaneous and chemically induced atherogenesis (Vesselinovitch, 1980; Jokinen *et al.*, 1985).

## *Homocysteine*

An elevated plasma homocysteine level is an established risk factor for atherosclerotic coronary heart disease (CHD), cerebrovascular disease (CVD), and lower extremity occlusive disease (LED), and is associated with death in patients with CHD, CVD, and LED (Taylor *et al.*, 1999). Several investigators have established a correlation between homocysteine, an intermediate in cellular methionine metabolism and inducer of oxidative stress, and the formation of oxLDLs and $H_2O_2$ in the presence of cuprous and ferrous ions (McCully, 1996). Homocysteine has also been linked to myointimal cellular proliferation in baboons (Harker *et al.*, 1983), and vSMC proliferation *in vitro* following up-regulation of cyclins D1 and A (Tsai *et al.*, 1994). Nishio and Watanabe (1997) examined the effects of homocysteine on rat vSMC proliferation *in vitro* and found that homocysteine was only weakly mitogenic compared with PDGF-BB. When combined with PDGF-BB, however, homocysteine enhanced vSMC proliferation fourfold compared with controls (Nishio and Watanabe, 1997). Interestingly, homocysteine decreased glutathione peroxidase activity, increased superoxide dismutase activity, and had no effect on catalase activity (Nishio and Watanabe, 1997). These results are consistent with the notion that mitogenic signaling in vSMCs involves alterations in cellular redox capacity.

During the initial stages of plaque formation, oxidized low-density lipoproteins circulating in blood are engulfed by macrophages in the subendothelial space, giving rise to foam cells that eventually become "fatty streaks." Oxidized LDLs also injure cells within the vessel wall (Ross, 1993), and modulate mitogenic signaling in vSMCs (Kusuhara *et al.*, 1997). Halvorsen and co-workers (1996) observed that normal homocysteine plasma concentrations (6 μM) had no effect on LDL oxidation, whereas higher concentrations (25–500 μM) protected lipid and protein modifications of LDL. Interestingly, in the presence of copper ions, homocysteine stimulated LDL oxidation, therefore in the absence of circulating copper ions homocysteine-induced atherosclerosis may be explained by mechanisms other than LDL oxidation (Halvorsen *et al.*, 1996). Treatment of elevated homocysteine levels by therapy with folate (Abby *et al.*, 1998; Hornstra *et al.*, 1998; Taylor *et al.*, 1999) and vitamins B6 and B12 has been suggested previously (Hornstra *et al.*, 1998; Taylor *et al.*, 1999).

### Hydrazinobenzoic acid

Hydrazinobenzoic acid is a nitrogen–nitrogen bonded chemical present in the cultivated mushroom *Agaricus bisporus*. McManus *et al.* (1987) reported that this hydrazine derivative causes smooth muscle cell tumors of the aorta and large arteries of mice when administered over the life span of the animals. These tumors showed the characteristic appearance and immunocytochemical features of vascular leiomyomas and leiomyosarcomas. Smooth muscle cell lysis with vascular perforation apparently precedes malignant smooth muscle cell growth. The ability of hydrazinobenzoic acid to cause vascular smooth muscle cell tumors is shared with other synthetic and naturally occurring hydrazines (Toth *et al.*, 1978). Recently, a role for hydrazine-derived alkyl radicals in cytotoxicity and transformation of mouse fibroblasts was reported by Gamberini *et al.* (1998). Although angiomyomas (or vascular leiomyomas) derived histogenetically from the media of blood and lymph vessels occur most commonly in the oral cavity and in the skin (Savage *et al.*, 1983), evidence that primary leiomyosarcomas occur in the abdominal aorta has been previously presented (Hernandez *et al.*, 1979; Milili *et al.*, 1981). These observations are particularly significant when considering that transformation of vSMCs is an uncommon event.

We have conducted *in vitro* studies to examine the direct cytotoxic effects of hydrazinobenzoic acid in cultured rat aortic smooth muscle cells. Exposure of smooth muscle cells to hydrazinobenzoic acid (0.1–100 μM) for various times was not lethal to the cells, as reflected by leakage of lactate dehydrogenase (Piron and K.S. Ramos, unpublished observations). However, significant fluctuations in cellular glutathione content upon exposure to hydrazinobenzoic acid were observed. The impact of such alterations to the *in vivo* toxicity of hydrazinobenzoic acid has not been defined. Bioactivation of hydrazines to mutagenic products is accomplished by enzymes such as mushroom tyrosinase (Walton *et al.*, 1997). Because free radicals can be generated from hydrazines by oxidizing systems, including metal-catalyzed auto-oxidation, prostaglandin synthetase, and cytochrome P450/NADPH (Kalyanaraman and Sinha, 1985), the modulation of glutathione by hydrazinobenzoic acid may be mediated by free radical formation. This suggestion is consistent with previous reports showing that hydrazines bind covalently to macromolecules, promote lipid peroxidation, and induce DNA damage (Whiting *et al.*, 1979; Noda *et al.*, 1986), as is the case with unsymmetrically alkylated hydrazines which cause lethal DNA lesions in repair-deficient strains (Poso *et al.*, 1995).

## Metals

Although epidemiologic and clinical reports regarding the vascular effects of metals have received some attention in past years (Beevers *et al.*, 1976; Voors *et al.*, 1982; Medeiros and Pellum, 1985), only a limited number of studies have been conducted to define the cellular and molecular mechanisms of metal-induced angiotoxicity. As in other systems, the vascular toxicity of food- and waterborne elements (selenium, chromium, copper, zinc, cadmium, lead, and mercury), as well as airborne elements (vanadium and lead), is thought to be due to non-specific reactions of metals with sulfhydryl, carboxyl, or phosphate groups. In addition, the ability of metals such as cobalt, magnesium, manganese, nickel, cadmium, and lead to interact with and block calcium channels has been recognized for some time (Carafoli, 1984). Evidence that intracellular calcium-binding proteins are biologically relevant targets of heavy metal toxicity has also been presented. Calmodulin, a ubiquitous calcium-binding protein in eukaryotes, serves as a major intracellular calcium receptor in the regulation of multiple cellular processes. Certain heavy metals, including mercury and lead, effectively substitute for calcium within the calmodulin molecule (Cheung, 1984). However, the contribution of this mechanism to the toxic effects of metals has been questioned based on the inability of beryllium, barium, cobalt, zinc, and cadmium to bind readily to calmodulin *in vitro* (Habermann and Richardt, 1986).

Most vascular toxicity studies have focused on the effects of cadmium. Cadmium is not preferentially located in blood vessels relative to other tissues. However, when present, cadmium localizes to the elastic lamina of large arteries, with particularly high concentrations at arterial branching points (Perry *et al.*, 1989). A large portion of cadmium accumulated in the body is tightly bound to hepatic and renal metallothionein, a detoxification mechanism (Webb, 1979; Georing and Klaassen, 1984). Thus, low metallothionein levels in vascular tissue may predispose to cadmium toxicity (Perry *et al.*, 1989). Long-term exposure of laboratory animals to low levels of cadmium has been associated with the development of atherosclerosis and hypertension in the absence of other toxic effects (Revis *et al.*, 1981). However, dietary cadmium has also been shown to reduce atherogenesis through suppression of free iron concentration (Meijer *et al.*, 1996). Although most experimental studies conducted to date have focused on the putative hypertensive effects of cadmium, some of the critical information required to establish a causal relationship remains elusive.

Schroeder and Vinton (1962) first reported that exposure of rats to 5 p.p.m. cadmium in the drinking water causes hypertension. This observation has been corroborated by several independent laboratories (Perry *et al.*, 1977; Kopp *et al.*, 1982) and refuted by others (Shukla and Singhal, 1984). To account for such discrepancies, Perry *et al.* (1989) suggested that cadmium-induced hypertension is only observed in a narrow concentration range of 0.1–5 p.p.m., above which toxicity without hypertensive effects is only observed. These investigators further proposed that failure to induce hypertension with chronic cadmium may be due to low levels of heavy metal contamination in the water or food supplies used in the course of experiments. This interpretation would be consistent with the observation that selenium and zinc inhibit (Perry *et al.*, 1980), whereas lead potentiates, the hypertensive effects of cadmium (Perry *et al.*, 1983). Concentrations of cadmium which increase blood pressure fail to raise blood pressure in the presence of calcium (Revis *et al.*, 1981). In contrast, the protective effects of zinc and selenium may be related to their ability to increase the synthesis of cadmium-binding proteins and, thus, enhance cadmium detoxification.

The mechanism of cadmium-induced vascular toxicity is not yet known. Cadmium has been reported to increase sodium retention (Doyle *et al.*, 1975), induce vasoconstriction (Perry and Yunice, 1965), increase cardiac output (Perry *et al.*, 1967), and produce hyper-reninemia (Perry *et al.*, 1979). At the cellular level, cadmium causes vesiculation, vacuolization, widened intercellular junctions, and fragmentation of vascular endothelium (Schlaepfer, 1971). *In vitro* exposure to cadmium decreases prostacyclin formation in aortic rings and reduces ADP clearance by arterial tissue (Togna *et al.*, 1985). The responsiveness of rabbit platelets to non-aggregating concentrations of arachidonic acid or collagen can be potentiated by prior exposure to cadmium chloride (Caprino *et al.*, 1979). Many questions regarding the angiotoxic effects of cadmium remain unanswered, particularly as it relates to the study of microvascular responses to cadmium.

Because hypertension is not commonly observed during clinical lead intoxication, many investigators consider existing evidence to be conflicting and inconclusive. Epidemiologic studies have shown that a large percentage of patients with essential hypertension have increased body stores of lead (Batuman *et al.*, 1983). Elevated blood pressure has also been observed during childhood lead poisoning (Jhaveri *et al.*, 1979; Needleman *et al.*, 1990). Although in these children the level of lead burden was not severe, a significant increase in blood pressure was seen on the 10th day of poisoning, which persisted for the remainder of the study. The direct vasoconstrictor effect of lead may be related to the putative hypertensive response (Chipino *et al.*, 1968). This effect can be complemented by lead's ability to activate the renin/angiotensin/aldosterone system (Fine *et al.*, 1988). Lead also stimulates the proliferation of cultured vSMCs via a calcium-dependent pathway (Fujiwara *et al.*, 1995).

A number of studies have focused on the toxic interactions of metals. For example, lead potentiates the vasopressor response to cadmium (Perry *et al.*, 1980). In contrast to the protective effects of calcium in cadmium-induced hypertension,

calcium is ineffective in reducing the toxic cardiovascular effects of lead (
*et al.*, 1981). However, magnesium promotes the atherosclerotic and hypert
effects of both lead and cadmium. Mercury and lead cause contraction of aortic
smooth muscle *in vitro*, whereas cadmium is without effect (Tomera and Harakal,
1986). Mercury added to platelet-rich plasma causes a marked increase in platelet
thromboxane $B_2$ production and increased platelet responsiveness to arachidonic
acid (Caprino *et al.*, 1983). Although it is unlikely that mercury and lead compete
with calcium for intracellular binding sites, their accessibility to the intracellular
compartment appears to be calcium dependent (Tomera and Harakal, 1986).
Several investigators have proposed that acute lead-induced neuropathy is due to
cerebral capillary dysfunction (Jhaveri *et al.*, 1979; Needleman *et al.*, 1990). This
hypothesis is consistent with recent *in vitro* studies showing that lead causes dose-
and time-dependent inhibition of cell division and glucose uptake in cerebral
microvessel endothelium (Maxwell *et al.*, 1986).

### *Nicotine*

Nicotine, an alkaloid found in various plants, mimics the actions of acetylcholine
at nicotinic receptors throughout the body. The cardiovascular effects of this toxin
have been studied within the context of tobacco-associated toxicities, as well as
its use as a botanical insecticide. Epidemiologic and experimental studies have
suggested that nicotine is a causative or aggravating factor in myocardial and
cerebral infarction, gangrene, and aneurysm. Bull *et al.* (1985) have shown that
repeated subcutaneous infusion of nicotine for 7 days is associated with reduced
prostacyclin production in aortic segments. Reduced prostacyclin production has
been observed in isolated rabbit hearts, rabbit aorta, human vein, rat aorta, and
umbilical arteries when incubated with nicotine *in vitro* (Wennmalm, 1978;
Sonnfield and Wennmalm, 1980; Stoel *et al.*, 1980; Alster and Wennmalm, 1983).
It has been suggested that the effects of nicotine are due to competitive inhibition
of cyclooxygenase, which precludes the formation of prostaglandin endoperoxides
*in vivo*. Alterations in the structural integrity of the aortic endothelium following
chronic oral administration of nicotine *in vivo* and upon exposure of cultured
aortic endothelial cells *in vitro* have also been noted (Tulloss and Booyse, 1978;
Zimmerman and McGeachie, 1985). Because nicotine stimulates catecholamine
release from sympathetic ganglia and nerve endings, as well as the adrenal medulla,
its toxicologic profile may share features in common with those described for
catecholamines.

At the cellular level, nicotine modulates the proliferation of vascular endothelial
and smooth muscle cells. Nicotine increases the synthesis of DNA in luminal
endothelial cells after *in vivo* administration (Zimmerman and McGeachie, 1985).
At concentrations lower than those present in blood after smoking, nicotine also
increases the rate of DNA synthesis in growth-arrested subcultures of smooth
muscle cells (Thyberg, 1986). This response appears to be independent of those
of other mitogens present in the medium, and additive to that of serum. Such

changes in smooth muscle cell proliferation are consistent with the enhanced rate of phenotypic modulation from a contractile to a synthetic state induced by nicotine. Increased numbers of lysosomes with incompletely degraded inclusions and/or inhibition of intralysosomal proteolysis in macrophages upon exposure to nicotine have been reported (Thyberg and Nilsson, 1982). Interestingly, the effect of nicotine on lysosomal structure is shared with other weak bases and amines and may be due to accumulation of the drug within lysosomes. Cytoskeletal changes have also been observed in cultured vascular cells upon exposure to nicotine (Csonka *et al.*, 1985). Although extensive circumstantial evidence is available, the mechanism by which nicotine causes vascular toxicity is not clear.

### *Polycyclic aromatic hydrocarbons*

The pioneering work of Benditt and Benditt in the early 1970s paved the way for much of the work focusing on the vascular toxicity of polycyclic aromatic hydrocarbons and their ability to promote the initiation and/or progression of atherosclerosis. These investigators first proposed that atherosclerotic lesions, such as benign smooth muscle tumors of the uterus, originate from the mutation of a single smooth muscle cell (Benditt and Benditt, 1973). This proposal was based on the observation that a normal section of the arterial wall contained cells expressing the A and B allele of the glucose-6-phosphate dehydrogenase gene, whereas most plaques were monotypic containing cells expressing only the A or B allele. Although this proposal was received with great skepticism, evidence implicating carcinogens (Albert *et al.*, 1977), radiation (Gold, 1961), and viruses (Benditt *et al.*, 1983) in atherosclerosis has continued to accumulate over the years. Exposure of avian species to benzo(a)pyrene and 7,12-dimethyl-benz(a,h)anthracene causes atherosclerosis without alterations in serum cholesterol levels (Albert *et al.*, 1977). The ability of these carcinogens to cause atherosclerotic lesions has been associated with cytochrome P450-mediated conversion of the parent compound to toxic metabolic intermediates. Microsomal monooxygenases, including P450 forms 2 and 6 and NADPH–cytochrome P450 reductase, have been identified in rabbit aortic vascular tissue (Serabjit-Singh *et al.*, 1985). Human fetal aortic smooth muscle cells metabolize benzo(a)pyrene and 7,12-dimethylbenz(a)anthracene via cytochrome P450-dependent mechanisms to phenols and 12-hydroxymethyl-7-methylbenz(a)anthracene, 7-hydroxymethyl-12-methylbenz(a)anthracene, 7,12-dihydroxymethyl benz(a)anthracene, and trans-8,9-dihydrodiol-7,12-dimethylbenz(a)anthracene respectively (Bond *et al.*, 1979). Pretreatment of chickens with Aroclor 1254, 3-methylcholanthrene and 5,6-benzoflavone, but not phenobarbital or pregnolone 16α-carbonitrile, increases the aortic monooxygenation of polycyclic aromatic hydrocarbons (Bond *et al.*, 1980). The majority of the activity responsible for the biotransformation of benzo(a)pyrene is associated with the smooth muscle layers of the aorta (Serabjit-Singh *et al.*, 1985). However, cytochrome P450-dependent monooxygenase activity, which can potentially bioactivate carcinogens, is also present in the aortic endothelium (Baird *et al.*, 1980; Pinto *et al.*, 1986). Interestingly, the activity of aortic aryl hydrocarbon hydroxylase has been correlated with the degree of susceptibility to atherosclerosis in avian species (Majesky *et al.*, 1983).

The generation of phase II metabolites via sulfoconjugation of 3-hydroxybenzo(a)pyrene has been demonstrated in aortic tissue (Yang *et al.*, 1986a). This reaction is important in the reduction of toxic phenolics. Sulfation takes place in cultured aortic smooth muscle cells and endothelial cells, aortic whole organ explants, and in cytosolic fractions of cell-free preparations. The conjugation capacity of avian aortic tissues is 10–20 percent of the total avian hepatic capacity to sulfoconjugate 3-hydroxybenzo(a)pyrene. Avian aortic tissues also contain active UDP-glucuronosyltransferase activity which catalyzes the glucuronidation of 3-hydroxybenzo(a)pyrene (Yang *et al.*, 1986b). In abdominal aortic segments, glucuronosyltransferase activity is eight- to ninefold higher than that of the thoracic aorta. Phenobarbital, but not 3-methylcholanthrene, increases the activity of microsomal fractions in both segments. Although glucuronidation of 3-hydroxybenzo(a)pyrene appears to be less active than sulfation in aortic tissues, the differential distribution of glucuronyltransferase activity may account for differences in the responses of abdominal versus thoracic regions of the aorta to benzo(a)pyrene. This concept is supported by studies showing that glucuronidation decreases the mutagenic and carcinogenic effects of polycyclic aromatic hydrocarbons in the Ames test (Owens *et al.*, 1978), but increases the generation of reactive intermediates in other preparations (Nemoto *et al.*, 1983).

Albert *et al.* (1977) and Penn and Snyder (1988) have reported that treatment with several polycyclic hydrocarbons increases the size, but not the frequency, of atherosclerotic lesions. These observations suggest that polycyclic aromatic hydrocarbons act as promoters of the atherosclerotic process, but do not initiate lesion formation. In contrast, Paigen *et al.* (1985) have shown that 3-methylcholanthrene increases both the number and size of lipid-staining lesions in the aorta of animals fed an atherogenic diet for 8 weeks. Furthermore, Majesky *et al.* (1985) have shown that focal proliferation of intimal smooth muscle cells can be produced by an initiation/promotion sequence using 7,12-dimethyl-benz(a)anthracene and the $\alpha_1$ selective adrenergic agonist methoxamine. The discrepancy in these studies may be accounted for by regional differences in the toxicologic response. Distal segments of aorta have been proposed as preferential sites for promotion, while initiation is thought to be confined to the thoracic region. Because hydrocarbons associate readily with plasma lipoproteins, Revis *et al.* (1984) have suggested that the atherogenic effect of polycyclic aromatic hydrocarbons is related to the mechanism by which these chemicals are transported in plasma. This proposal was based on the observation that carcinogens which do not associate with lipoproteins, such as 2,4,6-trichlorophenol, are not atherogenic. An interesting area of investigation which has not yet been rigorously addressed is the role of Ah receptor mechanisms in vascular toxicity of polycyclic aromatic hydrocarbons. In this regard, it is interesting to note that Ah-responsive mice are more susceptible to 3-methylcholanthrene-induced atherosclerosis than Ah-resistant mice (Paigen *et al.*, 1986). We have recently found that epigenetic disturbances in vSMCs by benzo(a)pyrene are absent in AhR nullizygous mice (Kerzee and Ramos, 1999).

*In vivo* exposure of quail to benzo(a)pyrene modulates phosphorylation of medial aortic proteins. Benzo(a)pyrene enhances basal phosphorylation of several cytosolic proteins, but inhibits C kinase-mediated protein phosphorylation in the particulate fraction (Ou and Ramos, 1992). This inhibition leads to disruption of mechanisms that regulate vascular smooth muscle cell phenotypes (Ou *et al.*, 1995). The profile of medial protein phosphorylation induced by benzo(a)pyrene is altered when *in vitro* phosphorylation measurements are carried out in the presence of endothelial cells. Increased phosphorylation of cytosolic proteins is observed in aortic homogenates containing endothelial and smooth muscle cell proteins (Ou and Ramos, 1992). Smooth muscle cells from benzo(a)pyrene-treated rats are characterized by increased abundance of phosphatidylinositol metabolites, primarily products of phosphatidylinositol-3-kinase activity (Ramos *et al.*, 1996). These observations suggest that multiple cell interactions may be critical to the expression of the toxic response. Because phosphorylation mechanisms are intimately involved with the regulation of vascular smooth muscle cell growth and differentiation, these results suggest that signal transduction pathways involved in the phosphorylation of proteins may be targeted by polycyclic aromatic hydrocarbons. More recently, we have shown that acute benzo(a)pyrene exposure causes enhanced expression of the c-*Ha-ras* oncogene in aortic smooth muscle cells (Sadhu and Ramos, 1993). This induction is regulated at the transcriptional level and involves multiple protein–protein/DNA–protein interactions, including binding of antioxidant/electrophile response element-binding proteins to the antioxidant/electrophile response element (Bral and Ramos, 1997) (Figure 15.2). Redox cycling of benzo(a)pyrene quinone metabolites may contribute to the gene induction response. This response may be relevant to loss of co-ordinated cell cycle expression leading to genomic instability and phenotypic modulation, as shown for fibroblasts by Stambrook and co-workers (Denko *et al.*, 1994).

### T-2 toxin

Trichothecene mycotoxins, commonly classified as tetracyclic sesquiterpenes, are naturally occurring cytotoxic metabolites of *Fusarium* species (Schiefer *et al.*, 1987). These mycotoxins, including T-2 toxin [$4\beta$,15-diacetoxy-$8\alpha$-(3-methylbutyryloxy)-$3\alpha$-hydroxy-12,13-epoxytrichothec-9-ene], are major contaminants of foods and animal feeds and may cause illness in animals and man. Although the carcinogenic effects of trichothecene mycotoxins has been documented for many years, little is known about the vascular toxicity of these agents. Acute parenteral administration of T-2 toxin to laboratory animals induces shock, hypothermia, and death due to cardiovascular and respiratory failure (Feuerstein *et al.*, 1985). Wilson *et al.* (1982) reported that intravenous infusion of T-2 toxin in rats causes an initial decrease in heart rate and blood pressure,

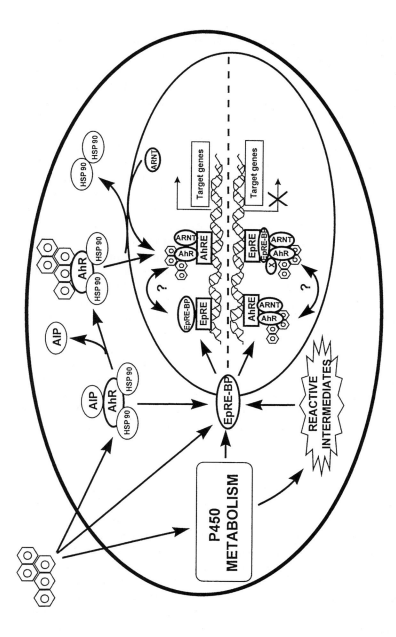

*Figure 15.2* Proposed mechanisms of benzo(a)pyrene-induced gene expression in vascular smooth muscle cells. BaP is metabolized by AhR-mediated P450 monooxygenases to various hydroxylated and epoxidated intermediates. These intermediates induce activation of electrophile response element-binding proteins (EpRE-BP) which interact with the electrophile-responsive element (EpRE) of *c-Ha-ras*. Concomitantly, BaP interacts with the AhR, inducing translocation to the nucleus, interaction with aryl hydrocarbon receptor nuclear translocator (ARNT) and association with the AhR response element (AhRE) element of *c-Ha-ras*. Possible interactions between the activated AhR and EpRE-BP could lead to positive, as well as negative, regulation of target genes. AIP, aryl hydrocarbon receptor-associated immunophilin-like protein.

followed by tachycardia and hypertension, and finally bradycardia and hypotension. These actions may be related to a central effect on blood pressure and catecholamine release (Siren and Feuerstein, 1986). Siren and Feuerstein (1986) also suggested that, although T-2 toxin reduces blood flow and increases vascular resistance in skeletal muscle and mesenteric and renal vascular beds, no changes in mean arterial pressure and heart rate could be detected. Acute T-2 toxin exposure causes extensive destruction of myocardial capillaries, while repeated dosing promotes thickening of large coronary arteries (Yarom *et al.*, 1983). A more generalized atherosclerosis and hypertension are delayed consequences of repeated T-2 toxin exposure (Schoenthal *et al.*, 1979).

At the cellular level, T-2 toxin is a potent inhibitor of protein synthesis (Ueno, 1977). T-2 toxin is thought to bind to the 60S subunit of the ribosome to interfere with peptidyl transferase activity. Inhibition of DNA synthesis is thought to be secondary to the interference with protein synthesis (Cannon *et al.*, 1976). A single large dose of 2 mg kg$^{-1}$ or four injections of 0.3 mg kg$^{-1}$ T-2 toxin causes necrosis of endothelial cells, accumulation of basement membrane-like material in the intima, and swelling and activation of smooth muscle cells in the media (Yarom *et al.*, 1987). Medial aortic smooth muscle cells decrease in number and increase in size upon exposure to T-2 toxin. Marked inhibition of smooth muscle cell growth is observed in explant cultures of smooth muscle cells. This is followed by stimulation of the proliferative capacity of smooth muscle cells *in vitro*. The fragmentation and increase in basement membrane-like material in these cells suggest that long-term changes occur even after the endothelium has returned to normal.

## Miscellaneous toxins

Exposure of factory workers in rayon plants to carbon disulfide has been associated with a significant increase in mortality from coronary heart disease. A cohort epidemiologic study conducted in Poland showed a statistically significant excess in deaths due to circulatory system diseases in carbon disulfide-exposed workers (Peplonska *et al.*, 1996). Although the mechanism of toxicity is not known, alterations of glucose and/or lipid metabolism and blood coagulation have been suggested (Kurppa *et al.*, 1984). Measurements of urinary 2-thiothiazotidine-4-carboxylic acid levels was shown to be a sensitive, precise, and selective marker to monitor carbon disulfide exposure in rats (Cox *et al.*, 1996). Studies have shown that 1,3-butadiene, a chemical used in the production of styrene butadiene, increases the incidence of cardiac hemangiosarcomas, rare tumors of endothelial origin (Huff *et al.*, 1984; Miller and Boorman, 1990). Penn and Snyder (1996) have shown that 1,3-butadiene, a component of the vapor phase of cigarette smoke, accelerates plaque formation at environmentally relevant concentrations in cockerels. Although hemangiosarcomas have also been observed in the liver, lung, and kidney, cardiac tumors are a major cause of death in animals exposed to this chemical.

Tetrachlorodibenzo-*p*-dioxin (TCDD), a widely studied polychlorinated hydrocarbon, induces hyperlipoproteinemia in animals and humans (Walker and Martin, 1979; Lovati *et al.*, 1984). In guinea pigs, a single dose of TCDD induces a nineteenfold increase in very-low-density lipoproteins, and a fourfold increase in low-density lipoproteins (Swift *et al.*, 1981). The ability of TCDD to modulate lipid metabolism may have serious consequences for the preservation of vascular function. Studies in our laboratory have shown that TCDD modulates protein phosphorylation in rat aortic smooth cells *in vivo* and *in vitro* (Weber *et al.*, 1991). Specifically, TCDD selectively alters the phosphorylation status at the $G_0/G_1$ transition by decreasing the activity of several protein kinase C isoforms, alpha, beta, and delta (Weber *et al.*, 1996). Although the significance of these observations is presently unclear, the vascular responses to TCDD resemble some of those described for benzo(a)pyrene. This parallelism raises the possibility that the vascular toxicities of these chemicals share common cellular and molecular pathways. Recent studies by Puga and co-workers showed that TCDD increased urinary levels of vasoactive eicosanoids, mediators of ischemic heart disease, and partitioned to lipoprotein particles, which may serve as a vehicle to deliver TCDD to atherosclerotic plaques (Dalton *et al.*, 1999). These effects may exacerbate the severity of ischemic heart disease. The vascular actions of TCDD may also involve deficits in vascular smooth muscle cell function as cells isolated from TCDD-treated mice consistently exhibit atherogenic phenotypes (Ramos *et al.*, unpublished observations).

Vitamin D hypervitaminosis causes medial degeneration, calcification of the coronary arteries, and smooth muscle cell proliferation in laboratory animals (Toda *et al.*, 1985; Koh *et al.*, 1988). The toxic effects of vitamin D may be related to its structural similarity to 25-hydroxycholesterol, a potent vascular toxin (Toda *et al.*, 1985). Koh *et al.* (1988) have shown that 1,25-dihydroxyvitamin D binds specifically to surface receptors of rat vSMCs to stimulate proliferation *in vitro*. The toxicity of vitamin D may be related to alterations in cyclic nucleotide metabolism. This suggestion is consistent with studies showing that cyclic nucleotides play a critical role in the regulation of vascular smooth muscle cell function (Murad, 1986). In this regard, phosphodiesterase inhibition has been associated with toxicity in medium-sized arteries of the mesentery, testis, and myocardium (Westwood *et al.*, 1990). Other reports showing that theophylline, an inhibitor of phosphodiesterase, causes cardiovascular lesions in mesenteric arterioles (Collins *et al.*, 1988), and that isomazole and indolidan cause periarteritis of the media and adventitia of small and medium-sized arteries have also been presented (Sandusky *et al.*, 1991).

From a toxicologic perspective, the recent demonstration that low-density lipoproteins are oxidized *in vitro* by oxygen free radicals released by arterial cells is of particular interest. Modified low-density lipoproteins attract macrophages and prevent their migration from the tissues (for a comprehensive review, see Gross *et al.*, 1983). Oxidation derivatives of cholesterol, such as cholestane-3β,5α,6β-triol and 25-hydroxycholesterol are potent inhibitors of 3-hydroxy-3-

methylglutaryl coenzyme A (HMG CoA) reductase, the rate-limiting enzyme in cholesterol biosynthesis (Naseem and Heald, 1987). Interestingly, many of the oxidized products of cholesterol formed spontaneously are identical to those formed enzymatically by the microsomal and mitochondrial cytochrome P450 systems (Hayaishi, 1969). However, although serum antioxidants may afford protection against oxidized lipoprotein injury, the atherogenicity of these products continues to be actively scrutinized.

Studies conducted in recent years have focused on the causative role of infectious agents in cardiovascular disease, in particular atherosclerotic plaque formation. These studies are based on the suggestion that early life experience and exposure to pathogens may influence adult risk of coronary heart disease (Mendall *et al.*, 1994). Although numerous studies have identified the presence of viral and bacterial pathogens in atheromatous plaques, an etiologic mechanism has yet to be identified. A possible mechanism of injury involves an immunologic response that enhances oxidation of LDLs through direct interactions on the vessel wall. Researchers have suggested that previous infection with *Chlamydia pneumoniae*, a common respiratory pathogen, is a major risk factor for stroke in young and middle-aged patients, possibly as a result of an enhanced hypercoagulable state that increases the risk of thrombosis (Valtonen, 1991). In clinical studies, seropositivity to *C. pneumoniae* has been independently associated with raised fibrinogen and malondialdehyde concentrations (Levy *et al.*, 1995). A role for chlamydial lipopolysaccharide (cLPS), a Gram-negative bacteria cell wall component, in the atherosclerotic process has been suggested by Kalayoglu and Byrne (1998a) in which *C. pneumoniae* induces macrophage foam cell formation in murine macrophage RAW-264.7 cells. Inhibition of cLPS prevented the uptake of cholesterol esters, suggesting that chronic exposure to cLPS may result in foam cell formation (Kalayoglu and Byrne, 1998a). Exposure of cultured macrophages to *C. pneumoniae* in combination with LDL resulted in foam cell formation that was not inhibited by the antioxidant butylated hydroxytoluene, suggesting that scavenger receptors are not involved in *Chlamydia*-induced LDL uptake (Kalayoglu and Byrne, 1998b). Furthermore, inhibition of LDL receptors blocked the uptake of LDL in macrophages, thus indicating that the mechanism of lipid accumulation was the result of unregulated LDL uptake and/or metabolism (Kalayoglu and Byrne, 1998b). It has also been suggested that chronic bacterial infection may aggravate pre-existing plaques by enhancing T-cell activation as well as other inflammatory responses that may participate in the destabilization of the intimal cap, resulting in plaque rupture, progression to acute ischemic syndromes, and ultimate enlargement of the atherosclerotic plaque (Muhlestein, 1998).

Human heat shock protein 60 (HSP 60) has previously been localized to atherosclerotic plaques, and a possible role for HSP 60 in atherogenesis has been proposed (Xu *et al.*, 1996; Birnie *et al.*, 1998). Kol and co-workers (1998) found that chlamydial and human HSP 60 co-localized in human atherosclerotic plaques. Furthermore, chlamydial HSP 60 can induce proinflammatory cytokines, such as tumor necrosis factor (TNF-$\alpha$) and matrix-degrading metalloproteinases (MMPs) (Kol *et al.*, 1998), which suggests a direct role for *C. pneumoniae* in the pathology of the vessel wall.

There are mixed reports in the literature regarding the role of *Helicobacter pylori*, a childhood-acquired bacterial infection, in cardiovascular disorders (Mendall *et al.*, 1994, Murray *et al.*, 1995; Blasi *et al.*, 1996; Markus and Mendall, 1998; Regnstrom *et al.*, 1998). Seropositivity to *H. pylori* has been independently associated with fibrinogen concentration and total leukocyte count (Levy *et al.*, 1995). The Atherosclerosis Risk In Communities (ARIC) study found that *H. pylori* seropositivity was associated with other cardiovascular disease risk factors, such as higher homocysteine levels, lower plasma pyridoxal 5′-phosphate, decreased vitamin supplement use, and seropositivity for cytomegalovirus and herpes simplex type I (Folsom *et al.*, 1998). Therefore, these investigators concluded that *H. pylori* is probably not a factor in coronary heart disease. In contrast, Pasceri *et al.* (1998) suggested that "low-grade" chronic exposure to *H. pylori* may influence atherosclerotic plaque formation, whereas Markus and Mendall (1998) suggested that *H. pylori* infection may be an independent risk factor for ischemic cerebrovascular disease. A proposed mechanism for *H. pylori*-induced cardiovascular disease involves decreases in folate bioavailability, resulting in decreased methionine synthase activity and increased homocysteine levels (Markle, 1997).

## Concluding remarks

The proposed mechanism of action for the vascular toxins surveyed in this chapter are summarized in Table 15.3. Although differences in cellular and subcellular targets are noted, many of these toxins share the ability to modulate growth and differentiation of vascular cells. Some of these chemicals require metabolic activation for the induction of toxicity, while others cause deleterious effects by virtue of their high chemical reactivity. Not discussed in this chapter were the vascular toxicities mediated by non-specific alterations of membrane function upon exposure to alcohols and solvents, and the hypertensive episodes induced by a variety of autonomic agents. As highlighted throughout the chapter, vasculotoxic insult is potentially associated with injury to one or more of the cell types within the vessel wall. Toxicity often involves the interplay of multiple cellular and non-cellular factors. The ultimate consequences of toxic challenge are influenced by the repair capacity of target cells and endocrine/paracrine influences on the tissue.

In recent years, the notion that toxic insult plays a significant role in the pathogenesis of vascular disorders, as well as various target organ-specific toxicities, has fueled interest in vascular toxicology. In attempting to unravel the cellular and molecular mechanisms of vasculotoxic insult, investigators must recognize the large degree of structural and functional heterogeneity that characterize the vascular system. Such differences add a level of complexity to the study of vascular toxicities which is often disregarded.

*Table 15.3* Selected chemicals with prominent vascular toxicity

| Chemical | Source | Putative mechanism of action |
|---|---|---|
| Allylamine | Synthetic precursor/ antifungal analogs | Bioactivation of parent compound by amine oxidase to acrolein and hydrogen peroxide; smooth muscle cell lysis |
| Butadiene | Synthetic precursor | Endothelial injury |
| Carbon disulfide | Fumigant, solvent | Metabolic disturbances in glucose/ lipid metabolism, protein cross-linking |
| Carbon monoxide | Environmental | Carboxyhemoglobin formation with resulting tissue hypoxia; modulation of second messenger systems in vascular smooth muscle cells |
| Catecholamines | Endogenous amines | Adrenergic receptor-mediated alterations of contractile and proliferative behavior in vascular endothelial and/or smooth muscle cells |
| Dinitrotoluene | Synthetic precursor | Bioactivation-related changes of DNA synthesis in vascular smooth muscle cells |
| Hydrazinobenzoic acid | Constituent of *Agaricus bisporus* | Unknown; potential involvement of free radical-mediated genotoxicity |
| Metals | Environmental | Interference with cellular sulfhydryl, amino and phosphate residues; interference with calcium-mediated cellular events |
| Nicotine | Tobacco smoke | Modulation of DNA synthesis in vascular endothelial and/or smooth muscle cells, altered signal transduction |
| Polycyclic aromatic hydrocarbons | Tobacco smoke/ environmental | Cytochrome P450-mediated bioactivation of reactive metabolic intermediates which bind to DNA in vascular smooth muscle cells |
| T-2 toxin | *Fusarium* mycotoxin | Endothelial and smooth muscle cell injury; modulation of smooth muscle cell proliferation |
| TCDD | Environmental | Modulation of lipid metabolism and hyperlipoproteinemia, altered signal transduction |
| Vitamin D | Dietary | Medial toxin, modulation of cyclic nucleotide metabolism |

## Acknowledgments

The authors' research cited in this chapter was supported in part by grants from the National Institute of Environmental Health Sciences (ES 04849, ES 09106) and from Research Development Funds by the Texas Agricultural Experiment Station. The contributions of present and past members of the laboratory are gratefully acknowledged.

## References

Abby, S.L., Harris, I.M., and Harris, K.M. 1998. Homocysteine and cardiovascular disease. *Journal of the American Board of Family Practitioners* 11: 391–398.

Ahlgren-Beckendorf, J.A., Maggio, W.W., Chen, F., and Kent, T.A. 1993. Neurofibromatosis 1 mRNA expression in blood vessels. *Biochemical and Biophysical Research Communications* 197: 1019–1024.

Albert, R.E., Vanderlaan, M., Burns, F.J., and Nishizumi, M. 1977. Effect of carcinogens on chicken atherosclerosis. *Cancer Research* 37: 2232–2235.

Alster, P. and Wennmalm, A. 1983. Effect of nicotine on prostacyclin formation in rat aorta. *European Journal of Pharmacology* 86: 441–446.

Astrup, P., Hellung-Larson, P., Kjeldsen, K., and Mellemgaard, K. 1966. The effect of tobacco smoking on the dissociation curve of oxyhemoglobin – investigations in patients with occlusive arterial diseases and in normal subjects. *Scandinavian Journal Clinical Laboratory Investigation* 18: 450–460.

Astrup, P., Kjeldson, K., and Wanstrup, J. 1967. Enhancing influence of carbon monoxide on the development of atheromatosis in cholesterol-fed rabbits. *Journal of Atherosclerotic Research* 7: 343–354.

Awasthi, S. and Boor, P.J. 1998. Allylamine and beta-aminopropionitrile-induced vascular injury: enhanced expression of high-molecular-weight protein. *Journal of Toxicology and Environmental Health* 53: 61–76.

Babior, B.M., Curnette, J.T., and McMurick, B.J. 1976. The particulate superoxide-forming system from human neutrophils: properties of the system and further evidence supporting its participation in the respiratory burst. *Journal of Clinical Investigation* 58: 989–996.

Baird, W.M., Chemerys, R., Grinspan, J.B., *et al.* 1980. Benzo(a)pyrene metabolism in bovine aortic endothelial and bovine lung fibroblast-like cell cultures. *Cancer Research* 40: 1781–1786.

Barhoumi, R., Mouneimme, Y., Ramos, K.S., *et al.* 1999. Analysis of benzo(a)pyrene partitioning and cytotoxicity in a rat liver cell line. *Toxocological Sciences* 53: 264–270.

Batuman, V., Landy, E., Maesaka, J.K., and Wedeen, R.P. 1983. Contribution of lead to hypertension with renal impairment. *New England Journal of Medicine* 309: 17–21.

Bauch, H.J., Grunwald, J., Vischer, P., *et al.* 1987. A possible role of catecholamines in atherogenesis and subsequent complications of atherosclerosis. *Experimental Pathology* 31: 193–204.

Beard, R.R. and Noe, J.T. 1981. Aliphatic and alicyclic amines. In *Patty's Industrial Hygiene and Toxicology*, Vol. II. Clayton, G.D., and Clayton, F.E. (eds), pp. 3135–3173. Wiley, New York.

Beckner, J.S., Hudgins, P.M., and Egle, J.L. 1974. Effects of acetaldehyde, propionaldehyde, formaldehyde and acrolein on contractility, $^{14}$C-norepinephrine and $^{45}$calcium binding in isolated smooth muscle. *Research Communications in Chemistry Pathology and Pharmacology* 9: 471–488.

Beevers, D.G., Campbell, B.C., Goldberts, A., *et al.* 1976. Blood cadmium in hypertensives and normotensives. *Lancet* 2: 12222–12224.

Benditt, E.P. 1974. Evidence for a monoclonal origin of human atherosclerotic plaque and some implications. *Circulation* 50: 650–652.

Benditt, E.P. and Benditt, J.M. 1973. Evidence for a monoclonal origin of human atherosclerotic plaques. *Proceedings of the National Academy of Sciences of the United States of America* 70: 1753–1756.

Benditt, E.P., Barrett, T., and McDougall, J.K. 1983. Viruses in the etiology of atherosclerosis. *Proceedings of the National Academy of Sciences of the United States of America* 80: 6386–6389.

Berk, B.C., Brock, T.A., Webb, R.C., *et al.* 1985. Epidermal growth factor, a vascular smooth muscle mitogen induces rat aortic contraction. *Journal of Clinical Investigation* 75: 1083–1086.

Berk, B.C., Alexander, R.W., Brock, T.A., *et al.* 1986. Vasoconstriction: A new activity for platelet-derived growth factors. *Science* 232: 87–90.

Birnie, D.H., Holme, E.R., McKay, I.C., *et al.* 1998. Association between antibodies to heat shock protein 65 and coronary atherosclerosis. Possible mechanism of action of *Helicobacter pylori* and other bacterial infections in increasing cardiovascular risk. *European Heart Journal* 19: 387–394.

Bishop, C.T., Mirza, Z., Crapo, J.D., and Freeman, B.A. 1985. Free radical damage to cultured porcine aortic endothelial cells and lung fibroblasts: Modulation by culture conditions. *In Vitro Cellular and Developmental Biology* 21: 21–25.

Blasi, F., Ranzi, M.L., Erba, M. *et al.* 1996. No evidence for the presence of Helicobacter pylori in the atherosclerotic plaques in abdominal aortic aneurysm specimens. *Atherosclerosis* 126: 339–340.

Boerth, N.J., Dey, N.B., Cornwell, T.L., and Lincoln, T.M. 1997. Cyclic GMP-dependent protein kinase regulates vascular smooth muscle cell phenotype. *Journal of Vascular Research* 34: 245–259.

Bond, J.A., Kocan, R.M., Benditt, E.P., and Juchau, M.R. 1979. Metabolism of benzo(a)pyrene and 7,12-dimethylbenz(a)anthracene in cultured human fetal aortic smooth muscle cells. *Life Sciences* 25: 425–430.

Bond, J.A., Hsueh-Ying, L.Y., Majesky, M.W., *et al.* 1980. Metabolism of benzo(a)pyrene and 7,12-dimethylbenz(a)anthracene in chicken aortas: Monooxygenation, bioactivation to mutagens, and covalent binding to DNA *in vitro*. *Toxicology and Applied Pharmacology* 52: 323–335.

Boor, P.J. 1985. Allylamine cardiovascular toxicity. V. Tissue distribution and toxicokinetics after oral administration. *Toxicology* 35: 167–177.

Boor, P.J., Moslen, M.J., and Reynolds, E.S. 1979. Allylamine cardiotoxicity. I. Sequence of pathologic events. *Toxicology and Applied Pharmacology* 50: 581–592.

Boor, P.J., Hysmith, R.M., and Sanduja, R. 1990. A role for a new vascular enzyme in the metabolism of xenobiotic amines. *Circulation Research* 66: 249–252.

Bral, C.M. and Ramos, K.S. 1997. Identification of benzo(a)pyrene-inducible *cis*-acting elements within *c-Ha-ras* transcriptional regulatory sequences. *Molecular Pharmacology* 52: 974–982.

Brune, B. and Ullrich, V. 1987. Inhibition of platelet aggregation by carbon monoxide is mediated by activation of guanylate cyclase. *Molecular Pharmacology* 32: 497–504.

Buffoni, F. 1983. Biochemical pharmacology of amine oxidases. *Trends in Pharmacological Sciences* 4: 313–315.

Bull, H.A., Pittilo, R.M., Blow, D.J., *et al*. 1985. The effects of nicotine on $PGI_2$ production by rat aortic endothelium. *Thrombosis and Haemostasis* 54: 472–474.

Campbell, G.R. and Campbell, J.H. 1985. Smooth muscle phenotypic changes in arterial wall homeostasis: implications for the pathogenesis of atherosclerosis. *Experimental and Molecular Pathology* 42: 139–162.

Campbell, G.R. and Chamley-Campbell, J.H. 1981. The cellular pathobiology of atherosclerosis. *Pathology* 13: 423–440.

Cannon, M., Smith, K.E., and Carter, C.J. 1976. Prevention, by ribosome-bound nascent polyphenylalanine chains, of the functional interaction of T-2 with its receptor site. *Biochemical Journal*. 156: 289–294.

Caprino, L., Togna, G., and Togna, A.R. 1979. Cadmium-induced platelet hypersensitivity to aggregating agents. *Pharmacological Research Communications* 11: 731–737.

Caprino, L., Togna, A.R., Cebo, B., *et al*. 1983. In vitro effects of mercury on platelet aggregation, thromboxane, and vascular prostacyclin production. *Archives of Toxicology* (Suppl.) 6: 48–51.

Carafoli, E. 1984. How calcium crosses plasma membrane including the sarcolemma. In *Calcium Antagonists and Cardiovascular Disease*. Opie, L.H. (ed.), pp. 29–41. Raven Press, New York.

Chadwick, R.W., Elizabeth George, E., Kohan, M.J., *et al*. 1993. Potentiation of 2,6-dinitrotoluene genotoxicity in Fischer-344 rats by pretreatment with Aroclor 1254. *Toxicology* 80: 153–171.

Cheung, W.Y. 1984. Calmodulin: its potential role in cell proliferation and heavy metal toxicity. *Federation Proceedings* 43: 2995–2999.

Chipino, G., Constantine, S., and Cirla, A.M. 1968. Changes induced by cadmium, zinc, and lead on renal and peripheral vascular resistance in the anesthetized rabbit. *Medicina del Lavoro* 59: 522–533.

Chrysant, S.G. 1998. Vascular remodeling: the role of angiotensin-converting enzyme inhibitors. *American Heart Journal* 135: S21–S30.

Cobarn, R.F. and Mayers, L.B. 1971. Myoglobin oxygen tension determined from measurements of carboxyhemoglobin in skeletal muscle. *American Journal of Physiology* 220: 66–74.

Collins, J.J., Elwell, M.R., Lamb, J.C., *et al*. 1988. Subchronic toxicity of orally administered (gavage and dosed-fed) theophylline in Fischer 344 rats and B6C3F$_1$ mice. *Fundamental and Applied Toxicology* 11: 472–484.

Cox, C., Que Hee, S.S., and Lynch, D.W. 1996. Urinary 2-thiothiazolidine-4-carboxylic acid (TTCA) as the major urinary marker of carbon disulfide vapor exposure in rats. *Toxicology and Industrial Health* 12: 81–92.

Cox, L.R. and Ramos, K. 1990. Allylamine-induced phenotypic modulation of aortic smooth muscle cells. *Journal of Experimental Pathology* 71: 11–18.

Cox, L.R., Murphy, S.K., and Ramos, K. 1990. Modulation of phosphoinositide metabolism in aortic smooth muscle cells by allylamine. *Experimental and Molecular Pathology* 53: 52–63.

Csonka, E., Somogyi, A., Augustin, J., *et al*. 1985. The effect of nicotine on cultured cells of vascular origin. *Virchows Archives* 407: 441–447.

Dalton, T.P., Dieter, M.Z., Miller, M., Yunker, R., Carty, M., Shertzer, H., Nebert, D.W., and Puga, A. 1999. TCDD increases the production of vasoactive eicosanoids and cofractionates with lipoprotein particles in hyperlipidemic mice. *The Toxicologist* 48: 219.

DeBlois, D., Schwartz, S.M., van Kleef, E.M., *et al.* 1996. Chronic alpha 1-adrenoreceptor stimulation increases DNA synthesis in rat arterial wall. Modulation of responsiveness after vascular injury. *Arteriosclerosis, Thrombosis, and Vascular Biology* 16: 1122–1129.

Delmolino, L.M. and Castellot, Jr., J.J. 1997. Heparin suppressed sgk, an early response gene in proliferating vascular smooth muscle cells. *Journal of Cellular Physiology* 173: 371–379.

Denko, N.C., Giaccia, A., Stringer, J.R., and Stambrook, P.J. 1994. The human Ha-ras oncogene induces genomic instability in murine fibroblasts within one cell cycle. *Proceedings of the National Academy of Sciences of the United States of America* 91: 5124–5128.

Dent, J.G., Schnell, S.R., and Guest, D. 1981. Metabolism of 2,4-dinitrotoluene in rat hepatic microsomes and cecal flora. In *Proceedings of the Second International Symposium on Biologically Reactive Intermediates: Chemical Mechanisms and Biologic Effects*, pp. 431–436. Plenum, New York.

Dhalla, N.S., Yates, J.C., Lee, S.L., and Singh, A. 1978. Functional and subcellular changes in the isolated rat heart perfused with oxidized isoproterenol. *Journal of Molecular and Cellular Cardiology* 10: 31–41.

Doyle, J.J., Bernhoft, R.A., and Sandstead, H.H. 1975. The effects of a low level of dietary cadmium on blood pressure, $^{24}$Na, $^{42}$K and water retention in growing rats. *Journal of Laboratory and Clinical Medicine* 86: 57–83.

Durante, W., Kroll, M.H., Christodoulides, N., and Peyton, K.J. 1997. Nitric oxide induces heme oxygenase-1 gene expression and carbon monoxide production in vascular smooth muscle cells. *Circulation Research* 80: 557–64.

Ellis, H.V., Hough, C.B., Dacre, Y.C., and Lee, C.C. 1978. Chronic toxicity of 2,4-dinitrotoluene in the rat. *Toxicology and Applied Pharmacology* 45: 245.

Escalante, B., Sessa, W.C., Falck, J.R., Yadagiri, P., and Schwartzman, M.L. 1990. Cytochrome P450-dependent arachidonic acid metabolites, 19- and 20-hydroxy-eicosatetraenoic acids enhance sodium–potassium ATPase activity in vascular smooth muscle. *Journal of Cardiovascular Pharmacology* 16: 438–443.

Ferrario, J.B., DeLeon, I.R., and Tracy, R.E. 1985. Evidence for toxic anthropogenic chemicals in human thrombogenic coronary plaques. *Archives of Environmental Contamination and Toxicology* 14: 529–534.

Feuerstein, G., Goldstein, D.S., Ramwell, R.O., *et al.* 1985. Cardiorespiratory, sympathetic and biochemical responses to T-2 toxin in the guinea pig and rat. *Journal of Pharmacology and Experimental Therapeutics* 232: 786–794.

Fine, B.P., Vetrano, T., Skurnick, J., and Ty, A. 1988. Blood pressure elevation in young dogs during low level lead poisoning. *Toxicology and Applied Pharmacology* 93: 388–393.

Folsom, A.R., Nieto, F.J., Sorlie, P., *et al.* 1998. *Helicobacter pylori* seropositivity and coronary heart disease incidence. Atherosclerosis Risk In Communities (ARIC) Study Investigators. *Circulation* 98: 845–850.

Frid, M.G., Dempsey, E.C., Durmowicz, A.G., and Stenmark, K.R. 1997. Smooth muscle cell heterogeneity in pulmonary and systemic vessels. Importance in vascular disease. *Arteriosclerosis, Thrombosis, and Vascular Biology* 17: 1203–1209.

Friedl, H.P., Till, G.O., Ryan, U.S., and Ward, P.A. 1989. Mediator-induced activation of xanthine oxidase in endothelial cells. *FASEB Journal* 3: 2512–2518.

Fujiwara, Y., Kaji, T., Yamamoto, C., *et al.* 1995. Stimulatory effect of lead on the proliferation of cultured vascular smooth-muscle cells. *Toxicology*. 98: 105–110.

Gamberini, M., Cidade, M.R., Valotta, L.A., *et al.* 1998. Contribution of hydrazine-derived alkyl radicals to cytotoxic transformation induced in normal c-myc-overexpression mouse fibroblasts. *Carcinogenesis* 19: 147–155.

Georing, P.L. and Klaassen, C.D. 1984. Zinc-induced tolerance to cadmium toxicity. *Toxicology and Applied Pharmacology* 74: 299–307.

Ghilarducci, D.P. and Tjeerdema, R.S. 1995. Fate and effects of acrolein *Reviews of Environmental Contamination and Toxicology* 144: 95–146.

Gold, H. 1961. Production of arteriosclerosis in the rat: Effect of x-ray and high-fat diet. *Archives of Pathology* 71: 46/268–51/273.

Gordon, D. and Schwartz, S.M. Arterial smooth muscle differentiation. 1987. In *Vascular Smooth Muscle in Culture*, Vol. I. Campbell, J.H., and Campbell, G.R. (eds), pp. 1–14. CRC Press, Boca Raton, FL.

Gran, C.M., Sadhu, D.N., and Ramos, K.S. 1996. Transcriptional activation of the c-Ha-Ras protooncogene in vascular smooth muscle cells by benzo(a)pyrene. *In Vitro Cellular and Developmental Biology* 32: 599–601.

Granger, H.J., Schelling, M.E., Lewis, R.E., *et al.* 1988. Physiology and pathobiology of the microcirculation. *American Journal of Otolaryngology* 9: 264–277.

Graser, T., Vedernikov, Y.P., and Li, D.S. 1990. Study on the mechanism of carbon monoxide induced endothelium-independent relaxation in porcine coronary artery and vein. *Biomedica et Biochimica Acta* 49: 293–296.

Grimm, M., Weidmann, P., Keusch, G., *et al.* 1980. Norepinephrine clearance and pressure effect in normal and hypertensive man. *Klinische Wochenschrift* 58: 1175–1181.

Gross, J.L., Moscatelli, D., and Rifkin, D.B. 1983. Increased capillary endothelial cell protease activity in response to angiogenic stimuli *in vitro*. *Proceedings of the National Academy of Sciences of the United States of America* 80: 2623–2627.

Grossman, S.L., Alipui, C., and Ramos, K. 1990. Further characterization of the metabolic activation of allylamine to acrolein in rat vascular tissue. *In Vitro Toxicology* 3: 303–307.

Grunwald, J., Schaper, W., Mey, J., and Hauss, W.H. 1982. Special characteristics of cultured smooth muscle cell subtypes of hypertensive and diabetic rats. *Artery* 11: 1–14.

Grunwald, J. and Haudenschild, C.C. 1984. Intimal injury *in vivo* activates vascular smooth muscle cell migration and explant outgrowth *in vitro*. *Arteriosclerosis* 4: 183–188.

Guzman, R.J., Loquvam, G.S., Kodama, J.K., and Hine, C.H. 1961. Myocarditis produced by allylamines. *Archives of Environmental Health* 2: 62–73.

Habermann, E. and Richardt, G. 1986. Intracellular calcium binding proteins as targets for heavy metal ions. *Trends in Pharmacological Sciences* 7: 298–300.

Halvorsen, B., Brude, I., Drevon, C.A., *et al.* 1996. Effect of homocysteine on copper ion-catalyzed, azo compound-initiated, and mononuclear cell-mediated oxidative modification of low density lipoprotein. *Journal of Lipid Research* 37: 1591–1600.

Hamet, P., deBlois, D., Dam, T.V., *et al.* 1996. Apoptosis and vascular wall remodeling in hypertension. *Canadian Journal of Physiology and Pharmacology* 74: 850–861.

Harker, L.A., Harlan, J.M., and Ross, R. 1983. Effect of sulfinpyrazanone on homocysteine-induced endothelial injury and arteriosclerosis in baboons. *Circulation Research* 53: 731–739.

Hayaishi, O. 1969. Enzyme hydroxylation. *Annual Review of Biochemistry* 38: 21–44.

Heinecke, J.W. 1987. Free radical modification of low-density lipoprotein: mechanisms and biological consequences. *Free Radical Biology and Medicine* 3: 65–73.

Helin, P., Lorenzen, I., Garbarsch, C., and Matthiessen, N.E. 1970. Arteriosclerosis in rabbit aorta induced by noradrenaline. *Atherosclerosis* 12: 125–132.

Hernandez, F.J., Stanley, J.M., Ranganath, K.A., and Rubinstein, A.I. 1979. Primary leiomyosarcoma of the aorta. *American Journal of Surgical Pathology* 3: 251–254.

Hiebert, L.M. and Liu, J.M. 1990. Heparin protects cultured arterial endothelial cells from damage by toxic oxygen metabolites. *Atherosclerosis* 83: 47–51.

Hine, C.H., Kodama, J.K., Guzman, R.J., and Loquvam, G.S. 1960. The toxicity of allylamines. *Archives of Environmental Health* 1: 343–352.

Hornstra, G., Barth, C.A., Galli, C., *et al.* 1998. Functional food science and the cardiovascular system. *British Journal of Nutrition* 80 (Suppl.) 1: S113–46.

Hu, Z.W., Shi, X.Y., Okazaki, M., and Hoffman, B.B. 1995. Angiotensin II induces transcription and expression of alpha1-adrenergic receptors in vascular smooth muscle cells. *American Journal of Physiology* 268: H1006–H1014.

Hu, Z.W., Shi, X.Y., and Hoffman, B.B. 1996. Insulin and insulin-like growth factor I differentially induce alpha1-adrenergic receptor subtypes expression in rat vascular smooth muscle cells. *Journal of Clinical Investigation* 98: 1826–34.

Hudlicka, O. 1980. Development of microcirculation: capillary growth and adaptation. In: *Handbook of Physiology: A Critical Comprehensive Presentation of Physiological Knowledge and Concepts*, Vol. IV. Bohr, D.R., Somlyo, A.P., Sparks, H.V., and Geiger, S.R. (eds), pp. 165–216. Waverly Press, Baltimore, MD.

Huff, J.E., Melnick, R.L., Solleveld, H.A., *et al.* 1984. Multiple organ carcinogenicity of 1,3-butadiene in B6C3F$_1$ mice after 60 weeks of inhalation exposure. *Science* 227: 548–549.

Hughes, A.D., Clumm, G.F., Refson, J., and Demoliou-Mason, C. 1996. Platelet-derived growth factor (PDGF): Actions and mechanisms in vascular smooth muscle. *General Pharmacology* 27: 1079–1089.

Hysmith, R.M. and Boor, P.J. 1985. Allylamine cardiovascular toxicity. VI. Subcellular distribution in rat aortas. *Toxicology* 35: 179–187.

Isner, J.M., Kearney, M., Bortman, S., and Passeri, J. 1995. Apoptosis in human atherosclerosis and restenosis. *Circulation.* 91: 2703–2711.

Jaffe, E.A. 1985. Physiologic functions of normal endothelial cells. *Annals of the New York Academy of Sciences* 454: 279–291.

Janes, S.M., Mu, D., Wemmer, D., *et al.* 1990. A new redox cofactor in eukaryotic enzymes: 6-hydroxydopa at the active site of bovine serum amine oxidase. *Science* 248: 981–987.

Jhaveri, R., Lavorgna, L., Dube, S.K., Glass, L., Khan, F., and Evans, H.E. 1979. Relationship of blood pressure to blood lead concentrations in small children. *Pediatrics* 63: 674–676.

Jokinen, M.P., Clarkson, T.B., and Prichard, R.W. 1985. Recent advances in molecular pathology. Animal models in atherosclerosis research. *Experimental and Molecular Pathology* 42: 1–28.

Kalayoglu, M.V. and Byrne, G.I. 1998a. A *Chlamydia pneumoniae* component that induces macrophage foam cell formation is chlamydial lipopolysaccharide. *Infection and Immunity* 66: 5067–5072.

Kalayoglu, M.V. and Byrne, G.I. 1998b. Induction of macrophage foam cell formation by *Chlamydia pneumoniae*. *Journal of Infectious Diseases* 177: 725–729.

Kalyanaraman, B. and Sinha, B.K. 1985. Free radical-mediated activation of hydrazine derivatives. *Environmental Health Perspectives* 64: 179–184.

Kerzee, K. and Ramos, S.R. 2000. Activation of c-H-ras by benzo(a)pyrene in vascular smooth muscle cells involves redox stress and aryl hydrocarbon receptor. *Molecular Pharmacology* 58: 152–158.

King, G.L. and Johnson, S.H. 1985. Receptor-mediated transport of insulin across endothelial cells. *Science* 227: 1583–1586.

Koh, E., Morimoto, S., Fukuo, K., *et al.* 1988. 1,25-Dihydroxyvitamin $D_3$ binds specifically to rat vascular smooth muscle cells and stimulates their proliferation *in vitro*. *Life Sciences* 42: 215–223.

Kol, A., Sukhova, G.K., Lichtman, A.H., and Libby, P. 1998. Chlamydial heat shock protein 60 localizes in human atheroma and regulates macrophage tumor necrosis factor-alpha and matrix metalloproteinase expression. *Circulation* 98: 300–307.

Kontos, H.A., Wei, E.P., Dietrich, W.D., *et al.* 1981. Mechanism of cerebral arteriolar abnormalities after acute hypertension. *American Journal of Physiology* 240: H511–H527.

Kopp, S.J., Glonek, T., Perry, Jr., H.M., *et al.* 1982. Cardiovascular actions of cadmium at environmental exposure levels. *Science* 217: 837–839.

Kourembanas, S., Morita, T., Liu, Y., and Christou, H. 1997. Mechanisms by which oxygen regulates gene expression and cell–cell interaction in the vasculature. *Kidney International* 51: 438–43.

Kroon, P.A. 1997. Cholesterol and atherosclerosis. *Australian and New Zealand Journal of Medicine* 27: 492–496.

Kukreja, R.S., Datta, B.N., and Chakravarti, R.N. 1981. Catecholamine-induced aggravation of aortic and coronary atherosclerosis in monkeys. *Atherosclerosis* 40: 291–298.

Kurppa, K., Hietanen, E., Klockars, M., *et al.* 1984. Chemical exposures at work and cardiovascular morbidity: Atherosclerosis, ischemic heart disease, hypertension, cardiomyopathy and arrhythmias. *Scandinavian Journal of Work, Environment and Health* 10: 381–388.

Kusuhara, M., Chait, A., Cader, A., and Berk, B.C. 1997. Oxidized LDL stimulates mitogen activated protein kinases in smooth muscle cells and macrophages. *Arteriosclerosis Thrombosis and Vascular Biology* 17: 141–148.

Kutzman, R.S., Wehner, R.W., and Haber, S.B. 1984. Selected responses of hypertension-sensitive and resistant rats to inhaled acrolein. *Toxicology* 31: 53–65.

Lalich, J.J., Allen, J.R., and Paik, W.C.W. 1972. Myocardial fibrosis and smooth muscle cell hyperplasia in coronary arteries of allylamine-fed rats. *American Journal of Pathology* 66: 225–233.

Leonard, T.B., Graichen, M.E., and Popp, J.A. 1987. Dinitrotoluene isomer-specific hepatocarcinogenesis in F344 rats. *Journal of the National Cancer Institute* 79: 1313–1319.

Levene, C.I., Barlet, C.P., Fornieri, C., and Heale, G. 1985. Effect of hypoxia and carbon monoxide on collagen synthesis in cultured porcine and bovine aortic endothelium. *British Journal of Experimental Pathology* 66: 399–408.

Levine, R.J. 1987. Dinitrotoluene: Human atherogen, carcinogen, neither or both? *Chemical Industry Institute of Toxicology* 7: 2–5.

Levine, R.J., Andjelkovich, D.A., Kersteter, S.L., *et al.* 1986. Heart disease in workers exposed to dinitrotoluene. *Journal of Occupational Medicine* 28: 811–816.

Levy, J., Blakeston, C., Seymour, C.A., and Camm, A.J. 1995. Association of *Helicobacter pylori* and *Chlamydia pneumoniae* infections with coronary heart disease and cardiovascular risk factors. *British Medical Journal* 311: 711–714.

Lin, H. and McGrath, J.J. 1988. Vasodilating effects of carbon monoxide. *Drug and Chemical Toxicology* 11: 371–385.

Little, T.L., Xia, J., and Duling, B.R. 1995. Dye tracers define differential endothelial and smooth muscle coupling patterns within the arteriolar wall. *Circulation Research.* 76: 498–504.

Long, R.M. and Rickert, D.E. 1982. Metabolism and excretion of 2,6-dinitro[$^{14}$C]toluene *in vivo* and in isolated perfused rat livers. *Drug Metabolism and Disposition* 10: 455–458.

Lovati, M.R., Galbussera, M., Franceschini, G., *et al.* 1984. Increased plasma and aortic triglycerides in rabbits after acute administration of 2,3,7,8-tetrachlorodibenzo-p-dioxin. *Toxicology and Applied Pharmacology* 75: 91–97.

Lu, K.P. and Ramos, K.S. 1998. Identification of genes differentially expressed in vascular smooth muscle cells following benzo(a)pyrene challenge: Implications for chemical atherogenesis. *Biochemical and Biophysical Research Communications* 253: 828–833.

Lyles, G.A. 1996. Mammalian plasma and tissue-bound semicarbazide-sensitive amine oxidases: biochemical, pharmacological and toxicological aspects. *International Journal of Biochemistry and Cell Biology* 28: 259–274.

McCord, J.M. 1985. Oxygen-derived free radicals in post ischemic tissue injury. *New England Journal of Medicine* 312: 159–163.

McCully, K.S. 1996. Homocysteine and vascular disease. *Nature Medicine* 2: 386–389.

McFaul, S.J. and McGrath, J.J. 1987. Studies on the mechanism of carbon monoxide-induced vasodilation in the isolated perfused rat heart. *Toxicology and Applied Pharmacology* 87: 464–473.

McGill, H.C. 1988. The pathogenesis of atherosclerosis. *Clinical Chemistry* 34: 33–39.

Machlin, L.J. and Bendich, A. 1987. Free radical tissue damage: protective role of antioxidant nutrients. *FASEB Journal* 1: 441–445.

McManus, B.M., Toth, B., and Patil, K.D. 1987. Aortic rupture and aortic smooth muscle tumors in mice: Induction by p-hydrazinobenzoic acid hydrochloride of the cultivated mushroom *Agaricus bisporus. Laboratory Investigation* 57: 78–85.

Majesky, M., Yang, H.Y., Benditt, E., and Juchau, M. 1983. Carcinogenesis and atherogenesis: differences in mono-oxygenase inducibility and bioactivation of benzo(a)pyrene in aortic and hepatic tissue of atherosclerosis-susceptible versus resistant pigeons. *Carcinogenesis* 4: 647–652.

Majesky, M.W., Reidy, M.A., Benditt, E.P., and Juchau, M.R. 1985. Focal smooth muscle proliferation in the aortic intima produced by an initiation–promotion sequence. *Proceedings of the National Academy of Sciences of the United States of America* 82: 3450–3454.

Markle, H.V. 1997. Coronary artery disease associated with *Helicobacter pylori* infection is at least partially due to inadequate folate status. *Medical Hypotheses* 49: 289–292.

Markus, H.S. and Mendall, M.A. 1998. *Helicobacter pylori* infection: a risk factor for ischemic cerebrovascular disease and carotid atheroma. *Journal of Neurology, Neurosurgery and Psychiatry* 64: 104–107.

Matsubara, T. and Ziff, M. 1986. Superoxide anion release by human endothelial cells: Synergism between a phorbol ester and a calcium ionophore. *Journal of Cellular Physiology* 127: 207–210.

Maxwell, K., Vinters, H.V., Berliner, J.A., *et al.* 1986. Effect of inorganic lead on some functions of the cerebral microvessel endothelium. *Toxicology and Applied Pharmacology* 84: 389–399.

Medeiros, D.M. and Pellum, L.K. 1985. Blood pressure and hair cadmium, lead, copper, and zinc concentrations in Mississippi adolescents. *Bulletin of Environmental Contamination and Toxicology* 34: 163–169.

Meijer, G.W., Beems, R.B., Janssen, G.B., *et al.* 1996. Cadmium and atherosclerosis in rabbit: reduced atherogenesis by superseding of iron? *Food and Chemical Toxicology* 34: 611–621.

Mendall, M.A., Goggin, P.M., Molineaux, N., *et al.* 1994. Relation of *Helicobacter pylori* infection and coronary heart disease. *British Heart Journal* 71: 437–439.

Miano, J.M., Tota, R.R., Niksa, V., *et al.* 1990. Early proto-oncogene expression in rat aortic smooth muscle cells following endothelial removal. *American Journal of Pathology* 137: 761–765.

Milili, J.J., LaFlare, R.G., and Nemir, P. 1981. Leiomyosarcoma of the abdominal aorta: a case report. *Surgery* 89: 631–634.

Miller, R.A. and Boorman, G.A. 1990. Morphology of neoplastic lesions induced by 1,3-butadiene in B6C3F$_1$ mice. *Environmental Health Perspectives* 86: 37–48.

Mirsalis, J.C., Hamm, T.E., Sherrill, J.M., and Butterworth, B.E. 1982. Role of gut flora in the genotoxicity of dinitrotoluene. *Nature* 295: 322–323.

Misra, P., Srivastava, S.K., Singhal, S.S., *et al.* 1995. Glutathione S-transferase 8–8 is localized in smooth muscle cells of rat aorta and is induced in an experimental model of atherosclerosis. *Toxicology and Applied Pharmacology* 133: 27–33.

Morey, A.K., Pedram, A., Razandi, M., *et al.* 1997. Estrogen and progesterone inhibit vascular smooth muscle proliferation. *Endocrinology* 138: 3330–3339.

Morita, T. and Kourembanas, S. 1995. Endothelial cell expression of vasoconstrictors and growth factors is regulated by smooth muscle cell-derived carbon monoxide. *Journal of Clinical Investigation* 96: 2676–2682.

Morita, T., Mitsialis, S.A., Koike, H., *et al.* 1997. Carbon monoxide controls the proliferation of hypoxic vascular smooth muscle cells. *Journal of Biological Chemistry* 272: 32804–32809.

Muhlestein, J.B. 1998. Bacterial infections and atherosclerosis. *Journal of Investigative Medicine* 46: 396–402.

Murad, F. 1986. Cyclic guanosine monophosphate as a mediator of vasodilation. *Journal of Clinical Investigations* 78: 1–5.

Murray, L.J., Bamford, K.B., O'Reilly, D.P., *et al.* 1995. *Helicobacter pylori* infection: relation with cardiovascular risk factors, ischemic heart disease, and social class. *British Heart Journal* 74: 497–501.

Murry, C.E., Gipaya, T.B., Benditt, E.P., and Schwartz, S.M. 1997. Monoclonality of smooth muscle cells in human atherosclerosis. *American Journal of Pathology* 151: 697–706.

Nabel, E.G., Yang, Z.Y., Plautz, G., *et al.* 1993. Recombinant fibroblast growth factor-1 promotes intimal hyperplasia and angiogenesis in arteries in-vivo. *Nature (London)* 362: 844–846.

Naftilan, A.J., Gilliland, G.K., Eldridge, C.S., and Kraft, A.S. 1990. Induction of the protooncogene c-jun by angiotensin II. *Molecular and Cellular Biology* 10: 5536–5540.

Nakaki, T., Nakayama, M., Yamamoto, S., and Kato, R. 1989. $\alpha_1$-Adrenergic stimulation and $\beta_2$-adrenergic inhibition of DNA synthesis in vascular smooth muscle cells. *Molecular Pharmacology* 37: 30–36.

Naseem, S.M. and Heald, F.P. 1987. Cytotoxicity of cholesterol oxides and their effects on cholesterol metabolism in cultured human aortic smooth muscle cells. *Biochemistry International* 14: 71–84.

Needleman, H.L., Schell, A.S., Bellinger, D., *et al.* 1990. The long-term effects of exposure to low doses of lead in childhood: An 11 year follow-up report. *New England Journal of Medicine* 322: 83–88.

Nemoto, N., Kawana, M., and Tokoyama, S. 1983. Effects of activation of UDP-glycuronyl transferase on metabolism of benzo(a)pyrene with rat liver microsomes. *Journal of Pharmacobiodynamics* 6: 105–113.

Nishida, K., Abiko, T., Ishihara, M., and Tomikawa, M. 1990. Arterial injury-induced smooth muscle cell proliferation in rats is accompanied by increase in polyamine synthesis and level. *Atherosclerosis* 83: 119–125.

Nishio, E. and Watanabe, Y. 1997. Homocysteine as a modulator of platelet-derived growth factor action in vascular smooth muscle cells: a possible role for hydrogen peroxide. *British Journal of Pharmacology* 122: 268–274.

Nishio, Y., Aiello, L.P., and King, G. 1994. Glucose induced genes in bovine aortic smooth muscle cells identified by mRNA differential display. *FASEB Journal* 8: 103–106.

Noda, A., Ishizawa, M., Ohino, K., *et al.* 1986. Relationship between oxidative metabolites of hydrazine and hydrazine-induced mutagenicity. *Toxicology Letters* 31: 131–137.

Ou, X. and Ramos, K.S. 1992. Modulation of aortic protein phosphorylation by benzo(a)pyrene: implications in PAH-induced atherogenesis. *Journal of Biochemical Toxicology* 7: 147–154.

Ou, X., Weber, T.J., Chapkin, R.S., and Ramos, K.S. 1995. Interference with protein kinase C-related signal transduction in vascular smooth muscle cells by benzo(a)pyrene. *Archives of Biochemistry and Biophysics* 318: 122–130.

Owens, G.K. and Schwartz, S.M. 1982. Alterations in vascular smooth muscle cells in the spontaneously hypertensive rat: Role of cellular hypertrophy, hyperploidy, and hyperplasia. *Circulation Research* 9: 264–277.

Owens, I.S., Koteen, G.M., Pelkonen, O., and Legraverend, C. 1978. Activation of certain benzo(a)pyrene phenols and the effect of some conjugating enzyme activities. In *Conjugation Reactions in Biotransformation*. Aito, A. (ed.), p. 39. Elsevier Biomedical, Amsterdam.

Paigen, B., Havens, M.B., and Morrow, A. 1985. Effect of 3-methylcholanthrene on the development of aortic lesions in mice. *Cancer Research* 45: 3850–3855.

Paigen, B., Holmes, P., Morrow, A., and Mitchell, D. 1986. Effects of 3-methylcholanthrene on atherosclerosis in two congenic strains of mice with different susceptibilities to methylcholanthrene-induced tumors. *Cancer Research* 46: 3321–3324.

Parrish, A.R. and Ramos, K.S. 1997. Differential processing of osteopontin characterizes the proliferative vascular smooth muscle cell phenotype induced by allylamine. *Journal of Cellular Biochemistry* 65: 267–275.

Pasceri, V., Cammarota, G., Patti, G., *et al.* 1998. Association of virulent *Helicobacter pylori* strains with ischemic heart disease. *Circulation* 97: 1675–1679.

Patel, J.M., Gordon, W.P., Nelson, S.D., and Leibman, K.C. 1983. Comparison of hepatic biotransformation and toxicity of allyl alcohol and [1,1–2H2] allyl alcohol in rats. *Drug Metabolism and Disposition* 11: 164–166.

Paule, W.J., Zemplenyi, T.K., Rounds, D.E., and Blankenhorn, D.H. 1976. Light and electron-microscopic characteristics of arterial smooth muscle cell cultures subjected to hypoxia or carbon monoxide. *Atherosclerosis* 25: 111–123.

Penn, A. and Snyder, C. 1988. Arteriosclerotic plaque development is "promoted" by polynuclear aromatic hydrocarbons. *Carcinogenesis* 9: 2185–2189.

Penn, A. and Snyder, C.A. 1996. 1,3 Butadiene, a vapor phase component of environmental tobacco smoke, accelerates arteriosclerotic plaque development. *Circulation* 93: 552–557.

Penn, A., Garte, S.J., Warren, L., *et al.* 1986. Transforming genes in human atherosclerotic plaque DNA. *Proceedings of the National Academy of Sciences of the United States of America* 83: 7951–7955.

Peng, S.-K., Taylor, C.B., Hill, J.C., and Morin, R.J. 1985. Cholesterol oxidation derivatives and arterial endothelial damage. *Atherosclerosis* 54: 121–133.

Peplonska, B., Szeszenia-Dabrowska, N., Sobala, W., and Wilczynska, U. 1996. A mortality study of workers with reported chronic occupational carbon disulfide poisoning. *International Journal of Occupational Medicine and Environmental Health* 9: 291–299.

Perry, H.M., Erlanger, M.W., and Perry, E.F. 1979. Increase in the systolic pressure of rats chronically fed cadmium. *Environmental Health Perspectives* 28: 251–260.

Perry, Jr., H.M. and Yunice, A. 1965. Acute pressor effects of intra-arterial cadmium and mercuric ions in anesthetized rats. *Proceedings of the Society for Experimental Biology and Medicine* 120: 805–808.

Perry, Jr., H.M., Erlanger, M., Yunice, A., and Perry, E.F. 1967. Mechanism of the acute hypertensive effect of intra-arterial cadmium and mercury in anesthetized rats. *Journal of Laboratory and Clinical Medicine* 70: 963–971.

Perry, Jr., H.M., Erlanger, M.W., and Perry, E.F. 1977. Elevated systolic pressure following chronic-level cadmium feeding. *American Journal of Physiology* 232: H114–H121.

Perry, Jr., H.M., Perry, E.F., and Erlanger, M.W. 1980. Possible influence of heavy metals in cardiovascular disease: An introduction and overview. *Journal of Environmental Pathology and Toxicology* 3: 195–203.

Perry, Jr., H.M., Erlanger, M.W., and Perry, E.F. 1983. Effect of a second metal on cadmium-induced hypertension. *Archives of Environmental Health* 8: 80–85.

Perry, H.M., Erlanger, M.W., Gustafsson, T.O., and Perry, E.F. 1989. Reversal of cadmium-induced hypertension by D-myo-inositol-1,2,6-triphosphate. *Journal of Toxicology and Environmental Health* 28: 151–159.

Pettersson, K., Bejne, B., Bjork, H., *et al.* 1990. Experimental sympathetic activation causes endothelial injury in the rabbit thoracic aorta via $\beta_1$-adrenoceptor activation. *Circulation Research* 67: 1027–1034.

Pinto, A., Abraham, N.G., and Mullane, K.M. 1986. Cytochrome P-450-dependent monooxygenase activity and endothelial-dependent relaxations induced by arachidonic acid. *Journal of Pharmacology and Experimental Therapeutics* 236: 445–451.

Poso, A., Wright, A.V., and Gynther, J. 1995. An empirical and theoretical study on mechanisms of mutagenic activity of hydrazine compounds. *Mutation Research* 332: 63–71.

Ramos, K. 1990. Cellular and molecular basis of xenobiotic-induced cardiovascular toxicity: Application of cell culture systems. In *Cellular and Molecular Toxicology and In Vitro Toxicology*. Acosta, D. (ed.), pp. 139–155. CRC Press, Boca Raton, FL.

Ramos, K., and Cox, L.R. 1987. Primary cultures of rat aortic endothelial and smooth muscle cells. I. An *in vitro* model to study xenobiotic-induced vascular cytotoxicity. *In Vitro Cell and Developmental Biology* 21: 495–504.

Ramos, K.S., and Thurlow, C.H. 1993. Comparative cytotoxic responses of cultured avian and rodent aortic smooth muscle cells to allylamine. *Journal of Toxicology and Environmental Health* 40: 61–76.

Ramos, K., Grossman, S.L., and Cox, L.R. 1988. Allylamine-induced vascular toxicity *in vitro*: Prevention by semicarbizide-sensitive amine oxidase inhibitors. *Toxicology and Applied Pharmacology* 96: 61–71.

Ramos, K.S., Lin, H., and McGrath, J.J. 1989. Modulation of cyclic guanosine monophosphate levels in cultured aortic smooth muscle cells by carbon monoxide. *Biochemical Pharmacology* 38: 1368–1370.

Ramos, K., McMahon, K.K., Alipui, C., and Demick, D. 1990. Modulation of smooth muscle cell proliferation by dinitrotoluene. In *Biologic Reductive Intermediates*, Vol. V. Witmer, C.M., Snyder, R.R., Jollow, D.J., Kaef, G.F., Kocsis, J.J., and Sipes, I.G. (eds), pp. 805–807. Plenum Press, New York.

Ramos, K.S., McMahon, K.K., Alipui, C., and Demick, D. 1991. Modulation of DNA synthesis in aortic smooth muscle cells by dinitrotoluene. *Cell Biology and Toxicology* 7: 111–128.

Ramos, K.S., Zhang, Y., Sadhu, D.N., and Chapkin, R.S. 1996. The induction of proliferative vascular smooth muscle cell phenotypes by benzo(a)pyrene is characterized by up-regulation of inositol phospholipid metabolism and *c-Ha-ras* gene expression. *Archives of Biochemistry and Biophysics* 332: 213–222.

Regnstrom, J., Jovinge, S., Bavenholm, P., *et al.* 1998. *Helicobacter pylori* seropositivity is not associated with inflammatory parameters, lipid concentrations and degree of coronary artery disease. *Journal of Internal Medicine* 243: 109–113.

Revis, N.W., Zinsmeister, A.R., and Bull, R. 1981. Atherosclerosis and hypertension induction by lead and cadmium ions: An effect prevented by calcium ion. *Proceedings of the National Academy of Sciences of the United States of America* 78: 6494–6498.

Revis, N.W., Bull, R., Laurie, D., and Schiller, C.A. 1984. The effectiveness of chemical carcinogens to induce atherosclerosis in the white carneau pigeon. *Toxicology* 32: 215–227.

Rhodin, J.A.G. 1980. Architecture of the vessel wall. In *Handbook of Physiology: A Critical Comprehensive Presentation of Physiological Knowledge and Concepts*, Vol. II. Bohr, D.F., Somlyo, A.P., Sparks, H.V., and Geiger, S.R. (eds), pp. 1–31. Waverly Press, Baltimore, MD.

Robinson, C.P., Baskin, S.I., and Franz, D.R. 1985. The mechanisms of action of cyanide on the rabbit aorta. *Journal of Applied Toxicology* 5: 372–377.

Roger White, C., Brock, T.A., Chang, L.Y., *et al.* 1994. Superoxide and peroxynitrite in atherosclerosis. *Proceedings of the National Academy of Sciences of the United States of America* 91: 1044–1048.

Rosenblum, W.I. and Bryan, D. 1987. Evidence that in vivo constriction of cerebral arterioles by local application of tert-butyl hydroperoxide is mediated by release of endogenous thromboxane. *Stroke* 18: 195–199.

Ross, R. 1986. The pathogenesis of atherosclerosis – an update. *New England Journal of Medicine* 314: 488–500.

Ross, R. 1993. The pathogenesis of atherosclerosis: a perspective for the 1990's. *Nature* 362: 801–809.

Ross, R. and Glomset, J. 1976. The pathogenesis of atherosclerosis. *New England Journal of Medicine* 295: 369–377.

Rubanyi, G.M. 1988. Vascular effects of oxygen-derived free radicals. *Free Radical Biology and Medicine* 4: 107–120.

Ryder, N.S. 1988. Mechanism of action and biochemical selectivity of allylamine antimycotic agents. *Annals of the New York Academy of Sciences* 544: 208–220.

Sadhu, D.N. and Ramos, K.S. 1993. Modulation by retinoic acid of spontaneous and benzo[a]pyrene-induced *c-Ha-ras* expression. *Basic Life Sciences* 61: 263–268.

Sadhu, D.N., Crum, S., and Ramos, K.S. 1991. Benzo(a)pyrene-induced alterations in [$^3$H]-thymidine incorporation in cultured aortic smooth muscle cells. *The Toxicologist* 11: 339.

Sandusky, G.E., Vodicnik, M.J., and Tamura, R.N. 1991. Cardiovascular and adrenal proliferative lesions in Fischer 344 rats induced by long-term treatment with type III phosphodiesterase inhibitors (positive inotropic agents), isomazole and indolidan. *Fundamental and Applied Toxicology* 16: 198–209.

Sappino, A.P., Schurch, W., and Gabbiani, G. 1990. Differentiation repertoire of fibroblastic cells: Expression of cytoskeletal proteins as markers of phenotypic modulations. *Laboratory Investigation* 63: 144–161.

Sarkar, R., Meinberg, E.G., Stanley, J.C., *et al.* 1996. Nitric oxide reversibly inhibits the migration of cultured vascular smooth muscle cells. *Circulation Research* 78: 225–230.

Savage, N.W., Adkins, K.F., Young, W.G., and Chapman, P.J. 1983. Oral vascular leiomyoma: review of the literature and report of 2 cases. *Australian Dental Journal* 28: 346–349.

Schiefer, H.B., Rousseaux, C.G., Hancock, D.S., and Blakley, B.R. 1987. Effects of low-level long-term oral exposure to T-2 toxin in CD-1 mice. *Food and Chemical Toxicology* 25: 593–601.

Schlaepfer, W.W. 1971. Sequential study of endothelial changes in acute cadmium intoxication. *Laboratory Investigations* 25: 556–564.

Schoenthal, R., Jaffe, A.Z., and Yagen, B. 1979. Cardiovascular lesions and various tumors found in rats given T-2 toxin, a trichothecene metabolite of Fusarium. *Cancer Research* 39: 2179–2189.

Schroeder, H.A. and Vinton, Jr., W.H. 1962. Hypertension in rats induced by small doses of cadmium. *American Journal of Physiology* 202: 515–518.

Serabjit-Singh, C.J., Bend, J.R., and Philpot, R.M. 1985. Cytochrome P-450 monooxygenase system localization in smooth muscle of rabbit aorta. *Molecular Pharmacology* 28: 72–79.

Shasby, M., Lind, S.E., Shasby, S.S., *et al.* 1985. Reversible oxidant-induced increases in albumin transfer across cultured endothelium: Alterations in cell shape and calcium homeostasis. *Blood* 65: 605–614.

Shi, R.J., Simpson Haidaris, P.J., Lerner, N.B., *et al.* 1998. Transcriptional regulation of endothelial cells tissue factor expression during *Rickettsia rickettsii* infection: Involvement of the transcription factor NF-κB. *Infection and Immunity* 66: 1070–1075.

Sholley, M.M., Gimbrone, M.A., and Cotran, R.S. 1976. Cellular migration and replication in endothelial regeneration. *Laboratory Investigations* 36: 18–25.

Shukla, G.S. and Singhal, R.L. 1984. The present status of biological effects of toxic metals in the environment: lead, cadmium, manganese. *Canadian Journal of Physiology and Pharmacology* 62: 1015–1031.

Siren, A.L and Feuerstein, G. 1986. Effect of T-2 toxin on regional blood flow and vascular resistance in the conscious rat. *Toxicology and Applied Pharmacology* 83: 438–444.

Sirois, M.G., Simons, M., and Edelman, E.R. 1997. Antisense oligonucleotide inhibition of PDGFR-beta receptor subunit expression directs suppression of intimal thickening. *Circulation* 95: 669–676.

Sonnfield, T. and Wennmalm, A. 1980. Inhibition by nicotine of the formation of prostacyclin-like activity in rabbit and human vascular tissue. *British Journal of Pharmacology* 71: 609–613.

Stoel, I., Biessen, W.J.vd., Zwolsman, E., *et al.* 1980. Direct effect of nicotine on prostacyclin in human umbilical arteries. *Acta Therapeutica* 6(4): 32–34.

Sutton, W.L. 1963. Aliphatic and alicyclic amines. In *Industrial Hygiene and Toxicology*, Vol. 2. Patty, F.A., Fassett, D.W., and Irish, D.O. (eds), pp. 2038. Interscience, New York.

Swift, L.L., Gasiewicz, T.A., Dunn, G.D., and Neal, R.A. 1981. Characterization of the hyperlipidemia in guinea pigs induced by 2,3,7,8-tetrachlorodi-benzo-p-dioxin. *Toxicology and Applied Pharmacology* 59: 489–499.

Taylor, Jr., L.M., Moneta, G.L., Sexton, G.J., *et al.* 1999. Prospective blinded study of the relationship between plasma homocysteine and progression of symptomatic peripheral arterial disease. *Journal of Vascular Surgery* 29: 8–21.

Thom, S.R. and Ishirpoulos, H. 1997. Mechanism of oxidative stress from low levels of carbon monoxide *Research Report – Health Effects Institute* 80: 1–9, discussion pp. 21–27.

Thyberg, J. 1986. Effects of nicotine on phenotypic modulation and initiation of DNA synthesis in cultured arterial smooth muscle cells. *Virchows Archives* 52: 25–32.

Thyberg, J. and Nilsson, J. 1982. Effects of nicotine on endocytosis and intracellular degradation of horseradish peroxidase in cultivated mouse peritoneal macrophages. *Acta Pathologica, Microbiologica, et Immunologica Scandinavica – Section A, Pathology* 90: 305–310.

Toda, T., Ito, M., Toda, Y., *et al.* 1985. Angiotoxicity in swine of a moderate excess of dietary vitamin $D_3$. *Food and Chemical Toxicology* 23: 585–592.

Togna, G., Togna, A.R., and Caprino, L. 1985. Vascular endothelium and platelet preparations for the prediction of xenobiotic effects on the vascular system. *Xenobiotica* 15: 661–664.

Tomera, J.F. and Harakal, C. 1986. Mercury and lead-induced contraction of aortic smooth muscle in vitro. *Archives Internationales de Pharmacodynamie et de Therapie* 283: 295–302.

Toth, B., Nagel, D., Patil, K., *et al.* 1978. Tumor induction with N1-acetyl derivative of 4-hydroxy methyl phenyl hydrazine, a metabolite of agaritine of *Agaricus bisporus*. *Cancer Research* 38: 177–180.

Tsai, J.-C., Perrella, M.A., Yoshizumi, M., *et al.* 1994. Promotion of vascular smooth muscle cell growth by homocysteine: A link to atherosclerosis. *Proceedings of the National Academy of Sciences of the United States of America* 91: 6369–6373.

Tulloss, J. and Booyse, F.M. 1978. Effect of various agents and physical damage in bovine endothelial cultures. *Microvascular Research* 16: 51–58.

Uchida, K., Kanematsu, M., Morimitsu, Y., *et al.* 1998. Acrolein is a product of lipid peroxidant reaction. Formation of free acrolein and its conjugate with lysine residues in oxidized low density lipoproteins. *Journal of Biological Chemistry* 273: 16058–16066.

Ueno, Y. 1977. Trichothecenes: an overview. In *Mycotoxins in Human and Animal Health*. Rodrickes, J.V., Hesseltine, C.W., and Mehlmann, M.A. (eds), pp. 189–207. Pathotox Publishers, Illinois.

Valtonen, V.V. 1991. Infection as a risk factor for infarction and atherosclerosis. *Annals of Medicine* 23: 539–543.

Vedernikov, Y.P., Graser, T., and Vanin, A.F. 1989. Similar endothelium-independent arterial relaxation by carbon monoxide and nitric oxide. *Biomedica et Biochimica Acta* 48: 601–603.

Verheij, M., Dewit, L.G.H., Boomgaard, M.N., *et al.* 1994. Ionizing radiation enhances platelet adhesion to the extracellular matrix of human endothelial cells by an increase in the release of von Willebrand Factor. *Radiation Research* 137: 202–207.

Vesselinovitch, D. 1980. Animal models and the study of atherosclerosis. *Archives of Pathology and Laboratory Medicine* 112: 1011–1017.

Voors, A.W., Johnson, W.D., and Shuman, M.S. 1982. Additive statistical effects of cadmium and lead on heart-related disease in a North Carolina autopsy series. *Archives of Environmental Health* 37: 98–102.

Walker, A.E. and Martin, J.V. 1979. Lipid profiles in dioxin-exposed workers. *Lancet* 1: 446–447.

Walton, K., Coombs, M.M., Walker, R., and Ioannides, C. 1997. Bioactivation of mushroom hydrazines to mutagenic products mammalian and fungal enzymes. *Mutation Research* 381: 131–139.

Webb, M. 1979. The metallothioneins. In *The Chemistry, Biochemistry and Biology of Cadmium*. Webb, M. (ed.), pp. 195–266. Elsevier/North Holland, Amsterdam.

Weber, T.J., Ou, X., Narasimham, T.R., *et al.* 1991. Modulation of protein phosphorylation in rat aortic smooth muscle cells by 2,3,7,8 tetrachlorodibenzo-p-dioxin (TCDD). *The Toxicologist* 11: 340.

Weber, T.J., Chapkin, R.S., Davidson, L.A., and Ramos, K.S. 1996. Modulation of protein kinase C-related signal transduction by 2,3,7,8-tetrachlorodibenzo-p-dioxin exhibits cell cycle dependence. *Archives of Biochemistry and Biophysics* 328: 227–232.

Wei, E.P., Kontos, H.A., Dietrich, W.D., *et al.* 1981. Inhibition by free radical scavengers and by cyclooxygenase inhibitors of pial arteriolar abnormalities from concussive brain injury in cats. *Circulation Research* 48: 95–103.

Wei, E.P., Christman, C.W., Kontos, H.A., and Povlishock, J.T. 1985. Effects of oxygen radicals on cerebral arterioles. *American Journal of Physiology* 248: H157–H162.

Wennmalm, A. 1978. Nicotine inhibits release of 6-keto prostaglandin $F_1$ from isolated perfused rabbit heart. *Acta Physiologica Scandinavica* 103: 107–109.

Westwood, F.R., Iswaran, T.J., and Greaves, P. 1990. Pathologic changes in blood vessels following administration of an inotropic vasodilator (ICI 153,110) to the rat. *Fundamental and Applied Toxicology* 14: 797–809.

Whiting, R.F., Wei, L., and Stich, H.F. 1979. Enhancement by transition metals of unscheduled DNA synthesis induced by isoniazid and related hydrazines in cultured normal and xeroderma pegmentosum human cells. *Mutation Research* 62: 505–510.

Wilson, C.A., Everard, D.M., and Schoental, R. 1982. Blood pressure changes and cardiovascular lesions found in rats given T-2 toxin, a trichothecene secondary metabolite of certain Fusarium microfungi. *Toxicology Letters* 10: 35–40.

Wolin, M.S. and Belloni, F.L. 1985. Superoxide anion selectivity attenuates catecholamine-induced contractile tension in isolated rabbit aorta. *American Journal of Physiology* 249: H1127–H1133.

Xin, X., Yang, N., Eckhart, A.D., and Faber, J.E. 1997. Alpha 1D-adrenergic receptors and mitogen-activated protein kinase mediate increased protein synthesis by arterial smooth muscle. *Molecular Pharmacology* 51: 764–75.

Xu, Q., Kleindienst, R., Schett, G., *et al.* 1996. Regression of arteriosclerotic lesions induced by immunization with heat shock protein 65-containing material in normo-cholesterolemic, but not hypercholesterolemic, rabbits. *Atherosclerosis* 123: 145–155.

Yang, H.Y.L., Namkung, M.J., Nelson, W.L., and Juchau, M.R. 1986a. Phase II biotransformation of carcinogens/atherogens in cultured aortic tissues and cells. I. Sulfation of 3-hydroxy-benzo(a)pyrene. *Drug Metabolism and Disposition* 14: 287–298.

Yang, H.Y.L., Majesky, M.W., Namkung, M.J., and Juchau, M.R. 1986b. Phase II biotransformation of carcinogens/atherogens in cultured aortic tissues and cells. II. Glucoronidation of 3-hydroxy-benzo(a)pyrene. *Drug Metabolism and Disposition* 14: 293–298.

Yarom, R., More, R., Sherman, Y., and Yagen, B. 1983. T-2 toxin-induced pathology in the hearts of rats. *British Journal of Experimental Pathology* 64: 570–577.

Yarom, R., Sherman, Y., Bergmann, F., *et al.* 1987. T-2 toxin effect on rat aorta: Cellular changes *in vivo* and growth of smooth muscle cells *in vitro*. *Experimental and Molecular Pathology* 47: 143–153.

Young, L.J. and Caughey, W.S. 1990. Pathobiochemistry of carbon monoxide poisoning. *FEBS Letters* 272: 1–6.

Yu, S.M., Tsai, S.Y., Guh, J.H., *et al.* 1996. Mechanism of catecholamine-induced proliferation of vascular smooth muscle cells. *Circulation* 94: 547–554.

Zhao, W., Parrish, A.R., and Ramos, K.S. 1998. Constitutive and inducible expression of cytochrome P450IA1 and P450IB1 in human vascular endothelial and smooth muscle cells. *In Vitro Cellular and Developmental Biology Animal* 34: 671–673.

Zimmerman, M. and McGeachie, J. 1985. The effect of nicotine on aortic endothelial cell turnover: An autoradiographic study. *Atherosclerosis* 58: 39–47.

# 16

# PATHOBIOLOGY OF THE VASCULAR RESPONSE TO INJURY

*Peter G. Anderson,\* Zadok Ruben,†*
*and Bernard M. Wagner‡*

*\*University of Alabama at Birmingham,*
*Birmingham, AL, USA; †Patoximed Consultants,*
*Westfield, NJ, USA; and ‡Short Hills, NJ, USA*

## Introduction

The vasculature performs the vital function of providing the nutrient supply to and waste removal from the tissues of the body. In this role, it serves as the interface between blood elements and tissues. Although simplistically thought of as purely a conduit, blood vessels are important regulators of normal physiologic activity within the body. Because of the varied functions of the vasculature, the divergent cell types that make up blood vessels, and the essential nature of their functions, blood vessels have evolved important and unique mechanisms for regulating and responding to their environment. Cardiovascular diseases, primarily atherosclerosis and hypertension, are leading causes of morbidity and mortality in developed countries around the world. The response of the vasculature to lipids, inflammatory mediators, xenobiotics, infectious agents, and mechanical injury all importantly contribute to vascular function and dysfunction. The vulnerability of blood vessels to injury by numerous chemicals and drugs is well recognized and has previously been reviewed (Ruben *et al.*, 1992; Boor *et al.*, 1995; Burke *et al.*, 1997; Feuerstein and Kerns, 1997). The impact that these influences have on health and disease and on biomedical research aimed at investigating these health problems makes the understanding of the vascular response to injury of paramount clinical significance. Recent advances in vascular pathobiology have elucidated unique signaling and regulatory mechanisms that enable blood vessels to respond to and adapt to a variety of stresses and insults. The purpose of this chapter is to review the general mechanisms by which blood vessels respond to insults, be they physiologic, toxicologic, or mechanical.

## Regulation of normal vascular structure and function

The structural components that make up blood vessels vary according to the type and caliber of the vessel. Blood vessels are composed of an endothelial layer, a medial layer consisting of primarily smooth muscle cells, and a fibrous connective tissue layer that makes up the adventitia. The endothelial cell layer serves as the interface between blood and tissues and plays a critical role in regulating blood flow, body fluids, and bidirectional traffic of humoral factors and cells. In the mid-nineteenth century, Virchow referred to the vascular endothelium as "a membrane as simple as any that is ever met with in the body." Today, the endothelial cell is regarded as a complex, active regulator of vascular integrity. Endothelium regulates plasma–interstitial fluid exchange and intimal lipids, maintains a non-thrombogenic surface, produces mitogenic factors, and is a crucial element in the inflammatory response. At a physical level, the endothelium is a structural barrier between underlying smooth muscle and substances in the blood (Noishiki *et al.*, 1994; Feuerstein and Kerns, 1997). The junctions between endothelial cells are important physical barriers, and if the space between endothelial cells widens fluid and particles may penetrate the vessel wall. Toxic compounds are among the circulating substances in the blood, and therefore the endothelium serves to protect the media from injury. The endothelial cell can bind and catabolize certain circulating vasoactive agents (serotonin, norepinephrine, bradykinin), convert inactive precursors into active products (angiotensin I), and directly synthesize a variety of potent autocoids (prostacyclins). To this repertoire, the endothelial cell has now been shown to modulate directly the adjacent smooth muscle cells by secreting second messengers in response to luminal stimuli. In fact, the 1998 Noble prize in physiology and medicine was awarded jointly to Robert Furchgott, Louis Ignarro, and Ferid Murad for their discoveries concerning nitric oxide as a signaling molecule in the cardiovascular system. These investigators as well as many others have show that nitric oxide is a major regulator of vascular function and structure (Furchgott, 1996, 1999; Ignarro *et al.*, 1999; Murad, 1999). Discovery of this simple signaling molecule has had a significant impact on our understanding of vascular function and dysfunction and these mechanisms will be discussed later in this chapter.

In most blood vessels, the endothelial cells overlie an internal elastic lamina. This elastic lamina is produced by smooth muscle cells (Noishiki *et al.*, 1994; Davis, 1995) and contains focal adhesion sites where filaments anchor endothelial cells to the subjacent elastic lamina (Plump *et al.*, 1992). The elastic lamina is porous and contains ovoid fenestrations of varying diameters which allow for vessel constriction and dilation and through which molecules can transit across the vessel barrier (Clark and Glagov, 1976; Crissman, 1986). The smooth muscle cells within the media function to maintain vascular tone. Smooth muscle cells normally have a "contractile phenotype," in which the cells contain abundant myofilaments and are primarily suited for contraction. After vessel injury or when placed in culture, smooth muscle cells can modulate to a "synthetic phenotype," in which the cells lose their myofilaments and contain abundant rough endoplasmic reticulum (Campbell *et al.*, 1988). This capacity to modulate from contractile to synthetic phenotype has a significant impact on how vessels respond to injury and is an important area of ongoing investigation (Boerth *et al.*, 1997; Anderson *et al.*, 2000).

The tunica adventitia has recently received considerable investigation because of its role in the remodeling that occurs after mechanical vascular intervention (Gibbons and Dzau, 1994; Shi *et al.*, 1996). The adventitia is also involved in vascular adaptation to pressure loads with significant thickening and fibrosis evident in models of increased intravascular pressure (Regan *et al.*, 1996, 1997). The vasa vasorum, which enters the vessel via the adventitia and supplies circulation to the outer two-thirds of the vascular wall, is also known to play an important role in vascular structure and function. One primary example of vasa vasorum alterations leading to significant pathology is in the case of syphilitic aortitis. Syphilis can cause endarteritis obliterans of the vasa vasorum, characterized by perivascular plasma cell and lymphocyte cuffing. This damage to the vasa vasorum leads to degeneration of the thoracic aorta and can result in ectasia and/or rupture of that aorta (Heggtveit, 1983). Additional studies have demonstrated the importance of the vasa vasorum in the pathogenesis of atherosclerosis and atherosclerotic plaque stability (Kwon *et al.*, 1998).

The discovery of nitric oxide (NO·) as the "endothelial-derived relaxing factor" has greatly enhanced our understanding of the signaling pathways and the control mechanisms responsible for regulating cardiovascular function (Ignarro *et al.*, 1987). The role of NO· in both the regulation of normal vascular function and as a major player in many pathologic states has generated extensive interest and investigation. The signaling pathways by which NO· affects cell function are protean and these effects are due in part to the high affinity of NO· for heme-containing enzymes. Perhaps the most important intracellular signaling role for NO· is its capacity to activate guanylate cyclase, which leads to rapid and robust increases in cyclic GMP (cGMP) levels in target cells. The increased cGMP levels and subsequent cGMP-dependent phosphorylation of proteins appears to be involved in intracellular calcium sequestration or removal, which results in smooth muscle cell relaxation and reduction in vascular tone (Johnson and Lincoln, 1985; Lincoln *et al.*, 1995; Anderson *et al.*, 2000).

## Vascular injury

The structural responses of the arterial wall to injury depends on the nature of the chemical agent, the degree of host exposure, and the duration of exposure at the site of injury (Boor *et al.*, 1995; Boor and Langford, 1997). Injury may be defined as direct or indirect depending on the access of the agent or its metabolites to the artery. When an injurious chemical enters the arterial wall – regardless of mode of entry – and directly combines with biologically important macromolecules to alter function, direct injury has occurred. If, however, a chemical sets in motion a series of reactions by the cellular components of the arterial wall that lead to injury through inflammatory cells, immune mediators, or altered homeostasis, then injury may be considered as indirect or secondary. Blood vessels constrict and dilate and alterations in this vasomotion play a role in determining the nature and severity of chemically induced injury. This critical property of the artery is under extensive control by the neuroendocrine system and local metabolism affecting the cellular components of the wall (endothelia, connective tissue, and smooth muscle cells), which are integrated functionally by a unique extracellular matrix, elastin, and collagen fibers.

Ergot and ergot derivative drugs are powerful vasoconstriction agents and, along with other groups of vasoactive compounds, can result in structural changes in the vasculature (Joseph *et al.*, 1997). These drugs have been used in the treatment of migraine, postural hypotension, inadequate venous tone, forms of senile dementia, and, with heparin, as prophylaxis against post-operative thrombo-embolism. Because of their effect on vascular smooth muscle, these chemicals are prototype vasoconstrictors. There is an extensive clinical literature demonstrating the adverse effects of repeated vascular smooth muscle constriction. While ergot-type agents produce arterial vasoconstriction, they also cause venospasm and can result in venous thrombosis. Of interest is the fact that the vasoconstrictor activity is of long duration and independent of drug plasma levels. There is evidence to suggest that these agents accumulate in smooth muscle and induce constriction through stimulation of 5-hydroxytryptamine (5-HT) receptors. However, constriction is maintained by sensitization of the smooth muscle to endogenous vasoconstrictors such as biogenic amines.

Vascular angiography (arteriography and venography) have been helpful in elucidating the pathology (i.e. structural changes) associated with these drugs. A common observation in arteries of patients with vascular complications is segmental stenosis. The vessels are described as having thread-like, thorny, or hour glass-like narrowing due to spasm. The stenotic arterial segments have smooth margins and no thrombi are present. Thus, the toxic effects of ergot drugs on the arterial system may take the form of acute or chronic stenosis but not obstruction. Careful study of serial angiograms and comparison with tissue specimens allow one to postulate a mechanism of drug-induced pathologic changes. With repeated vasoconstriction, there is progressive loss of smooth muscle cells and fragmentation of the internal elastic lamina. The connective tissue stroma condenses and fibroblast activity with increased collagen deposition is induced. At this point, the arterial wall is vulnerable to an arteritis-type response. In the absence of inflammatory cells, smooth muscle cell loss, collagen deposition, and fibroblast hyperplasia continue until a fixed stenosis results.

The segmental pattern of arterial stenosis is in keeping with the anatomy of the wall and the role of the longitudinal smooth muscle cells in constriction. The twisting motion of the longitudinal smooth muscle cells requires segmental anchor points, which are determined physiologically and by receptor density. At the point of maximal vasoconstriction, endothelial cell injury may result in release of other biologically active substances that act on adjacent smooth muscle cells. This serves to accentuate the segmental nature of the stenosis. Vasoconstriction may be a factor in the segmental pathology of polyarteritis nodosa and diseases of small, muscular arteries, as seen in human generalized scleroderma (Burke *et al.*, 1997). Recent studies have demonstrated that endothelin receptor distribution was not homogeneous throughout the coronary circulation of the dog (Louden *et al.*, 2000). The local distribution of endothelin receptors correlated nicely with the distribution of lesions observed after administration of an experimental endothelin receptor-blocking agent. These data along with other observations suggest that there is significant inhomogeneity within the vasculature and that the distribution of receptors and signaling molecules can have a significant impact on the propensity for lesion development.

## Nitric oxide and peroxynitrite in vascular disease

Peroxynitrite (ONOO⁻), formed by a diffusion-limited reaction with NO· and superoxide, is a powerful oxidant capable of oxidizing low-density lipoprotein *in vitro* to a form taken up by the macrophage scavenger receptor (Graham *et al.*, 1993). One stable product of peroxynitrite attack on proteins is the addition of a nitro group ($NO_2$) to the ortho position of tyrosine to form nitrotyrosine (Beckman *et al.*, 1992). The reaction occurs spontaneously, but is also catalyzed by low molecular weight transition metals as well as by superoxide dismutase. The presence of nitrotyrosine in tissues can be used as a biologic marker for peroxynitrite damage (Beckman, 1996). Oxidative modification of lipoproteins and their uptake via the scavenger receptor in endothelium and macrophages is an early event in the pathogenesis of atherosclerosis. The "reaction to injury hypothesis" that was championed by the late Russell Ross is widely accepted as a unifying hypothesis to help explain the pathogenesis of atherosclerosis (Ross, 1986, 1993). This hypothesis suggests that atherosclerotic lesions result from an excessive inflammatory/fibroproliferative response to various forms of insult to the endothelium and smooth muscle of the artery wall. Extensive research has demonstrated that this unifying hypothesis does explain much of the pathogenesis of this complex disease process. The chronic inflammatory process that occurs during development of atherosclerotic lesions causes release of cytokines and stimulation of nitric oxide synthase (NOS). This inducible NOS (iNOS or NOS III) leads to elevated levels of NO· in tissues. The inflammatory process also produces free radicals, including superoxide. The superoxide reacts with the NO·, producing peroxynitrite. One way to show peroxynitrite formation *in vivo* is to detect the presence of stable by-products of its reaction with various biologic compounds. 3-Nitrotyrosine is an example of such a product, and nitrotyrosine can be used as a stable marker of peroxynitrite formation *in vivo*. As peroxynitrite may play an integral role in the development of atherosclerosis, the stable marker of peroxynitrite activation – nitrotyrosine – should be present in atherosclerotic tissues. Studies from our laboratory (Beckman *et al.*, 1994) have shown that, in the aorta and coronary arteries from human patients with atherosclerosis, nitrotyrosine is present in macrophages of fatty streak lesions and in advanced atherosclerotic lesions (Figure 16.1).

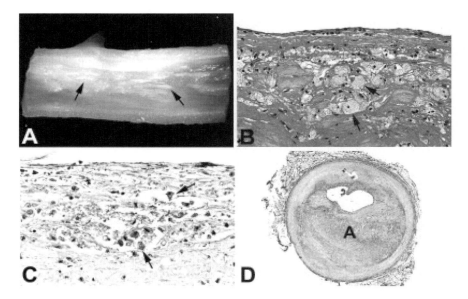

*Figure 16.1* Nitrotyrosine in human atherosclerosis. (A) The luminal surface of a section of coronary artery from a 32-year-old woman shows fatty streak lesions (arrows). (B) Histologically, these lesions are composed of foam cells (arrows). (C) Immunostaining with an antibody specific for nitrotyrosine demonstrates the presence of nitrotyrosine in the foam cells (arrows). (D) A cross-section of coronary artery from another patient with advanced atherosclerotic lesions demonstrates abundant nitrotyrosine staining.

## Pathology of vascular interventions

Direct mechanical injury to vessels elicits a wound-healing response similar to the response observed after any injury. The clinical importance of understanding this wound-healing process is vital for patient care. The challenge for investigators interested in vascular biology is to identify the mechanisms involved in vascular repair and remodeling in order to impact the problem of restenosis.

Percutaneous transluminal coronary angioplasty has become a frequently used clinically effective method for the revascularization of stenosed or occluded native arteries and vein grafts. However, the problem of restenosis continues to impact importantly on the clinical utility of this procedure. Data from retrospective and prospective studies of angioplasty, atherectomy, laser ablation, and endovascular stenting demonstrate that with all of these interventional techniques the restenosis rate ranges from 25 percent to 40 percent (Liu *et al.*, 1989; Windecker and Meier, 2000). Thus, any revascularization technique, which necessarily involves some degree of trauma to the vessel, may lead to restenosis in a certain cohort of patients. The specific factors that may lead to restenosis have not been well defined. The underlying basis for restenosis involves some form of vascular trauma with injury to endothelial and/or smooth muscle cells. Clinical and experimental studies have also shown that restenosis may result from other injurious procedures, such as electrical stimulation, freezing, alcohol perfusion, crush injury, or physical injury produced by placement of a constricting band around the outside of the vessel (Banai *et al.*, 1991; Stanley and Connett, 1991; Willerson *et al.*, 1991). The trophic factors, either bloodborne or locally produced and/or released during these interventions and which result in exuberant growth and phenotypic conversion of the smooth muscle cells after vascular injury, have been extensively studied with no clear consensus as to the specific factors responsible for restenosis (Liu *et al.*, 1989, 1996; Forrester *et al.*, 1991). It is clear that restenosis is a complex pathophysiologic process, and the unraveling of the specific factors leading to restenosis will require precise experimental design and appropriate model systems. Various *in vitro* and *in vivo* model systems have been used to study restenosis and to investigate methods for preventing restenosis. Intravascular irradiation after vessel injury (brachytherapy) has been effective and holds great promise for inhibiting or preventing restenosis. Yet the exact mechanisms responsible for the development of restenosis and the exact mechanism of action of brachytherapy still elude investigators. Results from these studies have elucidated many mechanisms involved in the restenosis process; however, there are some discrepancies in the efficacy of treatment protocols when comparative studies are performed on different animal species, including man. Thus, there appear to be significant species differences in the response to vascular injury that must be considered when performing and evaluating studies of restenosis (Ferrell *et al.*, 1992).

## Mechanical vascular injury: experimental models and study paradigms

The choice of model systems for studies of vascular biology and, specifically, studies of restenosis requires clear identification of the experimental end-point. It must be acknowledged from the outset that all model systems have limitations and that these experimental systems are just models of a process that occurs in humans. Thus, no experimental system can completely and accurately reproduce the restenosis phenomenon seen in an atherosclerotic coronary artery of human patients. However, it is possible by careful experimental design to answer specific questions related to the phenomenon of restenosis using *in vitro* systems or animal models (Anderson, 1992).

*In vitro* systems can be very precisely controlled and specific factors or processes can be isolated and studied (Blank and Owens, 1990; Dartsch *et al.*, 1990; Pukac *et al.*, 1991; Carere *et al.*, 1992). If a specific hypothesis is to be tested, *in vitro* systems can be manipulated in such a way that only one variable is examined. This will answer a specific question about a single variable. These studies are useful in studies of the cell and of the molecular biology of endothelial cells or smooth muscle cells. The information gleaned from these studies can be used to help better understand the complex situation seen *in vivo*. Although beneficial in basic scientific investigation, *in vitro* studies cannot be used to mimic or reproduce the restenosis process *in vivo*. The procedures used to isolate smooth muscle cells or endothelial cells and the techniques used to maintain them in culture are far removed from the milieu of an atherosclerotic coronary artery in a patient. Also, with *in vitro* techniques, it is impossible to maintain the interaction that occurs between the various cell types and the bloodborne factors that impact on the restenosis process *in vivo*. Studies of smooth muscle cells in culture demonstrate that, after passage and after transition from the contractile to the secretory phenotype, key regulatory signaling pathways are altered or lost (Lincoln *et al.*, 1994, 1998; Cornwell *et al.*, 1996). These studies suggest that using cultured or passaged smooth muscle cells in studies of the vascular response to injury may be problematic. Thus, data from *in vitro* studies should be used to evaluate specific mechanisms of the cell and the molecular biology of endothelial cells and smooth muscle cells and not to make definitive conclusions about the restenosis process *in vivo*.

Animal models are by far the most popular method for investigating restenosis. Investigators have utilized various animal species, different arteries or veins, and numerous types of interventions to induce restenosis. These model systems fall into three basic categories. In one group, models are designed to show a very reproducible neointimal reaction that can be easily quantitated. Examples of this type of model system include the rat aortic or carotid artery balloon injury model and rabbit models of femoral or iliac artery injury. In these systems, the degree of restenosis is predictable and uniform. Thus, experiments designed to modify neointimal growth can be easily tested in these models. The second type of model system often utilizes coronary arteries in larger animals with artery sizes similar to man. These model systems also endeavor to produce a consistent neointimal proliferative reaction; however, the reproducibility and ease of performing these experiments may be somewhat compromised in order to obtain the benefits of using a larger animal model. In these models, injury is produced in normal arteries, and the response to that injury is evaluated. Examples of models in this group include dog or pig coronary and carotid arteries. These models will be discussed in detail below. The third type of model system used to study restenosis attempts to reproduce the conditions seen in human atherosclerotic coronary arteries. These systems utilize artery injury and atherosclerotic diets to induce atherosclerotic lesions in arteries. After development of atherosclerotic lesions, mechanical interventions are performed (e.g. angioplasty, stents, atherectomy) and the response of the diseased artery to this intervention is evaluated. These types of model systems are good for testing new equipment or new techniques. These models are also useful for evaluating the response of the diseased artery to these insults and the ability of therapeutic techniques to diminish the restenosis phenomenon. Unfortunately, the complexity of these model systems makes it very difficult to obtain reproducible injury or reproducible restenosis; thus, statistical evaluation of the efficacy of therapeutic techniques is very difficult. In essence, trying to replicate human atherosclerosis makes these models so complex that these experiments have many of the same problems as human trials, i.e. large variability and large numbers of subjects needed to reach statistically significant end-points. Examples of these types of animal models are femoral or iliac artery injury plus atherosclerotic diet in rabbits, injury plus atherosclerotic diet in minipigs, and atherosclerosis in non-human primates. These models have distinct advantages and disadvantages that will be discussed below.

The primary factor to be considered when choosing animal models of restenosis is the end-point for the experiment. Each animal model has strengths and weaknesses that must be factored into the study plan. Each animal species has a slightly different anatomy and physiology, and these differences may or may not impact on the experimental results when compared with man. Thus, the model system should be carefully evaluated and pilot studies should be performed before undertaking a large study.

## Animal models in the study of vascular interventions

Numerous animal models are currently being used to investigate the pathogenesis of restenosis. This review will briefly discuss some of the more commonly used models and will describe the pros and cons of each model system.

### *Rodents*

Rats are by far the most commonly used rodent model of restenosis; however, transgenic mice have been used and their use has increased steadily. Transgenic mice have the benefit of allowing the investigator to modify specific genes and thus tailor-make the milieu of the restenosis process. Using these techniques, it is possible to investigate directly the role of specific factors on the restenosis process. Mice models of atherosclerosis also increase the utility of this model system for studies of vascular response to mechanical injury. Use of specific mouse stains, transgenic or knock-out mice, and special diets make it possible to induce the development of atherosclerotic lesions (Figure 16.2) (Paigen *et al.*, 1987; Breslow, 1996). The topographical locations of the lesions and the character of the atherosclerotic lesions in mice are quite variable depending on strain, diet, and which genes are knocked out. However, as in seen in Figure 16.2, there are intimal cholesterol deposits and a fibrous cap overlying these lesions. These model systems have been used extensively to study pathogenic mechanisms of atherosclerosis and are powerful tools for studying this important disease process. To date, studies of restenosis in transgenic mice and knock-out mice have been relatively few and the procedures used to induce mechanical injury are technically demanding; but, the utility and power of this model system suggests that these model systems will evolve and become important additions to our experimental armamentarium.

Rats have the advantage that they are relatively inexpensive to procure and maintain. They are also amenable to a variety of experimental manipulations and

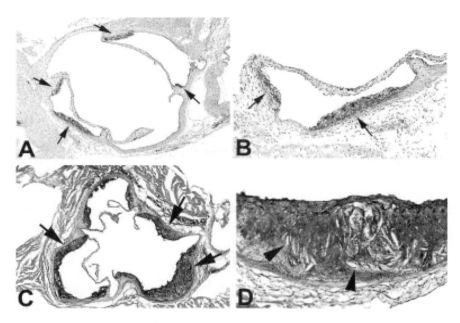

*Figure 16.2* Atherosclerosis in mice. (A and B) Sections from the aortic root of an atherosclerosis-prone mouse strain fed a high-cholesterol diet. Note the lesions (arrows) are rather modest and are primarily restricted to the aortic root. (C and D) Similar sections from an ApoE knock-out mouse demonstrating more severe lesions (arrows) with extensive cholesterol deposits within the lesions (arrowheads).

large numbers of animals can be utilized for complex experimental protocols. One disadvantage of rodents as models of restenosis is the small size of the arteries that are utilized. Also, the most commonly used vessels, the aorta and carotid arteries, are elastic arteries as opposed to muscular arteries and at least in the carotid artery there is no vasa vasorum (Sims, 1989). In addition, rats are relatively resistant to atherosclerosis and, although atherosclerosis can be induced in certain strains of rats (Wilgram and Ingle, 1965; Gross, 1985), there are no good models of atherosclerosis currently available in the rat. Despite these caveats, the rat is a very utilitarian model for studies of restenosis since it develops a very reproducible, rapid neointimal proliferative reaction.

Much of what we currently know about smooth muscle cell biology after vascular injury has been determined from studies utilizing the rat carotid balloon injury model (Fishman *et al.*, 1975; Clowes *et al.*, 1990; Fingerle *et al.*, 1990; Prescott *et al.*, 1991; Majesky *et al.*, 1992). In this model, a deflated Fogarty balloon is inserted into the carotid artery, the balloon is inflated and gently removed from the artery. This process results in dilation of the vessel wall and mechanical denudation of endothelial cells as the balloon is removed. The sequence of events after balloon injury, as initially described by Fishman *et al.* (1975) and expounded upon by others (Fingerle *et al.*, 1990; Prescott *et al.*, 1991; Majesky *et al.*, 1992), includes platelet adhesion and smooth muscle cell proliferation to form a neointima composed of almost 100 percent smooth muscle cells (Figure 16.3). The initial sequences of platelet adhesion and degranulation result in thrombus formation and the release of numerous growth factors. This process undoubtedly helps to initiate the neointimal proliferative response. If rats are made thrombocytopenic by injection of anti-platelet antibodies, the neointimal response is abrogated (Fingerle *et al.*, 1989). Medial injury by stretch and mechanical trauma also importantly impact on the neointimal proliferative response. Studies have demonstrated a significant loss of medial smooth muscle cells after balloon injury in this model. This has led many investigators to suggest that growth factors are released by the injured smooth muscle cells. In studies where the media was stretched by infusion of saline into the vessel lumen under pressure, resulting in little or no endothelial cell injury, the smooth muscle cell proliferation still occurred.

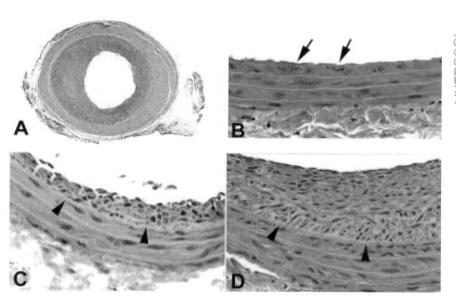

*Figure 16.3* Balloon injury model in the rat carotid artery. (A) Low-power photomicrograph demonstrating the concentric neointimal response with preservation of the media in this rat carotid artery 3 weeks after balloon injury. (B) High-power view of carotid artery wall 24 h after balloon injury. Note the absence of endothelial cells and the multiple breaks in the internal elastic membrane. There is also nuclear fragmentation in smooth muscle cells along the outermost layer of the vessel. (C) High-power view of carotid artery wall 4 days after balloon injury. Note the early formation of a neointima on the luminal side of the internal elastic membrane (arrowheads). (D) At 3 weeks after balloon injury, the neointima is well formed and has increased in thickness. Some of the smooth muscle cells have begun to develop a fusiform shape and line up circumferentially perpendicular to the direction of blood flow. Although difficult to appreciate at this magnification, the luminal surface of the neointima is covered with endothelial cells. The arrowheads outline the internal elastic membrane.

These data support the contention that medial injury *per se* also induces the neointimal proliferative response. Additional studies have further characterized the pathogenesis of restenosis after balloon injury in the rat. At 24–72 h after balloon injury, smooth muscle cells began to divide and migrate from the media into the intima (Clowes *et al.*, 1983). Approximately 50 percent of the cells that migrated into the intima did not divide; rather, they changed to the secretory phenotype (loss of myofilaments and increases in rough endoplasmic reticulum; Schwartz *et al.*, 1986; Campbell *et al.*, 1988; Manderson *et al.*, 1989) and began to produce extracellular matrix material. The cell division in the neointima continued for up to 8 weeks after injury in areas that were re-endothelialized and cell division in the neointima continued for up to 12 weeks in areas where endothelial cells did not regrow. In the balloon injury model, the central portion of the denuded artery segment may never have re-endothelialized (Clowes *et al.*, 1983) and the damage to the vessel wall limited pulsatile flow. It is evident that endothelial cell denudation plays a critical role in restenosis even without concurrent injury to the media. If a small region of the artery is denuded with a fine nylon thread which does not injure the underlying media, endothelial cells quickly grow over the denuded region and the proliferative process is greatly diminished (Clowes *et al.*, 1989; Fingerle *et al.*, 1990).

With the rat carotid artery balloon injury model, the neointimal proliferation is very reproducible, and accurate quantitation can be used to characterize the restenosis phenomenon. There are no breaks in the internal elastic membrane, thus the neointima is easily measured by morphometric techniques. This well-characterized model system, using animals that are relatively inexpensive and easy to handle, can be used to study specific pathogenic mechanisms in the restenosis process. This model system does have several caveats. First, the arteries are normal prior to the experimental manipulation. This is very different from that seen in atherosclerotic human coronary arteries which undergo angioplasty or other interventions. A more disturbing finding has been that many of the treatments that have been successful in preventing restenosis in the rat model have not been successful in large animal species and in man (Lafont and Faxon, 1998). Thus, there appear to be differences between rats and larger species that make it difficult to predict from rat studies the outcome of pharmacologic interventions on restenosis in man.

### Rabbits

Rabbits have been used extensively to study the pathogenic mechanisms of restenosis (Block *et al.*, 1980; Faxon *et al.*, 1982, 1984; Campbell *et al.*, 1988; Manderson *et al.*, 1989; Atkinson *et al.*, 1992; Carter *et al.*, 1999). Rabbits are relatively inexpensive to procure and maintain and they lend themselves well to laboratory experiments. Most studies have utilized the femoral or iliac arteries; however, studies of the carotid arteries and aorta have also been performed. Of these vessels, only the femoral artery is a muscular artery. After vascular injury, rabbits develop a neointimal proliferative response that is uniform and reproducible, and, as with rats, is composed primarily of smooth muscle cells. One advantage of the rabbit model over the rat is that the femoral and iliac arteries of an adult rabbit are similar in size to coronary arteries in man (Block *et al.*, 1980). Rabbits on a normal diet do not develop naturally occurring atherosclerotic lesions; however, with a high-cholesterol diet, serum cholesterol levels of greater than 2000 mg dl$^{-1}$ can be achieved (Gross, 1985). In these hyperlipemic animals, lipid-laden macrophages (foam cells) are deposited in the media and intima of large arteries as well as in the parenchyma of the spleen, liver, and lymph nodes. This vascular foam cell deposition does not resemble fibrocalcific atherosclerotic lesions in man. Other model systems in rabbits utilize a moderately high-cholesterol diet and some form of vessel injury, e.g. air drying or balloon injury (Faxon *et al.*, 1982, 1984). In these models, the arterial lesions consist of foam cells in the media and intima as well as a smooth muscle cell proliferative response similar to the type of response seen in human atherosclerotic arteries that have undergone balloon injury. This model system does not have the well-developed atheromatous lesion with a fibrous cap or areas of calcification that is seen in human arteries; however, the major components of the atherosclerotic process are present in the rabbit atherosclerotic model. A third rabbit model that may be used in restenosis research is the Watanabe rabbit. This strain of rabbit has an inherited deficiency in low-density lipoprotein receptors and the resultant hyperlipidemia predisposes the rabbits to atherosclerotic vascular disease (Oshima *et al.*, 1998). The pattern of atherosclerosis is similar to that found in patients with familial hyperlipidemia. Well-developed vascular lesions contain a cholesterol-filled necrotic core with areas of calcification and a fibrous cap. Recent studies have utilized heterozygous Watanabe rabbits fed a high-cholesterol diet (Atkinson *et al.*, 1992). This model may have advantages in that the morphology of the lesions more closely resembles human coronary artery disease as opposed to the foam cell lesions seen in normal rabbits fed high-cholesterol diets (Figure 16.4).

Non-atherosclerotic rabbits have been used in studies of restenosis (Consigny *et al.*, 1986); however, most studies have involved some experimental manipulation to induce atherosclerosis. The major utility of studies in atherosclerotic rabbits is that atherosclerosis is induced in the artery before the experimental intervention. In this way, the artery that is being investigated is already diseased, similar to the situation seen in patients who undergo vascular interventions. Even though the atherosclerotic lesion in rabbits is not identical to human atherosclerosis, there is intimal thickening, lipid accumulation (primarily foam cells) and fibrosis within the vessel wall, and some atrophy or degeneration of the media with adventitial thickening by fibrosis. Thus, any additional intervention (angioplasty, stent placement, or atherectomy) is performed in a diseased artery and not in a normal artery. This in itself may help to give credence to this model system as opposed to models in which injurious interventions are performed on normal arteries. One negative aspect of the atherosclerotic rabbit model is that the degree of atherosclerosis and the underlying vascular injury is not uniform in all animals

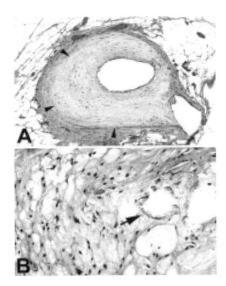

*Figure 16.4* Atherosclerotic lesion in an F1 Watanabe–New Zealand White rabbit fed a high-fat diet. (A) Low-power view of the atherosclerotic lesion in a coronary artery. The arrowheads outline the internal elastic membrane. (B) High-power view of the atheroma demonstrating an area of calcification (arrow).

that are studied. Thus, the starting point for all the experiments and the morphologic characteristics of the vessels prior to the experimental intervention are not uniform. This lack of uniformity in the vessel before the intervention is not pronounced, but it does tend to increase the scatter in the data and make it more difficult to demonstrate statistically significant differences between experimental groups. The atherosclerotic rabbit model is very good for investigations of new angioplasty balloons, intravascular stents, and atherectomy devices. Evaluation of new devices and accurate quantitation of the degree of restenosis can be accurately evaluated in large numbers of animals. Thus, for a small animal model, the atherosclerotic rabbit and possibly the Watanabe rabbit have many benefits for studies of restenosis.

### Non-human primates

Several species of non-human primates develop spontaneous atherosclerosis, and atherosclerosis can be induced by high-cholesterol diets (Coats, *et al.*, 1997; Clarkson, 1998; Giese *et al.*, 1999). The location and morphology of these atherosclerotic lesions is very similar to lesions seen in man. Both in spontaneously occurring atherosclerosis and in experimentally induced atherosclerosis there is species variability in the susceptibility to lesion formation and the character of lesions. The cost of procuring and maintaining non-human primates makes this an unattractive model for many investigators. However, there are many regional primate centers around the country where large numbers of primates are housed and bred. Collaboration with investigators at these primate centers can provide an excellent opportunity to evaluate restenosis in animals that are very similar to man.

## *Dogs*

Dogs are one of the most common large laboratory animals used for cardiovascular research. Their size, the relatively easy vascular access, and the ease of working with dogs in the research laboratory make them amenable to many types of acute and chronic experimental protocols. Coronary arteries of dogs are similar in size and morphology to human coronary arteries (Sims, 1989; Sims *et al.*, 1989). Dogs do not develop naturally occurring atherosclerosis and even with high-cholesterol diets there is little lipid accumulation within vessels. Models of atherosclerosis have been developed in dogs, but this model requires thyroidectomy and a high-lipid diet. In this model, the coronary arteries are not affected until late in the process and the lesions consist mainly of lipid-laden macrophages (foam cells) in the media (Geer and Guidry, 1962). Dogs also have a fibrinolytic system that is more active than in man (Bates *et al.*, 1991). Thus, studies of vascular devices and other interventions that may produce thrombosis may not receive adequate testing in the dog.

Despite these limitations, dog carotid, iliac, renal, and coronary arteries have been utilized in studies of restenosis and in trials to test interventional devices and intravascular stents (Roubin *et al.*, 1987; Schatz *et al.*, 1987; Bates *et al.*, 1991). Some studies have described the morphologic features and the time-course of neointimal proliferation after balloon angioplasty in normal vessels (Hehrlein *et al.*, 1991). These investigators noted endothelial cell denudation and platelet adhesion initially, followed by re-endothelialization and proliferation of smooth muscle cells to produce a smooth muscle cell-rich neointima. There was also a significant increase in DNA synthesis in the vessel wall for up to 2 weeks after angioplasty. These investigators also described in-growth of capillaries into the media of the vessel at the area of angioplasty injury. This morphologic description of the tissue reaction to angioplasty in the renal artery is similar to previous descriptions and to our own observations in coronary arteries after implantation of balloon-expandable coil stents. In our studies (P.G. Anderson, unpublished observations), coil stents were deployed by an angioplasty balloon, thus producing endothelial denudation and stretch injury to the vessel wall. Stents and delivery balloons were sized such that the fully inflated balloon was approximately 10–20 percent larger in diameter than the vessel. In previous studies (Roubin *et al.*, 1987) as well as in our own, dogs were treated with aspirin and dipyridamole. Despite this treatment, aggregates of platelets and fibrin attached to the denuded vessel surface and to the surface of the stent wires. This platelet/fibrin thrombotic material was most severe overlying the stent wires, reaching a maximum of 250–300 µm, and also extended intermittently along the entire length of the stented portion of the vessel, averaging 35–75 μm in thickness. The increased thickness of the thrombus over the stent wires was due to the indentation in the media produced by the stent wire and the "filling in" of this indentation by thrombotic material. With time, endothelial cells were observed overlying the thrombus, and smooth muscle cells grew into the thrombus. The smooth muscle cells were of the secretory phenotype. Ultrastructurally, they had lost most of their myofilaments and had abundant rough endoplasmic reticulum. Thus, the proliferative and migratory activities of medial smooth muscle cells as they leave the media and grow into the neointima cause them to overgrow the luminal thrombotic material and, in some cases, to grow down into the thrombus from the luminal surface. With time, the neointima becomes more cellular and little thrombotic material was visible. The neointima was composed of primarily smooth muscle cells, as evidenced by smooth muscle α-actin immunostaining, with only occasional fibroblasts and inflammatory cells. There was a moderate amount of amorphous eosinophilic extracellular matrix material surrounding the smooth muscle cells in the neointima.

At 6 months after stent placement, there was neointima covering the stent wires and this neointima was covered by endothelial cells (Figure 16.5). The neointima ranged in thickness from 100 to 250 μm. The vessel lumen was patent and the lumen contour was smooth. The neointima covering the stent wires was composed of smooth muscle cells with abundant eosinophilic cytoplasm and some small blood vessels (Figure 16.5B). These cells were primarily fusiform in shape along the luminal surface, as would be expected for mature smooth muscle cells of the contractile phenotype. Also, in deeper regions close to the stent wire, the smooth muscle cells were more irregular in appearance and there was more extracellular matrix material (secretory phenotype). In the areas between the stent wires, the neointimal proliferative reaction was less pronounced and the smooth muscle cells were primarily of the contractile phenotype. In many areas, the extracellular material in the neointima after 6 months was fibrillar in nature and stained positively for collagen with the trichrome stain; there was little elastic tissue present. Thus, in these specimens, the major portion of the extracellular matrix was composed of fibrous connective tissue. There was some rarefaction of the media underneath the stent wires and there was a minimal inflammatory response. In some sections, particularly sections where the stent wire had lacerated the internal and the external elastic membrane, there was a mild accumulation of macrophages, lymphocytes, and plasma cells adjacent to the stent wire.

In studies of angioplasty and stent placement in normal dog arteries, the neointimal proliferative response appears to be minimal and seldom produces significant compromise of the vessel lumen. The neointimal reaction does appear to contain some fibroblasts and, with time, collagen (fibrous tissue) is seen within the neointimal tissue. Compared with man, the dog appears to have a somewhat diminished response to vascular injury. This finding, along with the lack of a good atherosclerosis model in the dog, decreases the utility of this model system for studies of restenosis.

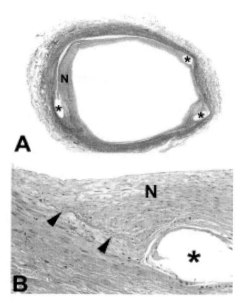

*Figure 16. 5* Dog coronary artery 6 months after stent placement. (A) Low-power view of the coronary artery after stent wires have been removed (asterisk). The neointima (N) is well formed but the thickness is variable. (B) High-power view of the vessel wall demonstrating the internal elastic membrane (arrowheads) that had been lacerated with the stent deployment. The neointima consists of primarily synthetic type smooth muscle cells with a mild to moderate amount of extracellular matrix.

## *Swine*

Swine models of vascular injury and restenosis are considered by most investigators to be the gold standard animal model for studies of vascular intervention. Pigs are relatively inexpensive to procure, are readily available, and are well suited for vascular research (Michel, 1966; Hughes, 1986; Swindle *et al.*, 1986). Juvenile farm pigs can be utilized for acute and short-term experiments of vascular injury. However, farm pigs grow rapidly and can reach an adult weight of greater than 400 kg. Thus, all studies in farm pigs must necessarily be of short duration. This problem of extreme size in pig models can be overcome by the use of specially bred mini- or micropigs (Gal *et al.*, 1990). These animals reach an adult weight of 30–40 kg. These animals are available commercially; however, the procurement costs are four to five times greater than farm pigs. This increased procurement cost is outweighed by the utility of using these specially bred laboratory animals, by the decreased cost of maintaining these animals, and by the ability to perform long-term experiments with these animals. Adult farm pigs develop naturally occurring atherosclerotic lesions (Gross, 1985; Vesselinovitch, 1988). Also, in both farm pigs and minipigs, high-cholesterol diets will produce an elevation in serum cholesterol and increased low-density lipoproteins. These serum lipid changes predispose to atherosclerosis. The lesions seen in the naturally occurring atherosclerosis closely resemble human atherosclerotic lesions, including lipid deposition, calcification, and development of a fibrous cap (Reitman et al., 1982; Weiner et al., 1985; Gal et al., 1990). Lesions from experimental models of atherosclerosis have some characteristics similar to man; however, the overall character of the lesions demonstrate little similarity to those commonly seen in human autopsy cases (Carter et al., 1996; Post et al., 1997).

Studies of balloon injury in pig coronary arteries involves overstretching and injury to the vessel wall (Anderson, 1992; Liu et al., 1996, 1997). The type of injury and the restenotic process is quite dissimilar to the classic rat carotid balloon injury model. In the rat, the vessel is denuded of endothelium and there is little or mild medial injury. However, in the pig coronary artery model, there must be significant medial injury before you elicit a restenotic reaction. As this model involves injury to a normal vessel, the type of lesion caused by the angioplasty balloon or the stent is somewhat different from that seen after interventional procedures in human atherosclerotic vessels. In man, it goes without saying that interventions are not usually performed unless there are underlying atherosclerotic lesions in the vessel. Work from our laboratory and from others (Farb et al., 1994; Anderson and Atkinson, 2001) has demonstrated that in atherosclerotic vessels balloon injury usually causes laceration at the "shoulder region" of the atherosclerotic plaque, with dissection between the plaque and media or the adventitia. In normal pig coronary arteries, there are no atherosclerotic plaques. Thus, as depicted in Figure 16.6, the angioplasty balloon stretches the vessel until there is laceration of the media with stretching of the external elastic lamina and the adventitia. Immediately after the balloon injury, a layer of platelets and thrombus form on the exposed external elastic lamina Figure 16.6C. Examination of vessel segments immediately after overstretch balloon injury demonstrate the laceration of the media and the exposed external elastic lamina (Figure 16.6D and E). Within 4 days after the injury, there is migration of smooth muscle cells into the thrombus that forms in the rent produced by the medial laceration (Figure 16.7A and B). Over time, the space produced by the overstretch injury is filled in as neointima forms (Figure 16.7C–F). Studies from our laboratory have shown that most of the neointima forms by 14 days after injury, with only a moderate increase in neointima between 14 and 28 days (Liu et al., 1997).

The response of pig coronary arteries to intravascular stenting in normal and atherosclerotic swine has been well characterized (Schwartz et al., 1990; Anderson, 1992; Cox et al., 1992). In these studies, vascular injury is induced by placement of wire stents which are deployed by an angioplasty balloon, thus producing endothelial denudation and stretch injury to the vessel wall. Stents and delivery balloons can be sized such that the size of the fully inflated balloon inside the vessel produces varying degrees of vessel wall stretch injury. In some studies, the balloons are purposely over stretched (50–100 percent oversizing, e.g. a 3.0-mm-diameter stent inside a 1.5- to 2.0-mm-diameter vessel) to produce significant neointimal proliferative reaction. It is also possible to use balloons and stents that

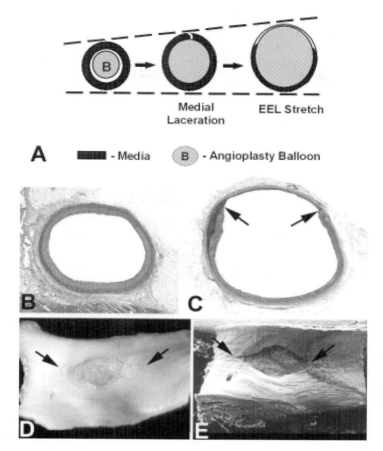

*Figure 16.6* Overstretch balloon injury in the pig. (A) Diagrammatic representation of overstretch balloon injury in the pig coronary artery. As the balloon [B] is inflated, the vessel stretches until finally there is a focal area of laceration in the vessel wall (center diagram). As the balloon is inflated further, the adventitia is stretched. (B) Low-power view of a normal pig coronary artery just proximal to the site of balloon injury. (C) Low-power view of pig coronary artery at the site of balloon injury. Note that the media is lacerated (arrows) and that there is an area of dissection between the media and the adventitia at both ends of the medial laceration. These focal areas of dissection are filled with thrombotic material. (D) Gross photographs of the luminal surface of a pig coronary artery immediately after overstretch balloon injury. Note the area of medial laceration (arrows) that exposes the external elastic membrane and the adventitia. (E) Scanning electron micrograph of the same section as seen in (D). Again note the area of medial laceration (arrows) running longitudinally along the vessel lumen.

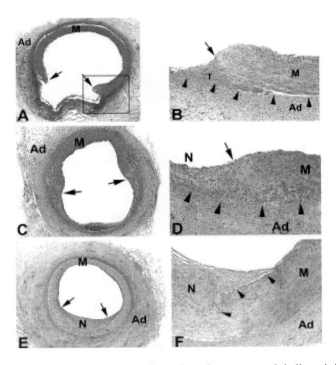

*Figure 16.7* Time-course of neointima formation after overstretch balloon injury in pig coronary arteries. (A) Low-power view of pig coronary artery 4 days after balloon injury. Note the laceration of the media with areas of dissection (arrows). (B) High-power view of an area of media (M) at the edge of the laceration (similar to the area outlined in A). The arrow points to the broken end of the internal elastic membrane. The arrowheads outline the external elastic membrane. Note that here is thrombotic material (T) adherent to the external elastic lamina. Near the surface of this thrombotic material, there are several smooth muscle cells beginning to form the neointima. Also note the abundance of inflammatory cells in the adventitia (Ad). (C and D) Similar sections of pig coronary artery 7 days after balloon injury. Again note areas of medial laceration (arrows). The neointima (N) is much larger and more organized. Note that there is still some thrombotic material trapped in the neointima present along the external elastic lamina (arrowheads). (E and F) Similar sections of pig coronary artery 14 days after balloon injury. Again note areas of medial laceration (arrows). The neointima (N) is even larger and more organized and slightly impinges on the vessel lumen. Note at high power (F) that the media and the neointima blend together and note the broken end of the internal elastic membrane (arrowheads).

produce less vessel wall injury (10–20 percent oversizing), which produces less neointimal reaction (Anderson, 1992; Schwartz *et al.*, 1990).

In our studies of the severe overstretching model of stent placement in the pig (Cox *et al.*, 1992; Waller and Anderson, 1998), we have observed frequent laceration of the internal elastic membrane with stent wires being embedded into the media or adventitia. Despite this degree of vessel injury, only one out of forty-five pigs demonstrated very mild extravasation of blood that was clinically insignificant. In pigs that were killed 28 days after stent implantation, there was a moderate thickening of the adventitia around the stented vessel segment and the degree of neointimal and adventitial reaction was clearly visible (Figure 16.9). The primary reaction within the vessel wall consisted of neointimal tissue which was found overlying the stent wires where the vessel wall had been indented and, to a lesser extent, around the entire circumference of the vessel (Figures 16.8 and 16.9). The neointimal tissue consisted of smooth muscle cells with varying amounts of eosinophilic extracellular material and occasional small blood vessels. Morphologically, the neointimal tissue is similar to human restenotic tissue seen after angioplasty or stenting (Anderson *et al.*, 1992; Farb *et al.*, 1994). In vessels

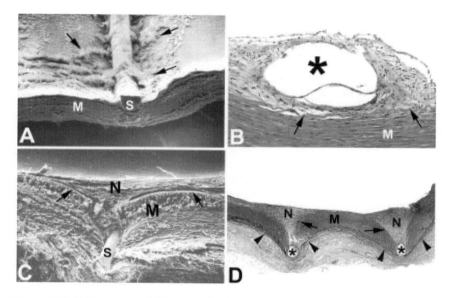

*Figure 16.8* Balloon-expandable stents in pig coronary arteries. (A) Scanning electron micrograph of a pig coronary artery 4 h after stent placement in which the stents were carefully deployed to minimize vessel stretching. Note that the stent wires only slightly indent the vessel media and that there is an accumulation of platelet-rich thrombotic material associated with the stent wires. (B) Three weeks after stent placement there is a well-formed neointima that has surrounded the stent (asterisk where stent wire was removed). (C) Scanning electron micrograph of a pig coronary artery 3 weeks after stents were placed using an overstretch technique to injure the vessel wall purposely. The stent wire (S) is deeply embedded into the media (M) and the wire is adjacent to the external elastic membrane. There is a well-formed neointima (N) that has filled in the indentation produced by the stent wire and is much thinner along the area of media between the stent wires. (D) Histology of a longitudinal section from the artery seen in (C). Note that the stent wires lacerated the internal elastic membrane (arrows) and completely lacerated the media (M). The stent wires (asterisk where wires were removed for processing) were contacting the external elastic lamina (arrowheads). Note that the contour of the vessel lumen is quite smooth. The neointima has "filled in" the indentations produced by the stent wires.

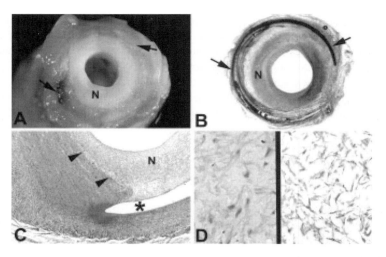

*Figure 16.9* Neointima formation 28 days after stent placement in pig coronary arteries. (A) Gross photograph of stented pig coronary artery demonstrating the well-developed concentric neointimal formation indicative of in-stent restenosis. Also note the marked thickening of the adventitia. (B) Low-power view of plastic embedded section of pig coronary artery showing the stent wire in the outer media and adventitial layer and the thick neointima. (C) Histologic section of vessel wall demonstrating the laceration of the internal elastic lamina (arrowheads) and the partial laceration of the media adjacent to the location of the stent wire (asterisk). Note the well-formed neointima (N). (D) High-power view of the neointima stained with hematoxylin and eosin (left) and immunostained for smooth muscle actin (right). Note the extensive extracellular matrix material that is especially evident in the section stained for smooth muscle actin (right). This morphology is virtually identical to that observed in human restenosis.

where the stent wires embedded deep into the media or into the adventitia, there is often a chronic inflammatory reaction consisting of macrophages, lymphocytes, plasma cells, and occasional eosinophils.

A significant neointimal proliferative reaction is seen in the oversized stent coronary artery model in the pig (Anderson, 1992; Cox *et al.*, 1992; Waller and Anderson, 1998). This neointimal reaction is morphologically similar to the reaction seen in humans after angioplasty; however, the degree of proliferation may be greater than that usually seen in man. This exuberant proliferative reaction may be so intense that pharmacologic means of preventing restenosis would be unable to ameliorate the neointimal proliferative response. Thus, studies utilizing compounds or techniques that may have promise in preventing restenosis could give a negative result. Further studies must be undertaken to characterize this model of restenosis better.

Investigations of restenosis in conjunction with atherosclerosis in pigs have utilized minipigs for these long-term studies. In one study (Rodgers *et al.*, 1990), minipigs were placed on an atherogenic diet consisting of 2 percent cholesterol, 15 percent fat, and 1.5 percent sodium cholate 2 weeks before balloon denudation of the coronary artery. Four to five months after the original vascular intervention, atherosclerotic lesions had developed at the area of denudation. These lesions were then used as sites for stent implantation to evaluate the response of a diseased artery to stent implantation. At sacrifice, there was a significant neointimal proliferative reaction within the stented region of the vessel. The character of these lesions was similar to that seen in the stented coronary arteries of pigs not on the atherogenic diet (described above), except that these arteries also contained foam cells and more fibrous connective tissue within the neointima. In additional studies with minipigs, stents were implanted in normal coronary arteries 2 weeks after the pigs had been started on an atherogenic diet (Santoian and King, 1992). In these studies, the character of the neointimal proliferation was similar to the non-atherogenic stented arteries described above and no mention was made of foam cells in these lesions.

It is apparent that swine models of vascular injury and restenosis are useful experimental tools for studies of the pathogenesis of restenosis. The neointimal proliferative response is very similar in character to that seen in man; however, as mentioned above, the proliferative response is very intense and may be more severe than the proliferative response seen in man. In addition, it is not apparent at this time what role the stent wire plays in producing the neointimal reaction seen in these animals. Further studies to characterize this restenosis reaction are needed to determine better the utility of these experimental systems as models for restenosis in man.

## Morphometric techniques in studies of restenosis

The various model systems described above all have inherent strengths and weaknesses. In all the animal model systems, the production of a neointimal response to a vascular insult is the primary goal of each experimental model. In an ideal experimental model, the degree of neointimal proliferation should be reproducible and consistent from animal to animal. Experimental manipulation of these model systems would result in an increase or decrease in the degree of neointimal proliferation that could be quantitated. Thus, for most experiments, accurate quantitation of the degree of neointimal proliferation is necessary to evaluate the experimental end-point. Accurate quantitation of the neointima requires correct utilization of morphometric techniques. Although simple in concept, valid morphometric evaluation of biologic tissues requires rigorous use of established morphometric techniques (Weibel, 1979, 1980; Elias and Hyde, 1980; Reid, 1980). The main tenant of morphometry is that the samples to be analyzed must be representative samples of the tissue reaction as a whole. This is especially germane to studies of restenosis in coronary arteries. In many of the models described above, focal areas of injury are produced in the vessel. A good example of this is the placement of stents in coronary arteries of pigs. In this instance, it is important to sample the entire region that is injured in order to evaluate properly the tissue response to injury. In many published studies of stent injury, tissue samples are taken from the stented region and a single sample is subjected to morphometric evaluation. In these studies, the one artery section with the most severe stenosis is evaluated. Picking the region with the most severe stenosis is a valid technique in clinical cardiology because the maximum blood flow to the distal myocardium is dictated by the most severe stenotic lesion. However, in experiments designed to evaluate tissue response to injury, it is important to take representative samples from the entire region of the vessel that was injured. The degree of restenosis for a specific experimental procedure should be the mean restenosis for the entire injured area, not the degree of restenosis in the most severely affected area of the vessel. This basic requirement of adequate tissue sampling for valid morphometric evaluation of biologic tissues is especially important in studies designed to compare the degree of restenosis after specific experimental interventions or treatment regimens. Accurate and valid morphometric techniques are a prerequisite for scientific experiments of restenosis.

In models of endothelial denudation and angioplasty with little distortion of the vessel wall (e.g. rat carotid model), the degree of restenosis can be readily quantitated. In these cases, the tissue inside (luminal to) the internal elastic membrane is easily identified as neointima. However, in experimental model systems in which the internal elastic membrane is ruptured or lacerated (balloon overstretching, stents, or lasers), it becomes more difficult to quantitate the neointima accurately. It is impossible to trace the internal elastic membrane for determinations of neointimal area in histologic sections if the internal elastic membrane is discontinuous. Estimations of where the internal elastic membrane "should have been" must be made by the investigator performing the morphometric evaluation. This raises some doubts about the validity and reproducibility of these measurements. We have developed protocols in our laboratory for evaluating restenosis in pig and dog arteries after angioplasty injury and stenting (Anderson, 1992; Cox et al., 1992; Liu et al., 1996, 1997). We have endeavored to use proper morphometric techniques to obtain reproducible measurements of restenosis after a variety of interventions. In our stented arteries, the stent wires lacerate the internal elastic membrane and, in some cases, also lacerate the external elastic membrane (see Anderson, 1992; Cox et al., 1992). In these cases, it is impossible to quantitate the neointima by simply tracing the internal elastic membrane and defining any material luminal to the internal elastic membrane as neointima. Because of these difficulties in accurately quantitating the tissue response to injury in the pig stent model, we developed the following technique.

In our studies with injured pig coronary arteries (angioplasty injury or stenting), the hearts were perfusion fixed with 10 percent buffered formalin or 2 percent glutaraldehyde at 60 mmHg. Segments of the coronary artery containing the injury were identified and were carefully dissected from the heart. Approximately 1–2 cm of normal coronary artery proximal and distal to the injury site was also included in this specimen. The fixed vessels were sectioned at 2- to 3-mm increments perpendicular to the vessel axis so that at least six serial sections of each artery segment were obtained, including one from the normal coronary artery proximal to and distal to the injury site or the stent. When present, stent wire coils were not removed before sectioning. The soft tissue of the stented artery was transected with a scalpel blade and the wire coils were cut with wire cutters. The pieces of wire embedded in the tissues were carefully removed with fine forceps to prevent distortion of the artery wall and neointima. The coronary artery sections were embedded in paraffin using standard histologic techniques, and 5-μm sections of each artery section were cut. Tissue sections were affixed to glass microscope slides, and two serial sections were stained with hematoxylin and eosin and aldehyde fuchsin Gomori's trichrome stain. With many types of intravascular stents, it is difficult or impossible to remove the stent wires from the vessels without causing undue distortion of the vessel architecture. In this case, stented vessel segments can be embedded in plastic and cut using techniques commonly used for processing of histology samples of orthopedic appliances (Carter et al., 1999).

Morphometric evaluation of coronary artery cross-sections was performed using techniques similar to those described previously (Anderson, 1992; Cox et al., 1992; Liu et al., 1996, 1997). A Graf/pen sonic digitizing system interfaced with a computer was used to evaluate light microscopic projected images of 5-μm trichrome-stained tissue sections. The external and internal perimeters of these vessel cross-sections were traced for each of the serial sections on each slide and a mean value was calculated. The external perimeter was measured by tracing the external elastic lamina when present, and when the external elastic lamina was disrupted by the stent wire the outer extent of the smooth muscle tissue was included in the tracing. The internal perimeter was determined by tracing the lumen of the vessel. Using standard mathematical formulae for a circle, these perimeter values were used to calculate the outer diameter of the vessel, the lumen diameter, the total vessel wall area, and the vessel lumen area. The vessel wall area of the control unstented vessel section was determined by subtracting the lumen area from the total vessel area. This calculation, therefore, derives the medial area of the unstented control region. The artery sections from the stented region contained media as well as neointima. Because of the disruption of the internal elastic lamina by the stent wires, it was impossible to separate accurately the media from the neointima by tracing with the digitizing system. To determine neointimal area in the stented region, the vessel wall area of the control unstented region (which consisted of only media) was subtracted from the vessel wall area of the stented region (which contained both media and neointima). This technique allowed us to obtain a direct measure of the mean neointimal area in the entire stented region of the vessel accurately.

Utilizing these morphometric techniques, we feel that we can accurately and reproducibly quantitate the degree of neointimal proliferation in vessel segments after experimental manipulation. Proper morphometric procedures must be utilized in studies of restenosis in animal models in order to allow investigators to make comparisons between different experiments and different treatment modalities.

## Concluding remarks

The endothelium, smooth muscle cells, and adventitia are the major structural components of the wall of blood vessels that are affected in the processes of chemically induced or mechanical injury. Connective tissue cells and the extracellular matrix produced by synthetic smooth muscle cells also play a role in the response of blood vessels to injury. Blood constituents, particularly platelets and components of the coagulation cascade, are also primary participants in vascular injury and repair.

Structural alterations are limited, whereas the mechanisms of injury are numerous, complex, and often poorly understood. Nonetheless, characterization of the morphologic changes often provide important directions for investigating the nature and mechanisms of injury. It is therefore essential that pathologists provide an anatomic/morphologic description of the changes observed that is as accurate as possible.

When evaluating the pathologic significance of morphologic changes observed in toxicologic evaluation studies, two general points should considered. (1) Not all the induced morphologic changes are a sign of toxicity (functional impairment). Structural alterations are limited, whereas the mechanisms of interaction for chemicals with cells and tissues are numerous, complex, and often poorly understood. This fundamental issue in toxicologic evaluation has been discussed in detail (Ruben and Rousseaux, 1991). An example is clear cytoplasmic vacuoles in muscle cells of coronary and other arteries in the dog induced by disobutamide. The morphologic change was remarkable, but no overt signs of toxicity were observed; the cytoplasmic vacuoles were a morphologic manifestation of intracellular drug storage (Ruben et al., 1993). (2) Background spontaneous lesions may present a problem in concluding that the observed changes in treatment animals are induced by the test article. Arteritis in beagle dogs or rats and some vascular neoplasms in rats are examples of this (Ruben et al., 1989, 1997, 2000).

These physiologic factors and the altered homeostasis in disease conditions should be taken into account when considering the mechanisms of toxic and mechanical injury to blood vessels. Furthermore, as just described, not all structural alterations induced by drugs or chemicals in toxicologic evaluation studies are signs of toxicity. The border between physiology (limits of normal functions) and toxicity (functional impairment) is not often clearly defined. This is a continuing important area of research that may lead to new insights and to understanding of the response of the vascular response to injury.

## References

Anderson PG. 1992. Restenosis: Animal models and morphometric techniques in studies of the vascular response to injury. *Cardiovasc Pathol* 1: 263–278.

Anderson PG, Atkinson JB. 2001. Atherosclerosis. In *Atlas of Cardiovascular Pathology*. McManus BM, Braunwald E (eds). Current Medicine, Philadelphia.

Anderson PG, Bajaj RK, Baxley WA, Roubin GS. 1992. Vascular pathology of balloon-expandable flexible coil stents in humans. *J Am Coll Cardiol* 19: 372–381.

Anderson PG, Boerth NJ, Liu MW, McNamara DB, Cornwell TL, Lincoln TM. 2000. Cyclic GMP-dependent protein kinase expression in coronary arterial smooth muscle in response to balloon catheter injury. *Arteriosclerosis Thromb Vasc Biol* 20: 2192–2197.

Atkinson JB, Swift LL, Virmani R. 1992. Watanabe heritable hyperlipidemic rabbits. Familial hypercholesterolemia. *Am J Pathol* 140: 749–753.

Banai S, Shou M, Correa R, Jaklitsch MT, Douek PC, Bonner RF, Epstein SE, Unger EF. 1991. Rabbit ear model of injury-induced arterial smooth muscle cell proliferation. Kinetics, reproducibility, and implications. *Circ Res* 69: 748–756.

Bates ER, McGillem MJ, Mickelson JK, Pitt B, Mancini GB. 1991. A monoclonal antibody against the platelet glycoprotein IIb/IIIa receptor complex prevents platelet aggregation and thrombosis in a canine model of coronary angioplasty. *Circulation* 84: 2463–2469.

Beckman JS. 1996. Oxidative damage and tyrosine nitration from peroxynitrite. *Chem Res Toxicol* 9: 836–844.

Beckman JS, Ischiropoulos H, Zhu L, van der Woerd M, Smith C, Chen J, Harrison J, Martin JC, Tsai M. 1992. Kinetics of superoxide dismutase- and iron-catalyzed nitration of phenolics by peroxynitrite. *Arch Biochem Biophys* 298: 438–445.

Beckman JS, Ye YZ, Anderson PG, Chen J, Accavitti MA, Tarpey MM, White CR. 1994. Extensive nitration of protein tyrosines in human atherosclerosis detected by immunohistochemistry. *Biol Chem Hoppe Seyler* 375: 81–88.

Blank RS, Owens GK. 1990. Platelet-derived growth factor regulates actin isoform expression and growth state in cultured rat aortic smooth muscle cells. *J Cell Physiol* 142: 635–642.

Block PC, Baughman KL, Pasternak RC, Fallon JT. 1980. Transluminal angioplasty: correlation of morphologic and angiographic findings in an experimental model. *Circulation* 61: 778–785.

Boerth NJ, Dey NB, Cornwell TL, Lincoln TM. 1997. Cyclic GMP-dependent protein kinase regulates vascular smooth muscle cell phenotype. *J Vasc Res* 34: 245–259.

Boor PJ, Langford SD. 1997. Pathology of chemically induced arterial lesions. In *Comprehensive Toxicology*. Sipes IG, McQueen CA, Gandolfi AJ (eds), pp. 309–332. Pergamon, New York.

Boor PJ, Gotlieb AI, Joseph EC, Kerns WD, Roth RA, Tomaszewski KE. 1995. Chemical-induced vasculature injury. Summary of the symposium presented at the 32nd annual meeting of the Society of Toxicology, New Orleans, Louisiana, March 1993. *Toxicol Appl Pharmacol* 132: 177–195.

Breslow JL. 1996. Mouse models of atherosclerosis. *Science* 272: 685–688.

Burke A, Mullick FG, Virmani R. 1997. Characterization of toxic and drug-induced cardiovascular lesions in humans. In *Comprehensive Toxicology*. Bishop SP, Kerns WD (eds), pp. 445–481. Pergamon, New York, NY.

Campbell GR, Campbell JH, Manderson JA, Horrigan S, Rennick RE. 1988. Arterial smooth muscle. A multifunctional mesenchymal cell. *Arch Pathol Lab Med* 112: 977–986.

Carere RG, Koo EWY, Liu PP, Gotlieb AI. 1992. Porcine coronary artery organ culture: A model for the study of angioplasty injury. *Cardiovasc Pathol* 1: 107–115.

Carter AJ, Laird JR, Kufs WM, Bailey L, Hoopes TG, Reeves T, Farb A, Virmani R. 1996. Coronary stenting with a novel stainless steel balloon-expandable stent: determinants of neointimal formation and changes in arterial geometry after placement in an atherosclerotic model, *J Am Coll Cardiol* 27: 1270–1277.

Carter AJ, Farb A, Gould KE, Taylor AJ, Virmani R. 1999. The degree of neointimal formation after stent placement in atherosclerotic rabbit iliac arteries is dependent on the underlying plaque. *Cardiovasc Pathol* 8: 73–80.

Clark JM, Glagov S. 1976. Luminal surface of distended arteries by scanning electron microscopy: eliminating configurational and technical artefacts. *Br J Exp Pathol* 57: 129–135.

Clarkson TB. 1998. Nonhuman primate models of atherosclerosis. *Lab Anim Sci* 48: 569–572.

Clowes AW, Reidy MA, Clowes MM. 1983. Mechanisms of stenosis after arterial injury. *Lab Invest* 49: 208–215.

Clowes AW, Clowes MM, Fingerle J, Reidy MA. 1989. Kinetics of cellular proliferation after arterial injury. V. Role of acute distension in the induction of smooth muscle proliferation. *Lab Invest* 60: 360–364.

Clowes AW, Clowes MM, Au YPT, Reidy MA, Belin D. 1990. Smooth muscle cells express urokinase during mitogenesis and tissue-type plasminogen activator during migration in injured rat carotid artery. *Circ Res* 67: 61–67.

Coats Jr. WD, Currier JW, Faxon DP. 1997. Remodelling and restenosis: insights from animal studies. *Semin Intervent Cardiol* 2: 153–158.

Consigny PM, Tulenko TN, Nicosia RF. 1986. Immediate and long-term effects of angioplasty-balloon dilation on normal rabbit iliac artery. *Arteriosclerosis* 6: 265–276.

Cornwell TL, Soff GA, Traynor AE, Lincoln TM. 1996. Regulation of cyclic GMP-dependent protein kinase by cell density in vascular smooth muscle cells. *J Vasc Res* 31: 330–337.

Cox DA, Anderson PG, Roubin GS, Chou C-Y, Agrawal SK, Cavender JB. 1992. Effect of local delivery of heparin and methotrexate on neointimal proliferation in stented porcine coronary arteries. *Coronary Artery Dis* 3: 237–248.

Crissman RS. 1986. SEM observations of the elastic networks in canine femoral artery. *Am J Anat* 175: 481–492.

Dartsch PC, Voisard R, Bauriedel G, Hofling B, Betz E. 1990. Growth characteristics and cytoskeletal organization of cultured smooth muscle cells from human primary stenosing and restenosing lesions. *Arteriosclerosis* 10: 62–75.

Davis EC. 1995. Elastic lamina growth in the developing mouse aorta. *J Histochem Cytochem* 43: 1115–1123.

Elias H, Hyde DM. 1980. An elementary introduction to stereology (quantitative morphology). *Am J Anat* 159: 412–446.

Farb A, Virmani R, Atkinson JB, Anderson PG. 1994. Long-term histologic patency after percutaneous transluminal coronary angioplasty is predicted by the creation of a greater lumen area. *J Am Coll Cardiol* 24: 1229–1235.

Faxon DP, Weber VJ, Haudenschild C, Gottsman SB, McGovern WA, Ryan TJ. 1982. Acute effects of transluminal angioplasty in three experimental models of atherosclerosis. *Arteriosclerosis* 2: 125–133.

Faxon DP, Sanborn TA, Weber VJ, Haudenschild C, Gottsman SB, McGovern WA, Ryan TJ. 1984. Restenosis following transluminal angioplasty in experimental atherosclerosis. *Arteriosclerosis* 4: 189–195.

Ferrell M, Fuster V, Gold HK, Chesebro JH. 1992. A dilemma for the 1990s. Choosing appropriate experimental animal model for the prevention of restenosis. *Circulation* 85: 1630–1631.

Feuerstein GZ, Kerns WD. 1997. Molecular pharmacology of arterial endothelium and smooth muscles. In *Molecular Pharmacology of Arterial Endothelium and Smooth Muscles*. Bishop SP, Kerns WD (eds), pp. 43–54. Pergamon, New York.

Fingerle J, Johnson R, Clowes AW, Majesky MW, Reidy MA. 1989. The role of platelets in smooth muscle cell proliferation and migration after vascular injury in the rat carotid artery. *Proc Natl Acad Sci USA* 86: 8412–8416.

Fingerle J, Au YPT, Clowes AW, Reidy MA. 1990. Intimal lesion formation in rat carotid arteries after endothelial denudation in absence of medial injury. *Arteriosclerosis* 10: 1082–1087.

Fishman JA, Ryan GB, Karnovsky MJ. 1975. Endothelial regeneration in the rat carotid artery and the significance of endothelial denudation in the pathogenesis of myointimal thickening. *Lab Invest* 32: 339–351.

Forrester JS, Fishbein M, Helfant R, Fagin J. 1991. A paradigm for restenosis based on cell biology: clues for the development of new preventive therapies. *J Am Coll Cardiol* 17: 758–769.

Furchgott RF. 1996. The 1996 Albert Lasker Medical Research Awards. The discovery of endothelium-derived relaxing factor and its importance in the identification of nitric oxide. *J Am Med Assoc* 276: 1186–1188.

Furchgott RF. 1999. Endothelium-derived relaxing factor: discovery, early studies, and identification as nitric oxide. *Biosci Rep* 19: 235–251.

Gal D, Rondione AJ, Slovekai GA, DeJesus ST, Lucas A, Fields CD, Isner JM. 1990. Atherosclerotic Yucatan microswine: an animal model with high-grade fibrocalcific, nonfatty lesions suitable for testing catheter-based interventions. *Am Heart J* 119: 291–300.

Geer JC, Guidry MA. 1962. Experimental canine atherosclerosis. In *Comparative Atherosclerosis: the Morphology of Spontaneous and Induced Atherosclerotic Lesions in Animals and Its Relation to Human Disease*. Roberts Jr. JC, Straus R (eds), pp. 170–185. Harper & Row, New York.

Gibbons GH, Dzau VJ. 1994. The emerging concept of vascular remodeling. *N Engl J Med* 330: 1431–1438.

Giese NA, Marijianowski MM, McCook O, Hancock A, Ramakrishnan V, Fretto LJ, Chen C, Kelly AB, Koziol JA, Wilcox JN, Hanson SR. 1999. The role of alpha and beta platelet-derived growth factor receptor in the vascular response to injury in nonhuman primates. *Arteriosclerosis Thromb Vasc Biol* 19: 900–909.

Graham A, Hogg N, Kalyanaraman B, O'Leary V, Darley-Usmar V, Moncada S. 1993. Peroxynitrite modification of low-density lipoprotein leads to recognition by the macrophage scavenger receptor. *FEBS Lett* 330: 181–185.

Gross DR. 1985. *Animal Models in Cardiovascular Research*, pp. 537–547. Martinus Nijhoff, Boston.

Heggtveit HA. 1983. Nonatherosclerotic diseases of the aorta. In *Cardiovascular Pathology*. Silver MD (ed.), pp. 707–737. Churchill Livingstone, New York.

Hehrlein C, Chuang CH, Tuntelder JR, Tatsis GP, Littmann L, Svenson RH. 1991. Effects of vascular runoff on myointimal hyperplasia after mechanical balloon or thermal laser arterial injury in dogs. *Circulation* 84: 884–890.

Hughes HC. 1986. Swine in cardiovascular research. *Lab Anim Sci* 36: 348–350.

Ignarro LJ, Buga GM, Wood KS, Byrns RE, Chaudhuri G. 1987. Endothelium-derived relaxing factor produced and released from artery and vein is nitric oxide. *Proc Natl Acad Sci USA* 84: 9265–9269.

Ignarro LJ, Cirino G, Casini A, Napoli C. 1999. Nitric oxide as a signaling molecule in the vascular system: an overview. *J Cardiovasc Pharmacol* 34: 879–886.

Johnson RM, Lincoln TM. 1985. Effects of nitroprusside, glyceryl trinitrate, and 8-bromo cyclic GMP on phosphorylase a formation and myosin light chain phosphorylation in rat aorta. *Mol Pharmacol* 27: 333–342.

Joseph EC, Mesfin G, Kerns WD. 1997. Pathogenesis of arterial lesions caused by vasoactive compounds in laboratory animals. In *Comprehensive Toxicology*. Bishop SP, Kerns WD (eds), pp. 279–307. Pergamon, New York.

Kwon HM, Sangiorgi G, Ritman EL, McKenna C, Holmes Jr. DR, Schwartz RS, Lerman A. 1998. Enhanced coronary vasa vasorum neovascularization in experimental hypercholesterolemia. *J Clin Invest* 101: 1551–1556.

Lafont A, Faxon D. 1998. Why do animal models of post-angioplasty restenosis sometimes poorly predict the outcome of clinical trials? *Cardiovasc Res* 39: 50–59.

Lincoln TM, Komalavilas P, Cornwell TL. 1994. Pleiotropic regulation of vascular smooth muscle tone by cyclic GMP-dependent protein kinase. *Hypertension* 23: 1141–1147.

Lincoln TM, Komalavilas P, Boerth NJ, MacMillan-Crow LA, Cornwell TL. 1995. cGMP signaling through cAMP- and cGMP-dependent protein kinases. In *Nitric Oxide: Biochemistry, Molecular Biology and Therapeutic Implications*. Ignarro L, Murad F (eds), pp. 305–322. Academic Press, San Diego.

Lincoln TM, Dey NB, Boerth NJ, Cornwell TL, Soff GA. 1998. Nitric oxide–cyclic GMP pathway regulates vascular smooth muscle cell phenotypic modulation: implications in vascular diseases. *Acta Physiol Scand* 164: 507–515.

Liu MW, Roubin GS, King III SB. 1989. Restenosis after coronary angioplasty. Potential biologic determinants and role of intimal hyperplasia. *Circulation* 79: 1374–1387.

Liu MW, Hearn JA, Luo JF, Anderson PG, Roubin GS, Iyer, S, Bilodou L. 1996. Reduction of thrombus formation without inhibiting coagulation factors does not inhibit intimal hyperplasia after balloon injury in pig coronary arteries. *Coronary Artery Dis* 7: 667–671.

Liu MW, Anderson PG, Luo JF, Roubin GS. 1997. Local delivery of ethanol inhibits intimal hyperplasia in pig coronary arteries after balloon injury. *Circulation* 96: 2295–2301.

Louden CS, Nambi P, Pullen MA, Thomas RA, Tierney LA, Solleveld HA, Schwartz LW. 2000. Endothelin receptor subtype distribution predisposes coronary arteries to damage. *Am J Pathol* 157: 123–134.

Majesky MW, Giachelli CM, Reidy MA, Schwartz SM. 1992. Rat carotid neointimal smooth muscle cells reexpress a developmentally regulated mRNA phenotype during repair of arterial injury. *Circ Res* 71: 759–768.

Manderson JA, Mosse PRL, Safstrom JA, Young SB, Campbell GR. 1989. Balloon catheter injury to rabbit carotid artery. I. Changes in smooth muscle phenotype. *Arteriosclerosis* 9: 289–298.

Michel G. 1966. *Swine in Biomedical Research*, p 421. Frayn Printing Co., Seattle.

Murad F. 1999. Discovery of some of the biological effects of nitric oxide and its role in cell signaling. *Biosci Rep* 19: 133–154.

Noishiki Y, Yamane Y, Tomizawa Y, Okoshi T, Satoh S, Takahashi K, Yamamoto K, Ichikawa Y, Imoto K, Tobe M, *et al.* 1994. Rapid neointima formation with elastic laminae similar to the natural arterial wall on an adipose tissue fragmented vascular prosthesis. *Asaio J* 40: 267–72.

Oshima R, Ikeda T, Watanabe K, Itakura H, Sugiyama N. 1998. Probucol treatment attenuates the aortic atherosclerosis in Watanabe heritable hyperlipidemic rabbits. *Atherosclerosis* 137: 13–22.

Paigen B, Morrow A, Holmes PA, Mitchell D, Williams RA. 1987. Quantitative assessment of atherosclerotic lesions in mice. *Atherosclerosis* 68: 231–240.

Plump AS, Smith JD, Hayek T, Aalto-Setala K, Walsh A, Verstuyft JG, Rubin EM, Breslow JL. 1992. Severe hypercholesterolemia and atherosclerosis in apolipoprotein E-deficient mice created by homologous recombination in ES cells. *Cell* 71: 343–353.

Post MJ, de Smet BJ, van der HY, Borst C, Kuntz RE. 1997. Arterial remodeling after balloon angioplasty or stenting in an atherosclerotic experimental model. *Circulation* 96: 996–1003.

Prescott MF, Webb RL, Reidy MA. 1991. Angiotensin-converting enzyme inhibitor versus angiotensin II, AT1 receptor antagonist. Effects on smooth muscle cell migration and proliferation after balloon catheter injury. *Am J Pathol* 139: 1291–1296.

Pukac LA, Hirsch GM, Lormeau J-C, Petitou M, Choay J, Karnovsky MJ. 1991. Antiproliferative effects of novel, nonanticoagulant heparin derivatives on vascular smooth muscle cells in vitro and in vivo. *Am J Pathol* 139: 1501–1509.

Regan CP, Anderson PG, Bishop SP, Berecek KH. 1996. Captopril prevents vascular and fibrotic changes but not cardiac hypertrophy in aortic-banded rats. *Am J Physiol* 271: 906–913.

Regan CP, Anderson PG, Bishop SP, Berecek KH. 1997. Pressure-independent effects of AT1-receptor antagonism on cardiovascular remodeling in aortic-banded rats. *Am J Physiol* 272: 2131–2138.

Reid IM. 1980. Morphometric methods in veterinary pathology: A review. *Vet Pathol* 17: 522–543.

Reitman JS, Mahley RW, Fry DL. 1982. Yucatan miniature swine as a model for diet-induced atherosclerosis. *Atherosclerosis* 43: 119–132.

Rodgers GP, Minor ST, Robinson K, Cromeens D, Woolbert SC, Stephens LC, Guyton JR, Wright K, Roubin GS, Raizner AE. 1990. Adjuvant therapy for intracoronary stents. Investigations in atherosclerotic swine. *Circulation* 82: 560–569.

Ross R. 1986. The pathogenesis of atherosclerosis – an update. *N Engl J Med* 314: 488–500.

Ross R. 1993. The pathogenesis of atherosclerosis: a perspective for the 1990s. *Nature* 362: 801–808.

Roubin GS, Robinson KA, King III SB, Gianturco C, Black AJ, Brown JE, Siegel RJ, Douglas JS. 1987. Early and late results of intracoronary arterial stenting after coronary angioplasty in dogs. *Circulation* 76: 891–897.

Ruben Z, Rousseaux CG. 1991. The limitations of toxicologic pathology. In *Handbook of Toxicologic Pathology*. Hasdai D, Rousseau CG (eds), pp. 131–142. Academic Press, Orlando.

Ruben Z, Deslex P, Nash G, Redmond NI, Poncet M, Dodd DC. 1989. Spontaneous disseminated panarteritis in laboratory beagle dogs in a toxicity study: a possible genetic predilection. *Toxicol Pathol* 17: 145–152.

Ruben Z, Arceo RJ, Wagner BM. 1992. Chemically induced injury of blood vessels. In *Cardiovascular Toxicology*, 2nd edn. Acosta D (ed.), pp. 517–541. Raven Press, New York.

Ruben Z, Rorig KJ, Kacew S. 1993. Perspectives on intracellular storage and transport of cationic–lipophilic drugs. *Proc Soc Exp Biol Med* 203: 140–149.

Ruben Z, Arceo RJ, Bishop SP. 1997. Proliferative lesions of the heart and vasculature in rats. In *Guides for Toxicologic Pathology*. STP/ARP/AFIP, Washington.

Ruben Z, Arceo RJ, Bishop SP. 2000. Proliferative lesions of the heart and vasculature in rats. In *Guides for Toxicologic Pathology*. STP/ARP/AFIP, Washington.

Santoian EC, King III SB. 1992. Intravascular stents, intimal proliferation and restenosis. *J Am Coll Cardiol* 19: 877–879.

Schatz RA, Palmaz JC, Tio FO, Garcia F, Garcia O, Reuter SR. 1987. Balloon-expandable intracoronary stents in the adult dog. *Circulation* 76: 450–457.

Schwartz SM, Campbell GR, Campbell JH. 1986. Replication of smooth muscle cells in vascular disease. *Circ Res* 58: 427–444.

Schwartz RS, Murphy JG, Edwards WD, Camrud AR, Vlietstra RE, Holmes DR. 1990. Restenosis after balloon angioplasty. A practical proliferative model in porcine coronary arteries. *Circulation* 82: 2190–2200.

Shi Y, O'Brien Jr. JE, Fard A, Mannion JD, Wang D, Zalewski A. 1996. Adventitial myofibroblasts contribute to neointimal formation in injured porcine coronary arteries. *Circulation* 94: 1655–1664.

Sims FH. 1989. A comparison of structural features of the walls of coronary arteries from 10 different species. *Pathology* 21: 115–124.

Sims FH, Gavin JB, Vanderwee MA. 1989. The intima of human coronary arteries. *Am Heart J* 118: 32–38.

Stanley WC, Connett RJ. 1991. Regulation of muscle carbohydrate metabolism during exercise. *FASEB J* 5: 2155–2159.

Swindle MM, Horneffer PJ, Gardner TJ, Gott VL, Hall TS, Stuart RS, Baumgartner WA, Borkon AM, Galloway E, Reitz BA. 1986. Anatomic and anesthetic considerations in experimental cardiopulmonary surgery in swine. *Lab Anim Sci* 36: 357–361.

Vesselinovitch D. 1988. Animal models and the study of atherosclerosis. *Arch Pathol Lab Med* 112: 1011–1017.

Waller BF, Anderson PG. 1998. The pathology of interventional coronary artery techniques and devices. In *Textbook of Interventional Cardiology*. Topol EJ (ed.). W.B. Saunders Company, Philadelphia.

Weibel ER. 1979. *Stereological Methods*. Vol. 1. *Practical Methods for Biological Morphometry*. Academic Press, London.

Weibel ER. 1980. *Stereological Methods*. Vol. 2. *Theoretical Foundations*. Academic Press, London.

Weiner BH, Ockene IS, Jarmolych J, Fritz KE, Daoud AS. 1985. Comparison of pathologic and angiographic findings in a porcine preparation of coronary atherosclerosis. *Circulation* 72: 1081–1086.

Wilgram GF, Ingle DJ. 1965. "Spontaneous" cardiovascular lesions in rats. In *Comparative Atherosclerosis: the Morphology of Spontaneous and Induced Atherosclerotic Lesions in Animals and Its Relation to Human Disease*. Roberts Jr. JC, Straus R (eds), pp. 87–91. Harper & Row, New York.

Willerson JT, Eidt JF, McNatt J, Yao S-K, Golino P, Anderson HV, Buja LM. 1991. Role of thromboxane and serotonin as mediators in the development of spontaneous alterations in coronary blood flow and neointimal proliferation in canine models with chronic coronary artery stenoses and endothelial injury. *J Am Coll Cardiol* 17: 101B–110B.

Windecker S, Meier B. 2000. Intervention in coronary artery disease. *Heart* 83: 481–490.

# 17

# THE ARTERIAL MEDIA AS A TARGET OF INJURY BY CHEMICALS

*Paul J. Boor*

*Department of Pathology,*
*University of Texas Medical Branch, Galveston, TX, USA*

## Introduction

The vasculature of the mammalian body forms a vast, interconnected system. Each blood vessel performs a discrete and unique function, and each vessel's structure is uniquely suited to its job within the vasculature. Despite this, the cellular make-up of blood vessels is remarkably simple. All vessels – from the largest vessels, such as aorta and great veins, to the microscopic capillaries – are composed entirely of two basic cell types: the endothelial cell and the vascular smooth muscle cell (Rhodin, 1974).

Endothelial cells form a vast surface that is a "barrier" between blood vessel and blood (Ettenson and Gotlieb, 1993). The endothelial cells sit on a basement membrane (the "internal elastic lamina") and a scant amount of matrix to form the thin intima. Immediately adjacent is the media, which constitutes the major part of arteries but is less prevalent in veins. The media, which is composed of varying thicknesses of vascular smooth muscle cells and extracellular or structural elements such as collagen, elastin, and other proteins, is responsible for the mechanical function of blood vessels. The largest blood vessels are the elastic arteries, so-called because elastin arranged in thick, concentric layers is the main part of their extracellular matrix. The function of elastic arteries is to recoil, i.e. they absorb pulsatile energy transmitted from the left ventricle, converting blood flow to a smoother, more continuous flow. Their medial smooth muscle cells produce and maintain the elastin that is critical to their recoil, as well as other structural and matrix proteins of the vessel wall. These cells are capable of contraction, but this is not their primary function in elastic arteries.

As the large arteries taper to medium-sized arteries, the muscular component of the media increases relative to the amount of elastin; accordingly, the function of the media becomes more contractile. Even muscular arteries such as coronary arteries are capable of significant contraction – a function that is important in the pathophysiology of ischemic heart disease, which today is still the major cause of death in the USA (Ross, 1997).

The smallest muscular arteries are the arterioles. These microscopic vessels are the "valves" of the vascular system, tightly controlling flow to peripheral tissues through the contraction and relaxation of the vascular smooth muscle cells of their media. Thus, the smaller muscular arteries and arterioles – known as "peripheral resistance vessels" – are part of a complex interplay among peripheral tissues, the heart, and the kidney. These vessels are essential to the control of blood pressure, cardiac output, and fluid balance.

As can be determined from the above information, the media is an important part of all arteries – from the largest to the smallest. In this chapter, chemicals that cause vascular injury by damaging the arterial media will be discussed. These chemicals may exert their deleterious effects predominantly on the medial smooth muscle cell, or they may damage both the endothelium and the media. In some cases, these chemicals have major pathophysiologic effects on blood pressure and the flow of blood in the vasculature, whereas in other instances physiologic effects are minimal or unknown. Chemicals may also target the extracellular matrix, altering the structure of the blood vessel wall and causing the vessel to weaken and dilate, eventually forming an aneurysm that bursts. In every example chosen, the focus of this chapter will be on the vascular media as a target of injury caused by chemicals, and wherever possible the structural changes and the mechanisms of injury that underlie these unique toxic lesions will be emphasized.

## Vasoactive chemicals

The small muscular arteries, and especially the arterioles, are the peripheral vessels that (through contraction and dilatation) control blood pressure and the flow of blood to the peripheral tissues. "Vasoactive" chemicals are those that either lower or raise blood pressure by acting on these peripheral vessels. In toxicology, "The right dose differentiates a poison from a remedy" (attributed to Paracelsus, 1493–1541). This axiom is especially true of vasoactive chemicals that have beneficial effects at lower doses but that injure the vessel wall at higher doses. Many clinically useful drugs either lower or raise blood pressure in treating shock, heart failure, or hypertension. But at high doses, these same drugs may injure the media of peripheral resistance vessels.

### Vasopressors, catecholamines

The first family of vasoactive chemicals is the catecholamines. This group includes endogenous catecholamines produced by the adrenal gland, and an array of drugs that raise blood pressure ("vasopressors") by constricting peripheral arteries and arterioles. (Hence, they are also known as "vasoconstrictors.")

In high or repeated doses, catecholamines injure the media of arteries and arterioles. This has been known since the early 1900s, when scientists first described medial degeneration, necrosis, and calcification in experimental animals given large cumulative doses of the endogenous catecholamines epinephrine and norepinephrine (Szakacs and Mehlman, 1960). Experimental work in the latter half of the last century showed that a host of vasopressors, including many that have enjoyed extensive clinical usage, cause necrosis of medial vascular smooth muscle cells (Rona *et al.*, 1959, 1977). When severe, areas of medial damage are associated with overlying loss of endothelium; exposure of the basement membrane and subintimal matrix then results in a platelet–fibrin thrombus on the intimal surface. Injurious catecholamines and closely related amines include dopamine, isoproterenol, tyramine, and 5-hydroxytryptamine. Many other vasoconstrictors cause systemic hypertension and lesions of small muscular arteries and arterioles; these include, among others, vasopressin, methoxamine, and angiotensin II (Kerns *et al.*, 1989; Joseph *et al.*, 1997).

Exactly how vasopressors cause medial damage has been the topic of many experimental investigations for over 60 years. Earlier experiments, such as those by Waters and DeSoto-Nagy (1950) and the classic studies of renal-induced hypertension by Goldblatt (1938) showed that hypertension of severe enough degree and long enough duration will universally cause damage to peripheral resistance vessels, and even larger muscular arteries. Vasopressors directly applied to – or perfused through – isolated peripheral vessels, however, also cause contraction and medial damage that is often accompanied by endothelial dysfunction and disruption (Kobori *et al.*, 1979; Vitullo *et al.*, 1985). Thus, although we know that severe hypertension – no matter the cause – is injurious to vessels, it appears that vasopressors may also be directly toxic to the media and endothelium, or to the intima.

### *Vasodilators*

Vasodilators are a second family of vasoactive chemicals that injure arteries. Many vasodilators are useful drugs because they lower blood pressure in patients with severe hypertension; others were developed for the treatment of congestive heart failure. Minoxidil, for example, is a useful drug in two distinctly different clinical settings: it is used to treat severe hypertension and is applied topically for the treatment of baldness in men. In extremely high doses, and especially when given intravenously, minoxidil causes hemorrhagic necrosis of small muscular branches of the coronary arteries in dogs and pigs; similar lesions are found in the mesenteric – or splanchnic – arteries of rats (Herman *et al.*, 1979; Van Vleet *et al.*, 1995). Lesions of coronary arteries are also caused by experimental vasodilator drugs that act by inhibiting the specific type III isozyme of phosphodiesterase (Issacs *et al.*, 1989). Fenoldopam was another drug developed for the treatment of hypertensive patients, but when medial hemorrhage and necrosis was found in renal and splanchnic arteries of rats given the drug, preclinical trials in humans were stopped (Kerns *et al.*, 1989). Thus, there are several examples of vasodilators – both drugs and experimental drugs – that injure the media of arteries.

Vasoconstrictors and vasodilators cause morphologically different medial lesions, in different vessels. In general, vasopressors cause necrosis of the vascular smooth muscle cells of the media, characterized by bright pink, homogeneous areas of media in routine histologic preparations stained with hematoxylin and eosin. These bland pink areas, known as fibrinoid necrosis, are not associated with hemorrhage, but are widespread in small muscular arteries and arterioles. The catecholamine vasopressors also affect much larger arteries, including the aorta, and – when given chronically – result in calcification of the media and degeneration of elastic fibers.

Vasodilators – on the other hand – typically affect muscular arteries such as splanchnic, renal, and coronary arteries. Vasodilators cause medial necrosis, generally without overt endothelial damage, and the necrotic areas within the media are extremely hemorrhagic. The reader will find a more thorough discussion of arterial lesions caused by other vasoactive chemicals in the excellent review by Joseph et al. (1997).

### Nitric oxide-associated medial injury

The discovery that nitric oxide (NO) is a major endothelial-derived vasodilator of peripheral arteries has given new insights into how the endothelium plays a role in the control of vascular tone and blood pressure. The release of the highly diffusible NO from endothelium to relax adjacent vascular smooth muscle cells by stimulating guanylate cyclase to generate cGMP is an exciting example of paracrine control within the vascular wall. Virtually thousands of experimental studies have now defined other roles for NO; it is now known to be a major player in the vascular pathophysiology of cigarette smoking (Campisi et al., 1998).

It does not appear, however, that drugs causing vasodilation through release of NO are capable of causing morphologically detectable medial injury. For instance, commonly used drugs – such as the organic nitrates (which have been used to treat angina pectoris since 1857) or nitroprusside (a major therapeutic used in the treatment of acute, severe hypertension) – do not cause any vascular lesions whatsoever (Needleman et al., 1985). This is unlike other vasodilators (discussed above) that cause medial necrosis characterized by extensive hemorrhage into the vessel wall, accompanied by little endothelial damage.

A few experiments indicate that chemicals which interfere with NO metabolism, however, may be injurious to the vascular wall. Specifically, large doses of inhibitors of NO synthase (NOS), the enzyme responsible for generating NO from L-arginine, cause hypertension and have widespread toxic effects on arteries. Two independent groups of researchers have described coronary vascular lesions – including perivascular fibrosis, medial hypertrophy and intramedial fibrosis, and vascular smooth muscle proliferation – in rats treated with the NOS inhibitor $N^{\omega}$-nitro-L-arginine methyl ester (L-NAME) (Kristek et al., 1995; Numaguchi et al., 1995). These investigators also described sustained hypertension in animals treated with L-NAME, and severe myocardial hypertrophy and fibrosis, consistent with hypertension and previous myocardial infarcts. Others have documented acute myocardial necrosis and hyperplasia of the arterial media in rats following chronic L-NAME treatment (Moreno *et al.*, 1995; Babal *et al.*, 1997).

Another group of scientists found spinal cord infarcts in rats treated with long-term L-NAME (Blot *et al.*, 1994). Hitchon and co-workers (1996), using a similar NOS inhibitor (L-$N^\omega$-nitroarginine), then showed that inhibiting NOS causes systemic hypertension and reduces blood flow to the spinal cord; these observations confirm that spinal cord infarcts are likely due to constriction of small spinal cord vessels. Surprisingly, however, Hitchon *et al.* (1996) found that, in traumatized spinal cords, blood flow was actually increased by NOS inhibition. Based on their studies, they suggest that NOS inhibition could be potentially therapeutic following spinal cord trauma (Hitchon *et al.*, 1996).

Our laboratory has recently concluded similar experiments with NOS inhibitors. Although these experimental compounds caused moderate rises in systemic blood pressure, the necrotizing lesions that we found diffusely in myocardium, and the fibrinoid necrosis and medial hypertrophy seen in coronary arteries, suggest to us that these chemicals induce severe vasoconstriction and injury in muscular arteries of several sizes (see Figure 17.1). Also, the severity of these heart and coronary

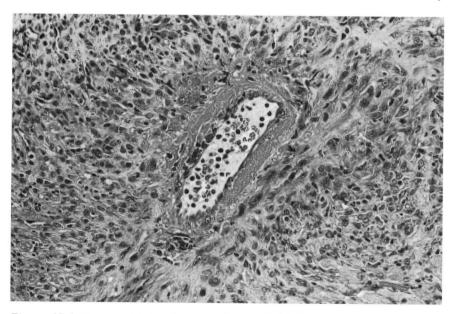

*Figure 17.1* Vasoconstrictor, hypertensive medial injury. Acute necrosis of an intramyocardial coronary artery caused by inhibition of NO synthase (NOS), usually associated with systemic hypertension. The term "hyaline" necrosis has been used to describe the media because of its homogeneous pink appearance and loss of cell detail. Acute medial necrosis such as this can be caused by NOS inhibitors such as L-NAME (Moreno *et al.*, 1995; Babal *et al.*, 1997) and also by pressor agents that cause severe hypertension (hematoxylin and eosin stain; 210×).

artery lesions seemed out of proportion to the moderate hypertension developed (10–20 mmHg rises).

In our studies, we also found spinal cord infarcts in rats treated with NOS inhibitors (Blot *et al.*, 1994; Hitchon *et al.*, 1996) and noted focal infarct-like lesions in skeletal muscle as well, consistent with necrosis due to vasospasm of peripheral resistance vessels (P. J. Boor and S. Stofanski, unpublished data). Thus, it appears that inhibition of NOS by different chemicals results in variable lesions, affecting different vessels. There clearly are several subtypes of NOS, and perhaps these subtypes are localized in different vessels. Whatever the vessel subtype, however, it appears that interfering with the normal homeostasis of NO metabolism may result in severe injury to the vascular media.

## *Ergot alkaloids*

One final example is a family of vasoconstrictive toxins that cause severe injury of small muscular arteries without changes in systemic blood pressure – the ergot alkaloids. These naturally occurring chemicals have sporadically intoxicated human populations for centuries, causing epidemic outbreaks of great historical importance. These extremely potent toxins are elaborated by an endophytic fungus of the species *Acremonium* that infests the aerial portion of grasses, such as rye or tall fescue, that are commonly grazed upon by cattle. *Acremonium* produces several ergopeptine alkaloids, or ergot alkaloids, including lysergic acid amide (ergine), ergovaline, ergotamine, the clavine class of alkaloids, and pyrrolizidine alkaloids such as permine (Porter, 1995). Contamination of livestock grazing grasses with the ergot-forming fungi causes a well-known cattle toxicosis of great economic importance (Woods *et al.*, 1966; Hoveland, 1993). As in human cases of ergot overdose, intoxicated cattle develop gangrene of hoofs and extremities as a result of vasoconstriction or "arteriospasm" (Oliver *et al.*, 1993).

Of the many compounds made by *Acremonium*, ergotamine is the only one that has been used as a drug, beginning in the late 1800s when it was used in obstetrical practice. Following its isolation from ergot extract in 1918, ergotamine began to be used for migraine headaches (in 1925). Today, it is the most common drug prescribed for the treatment of migraine headache (Silberstein and Young, 1995). The drug is thought to have a complex effect on intracerebral blood flow via selective vasoconstriction of the carotid artery (Saxena and de Vlaam-Schluter, 1974). Although the clinical use of ergotamine is generally safe, excessive usage by patients, or purposeful overdose, results in severe arterial vasospasm in a variety of vascular beds with serious complications of ischemia and necrosis of limbs, bowel, face, and – rarely – overt myocardial infarction (for a review, see Silberstein and Young, 1995).

Human populations have been exposed to ergot alkaloids through contamination of flour and bread during outbreaks of *Acremonium* infestation of grains such as rye. During such outbreaks, there is some evidence that bizarre societal behavior has occurred, including medieval witch-hunts in Europe and religious revivals in

America (Fuller, 1968; Matossian, 1982a). Indeed, major epidemics of so-called ergotism, known as Saint Anthony's fire, are presumed to have occurred in Europe throughout recorded history.

As there are many biologically active compounds produced by contaminating grass endophytes, it is thought that a variety of central nervous system effects, as well as the peripheral manifestations caused by vasospasm of peripheral arteries, occur during such outbreaks. It has been postulated that the witch trials of 1692 in Salem, Massachusetts, took place during an outbreak of convulsive ergotism in which hallucinations, bizarre convulsant disorders, and necrosis (or gangrene) of extremities affected a series of young women who were, accordingly, accused of practicing witchcraft (Spanos and Gottlieb, 1976; Matossian, 1982b). Because a whole community would be affected by the bread produced from contaminated grains, it is likely that all community members – including the judges involved – suffered similar central nervous system effects. It is disconcerting that contamination of foodstuffs by ergot continues today, even in highly industrialized countries (Scott and Lawrence, 1980; Scott et al., 1992).

Only a few experimental studies have examined the mechanism by which ergot alkaloids exert their extreme vascular toxic effects. Ergotamine is an extremely powerful constrictor of vascular smooth muscle of the media, constricting even veins, presumably through serotonin receptors (Silberstein and Young, 1995). Ergotamine itself probably causes a complex interplay of direct vasoconstrictive action, central nervous system effects, and inhibition of vascular reflexes to result in vasospasm of peripheral blood vessels, vascular injury, and necrosis of widespread tissues as a consequence. Few research studies have addressed the mechanism of action of the other ergot alkaloids.

## Lesions secondary to endothelial injury

Besides working in concert to control blood flow to the peripheral tissues, the intima and media also depend on each other to maintain the integrity of the blood vessel wall. Atherosclerosis – the nearly universal vascular disease that is the major cause of death and suffering in the Western world – illustrates this interdependence. The atherosclerotic plaque is thought to begin with subtle endothelial injury that results in the recruitment of both circulating cells (macrophages and T lymphocytes) and aberrant, proliferative smooth muscle cells that migrate to the plaque from the vascular media (Ross, 1997). A tremendous amount of experimental work is now defining the pathophysiologic events that begin the atherosclerotic plaque and support its progression.

Thus, the media contributes phenotypically altered, proliferating cells to the early atherosclerotic plaque. The media further adds to plaque progression by supporting growth of new blood vessels into the plaque, allowing further cellular influx, and leading to late complications of the plaque including plaque hemorrhage and rupture (Moulton et al., 1999). Eventually, as plaque burden in the vessel wall advances, the atherosclerotic plaque impinges on the media, causing it to degenerate, to scar, and eventually to disappear. The loss of media is especially evident in advanced atherosclerotic abdominal aorta or coronary artery, where large expanses of vessel may have only scattered remnants of media remaining and large areas of vessel wall are replaced by fibrous tissue (P. J. Boor, unpublished observation).

Homocysteine is an excellent example of a chemical that severely damages blood vessels through initial endothelial injury. It has been known since 1975 that children with inborn metabolic defects resulting in high serum levels of homocysteine (homocysteinemia) develop severe, fatal occlusive and thrombotic vascular disease with many similarities to atherosclerosis (McCully, 1969). High serum homocysteine has now been established as an independent risk factor for the development of atherosclerosis in humans (Clark et al., 1991).

Experiments in rabbits, baboons, rhesus monkeys, pigs, and rats have confirmed that administration of homocysteine severely injures endothelium in large blood vessels such as the aorta. Administration of methionine, which is degraded in vivo to homocysteine, also results in hyperhomocysteinemia and endothelial cell lysis and dysfunction accompanied by superficial smooth muscle damage of the media (Matthias et al., 1996; Upchurch, et al., 1996). Homocysteine may interfere with normal physiologic regulation by NO because homocysteine rapidly binds NO to form S-nitroso-homocysteine. Homocysteine in the blood also may directly damage endothelium by generating oxygen-derived free radicals that target intracellular sites such as DNA and $NAD^+$ (Blundell et al., 1996). Although its most important action as a vascular toxin is to act as an atherogen, as the lesions it causes are so dramatically destructive to arteries, homocysteine should be considered injurious to the entire vascular wall, including the media.

Many other chemicals, including a multitude of toxins in cigarette smoke, have been implicated in initiating the atherosclerotic plaque through endothelial injury. The medial involvement in atherosclerosis should be viewed as secondary to that initial injury of endothelium. However, it is not the purpose of this chapter to address atherosclerosis in depth; the reader is referred to other reviews and discussions in this volume for more on atherosclerosis (Ross, 1997).

The media is injured and restructured following other more subtle types of initial endothelial insult. Several of the best examples of this are found in the pulmonary vasculature. For instance, the seeds of plants of Crotalaria species contain a pyrralizidine alkaloid known as monocrotaline that is highly toxic to the liver and the pulmonary vasculature. Monocrotaline is metabolized in the liver by P450 oxidative enzymes to a highly reactive pyrrolic derivative, which is extremely unstable and exists only long enough to circulate from the liver via hepatic veins to the pulmonary arteries. Thus, monocrotaline targets the small arteries and capillaries of the lung. Remarkably, a single intraperitoneal dose of monocrotaline results in permanent elevation of the pulmonary arterial pressure 2–3 weeks later. The pathologic picture closely resembles primary pulmonary hypertension in man, a fatal disease without known cause.

Monocrotaline toxicity begins with degeneration of pulmonary endothelium induced by covalent binding of the highly reactive monocrotaline pyrrole metabolite to macromolecules of the lung endothelium. The critical barrier function of the intima is thus breached, resulting in vascular leakage with rapidly accumulating pulmonary interstitial edema and formation of platelet thrombin in lung capillaries.

Following these events of the first 2 or 3 days of monocrotoline intoxication, the small pulmonary arteries undergo structural remodeling, with smooth muscle hypertrophy, hyperplasia, and periarterial fibrosis developing along with a marked rise in pulmonary arterial pressure. These changes are not those of acute cell death in the wall of the artery, but reflect the development of advanced, end-stage pulmonary hypertension a few weeks after monocrotoline administration. This essentially fatal condition is characterized both in humans and in experimental animals by severely elevated intravascular pressure, secondary failure of the right ventricle, and terminal pulmonary parenchymal hemorrhage.

We know the details of this scenario because for over 20 years scientists such as Huxtable, Meyrick, and Roth and his co-workers (Huxtable *et al.*, 1978; Meyrick *et al.*, 1980; Boor *et al.*, 1995) have defined the mechanisms through which monocrotoline causes pulmonary vascular injury and hypertension. It is tempting to speculate that unknown toxins may play a similar role in at least some cases of idiopathic or primary pulmonary hypertension, a human disorder that remains enigmatic (Galie *et al.*, 1998).

A similar problem with much greater human relevance is the clinical and pathologic complications of the commonly used diet pill known as "fen-phen." Fenfluramine ("fen") and phentermine ("phen") are two appetite suppressants that are effective when given alone, but were prescribed in combination (fen-phen) in the early part of the 1990s. Use of the combination diet pill rose dramatically, so that in 1996 the total number of prescriptions was greater than 18 million (Connolly *et al.*, 1997). Combined therapy with the drug mixture was also used to reduce the consumption of alcohol by alcoholics and to quell cocaine craving (Hitzig, 1993, 1994). Early clinical reports of pulmonary hypertension developing in patients on either drug alone (McMurray *et al.*, 1986; Brenot *et al.*, 1993) were followed by extensive clinical studies indicating that either of these drugs alone, the drugs in combination, or a similar appetite suppressant (dexfenfluramine) caused pulmonary hypertension and fibrosing lesions of the cardiac valves (Abenhaim *et al.*, 1996; Connolly *et al.*, 1997; McCann *et al.*, 1997). These problems appear to regress after the drugs are stopped, further supporting a cause–effect relationship (Smith and Shuster, 1962).

In experiments with cultured pulmonary arterial smooth muscle cells and whole lungs isolated from rats, these agents inhibit specific voltage-gated $K^+$ channels (Weir *et al.*, 1996). In patients with pulmonary hypertension, similar $K^+$ channel dysfunction has been documented to result in membrane depolarization and calcium influx – phenomena that are presumably associated with vasoconstriction and subsequent proliferation of medial smooth muscle cells as the vessel wall thickens and pulmonary hypertension develops (Yuan *et al.*, 1998). This pathogenetic sequence bears some resemblance to the experimental pulmonary hypertension caused by monocrotoline, except that these diet-suppressing drugs appear to have a more direct effect on the vascular media. Endothelial injury has not been postulated to occur in "diet pill" pulmonary hypertension; however, it is fair to say that not many experimental studies have examined this form of medial injury.

## Structural injury to the media: lathyrism

The term "lathyrism" was coined in 1873 by Contani to describe a human disease characterized by the sudden onset of lower extremity spasticity that progresses to paralysis (Contani, 1873). The disease was again described in 1892 by Erb; hence the later term "Erb's paralysis" (Minchin, 1940). The neurologic component of lathyrism is clinically overt; however, "neurolathyrism" is the term best used to distinguish lathyrism's neurologic deficits from the bone pathology ("osteo-lathyrism") and aortic aneurysm ("angiolathyrism") that are also part of the disease in humans and in experimental animals.

By the 1800s, when it was first defined, the syndrome of neurolathyrism had already long been recognized to be caused by eating the seeds (or the flour made from these pea-like seeds) from plants of the genus *Lathyrus*. People consume *Lathyrus sativus*, *Lathyrus odoratus*, or the related *Ervum ervilia* as an alternative foodstuff during times of famine or extreme hardship. For instance, the disease was documented in World War II prisoner of war camps, and it has occurred in Europe, Syria, and India during times of famine. Ancient Hindu texts recognized the disease, and Hippocrates described the neurologic syndrome and associated it with *Lathyrus* consumption (Denny-Brown, 1947; Paissios and Demopoulos, 1962). Neurolathyrism occurs in domesticated animals such as cattle, chickens, horses and even elephants (Selye, 1957). The toxicity of *Lathyrus* is still an alarmingly real problem for both domestic animals and humans today, especially in India where a growing market for *Lathyrus sativus* as an adulterant of more expensive peas has resulted in commercial exportation of the toxic peas from the area where they grow (Gopalan, 1992).

Over 50 years ago, scientists began to study how *Lathyrus* causes such varied tissue lesions. This research is an example of how basic experiments, beginning with a complex plant toxin, can lead to a much deeper understanding of both physiologic and pathologic processes now known to be important in all connective tissues, and especially in the blood vessel wall. In the earliest experiments, the human syndrome of neurolathyrism was reproduced in rats fed *Lathyrus* plants (Stockman, 1929). Researchers observed the typical spastic paralysis of the lower limbs, but found that rats also developed severe skeletal deformities and frequently died of ruptured aortic aneurysms (Vivanco and Diaz, 1951; Ponseti, 1957; Dastur and Iyler, 1959). It was originally thought that these lesions of bone and aorta in the rat and other species did not occur in humans. Although there is some degree of species variation in the response to intoxication with *Lathyrus*, it is now known that humans also develop connective tissue pathology in addition to the more evident problems associated with neurolathyrism (Schulert and Lewis, 1952; Paissios and Demopoulos, 1962; Yeager *et al.*, 1985).

*Lathyrus* plants were then shown to contain several toxic chemicals. One component, the amino acid β-*N*-oxalylamine-L-alanine, is an extraordinarily powerful toxin to neurons in culture, and shows selective toxicity to thalamus and brain stem *in vivo* (Pai *et al.*, 1993). Accordingly, neurolathyrism is now thought to be due to direct neuronal toxicity of such components of *Lathyrus*, as well as to vascular compromise of small arteries to the spinal cord, or to true infarcts that are characteristic of the sudden onset of neurologic symptoms (Denny-Brown, 1947).

During the early studies of *Lathyrus* toxicity in animals, scientists found that the majority of animals fed the toxic seeds for extended periods (weeks to months) died of ruptured thoracic aortic aneurysms. This was universally true when immature, growing animals were fed *Lathyrus* (Ponseti, 1954; Bean and Ponseti, 1955; Lalich and Ishida, 1966; Lalich, 1967; Lalich *et al.*, 1971; Boor, 1985). The aneurysms were recognized as "dissecting" aneurysms, i.e. the media of the aorta degenerates and splits so that blood dissects all through the media, eventually rupturing the vessel. These pathologic findings bear many similarities to human conditions such as aneurysms of the cerebral circulation (Hazama and Hashimoto, 1987; Hashimoto *et al.*, 1987; Kim *et al.*, 1989), cystic medial necrosis of the aorta, and the aortic aneurysms seen in Marfan's or Menke's syndromes and idiopathic juvenile kyphoscoliosis (Ponseti and Baird, 1952). Scientists coined the term "angiolathyrism" to describe this remarkable toxic effect of *Lathyrus*, then turned their attention to how these plants exerted their remarkable toxic effects on the aorta (Lalich and Ishida, 1966; Lalich, 1967).

Dupuy and Lee (1954) isolated biologically active crystals from *Lathyrus pusillus*, and within a year the active component of plants causing angiolathyrism was identified as β-aminopropionitrile (β-APN) (Bachhuber and Lalich, 1954; Dasler, 1954; Schilling and Strong, 1954; Wawzonek *et al.*, 1955). The isolation of β-APN began a new era of experimental work on the mechanisms of vascular damage by organic nitriles and other chemicals. Martin and co-workers extracted abnormal collagen fractions from lathyritic tissues, especially bone, and recognized that the defect in insoluble collagen was due to abnormal cross-linking of the collagen molecule (Martin *et al.*, 1961, 1963). Page and Benditt (1967) defined the specific enzyme that cross-links precollagen molecules at lysine residues; this enzyme later became known as lysyl oxidase (protein-lysine 6-oxidase; EC 1.4.3.13). It is now generally accepted that the basis of the toxic action of β-APN is its property of inhibiting lysyl oxidase, resulting in abnormal, weakened collagen and elastin.

In this way, the investigation of a plant toxin led to a major breakthrough in understanding a critical biochemical step in the formation of structural proteins essential to all blood vessels. It is now well accepted that lysyl oxidase deaminates amino groups of lysine and hydroxylysine residues to yield aldehyde derivatives that subsequently form intermolecular bonds with other aldhydic residues in the mature collagen molecule. Similar bonds form through the action of lysyl oxidase on desmosine and isodesmosine, amino acids that are specific for elastin. These bonds impart great tensile strength to these critical structural proteins and are essential for their maturation and maintenance.

The reason, therefore, that β-APN has its greatest toxic effect on immature animals is because during periods of rapid growth these proteins are most actively synthesized and cross-linked by lysyl oxidase. Similarly, the aorta is a target of the toxic action of β-APN because – as the major elastic artery – it contains the highest percentage of elastin of any tissue. Other tissues that are deformed in lathyrism, such as bone and cartilage, also contain large amounts of collagen or elastin.

Utilizing β-APN as a tool, scientists have revealed much about the basic biology of connective tissue metabolism. The biochemistry of lysyl oxidase has been extensively characterized and its gene has been cloned and sequenced in several species and in man. The enzyme contains copper and also contains a second cofactor that is likely to have a reactive carbonyl group to transfer an electron from the amine of the lysyl (or other) residue to molecular oxygen. The cofactor of lysyl oxidase is likely to be pyrroloquinoline quinone (PQQ) or a PQQ-like moiety (Levene et al., 1988; Gacheru et al., 1989; Kagan and Trackman, 1991); other cofactors that have been proposed include 6-hydroxydopa or pyridoxal phosphate (Lyles, 1996).

Lysyl oxidase is a 32-kDa protein that exhibits distinct variants among species and tissues (Kagan et al., 1979; Kuivaniemi et al., 1984; Cronlund and Kagan, 1986). The human lysyl oxidase gene was first cloned and sequenced by Kagan and co-workers. Boyd et al. (1995) then defined seven exons of the gene, but the heterogeneity of lysyl oxidase mRNA was not thought to be the result of alternate exon usage. Instead, these scientists hypothesized that expression of multiple lysyl oxidase proteins was due to variable expression of multiple polyadenylation sites found within exon 7. A similar mechanism was reported for the mouse lysyl oxidase gene, partially explaining how lysyl oxidase exhibits such varied interactions with multiple forms of procollagen and tropoelastin and serves several different functions within the extracellular matrix (Contente et al., 1993).

Lysyl oxidase is now thought to be involved in many important cell processes. The enzyme is down-regulated in cells transformed by the ras oncogene, indicating that as cells transform to a malignant state they allow the surrounding extracellular matrix to degrade in order to form tumor masses more easily and to metastasize (Hajnal, 1993). Conversely, marked up-regulation of lysyl oxidase genes occurs in tissues during pathologic fibrosis or scarring. For instance, vascular smooth muscle cells up-regulate lysyl oxidase if stimulated by platelet-derived growth factor (Green et al., 1995). This experimental finding suggests that proliferating cells within the atherosclerotic plaque are stimulated by growth factors to lay down an extensive pathologic plaque matrix through the action of lysyl oxidase.

Similar mechanisms have been found in an experimental model of toxin-induced vascular injury that several laboratories, including our own, have utilized in recent years. Allylamine (3-aminopropene), when given to a variety of species for a period of weeks, results in proliferative intimal lesions that in many ways mimic the human atherosclerotic plaque (Boor *et al.*, 1979). Ramos and co-workers showed that the phenotype of vascular smooth muscle cells cultured from the aortic media of rats given allylamine *in vivo* modulates to a proliferative state characterized by rapid growth and production of extracellular matrix (Ramos *et al.*, 1993; Ramos and Ou, 1994). This phenotypic change is accompanied by enhanced protein kinase C-mediated protein phosphorylation and expression of aberrant matriceal proteins – these events are believed also to be important occurrences in the development of early atherosclerotic plaques in humans (Ross and Glomset, 1976). The fact that β-APN experimentally inhibits intimal proliferation and luminal narrowing supports a role for lysyl oxidase in atherosclerosis.

Historically, then, the term "lathyrism" was originally used for the human syndrome of neurotoxicity; scientists and clinicians then added the concepts of "osteolathyrism," and the remarkable medial degeneration of the aorta leading to aneurysm and death, i.e. "angiolathyrism." Through basic science investigations aimed at understanding connective tissue metabolism, the term "lathyrism" quickly came to be applied to abnormal collagen formation, usually through inhibition of lysyl oxidase.

Indeed, for a period of time there was great interest in developing therapeutic lathyrogenic chemicals to prevent scarring or the deposition of connective tissue. The list of disorders for which β-APN has been given in clinical or experimental attempts to alter the course of collagen formation in a scarring process is impressive, and includes Peyronie's disease, urethral stricture, scleroderma, systemic silicosis, Bleomycin-induced pulmonary fibrosis, and, post-operatively, following tendon grafts or ophthalmic procedures (Keiser and Sjoerdsma, 1967; Peacock and Madden, 1978; Riley *et al.*, 1982, 1987; Gelbard *et al.*, 1983; Chvapil *et al.*, 1984; Speer *et al.*, 1985; Busin *et al.*, 1986; Geismar *et al.*, 1988). Although β-APN therapies have been abandoned, the search for similar manipulations of connective tissue metabolism continues, especially with regard to vascular remodeling following injury such as that occurring after angioplasty.

"Lathyrogenic" has been applied to literally hundreds of compounds that interfere with collagen metabolism, but only a small fraction of these are true angiolathyrogens. Therefore, for clarity, the term "angiolathyrism" has been used in this chapter for vascular medial injury that has been clearly demonstrated *in vivo*. Chemicals which cause such medial injury are quite few. Nitriles such as β-APN itself and also aminoacetonitrile appear to be best documented as true angiolathyrogens. Several sulfhydryl-containing compounds, including β-mercaptoethylamine and cystamine, cause less dramatic vascular lesions, as does semicarbazide given in several different forms to experimental animals (Wawzonek *et al.*, 1955; Levene, 1960, 1961; Levene and Carrington, 1985; Noda *et al.*, 1987). Several powerful *in vitro* lathyrogens – including D-penicillamine, which has been tested clinically as an antifibrotic agent (Harris and Sjoerdsma, 1966) – do not injure blood vessels *in vivo*. Connective tissue metabolism is apparently complex, so that an effect shown in isolated cell or biochemical systems does not necessarily correlate with an *in vivo* action. For a more detailed account of angiolathyrogens, the reader is referred to the review by Boor and Langford (1997).

Our laboratory has studied the vascular toxic effects of the simple, non-catechol allylamine (3-aminopropene). This aliphatic amine causes myocardial necrosis that may be related to pathophysiologic contractions, or "vasospasm," of coronary artery (Boor and Hysmith, 1987; Boor *et al.*, 1995; Conklin and Boor, 1998), but allylamine is not – in a strict sense – a vasoactive amine because it does not alter blood pressure. Long-term treatment of several mammalian species with allylamine causes focal, individual necrosis of medial smooth muscle cells of aorta, but not broad areas of medial degeneration, connective tissue degeneration, or aneurysm. Hence, allylamine is not an angiolathyrogen to the degree that β-APN is (Kumar *et al.*, 1990, 1998).

In more recent experiments, we followed the lead set by other investigators who made the puzzling observations that a single chemical – hydralazine – protected the myocardium from allylamine-induced injury but increased the severity of β-APN-induced aortic aneurysm (Lalich and Paik, 1974; Simpson, 1982; Simpson and Taylor, 1982). We found that allylamine and β-APN were truly synergistic toxins in the aortic wall, causing striking degeneration and necrosis of vascular smooth muscle cells when given together for 10 days (see Figure 17.2), whereas their individual toxicity was minimal (Kumar *et al.*, 1990). We then found that other chemicals, when given in combination with allylamine, caused similar synergistic medial toxicity (Kumar *et al.*, 1998). Our working hypothesis is now that allylamine is the primary medial toxin in these combined protocols, and that the metabolism of allylamine is rendered more toxic to the media by other compounds. The combined treatment protocols in these experiments are excellent examples of angiolathyrism. Smooth muscle cells die within days of treatment, do not appear to repopulate the media, and the long-term structural damage is morphologically striking (see Figures 17.2 and 17.3).

### Human relevance

Do these experimental lesions have parallels in human disease? This question has been asked by scientists for over 90 years, because the earliest investigators of catecholamine-induced medial injury likened those experimental lesions to atherosclerosis or to Monckeberg's sclerosis, a disease characterized by destruction and calcification of the media of large arteries of head, neck, and extremities.

Degeneration of the media has long been recognized as a part of the so-called "connective tissue disorders" such as Marfan's or Menke's syndromes. Patients with these syndromes frequently die of aortic aneurysms caused by the degeneration of media morphologically similar to that seen in angiolathyrism due to chemicals (Pasquali-Ronchetti *et al.*, 1994). "Cystic medial necrosis" refers to

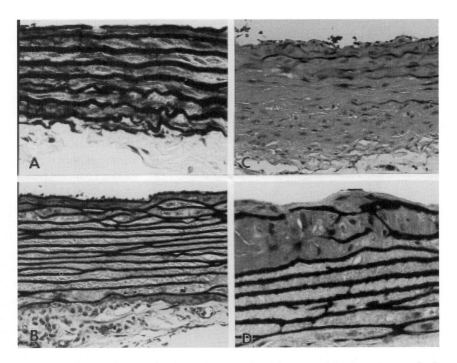

*Figure 17.2* Experimental lathyrism. (A) Normal architecture of the thoracic aorta in the rat shows dark elastic layers alternating with vascular smooth muscle cells (Movat's pentachrome stain; 210×). (B) Rats treated with substances that cause lathyrism exhibit relatively acute (occurring in 10 days) necrosis of medial smooth muscle cells. Note the absence of inflammatory infiltrate of any type in the media. The integrity of the elastic lamellae is maintained. Lathyrogenic chemicals include β-aminoproprionitrile, other nitriles such as aminoacetonitrile, sulfhydryl-containing compounds such as β-mercaptoethylamine and cystamine, and combinations of chemicals such as allylamine with β-amino-proprionitrile and/or phenelzine. For more details, see text and selected references (Kumar *et al.*, 1990, 1998) (Movat's pentachrome stain; 210×). (C) Six months after the initial injury by lathyrogens, media is not repopulated with smooth muscle cells, but has undergone fibrosis. Note the loss of elastic lamellae (Movat's pentachrome stain; 210×). (D) Six months after the initial injury by lathyrogens, focal areas of media undergo cartilaginous metaplasia, evidenced by large areas of amorphous, dark chondroid matrix surrounding chondrocytes. Elastic lamellae are present but are swollen and irregular. Note that the inter-elastic areas have not repopulated with vascular smooth muscle, nor with any other type of cell (Movat's pentachrome stain; 210×).

focal smooth muscle cell drop out and connective tissue degeneration that may be seen in these syndromes, as well as in aortas with dissecting aneurysm unrelated to these distinct genetic disorders. Dissecting aneurysms often sporadically affect young persons, and although the medial degeneration is morphologically similar to chemical-induced experimental models of angiolathyrism, the etiology of this

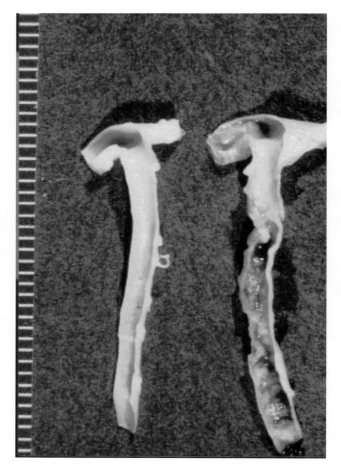

*Figure 17.3* Chronic medial injury; experimental lathyrism. Chronic injury of rat aorta by lathyrogen results in metaplasia of aorta (for histopathology, see Figure 17.2) and markedly thinned, irregular contour (left, control). Note the relative dilatation of distal aorta, similar to aneurysm formation in man (rule, mm). Reprinted with permission from Kumar *et al.* (1990).

fatal disorder remains unknown (Wilson and Hutchins, 1982). Rarely, coronary arteries may undergo spontaneous dissection, resulting in sudden death owing to acute occlusion of an otherwise normal-appearing artery (see Figure 17.4) (Virmani and Forman, 1989). Such coronary arterial dissections do not appear to be associated with overt degenerative changes, although they are more prevalent in women in the post-partum period, when hypertension or pregnancy-associated structural changes in the media may play a role (Manalo-Estrella and Barker, 1967).

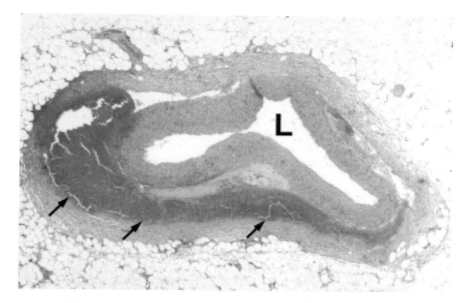

*Figure 17.4* Human coronary arterial-dissecting aneurysm. Spontaneous coronary arterial dissection occurring in an otherwise healthy 38-year-old woman who died suddenly. Note the dissection of blood into the outer layers of the media (arrows) and the consequent luminal occlusion (L, lumen). This rare, spontaneous occurrence of unknown etiology points out our lack of knowledge of medial biology and pathobiology, and the potential role that toxins may play in such lesions (Virmani and Forman, 1989) (hematoxylin and eosin stain; ~40×).

Although dissecting aneurysms affect the aorta diffusely, often being found in the thoracic aorta, abdominal aortic aneurysms are a much more common disease in older men. These aneurysms are associated with increasing age, smoking, and hypertension. However, a distinct familial incidence, as well as associated changes in elastin and collagen, suggests underlying derangements in the vascular media that are analogous to those described in angiolathyrism (Dobrin, 1989; Reilly and Tilson, 1989; Anidjar *et al.*, 1990; Tilson, 1992; Herron *et al.*, 1995). Thus, there are similarities between these significant human disorders and experimental angiolathyrism, although by no means have all the similarities or differences been defined.

## Nutritional deficiencies; genetic errors

Several experimental nutritional deficiencies result in vascular changes that are similar to the medial injury caused by chemicals that has been discussed above. Foremost is copper deficiency, which for over 30 years has been known to result in elastin and collagen abnormalities and dissecting aortic aneurysm (O'Dell *et al.*, 1961, 1978; Shields *et al.*, 1962; Harris and O'Dell, 1974). More recently, dietary deficiency of pyridoxine, or vitamin $B_6$, has been shown to result in similar degeneration of and disorganization of medial connective tissue, with resultant aortic aneurysm (Murray and Levene, 1977; Murray et al., 1978). These vascular medial lesions were correlated with decreased lysyl oxidase activity in connective tissues systemically. As both copper and pyridoxal or pyridoxal-related quinones have been suggested as essential cofactors for lysyl oxidase – as with inhibitors of the enzyme – the deficiency of these cofactors is thought to result in aberrant collagen and elastin cross-linking.

Similar in etiology is the known genetic human disorder originally described as a fatal disease of childhood. This sex-linked disease – known as Menke's kinky hair syndrome because of peculiar hair shaft deformities – is characterized by variegated hypopigmentation, skeletal deformities and aortic aneurysm, and progressive cerebellar degeneration. Over 20 years ago, the syndrome was associated with abnormal copper absorption from the gut and depressed lysyl oxidase activity (Danks et al., 1972; Rowe et al., 1977).

Scientists soon made an analogy between Menke's syndrome and mice with alleles at the Mottled (Mo) locus of the X chromosome. Mutations of Mo result in several different phenotypes in the hemizygous males, ranging from coat color changes (pewter, $Mo^{pew}$) to the severe connective tissue abnormalities that include aneurysms primarily of the thoracic aorta (in blotchy, $Mo^{blo}$, and the more viable brindled, $Mo^{vbr}$, mice) and to severe neurologic degeneration resulting in perinatal death (in brindled, $Mo^{br}$, and macular, $Mo^{dp}$, mice). The least viable alleles are the dappled ($Mo^{dp}$) and tortoiseshell ($Mo^{br}$) mice. The female tortoiseshell mice die in utero of ruptured aortic aneurysms; the males also have arterial aneurysm before birth (Grahn et al., 1969; Rowe et al., 1974; Andrews et al., 1975).

The complete sequencing of the human Menke's disease gene predicted a protein with homology to a P-type ATPase similar to the copper-exporting enzyme of the bacterium Enterococcus hirae. The human Menke's gene, ATP7A, is now thought to be homologous to the mouse mottled gene, and in both species the underlying pathogenetic mechanism is thought to be defective copper metabolism (Levinson et al., 1994; Mercer et al., 1994). Cells from tissues in these patients have an aberrant copper exporter that results in cytosolic accumulation of copper at the same time that copper-dependent enzymes have reduced activity. Because lysyl oxidase is dependent on copper, its decreased activity has long been thought to be the reason for markedly abnormal cross-linking of collagen and elastin, with resultant aortic aneurysms. However, other enzymes of major importance are also defective, including cytochrome oxidase, dopamine β-hydroxylase, and superoxide dismutase. Thus, although the genetic abnormality and associated biochemical defects of both the human disease and the homologous disorder in the mouse have been well studied, the complex pathophysiology occurring in the aortic wall, or other tissues, of Menke's syndrome patients is still not completely defined.

## Conclusions

From the largest elastic arteries to the microscopic arterioles, the media is the frequent target of injury by a variety of exogenous chemicals. Some are vasoactive chemicals, causing pronounced physiologic effects on blood pressure or flow; others act locally as constrictors or dilators of arteries and arterioles; still others have no discernible hemodynamic effect. Many examples of medial injury represent a more subtle, long-term disruption of maintenance or development of medial structure, with the result that the vessel wall deteriorates, weakens, and is eventually disrupted.

The current emphasis on atherosclerosis research has greatly improved our understanding of the role of the intima, and endothelial cells, in vascular injury. However, the intima and the media clearly depend on each other for normal physiologic regulation of vascular function, and are intimately associated during vascular injury. Through a better understanding of the pathologic mechanisms of cellular and structural injury and repair in the media, we will become more able to manipulate these processes therapeutically to strengthen the vascular wall, improve its function, and protect it against the ravages of the environment and of time.

## References

Abenhaim, L., Moride, Y., Brenot, F., Rich, S., Benichou, J., Kurz, X., Higenbottam, T., Oakley, C., Wouters, E., Aubier, M., Simonneau, G., and Begaud, B. 1996. Appetite suppressant drugs and the risk of primary pulmonary hypertension. *N Engl J Med* 335: 609–616.

Andrews, E.J., White, W.J., and Bullock, L.P. 1975. Spontaneous aortic aneurysms in *blotchy* mice. *Am J Pathol* 78: 199–210.

Anidjar, S., Salzmann, J.-L., Gentric, D., Lagneau, P., Camilleri, J-P., and Michel, J-B. 1990. Elastase-induced experimental aneurysms in rats. *Circulation* 82: 973–981.

Babal, P., Pechanova, O., Bernatova, I., and Stvrtina, S. 1997. Chronic inhibition of NO synthesis produces myocardial fibrosis and arterial hyperplasia. *Histol Histopathol* 12: 623–629.

Bachhuber, T.E. and Lalich, J.J. 1954. Production of dissecting aneurysms in rats fed *Lathyrus odoratus*. *Science* 120: 712.

Bean, W.B. and Ponseti, I.V. 1955. Dissecting aneurysm produced by diet. *Circulation* 12: 185–192.

Blot, S., Arnal, J.-F., Xu, Y., Gray, F., and Michel, J.-B. 1994. Spinal cord infarcts during long-term inhibition of nitric oxide synthase in rats. *Stroke* 25: 1666–1673.

Blundell, G., Jones, B.G., Rose, F.A., and Tudball, N. 1996. Homocysteine mediated endothelial cell toxicity and its amelioration. *Atherosclerosis* 122: 163–172.

Boor, P.J. 1985. Allylamine cardiovascular toxicity. V. Tissue distribution and toxicokinetics after oral administration. *Toxicology* 35: 167.

Boor, P.J. and Hysmith, R.M. 1987. Allylamine cardiovascular toxicity. *Toxicology* 44: 129–145.

Boor, P.J. and Langford, S.D. 1997. Pathogenesis of medial lesions caused by chemical agents. In *Comprehensive Toxicology*, ed. by I.G. Sipes, C.A. McQueen, and A.J. Gandolfi, pp. 309–332. Elsevier Science, New York.

Boor, P.J., Moslen, M.T., and Reynolds, E.S. 1979. Allylamine cardiotoxicity: I. Sequence of pathologic events. *Toxicol Appl Pharmacol* 50: 581.

Boor, P.J., Gotlieb, A.I., Joseph, C., Kerns, W.D., Roth, R.A., and Tomaszewski, K.E. 1995. Contemporary issues in toxicology: Chemical-induced vascular injury. *Toxicol Appl Pharmacol* 132: 177–195.

Boyd, C.D., Mariani, T.J., Kim, Y., and Csiszar, K. 1995. The size heterogeneity of human lysyl oxidase mRNA is due to alternate polyadenylation site and not alternate exon usage. *Mol Biol Rep* 21: 95–103.

Brenot, F., Herve, P., Petitpretz, P., Parent, F., Duroux, P., and Simonneau, G. 1993. Primary pulmonary hypertension and fenfluramine use. *Br Heart J* 70: 537–541.

Busin, M., Yau, C.-W., Yamaguchi, T., McDonald, M.B., and Kaufman, H.E. 1986. The effect of collagen crosslinkage inhibitors on rabbit corneas after radial keratotomy. *Invest Ophthalmol Vis Sci* 27: 1001–1005.

Campisi, R., Czernin, J., Schoder, H., Sayre, J.W., Marengo, F.D., Phelps, M.E., and Schelbert, H.R. 1998. Effects of long-term smoking on myocardial blood flow, coronary vasomotion, and vasodilator capacity. *Circulation* 98: 119–125.

Chvapil, M., Weinstein, P.R., Misiorowski, R., Telles, D., and Rankin, L. 1984. Development of topical βAPN delivery system for acute spinal cord injury in dogs. *J Biomed Materials Res* 18: 757–769.

Clark, R.L., Daly, K., Robinson, E., Naughten, E., Cahalane, B., Fowler, B., and Graham, I. 1991. Hyperhomocysteinemia: an independent risk factor for vascular disease. *N Engl J Med* 324: 1149–1155.

Conklin, D.J. and Boor, P.J. 1998. Allylamine cardiovascular toxicology: evidence for aberrant vasoreactivity in rats. *Toxicol Appl Pharmacol* 148: 245–251.

Connolly, H.M., Crary, J.L., McGoon, M.D., Hensrud, D.D., Edwards, B.S., and Edwards, W.D. 1997. Valvular heart disease associated with fenfluramine-phentermine. *N Engl J Med* 337: 581–588.

Contani, A. 1873. Latirismo (lathyrismus) illustrato di tre casi clinici. *Il Morgagni* 15: 745–785.

Contente, S., Csiszar, K., Kenyon, K., and Friedman, R.M. 1993. Structure of the mouse lysyl oxidase gene. *Genomics* 16: 395–400.

Cronlund, A.L. and Kagan, H.M. 1986. Comparison of lysyl oxidase from bovine lung and aorta. *Connect Tissue Res* 15: 173–185.

Danks, D.M., Campbell, P.E., Stevens, B.J., Mayne, V., and Cartwright, E. 1972. Menke's kinky hair syndrome: an inherited defect in copper absorption with widespread effects. *Pediatrics* 50: 188–201.

Dasler, W. 1954. Isolation of toxic crystals from sweet peas (*Lathyrus odoratus*). *Science* 120: 307–308.

Dastur, D.K. and Iyler, C.G.S. 1959. Lathyrism versus odoratism. *Nutr Rev* 17: 33.

Denny-Brown, D. 1947. Neurological conditions resulting from prolonged and severe dietary restriction. *Medicine* 26: 41–113.

Dobrin, P.B. 1989. Pathophysiology and pathogenesis of aortic aneurysms. *Surg Clin North Am* 69: 687–703.

Dupuy, H.P. and Lee, J.G. 1954. The isolation of a material capable of producing experimental lathyrism. *J Am Pharm Assoc* 43: 61–62.

Ettenson, D.S. and Gotlieb, A.I. 1993. Role of endothelial cells in vascular integrity and repair in atherosclerosis. *Adv Pathol Lab Med* 6: 285–309.

Fuller, J.G. 1968. *The Day of Saint Anthony's Fire*. Macmillan, New York.

Gacheru, S.N., Trackman, P.C., Calaman, S.D., Greenaway, F.T., and Kagan, H.M. 1989. Vicinal diamines as pyrroloquinoline quinone-directed irreversible inhibitors of lysyl oxidase. *J Biol Chem* 264: 12963–12969.

Galie, N., Manes, A., Uguccioni, L., Serafini, F., De Rosa, M., Branzi, A., and Magnani, B. 1998. Primary pulmonary hypertension: Insights into pathogenesis from epidemiology. *Chest* 114: 184S–194S.

Geismar, L.S., Kerr, J.S., Trelstad, R.L., and Riley, D.J. 1988. Treatment of experimental silicosis with antifibrotic agents. *Toxicology* 53: 331–344.

Gelbard, M., Lindner, A., Chvapil, M., and Kaufman, J. 1983. Topical beta-aminopropionitrile in the treatment of peyronie's disease. *J Urol* 129: 746–748.

Goldblatt, H.F. 1938. Studies on experimental hypertension: production of the malignant phase of hypertension. *J Exp Med* 67: 809–827.

Gopalan, C. 1992. The contribution of nutrition research to the control of undernutrition: The Indian experience. *Annu Rev Nutr* 12: 1–17.

Grahn, D., Fry, R.J.M., and Hamilton, K.F. 1969. Genetic and pathological analysis of of the sex-linked allelic series, mottled, in the mouse. *Genetics* 61, S22–S23.

Green, R.S., Lieb, M.E., Weintraub, A.S., Gacheru, S.N., Rosenfield, C.L., Shah, S., Kagan, H.M., and Taubman, M.B. 1995. Identification of lysyl oxidase and other platelet-derived growth factor-inducible genes in vascular smooth muscle cells by differential screening. *Lab Invest* 73: 476–482.

Hajnal, A. 1993. Up-regulation of lysyl oxidase in spontaneous revertants of H-ras-transformed rat fibroblasts. *Cancer Res* 53: 4670–4675.

Harris, E.D. and O'Dell, B.L. 1974. Copper and amine oxidases in connective tissue metabolism. *Adv Exp Med Biol* 48: 267–284.

Harris, E.D. and Sjoerdsma, A. 1966. Effect of penicillamine on human collagen and its possible application to treatment of scleroderma. *Lancet* November: 996–999.

Hashimoto, N., Kim, C., Kikuchi, H., Kojima, M., Kang, Y., and Hazama, F. 1987. Experimental induction of cerebral aneurysms in monkeys. *J Neurosurg* 67: 903–905.

Hazama, F. and Hashimoto, N. 1987. An animal model of cerebral aneurysms. *Neuropathol Appl Neurobiol* 13: 77–90.

Herman, E.H., Balazs, T., Young, R., Earl, F.L., Krap, S., and Ferrans, V.J. 1979. Acute cardiomyopathy induced by the vasodilating antihypertensive agent minoxidil. *Toxicol Appl Pharmacol* 47: 493–503.

Herron, G.S., Unemori, E.N., and Stoney, R.J. 1995. Proteinases and inhibitors in aortic aneurysms. In *Wound Healing in Cardiovascular Disease*, ed. by K.T. Weber, pp. 195–209. Futura Publishing Company, Armonk, NY.

Hitchon, P.W., Mouw, L.F., Rogge, T.N., Torner, J.C., and Miller, A.K. 1996. Response of spinal cord blood flow to the nitric oxide inhibitor nitroarginine. *Neurosurgery* 39: 795–803.

Hitzig, P. 1993. Combined dopamine and serotonin agonists: a synergistic approach to alcoholism and other addictive behaviors. *Md Med J* 42: 153–156.

Hitzig, P. 1994. Combined serotonin and dopamine indirect agonists correct alcohol craving and alcohol-associated neuroses. *J Subst Abuse Treat* 11: 489–490.

Hoveland, C.S. 1993. Importance and economic significance of the *Acremonium* endophytes to performance of animals and grass plant. *Agric Ecosyst Environ* 44: 3.

Huxtable, R.J., Ciaramitaro, D., and Eisenstein, D. 1978. The effect of a pyrralaizidine alkaloid, monocrotaline, and a pyrrole, dehydroretronecine, on the biochemical functions of the pulmonary endothelium. *Mol Pharmacol* 14: 1189–1203.

Issacs, K.R., Joseph, E.C., and Betton, G.R. 1989. Coronary vascular lesions in dogs treated with phosphodiesterase III inhibitors. *Toxicol Pathol* 17: 153–163.

Joseph, E.C., Mesfin, G., and Kerns, W.D. 1997. Pathogenesis of arterial lesions caused by vasoactive compounds in laboratory animals. In *Cardiovascular Toxicology*, ed. by S.P. Bishop, and W.D. Kerns, pp. 279–305. Elsevier Science, New York.

Kagan, H.M. and Trackman, P.C. 1991. Properties and function of lysyl oxidase. *Am J Respir Cell Mol Biol* 5: 206–210.

Kagan, H.M., Sullivan, K.A., Olsson, III, T.A., and Cronlund, A.L. 1979. Purification and properties of four species of lysyl oxidase from bovine aorta. *Biochem J* 177: 203–214.

Keiser, H.R. and Sjoerdsma, A. 1967. Studies on beta-aminopropionitrile in patients with scleroderma. *Clin Pharm Ther* 8: 593–602.

Kerns, W.D., Arena, E., Macia, R.A., Bugelski, P.J., Mathews, W.D., and Morgan, D.G. 1989. Pathogenesis of arterial lesions induced by dopaminergic compounds in the rat. *Toxicol Pathol* 17: 203–213.

Kim, C., Kikuchi, H., Hashimoto, N., and Hazama, F. 1989. Histopathological study of induced cerebral aneurysms in primates. *Surg Neurol* 32: 45–50.

Kobori, K., Suzuki, K., Yoshida, Y., and Ooneda, G. 1979. Light and electron microscopic studies on rat arterial lesions induced by experimental arterial contraction. *Virchows Arch A* 385: 29–39.

Kristek, F., Gerova, M., Devat, L., and Varga, I. 1995. Cardiac hypertrophy and vascular remodeling in nitric oxide-deficient hypertension. *Endothelium* 3 (Suppl.): 94.

Kuivaniemi, H., Savolainen, E.R., and Kivirikko, K.I. 1984. Human placental lysyl oxidase. Purification, partial characterization, and preparation of two specific antisera to the enzyme. *J Biol Chem* 259: 6996–7002.

Kumar, D., Hysmith, R.M., and Boor, P.J. 1990. Allylamine and β-aminopropionitrile-induced vascular injury: An *in vivo* and *in vitro* study. *Toxicol Appl Pharmacol* 103: 288–302.

Kumar, D., Trent, M.B., and Boor, P.J. 1998. Allylamine and β-aminopropionitrile-induced aortic medial necrosis: mechanisms of synergism. *Toxicology* 125: 107–115.

Lalich, J.J. 1967. Aortic aneurysms in experimental lathyrism. *Arch Pathol* 84: 528–535.

Lalich, J.J. and Ishida, K. 1966. Alteration in elastin and orientation of collagen in angiolathyrism. *Arch Pathol* 82: 129–137.

Lalich, J.J. and Paik, W.C.W. 1974. Influence of hydralazine consumption on allylamine induced myocardial fibrosis and hypertrophy in rats. *Exp Mol Pathol* 21: 29.

Lalich, J.J., Paik, W.C.W., and Allen, J.R. 1971. Production of arterial hemosiderosis in rhesus monkeys following the ingestion of β-aminopropionitrile. *Lab Invest* 25: 302–308.

Levene, C.I. 1960. The lathyrogenic effect of isonicotinic acid hydrazide (INAH) on the chick embryo and its reversal by pyridoxyl. *J Exp Med* 113: 795–811.

Levene, C.I. 1961. Structural requirements for lathyrogenic agents. *J Exp Med* 114: 295–310.

Levene, C.I. and Carrington, M.J. 1985. The inhibition of protein-lysine 6-oxidase by various lathyrogens: evidence for two different mechanisms. *Biochem J* 232: 293–296.

Levene, C.I., O'Shea, M.P., and Carrington, M.J. 1988. Protein lysine 6-oxidase (lysyl oxidase) cofactor: methoxatin (PQQ) or pyridoxal? *Int J Biochem* 20: 1451–1456.

Levinson, B., Vulpe, C., Elder, B., Martin, C., Verley, F., Packman, S., and Gitschier, J. 1994. The mottled gene is the mouse homologue of the Menkes disease gene. *Nature Genetics* 6: 369–373.

Lyles, G.A. 1996. Mammalian plasma and tissue-bound semicarbazide-sensitive amine oxidases: biochemical, pharmacological and toxicological aspects. *Int J Biochem Cell Biol* 28: 259–274.

McCann, U.D., Seiden, L.S., Rubin, L.J., and Ricaurte, G.A. 1997. Brain serotonin neurotoxicity and primary pulmonary hypertension from fenfluramine and dexfenfluramine. *J Am Med Assoc* 278: 666–672.

McCully, K.S. 1969. Vascular pathology of homocysteinemia: Implications for the pathogenesis of arteriosclerosis. *Am J Pathol* 56: 111–128.

McMurray, J., Bloomfield, P., and Miller, H.C. 1986. Irreversible pulmonary hypertension after treatment with fenfluramine. *Br Med J* 292: 239–240.

Manalo-Estrella, P. and Barker, A.E. 1967. Histopathologic findings in human aortic media associated with pregnancy. *Arch Pathol* 83: 336.

Martin, G.R., Gross, J., Piez, K.A., and Lewis, M.S. 1961. On the intramolecular cross-linking of collagen in lathyritic rats. *Biochim Biophys Acta* 53: 599–601.

Martin, G.R., Piez, K.A., and Lewis, M.S. 1963. The incorporation of [$^{14}$C]glycine into the subunits of collagens from normal and lathyritic animals. *Biochim Biophys Acta* 69: 472–479.

Matossian, M.K. 1982a. Religious revivals and ergotism in America. *Clio Med* 16: 185–192.

Matossian, M.K. 1982b. Ergot and the Salem witchcraft affair: An outbreak of a type of food poisoning known as convulsive ergotism may have led to the 1692 accusations of witchcraft. *Am Sci* 70: 355–357.

Matthias, D., Becker, C.H., Riezler, R., and Kindling, P.H. 1996. Homocysteine induced arteriosclerosis-like alterations of the aorta in normotensive and hypertensive rats following application of high doses of methionine. *Atherosclerosis* 122: 201–216.

Mercer, J.F.B., Grimes, A., Ambrosini, L., Lockhart, P., Paynter, J.A., Dierick, H., and Glover, T.W. 1994. Mutations in the murine homologue of the Menkes gene in dappled and blotchy mice. *Nature Genetics* 6: 374–378.

Meyrick, B., Gamble, W., and Reid, L. 1980. Development of crotalaria pulmonary hypertension: hemodynamic and structural study. *Am J Physiol* 239: H692–H702.

Minchin, R.L.H. 1940. Primary lateral sclerosis of south India. *Br Med J* 17 February: 253–255.

Moreno, H., Nathan, L.P., Costa, S.K.P., Metze, K., Antunes, E., Zatz, R., and DeNucci, G. 1995. Enalapril does not prevent the myocardial ischemia caused by the chronic inhibition of nitric oxide synthesis. *Eur J Pharmacol* 287: 93–96.

Moulton, K.S., Heller, E., Konerding, M.A., Flynn, E., Palinski, W., and Folkman, J. 1999. Angiogenesis inhibitors endostatin or TNP-470 reduce intimal neovascularization and plaque growth in apolipoprotein E-deficient mice. *Circulation* 99: 1726–1732.

Murray, J.C. and Levene, C.I. 1977. Evidence for the role of vitamin B-6 as a cofactor of lysyl oxidase. *Biochem J* 167: 463–467.

Murray, J.C., Fraser, D.R., and Levene, C.I. 1978. The effect of pyridoxine deficiency on lysyl oxidase activity in the chick. *Exp Mol Pathol* 28: 301–308.

Needleman, P., Corr, P.B., and Johnson, E.M. 1985. Drugs used for the treatment of angina: organic nitrates, calcium channel blockers, and beta-adrenergic antagonists. In *The Pharmacological Basis of Therapeutics*, ed. by A.G. Gilman, L.S. Goodman, T.W. Rall, and F. Murad, pp. 806–816. Macmillan Publishing Company, New York.

Noda, A., Sendo, T., Ohno, K., Noda, H., and Goto, S. 1987. Metabolism and cytotoxicity of hydrazine in isolated rat hepatocytes. *Chem Pharm Bull* 35: 2538–2544.

Numaguchi, K., Egashira, K., Takemoto, M., Kadokami, T., Shimokawa, H., Sueishi, K., and Takeshita, A. 1995. Chronic inhibition of nitric oxide synthesis causes coronary microvascular remodeling in rats. *Hypertension* 26: 957–962.

O'Dell, B.L., Hardwick, B.C., Reynolds, G., and Savage, J.E. 1961. Connective tissue defect in the chick resulting from copper deficiency. *Proc Soc Exp Biol Med* 108: 402–405.

O'Dell, B.L., Kilburn, K.H., McKenzie, W.N., and Thurston, R.J. 1978. The lung of the copper-deficient rat: A model for developmental pulmonary emphysema. *Am J Pathol* 91: 413–431.

Oliver, J.W., Abney, L.K., Strickland, J.R., and Linnabary, R.D. 1993. Vasoconstriction in bovine vasculature induced by the tall fescue alkaloid lysergamide. *J Anim Sci* 71: 2501–2509.

Page, R.C. and Benditt, E.P. 1967. A molecular defect in lathyritic collagen. *Proc Soc Exp Biol Med* 124: 459–465.

Pai, K.S., Shankar, S.K., and Ravindranath, V. 1993. Billionfold difference in the toxic potencies of two excitatory plant amino acids, L-BOAA and L-BMAA: biochemical and morphological studies using mouse brain slices. *Neurosci Res* 17: 241–248.

Paissios, C.S. and Demopoulos, T. 1962. Human lathyrism. A clinical and skeletal study. *Clin Orthop* 23: 236–249.

Pasquali-Ronchetti, I., Baccarani-Contri, M., Young, R.D., Vogel, A., Steinmann, B., and Royce, P.M. 1994. Ultrastructural analysis of skin and aorta from a patient with Menkes disease. *Exp Mol Pathol* 61: 36–57.

Peacock, Jr., E.E. and Madden, J.W. 1978. Administration of beta-aminopropionitrile to human beings with urethral strictures: A preliminary report. *Am J Surg* 136: 600–605.

Ponseti, I.V. 1954. Lesions of the skeleton and of other mesodermal tissues in rats fed sweet pea (*Lathyrus odoratus*) seeds. *J Bone Jt Surg* 36A: 1031–1058.

Ponseti, I.V. 1957. Skeletal lesions produced by aminonitriles. *Clin Orthop* 9: 131–144.

Ponseti, I.V. and Baird, W.A. 1952. Scoliosis and dissecting aneurysm of the aorta in rats fed with *Lathyrus odoratus* seeds. *Am J Pathol* 28, 1059–1077.

Porter, J.K. 1995. Analysis of endophyte toxins: fescue and other grasses toxic to livestock. *J Anim Sci* 73: 871–880.

Ramos, K.S. and Ou, X. 1994. Protein kinase C (PKC)-mediated protein phosphorylation in rat aortic smooth muscle cells is enhanced by allylamine. *Toxicol Lett* 73: 123–133.

Ramos, K., Weber, T.J., and Liau, G. 1993. Altered protein secretion and extracellular matrix deposition is associated with the proliferative phenotype induced by allylamine in aortic smooth muscle cells. *Biochem J* 289: 57–63.

Reilly, J.M. and Tilson, M.D. 1989. Incidence and etiology of abdominal aortic aneurysms. *Surg Clin North Am* 69: 705–711.

Rhodin, J.A.G. 1974. Cardiovascular system. In *Histology: A Text and Atlas*, ed. by J.A.G. Rhodin, pp. 340–352. Oxford University Press, New York.

Riley, D.J., Kerr, J.S., Berg, R.A., Ianni, B.D., Pietra, G.G., Edelman, N.H., and Prockop, D.J. 1982. Beta-aminopropionitrile prevents bleomycin-induced pulmonary fibrosis in the hamster. *Am Rev Respir Dis* 125: 67–73.

Riley, D.J., Kramer, M.J., Kerr, J.S., Chae, C.U., Yu, S.Y., and Berg, R.A. 1987. Damage and repair of lung connective tissue in rats exposed to toxic levels of oxygen. *Am Rev Respir Dis* 135: 441–447.

Rona, G., Chappell, C.I., and Balaz, T. 1959. An infarct-like myocardial lesion and other toxic manifestations produced by isoproterenol. *Arch Pathol Lab Med* 67, 443–455.

Rona, G., Huttner, I., and Boutet, M. 1977. Microcirculatory changes in myocardium with particular reference to catecholamine-induced cardiac muscle cell injury. In *Handbuch der Allgemeinen Pathologie*, ed. by H. Meessen. Springer-Verlag, New York.

Ross, R. 1997. The pathogenesis of atherosclerosis. In *Heart Disease. A Textbook of Cardiovascular Medicine*, ed. by E. Braunwald, pp. 1105–1116. W.B. Saunders Company, Philadelphia, PA.

Ross, R. and Glomset, J.A. 1976. The pathogenesis of atherosclerosis (first of two parts). *N Engl J Med* 295: 369–377.

Rowe, D.W., McGoodwin, E.B., Martin, G.R., Sussman, M.D., Grahn, D., Faris, B., and Franzblau, C. 1974. A sex-linked defect in the cross-linking of collagen and elastin associated with the mottled locus in mice. *J Exp Med* 139: 180–192.

Rowe, D.W., McGoodwin, E.B., Martin, G.R., and Grahn, D. 1977. Decreased lysyl oxidase activity in the aneurysm-prone, mottled mouse. *J Biol Chem* 252: 939–942.

Saxena, P.R. and de Vlaam-Schluter, G.M. 1974. Role of some biogenic substances in migraine and relevant mechanism in antimigraine action of ergotamine – studies in an experimental model for migraine. *Headache* 1: 142–163.

Schilling, E.D. and Strong, F.M. 1954. Isolation, structure and synthesis of a lathyrus factor from *L. odoratus*. *J Am Chem Soc* 76: 2848.

Schulert, A.R. and Lewis, H.B. 1952. Experimental lathyrism. *Proc Soc Exp Biol Med* 81: 86–89.

Scott, P.M. and Lawrence, G.A. 1980. Analysis of ergot alkaloids in flour. *J Agric Food Chem* 28: 1258.

Scott, P.M., Lombaert, G.A., Pellaers, P., and Bacler, S., and Lappi, J. 1992. Ergot alkaloids in grain foods sold in Canada. *J Agric Food Chem* 28:1258–1261.

Selye, H. 1957. Lathyrism. *Rev Can Biol* 16: 1–82.

Shields, G.S., Coulson, W.F., Kimball, D.A., Carnes, W.H., Cartwright, G.E., and Wintrobe, M.M. 1962. Studies on copper metabolism. XXXII. Cardiovascular lesions in copper-deficient swine. *Am J Pathol* 41: 603–621.

Silberstein, S.D. and Young, W.B. 1995. Safety and efficacy of ergotamine tartrate and dihydroergotamine in the treatment of migraine and status migrainosus. *Neurology* 45: 577–584.

Simpson, C.F. 1982. Coronary and thyroid arteriopathy induced by allylamine and β-aminoproprionitrile. *Exp Mol Pathol* 37: 382–392.

Simpson, C.F. and Taylor, W.J. 1982. Effect of hydralazine on aortic rupture induced by β-aminoproprionitrile in turkeys. *Circulation* 65: 704–708.

Smith, D.J. and Shuster, R.C. 1962. Biochemistry of lathyrism. I. Collagen biosynthesis in normal and lathyritic chick embryos. *Arch Biochem Biophys* 98: 498–501.

Spanos, N.P. and Gottlieb, J. 1976. Ergotism and the Salem village witch trials: Records of the events of 1692 do not support the hypothesis that ergot poisoning was involved. *Science* 194: 1390–1394.

Speer, D.P., Feldman, S., and Chvapil, M. 1985. The control of peritendinous adhesions using topical β-aminopropionitrile base. *J Surg Res* 38: 252–257.

Stockman, R. 1929. Lathyrism. *J Pharm Exp Ther* 37: 43–53.

Szakacs, J.E. and Mehlman, B. 1960. Pathologic changes induced by L-norepinephrine. *Am J Cardiol* 5: 619–627.

Tilson, M.D. 1992. Aortic aneurysms and atherosclerosis. *Circulation* 85: 378–379.

Upchurch, Jr., G.R., Welch, G.N., and Loscalzo, J. 1996. Homocysteine, EDRF, and endothelial function. *J Nutr* 126: 1290S–1294S.

Van Vleet, J.F., Herman, E.H., and Ferrans, V.J. 1995. Cardiac morphologic alterations in acute minoxidil cardiotoxicity in miniature swine. *Exp Mol Pathol* 41: 10–25.

Virmani, R. and Forman, M.B. 1989. Coronary artery dissections. In *Nonatherosclerotic Ischemic Heart Disease*, ed. by R. Virmani and M.B. Forman, pp. 325–354. Raven Press, New York.

Vitullo, J.C., Gerrity, R., and Khairallah, P.A. 1985. Cellular changes in mesenteric arteries and veins after acute perfusions of angiotensin II and vasoactive amines. *Blood Vessels* 22: 286–300.

Vivanco, F. and Diaz, C.J. 1951. Nuevos estudios sobre los affectos de las proteines de las legnumbres (Leguminismos). *Rev Clin Esp* 40: 157.

Waters, L.L. and deSoto-Nagy, G.I. 1950. Circulatory factors in the pathogenesis of experimental arteriolar necrosis. *Yale J Biol Med* 22: 751–766.

Wawzonek, S., Ponseti, I.V., Shepard, R.S., and Wiedenman, L.G. 1955. Epiphyseal plate lesions, degenerative arthritis, and dissecting aneurysm of the aorta by aminonitriles. *Science* 121: 63–65.

Weir, E.K., Reeve, H.L., Huang, J.M.C., Michelakis, E., Nelson, D.P., Hampl, V., and Archer, S.L. 1996. Anorexic agents aminorex, fenfluramine and dexfenfluramine inhibit potassium current in rat pulmonary vascular smooth muscle and cause pulmonary vasoconstriction. *Circulation* 94: 2216–2220.

Wilson, S.K. and Hutchins, G.M. 1982. Aortic dissecting aneurysms. *Arch Pathol Lab Med* 106: 175–180.

Woods, A.J., Jones, J.B., and Mantle, P.G. 1966. An outbreak of gangrenous ergotism in cattle. *Vet Rec* 78: 742–749.

Yeager, V.L., Buranarugsa, M.W., and Arunatut, O. 1985. Lathyrism: Mini-review and a comment on the lack of effect of protease inhibitors on osteolathyrism. *J Exp Pathol* 2: 1–11.

Yuan, J.X-J., Aldinger, A.M., Juhaszovia, M., Wang, J., Conte, J.V., Gaine, S.P., Orens, J.B., and Rubin, L.J. 1998. Dysfunctional voltage-gated potassium channels in pulmonary artery smooth muscle cells of patients with primary pulmonary hypertension. *Circulation* 98: 1400–1406.

# INDEX

'accidental' cell death 154
acid–base balance 43
aconitine 331
acrolein 489
adrenergic receptor mechanism changes 280
adrenochrome 297–301
adrenoxyl 298–9
adult cardiac myocytes 67
adult rat cultures 6–7
agatoxin (AgTX) 335, 338, 340
allylamine 488–90, 508, 569, 570
α-adrenergic blocking agents 282, 283
α-scorpion toxin 329, 332
amikacin 211
amiloride 334, 356–7
aminochrome formation 301
aminoglycoside antibiotics 187, 192–3, 195–7, 199–200, 208–9, 210–11
4-aminopyridine (4-AP) 336
amiodarone 350
amphetamines 322–3
amphotericin B 206–7, 213
amsacrine (AMSA) 388–9
anabolic steroids 426, 434–6, 440–3, 453–7
anaerobic glycolysis 122
analogs of anthracycline 381
androgens 426, 434–6, 440–3, 453–7
angiolathyrism, experiments in 566–73
angiotensin-converting enzyme inhibitors 282, 284
animal models: cardiac disease 237; cardiovascular toxicity of drugs 51; pathobiology of vascular response to injury 533–47
anthracyclines 374–9
anti-arrhythmic drugs 282, 284
antibacterial antibiotics: aminoglycoside

antibiotics 195–204, 210–11; autonomic effects 193–4; cardiovascular actions, introduction 187–8; cardiovascular effects 194–208; clinical aspects 209; clinical reports 188–91; direct depressant actions of 188; macrocyclics 208, 212–13; macrolides 204–6, 212; mechanisms of 208–9; myocardium, aminoglycosides and the 199–204; pharmacodynamic profiles of 187; polyene antifungal agents 206–7, 213; respiratory depressant actions 191–3; studies *in vivo*, aminoglycoside antibiotics 196–7; tetracyclines 207–8, 212; VSM, aminoglycosides and the 197–9
anticonvulsants 323
antidepressant agents 319–20
antineoplastic agents: amsacrine (AMSA) 388–9; analogs of anthracycline 381; anthracyclines 374–9; cardioprotectants 379–80; cisplatin 386; cyclophosphamide 385; cytosine arabinoside (Ara-C) 387; dexrazoxane 380; 4′-epidoxorubicin 381–3; epirubicin 381–3; esorubicin 381; 5-fluorouracil (5-FU) 386–7; idarubicin 383–4; interferon 389; interleukin-2 (IL-2) 390; liposomal doxorubicin/daunorubicin 380–1; lymphokine-activated killer cells (LAK) 390; mitoxantrone 384; paclitaxel 387–8
antipsychotic agents 320
apamin 341
apoptosis: apoptotic bodies 135–6; apoptotic death, a normal process 4; of cardiac myocytes 16–22; cytochrome *c* microinjection and 134–6, 139, 142;

effectors 22; emerging research area 4; events leading to 127; *in vitro* model systems for study of 4–7; injuries leading to 146–8; in kidneys 133–4; kinetics and stages of 135–40; mechanisms not well understood 134; mechanisms of 140–6; myocardial 171–2; pathway to cell death 106; phenomenon of 133–40; signaling pathways 20–22; stimuli 17–19; targets 19–20; toxicant induced 22; *see also* myocytes
apoptotic necrosis: cell injury and 140, 145–6; normal process 4; stages of 150
argiotoxin-636 346; *see also* necrosis
arrhythmogenesis 172
arterial media: angiolathyrism, experiments in 566–73; arterioles 558; catecholamines 558–9; dissecting aneurysm 573; endothelial cells 557–8; endothelial injury, lesions secondary to 563–6; ergot alkaloids 562–3; experimental angiolathyrism, human relevance 570–3; genetic errors 574; lathyrism 566–73; lesions secondary to endothelial injury 563–6; lysyl oxidase 568; nitric oxide-associated medial injury 560–2; nutritional deficiencies 573–4; structural injury 566–73; vascular SMCs 557–8; vasoactive chemicals 558–63; vasodilators 559–60; vasopressors 558–9
arterial pressure: large animals 80–3; small animals 90–1
arterial stenosis 528–9
arterioles 480, 558
arylaminobenzoates 346
aspartate aminotransferase (AST) 275, 283
atherosclerosis: atherosclerotic lesion in rabbit 538; atherosclerotic plaque 164; chronic cycles of injury/repair and 482–3; medial involvement 564; in mice 534; passive smoking and 406–9; pathogens implicated in 190–1
ATPase activity 276, 299
ATP depletion 168–9, 172, 176
ATP-sensitive $K^+$ channel 341
ATP synthesis/regeneration 167, 171
autonomic alterations, myocardial ischemic injury 172

autonomic effects, antibacterial antibiotics 193–4
autophagocytosis 152–3
azithromycin 190

$Ba^{2+}$ ions 336–7
bacterial lipopolysaccharide *see* endotoxemia
bacterial pathogens 506
balloon injury: pig coronary arteries 542–3; rat carotid artery 535–6
balloon-expandable stents, pig coronary arteries 545
barbiturates 323
baseline values, cardiac toxicity in animals 52
batrachotoxin (BTX) 329, 331
*Bcl-2* gene family 143–5, 148
benzo(a)pyrene-induced gene expression 503
benzodiazepines 323
bepridil 334
β-adrenergic blocking agents 282, 283
β-adrenergic function 248
β-APN 568, 569, 570
β-scorpion toxin 329, 332
bile acids 430
biochemical change, catecholamine-induced cardiomyopathy 274, 275–6
biology of vascular cells 481–3
biventricular failure 226
blood flow measurement 39–40, 83
blood vessel walls 479–80
brevetoxin (PbTx) 330
brevetoxin-B (GbTX-B) 332–3
bronchodilators 48
butadiene 508

cadmium 336, 497–9
calcicludine 335
calcium: background ratios 116; $Ca^{2+}$-activated $Cl^-$ channels 346; $Ca^{2+}$-activated $K^+$ channels 340–1; $Ca^{2+}$ channel inhibiting toxins 335; $Ca^{2+}$ channels, fast/slow 334–6; $Ca^{2+}$ measurements, nanomolar calibration of 117, 118; Ca pumps 351–4; cell injury/death 114–18; channel blockers 282, 284; cytosolic, effect of injury on 119; homeostasis 72; intracellular concentration 169; intracellular free homeostasis 12; role of 169; vascular toxin 498, 499

calmodulin 497
cAMP-activated Cl⁻ channels 344–5
cAMP-dependent Cl⁻ channels 346
cAMP-modulated allylamine cells 490
candicidin 206–7, 213
capsaicin 343
carbamazepine 323
carbon disulfide 504, 508
carbon monoxide 490–2, 508
carcinogens in smoke 409
cardiac damage, major classes
    differentiated (by serum enzyme
    findings) 45
cardiac effects, steroidal agents 450–61
cardiac glycosides 349–50
cardiac hypertrophy see hypertrophic
    growth
cardiac myocytes see myocytes
cardiac output 91–2
cardiac steroid receptors 451
cardiodepressant toxins, circulating 242–
    3
cardiomyopathy, pathology of 47–9
cardioprotectants 379–80
cardiotoxicity: evaluation of drugs 33–4;
    relative infrequency in humans 47
cardiovascular actions, antibacterial
    antibiotics 187–8
cardiovascular dynamics: arterial
    pressure, small animals 90–1; arterial
    pressures, large animals 80–3; blood
    flow measurements 83; cardiac output
    91–2; Doppler ultrasonic flow
    technique 83–5; electromagnetic flow
    technique 83; future refinements 94–5;
    heart rate 92–3; physiologic
    techniques 79; respiratory rate 93–4;
    in smaller species 79–80, 90–5;
    telemetry 88–9; toxins, role of 79;
    ultrasonic transit time/flow velocity
    85–6; vascular dimensions 87–8;
    ventricular dimensions 86–7;
    ventricular function 94; ventricular
    pressures, large animals 80–3
cardiovascular effects, antibacterial
    antibiotics 194–208
cardiovascular observation, studies in
    humans 79
cardiovascular toxicology, concerns of 3
cariporide 357
caspases 146
catecholamine-induced cardiomyopathy:
    adrenochrome 297–301; adrenoxyl,

effect of 298–9; α-adrenergic blocking
    agents 283; angiotensin-converting
    enzyme inhibitors 284; anti-
    arrhythmic drugs 284; β-adrenergic
    blocking agents 283; biochemical
    change 274, 275–6; calcium channel
    blockers 284; cardiotoxic effect
    mechanisms 297, 302; characteristics
    271–81; comparison of effects of
    different catecholamines 271; complex
    effects of catecholamines 269–70;
    coronary spasm 281, 289–90; drugs,
    effects of 282; electrolyte change 276–
    7; electrolyte interventions 284–6;
    electrolyte shifts 293–7; epinephrine
    270; hemodynamic change 287–9;
    hemodynamic effects, coronary
    spasms and 289–90; histologic/
    histochemical change 273–5;
    hormonal interventions 284–6;
    intercellular Ca²⁺ overload 293–7;
    isoproterenol 271; lipid mobilization
    291; mechanisms 287–301; membrane
    change 277–81; metabolic effects
    290–3; metabolic interventions 284–6;
    monoamine oxidase inhibitors 281–3;
    norepinephrine 270–1; oxidation
    products 297–301; oxidized
    epinephrine, effect of 298–9;
    pharmacologic interventions 281–4;
    post-ganglionic blockers 284;
    psychosedative drugs 284; relative
    hypoxia 287–9; serum levels of
    electrolytes 277; sympathoadrenal
    system 269; tissue cation contents
    276–7; ultrastructural change 272–3;
    vasodilators 284
catecholamines 269–301, 492–4, 508,
    558–9
cell apoptosis: injuries leading to 146–7;
    kinetics and stages of 135–40;
    mechanisms of 140–6; necrosis 140,
    146, 150, 152; phenomenon of 133–40
cell deregulation, post injury: of calcium
    117–18; of magnesium 122; of
    potassium 121; of pH 120–1; of
    sodium 120
cell injury/death: autophagocytosis 152–
    3; Bcl-2 gene family 143–5; calcium
    114–18; caspases 145; cell death 148;
    cell necrosis 149–52; cell volume
    140–1; cytochrome c 142–3;
    cytoskeleton 128–29, 146; cytosolic

calcium of rabbit PTE cells, effect of injury on 119; diagram of stages of cell injury 108; endoplasmic reticulum, calcium and the 116–17; energy metabolism 122–3; gene activation 130–3; gene expression, alteration in 123–6; hypothesis, role of $Ca^{2+}$ and oncosis 126–33; immediate–early genes 123–5, 145; instantaneous cell death 152; ion homeostasis 113–14; ion regulation 140–1; junction changes 130; kinase pathways 145; magnesium 121–2; membrane changes 133; mitochondrial calcium uptake/release 115–16; mitochondrial function, alterations of 145; p53 induction 142; p53 tumor-suppressor genes 126; pH 120–1; phases of 63; phospholipases 146; plasmalemmal calcium regulation 115; potassium 121; programmed cell death 153; rates of, screening with multiple time points 64; regulation of $Ca^{2+}$ 114–5, 127, 141–2; response to lethal injury 105–7; signaling, role of $Ca^{2+}$ and oncosis 128; sodium 118–20; stress genes 125–6; terminal differentiation 153–4
cell oncosis: hypothesis of $Ca^{2+}$ and 126–33; injuries leading to 146–8; mechanisms of 112–22; necrosis, stages of 150–2; signaling role of $Ca^{2+}$ 128; stages of 107–12
cellular energy supply 69–70
cellular ion shift 109
cellular perspective *see* vascular toxicology
central nervous system (CNS) *see* drugs, centrally acting
c-*fos* 123–5, 145
charybdotoxin (ChTX) 337, 338–9, 340, 341
*Chlamydia pneumoniae* 506
chloral hydrate 323
chloramphenicol 194, 195, 212
chlorotoxin 348
cholesterol 430
chromium 497
chronic cardiomyopathy 48–9
ciguatoxin 330, 333
circulatory disturbance/collapse 188–9
circulatory shock 222–3
cisplatin 386
Cl⁻ channels 344–8

clinical aspects, antibacterial antibiotics 209
clinical pathology 41–6
clinical reports, antibacterial antibiotics 188–91
cobalt 497
cobra venom cardiotoxin 353
cocaine 320–2
colymycin 195
conclusions *see* summaries/conclusions
congestive cardiomyopathy 47–9
conotoxins 333, 335
continuous wave (CW) flowmeters 84–5, 88
contractile activity, modeling cytotoxicity 69
copper 497
coronary alterations: clinical correlates 166–7; observations 164–6
coronary occlusion 173, 176–7
coronary spasm 281, 289–90
creatine phosphokinase (CPK) 44, 275
cultured cell models 54
cyclophosphamide 385
cyclopiazonic acid 353
cyclosporine A 347
cytochrome *c* 134–7, 139, 142, 142–3
cytochrome P450 487, 497, 500
cytokines 462
cytoplasmic blebs 109, 128–30, 135
cytoplasmic vacuoles 109–10
cytosine arabinoside (Ara-C) 387
cytoskeleton 128–30, 146, 171, 500
cytosolic calcium, effect of injury on 119
cytosolic enzyme release 68
cytotoxic injury 48–9
cytotoxic lesions 187
cytotoxicity, modeling *in vitro*: adult cardiac myocytes 67; approaches 61–5; assays 61; assessment criteria, definition problems 60–1; assessment practice 67–73; assessment, *in vitro* approaches 62; calcium homeostasis 72; cellular energy supply 69–70; contractile activity 69; credence 59–60; cytosolic enzyme release 68; dye exclusion assays 67–8; hydrogen ion gradients 71–2; mechanistic investigations 69–72; mitochondrial membrane potential 70–1; MTT assay (succinate dehydrogenase activity) 70; neonatal cardiac myocytes 66; permeability assays, data evaluation

68–9; primary heart cell cultures for screening 65–7; rationale 59; sarcolemma breakdown 67–8

DCDPG (3′,5-dichlorodiphenylamine-2-carboxylate) 346
delayed rectifier K⁺ channels 338–9
δ-atracotoxins 332
dendrotoxin (DTX) 339, 340
depressants 323
deregulation, post injury: of calcium 117–18; of magnesium 122; of pH 120–1; of potassium 121; of sodium 120
dexrazoxane 380
diacetyl monoxime (DAM/BDM) 358
diastoloc properties after LPS and sepsis 234–5
DIDS (stilbene derivative) 345–7
dihydropyridine BayK8644 334
dihydrostreptomycin 194, 210
diltiazem 334
dinitrotoluene 494–5, 508
diphenylamine-2-carboxylate (DPC) 342, 345, 346
direct effects on vasculature, steroidal agents 440–50
DNA: damage 125, 126, 130, 135, 143, 154; fragmentation 171–2; synthesis 492, 494, 495
dogs, vascular intervention in 539–41
Doppler ultrasonic flow technique 83–5
doxorubicin 70, 350–1
DPI201–106 333
drug–exogenous steroid interactions 462
drugs, cardiovascular toxicity of: acid–base balance 43; animal models 51; blood flow measurement 39–40; cardiac hypertrophy 49; cardiomyopathy 47–9; clinical pathology 41–6; clinical signs/observations 41; creatine phosphokinase 44; dose–response curves 65; effects on catecholamine-induced cardiomyopathy 282; electrocardiograms 37–9; electrolytes 42–3; enzymes 43–4; evaluation of 33–4; heart rate 39; hemorrhage 50; in vitro models 51–6; lactate dehydrogenase 44; lipids 46; magnetic resonance imaging 40–1; osmolality 43; pathology 46–50; pharmacologic profiling 34–41; plasma albumin/myoglobin/fibrinogen 45–6; serum

transaminase (glutamic-oxaloacetic/pyruvic) 45; standard toxicity studies, in vivo evaluations 35–7; vasculature 49–50
drugs, centrally acting: amphetamines 322–3; anticonvulsants 323; antidepressant agents 319–20; antipsychotic agents 320; barbiturates 323; benzodiazepines 323; cocaine 320–2; depressants 323; non-barbiturate depressants 323; stimulants 320–3
dye exclusion assays 67–8

effectors in apoptosis 22
efonidipine 342
EGIS-7229 336
electrocardiograms 37–9
electrolyte: change 276–7; interventions 284–6; shifts 293–7; toxicity 42–3
electromagnetic flow technique 83
endotoxemia, pathophysiology of: circulating cardiodepressant toxins 242–3; circulatory shock 222–3; diastoloc properties after LPS and sepsis 234–5; endothelial mediators 245–50; free radical-induced injury 243–5; isolated cell/subcellular preparations 235–41; isolated tissue studies 231–5; LPS and sepsis models, experiments with 231–41; LPS and sepsis models, in vivo studies 226–31; LPS and sepsis syndromes, clinical studies 223–6; mediators of toxicity, LPS and sepsis 241–50; nitric oxide synthase (NOS) 246–50; platelet-activating factor (PAF) 245–6; septic shock 223; systolic properties after LPS and sepsis 231–4
endothelial cells 557–8
endothelial mediators 245–50
endoplasmic reticulum (ER) 116–7, 328
endothelial function 406
endothelial injury, lesions secondary to 563–6
energy metabolism 122–3
energy-dispersive X-ray microanalysis 114, 115, 116
enzymes 43–4
eosin 353–4
epidemiologic studies: interpretation of 413–14; passive smoking 411–16

epinephrine 270; *see also* catecholamine-induced cardiomyopathy
4′-epidoxorubicin 381–3
epirubicin 381–3
ergot/ergot derivatives 528, 562–3
erythrinin B 358
erythromycin 195, 204, 206, 212, 189
*Escherichia coli* 232, 236
esorubicin 381
estrogens 428, 436–8, 443–6, 457–9
ethanol 336
ethaverine 336
etiologic mechanisms 241
euchrenone-b10 358
eurocidine 206
evaluations of cardiotoxicity 34
exercise and passive smoking 403
experimental angiolathyrism, human relevance 570–3
experimental models: mechanical vascular injury 531–3; observations in myocardial ischemic injury 165–6

fenfluramine 565
fibroblast growth factor (FGF) 178
flufenamic acid 342–3, 346
flunarizine 334
5-fluorouracil (5-FU) 386–7
free radicals: generation of 170; passive smoking and 410–11; injury induced by 243–5
FTX polyamine 335
fungichromin 206
future refinements, cardiovascular dynamics 94–5

GABA (gamma-amino butyric acid) 346, 347–8
gadolinium 343
gene activation, cell injury/death cell 130–3
gene expression: alteration in cell injury/death 123–6; hypertrophy in 13–14
genetic errors 574
genomic mechanism 430–1
gentamicin 192, 198, 200–4, 205, 211
glucocorticoids steroidal 429, 438–40, 447–50, 460–1
glutamate–pyruvate transaminase (GPT) 275
glycosides, cardiac 430
G protein signaling 128
grayanotoxin (GTX) 329, 331–2
guanosine triphosphate (GTP) 482

hanatoxin (HaTX) 340
heart: disease and passive smoking 402; effects of exogenous steroids on 453; rate and cardiovascular dynamics 92–3; rate and toxic drugs 39; response to androgens 455–6; target for steroidal agents 450–3
heat shock proteins 125–6, 506–7
*Helicobacter pylori* 507
hemodynamic change 287–9
hemodynamic effects, coronary spasms and 289–90
hemodynamic pattern, septic shock 224–6
hemorrhage 50
hepatic triglyceride lipase (HTGL) 434–6, 437–8
histologic change: catecolamine-induced cardiomyopathy 273–5; myocardial infarction 173–5
HOE-694 357
homocysteine 495–6, 564
hormonal interventions 284–6
hydrazinobenzoic acid 496–7, 508
hydrogen ion gradients 71–2
hyperpolarization-activated channels 342
hypertension 483
hypertrophic growth: cardiac dysfunction and 14–16; defining *in vitro* 7–8; investigative focus 4; models *in vitro* 4–7; pathology 49; stimuli 9; toxicant induced 15; *see also* myocytes
hypertrophic signaling pathways 9–13
hypertrophic stimuli 8–9
hypotension 189
hypoxia due to isoproterenol 288

idarubicin 383–4
immediate–early genes 123–5, 145
immunologic mechanisms 187
*in vitro* models: cardiotoxicity 54–6; cardiovascular toxicity of drugs 51–6; systems for study of apoptosis 4–7; testing systems 51–6
indirect steroidal effects on vasculature 432–40
industrial toxicologists, concerns of 33
instantaneous cell death 152
intercellular $Ca^{2+}$ overload 293–7
interferon 389
interleukin-2 (IL-2) 390
inward rectifier $K^+$ channels 341–2
ion channels/pumps/exchangers: amiloride 356–7; amiodarone 350
ion Ca pumps 351–4; $Ca^{2+}$-activated $Cl^-$

channels 346; Ca$^{2+}$-activated K$^+$ channels 340–1; Ca$^{2+}$ channels, fast/slow 334–6; cAMP-dependent Cl$^-$ channels 346; cardiac glycosides 349–50; cariporide 357; Cl$^-$ channels 344–8; cobra venom cardiotoxin 353; cyclopiazonic acid 353; delayed rectifier K$^+$ channels 338–9; diacetyl monoxime (DAM) 358; doxorubicin 350–1; eosin 353–4; erythrinin-B 358; euchrenone-b10 358; HOE-694 357; hyperpolarization-activated channels 342; inward rectifier K$^+$ channels 341–2; K$^+$ channels 336–42; KB-R7943 356; lysophosphatidylcholine 353; maitotoxin 351 monensin 355–6; Na channels, fast 328–33; Na/Ca exchanger 354–6; Na/H exchanger 356–8; Na/K pump 349–51; neurotransmitter-activated Cl$^-$ channels 347–8; non-selective cation channels 342–3; opioids 358; palytoxin (PTX) 357–8; sea anemone toxins 355; stretch-activated channels 343–4; swelling-activated Cl$^-$ channels 346–7; target channels 328–48; target pumps/exchangers 349–58; 1,3,5-trihydroxy-4-(3-methylbut-2-enyl)xanthen-9-one 358; thapsigargin 353; transient outward current (K$^+$ channels) 339–40; vanadate 350; voltage-dependent Cl$^-$ channels 345–6; volvatoxin A 352–3; VX compound 351
ion homeostasis 112–14, 168–9
ion regulation 141–2
ischemic damage, passive smoking 410–11
ischemic heart disease, pathogenic mechanisms 165
isolated cell/subcellular preparations 235–41
isolated organ preparation 54
isolated tissue studies 231–5
isoproterenol 271; see also catecholamine-induced cardiomyopathy
JAK hypertrophic signaling pathways 12–13
junction changes, cell injury/death 130

K$^+$ channels: ATP-sensitive 341; Ca$^{2+}$ activated 340–1; delayed rectifier 338–9; diversity of 337; functionality

336–42; inward rectifier 341–2; molecular clones and inhibitors 340; toxins and targets 338; transient outward current 339–40
kalicludine (AsKC) 339
kaliotoxin (KTX) 338
kaliseptine (AsKS) 339
kanamycin 195, 210
KB-R7943 356
kinase pathways 145

lactate dehydrogenase (LDH) 44, 275, 283
lathyrism: concept of 566–73; experimental 571, 572
lathyrogenic compounds 569–70
lead 497, 498, 499
leiurotoxin (LeTX) 341
leucomycin 195
limbatustoxin (LbTX) 341
lincomycin 190, 206, 209, 212
lincosamide antibiotics 193
lipid cardiovascular toxicity 46
lipid metabolism 432–40
lipid mobilization, catecholamine-induced cardiomyopathy 292
lipopolysaccharide (LPS), bacterial see endotoxemia
lipoprotein: HDL/LDL 432–9, 496; metabolism, effects of exogenous steroids on 440; VLDL 432, 434, 436
liposomal doxorubicin/daunorubicin 380–1
logit analysis for doxorubicin 70
LPS and sepsis models: experiments with 231–41; in vivo studies 226–31
LPS and sepsis syndromes, clinical studies 223–6
LV stroke work index (LVSWI) 224, 225
lymphokine-activated killer cells (LAK) 390
lysophosphatidylcholine 353
lysosomal hydrolases 152
lysyl oxidase 568

macrocyclics 208, 212–13
macrolide antibiotics 195, 204–6, 212
magnesium 121–2, 497, 499
magnetic resonance imaging 40–1
maitotoxin 351
manganese 497
MAPK hypertrophic signaling pathway 12, 13
margatoxin (MgTX) 338

MDF (myocardial depressant factor) 242–3

mechanical vascular injury 531–47

mechanisms: antibacterial antibiotics 208–9; catecholamine-induced cardiomyopathy 287–301; investigations in cytotoxicity 69–72; myocardial ischemic injury 167–72; steroidal action 430–2

mechanosensitive channels 343

mediators of toxicity, LPS and sepsis 241–50

mefenamic acid 347

membrane change: catecholamine-induced cardiomyopathy 277–81; cell injury/death 133; progressive damage in myocardial ischemic injury 170–1

Menke's syndrome 574

mercury 497, 499

metabolic alterations, myocardial ischemic injury 167–8

metabolic effects, catecholamine-induced cardiomyopathy 290–3

metabolic interventions, catecholamine-induced cardiomyopathy 284–6

metals, molecular perspective on 497–9, 508

methacholine (MC) 442

mibefradil 334

microscopy, new methodologies in 114

mineralocorticoids 429, 447–50, 460–1

mitochondrial: ATP synthesis 122–3, 145; calcification 149–50; calcium uptake/release 115–16; compartments, condensation of 109–12; function, alterations in cell injury 145; membrane potential 70–1; permeability 112; profiles following cell injury 151

mitogen-activated protein kinase (MAPK) 458

mitoxantrone 384

modulation of myocardial ischemic injury 176–8

molecular perspective see vascular toxicology, cellular/molecular perspective

monensin 355–6

monoamine oxidase (MAO) 295

monoamine oxidase inhibitors (MAOIs) 281–3, 296

monocrotaline toxicity 564–5

MTT assay (succinate dehydrogenase activity) 70

multiple cardiac disease states 238

muscular venules 480

myocardial cell injury, morphologic features 174

myocardial hypoxia 48

myocardial infarct size 175

myocardial infarction: diagnostic tests for 175; evolution of 173–5; passive smoking and 411

myocardial ischemic injury, pathobiology of: apoptosis 171–2; arrhythmogenesis 172; autonomic alterations 172; calcium, role of 169; coronary alterations, clinical correlates 166–7; coronary alterations, observations 164–6; experimental models, observations in 165–6; histologic change, myocardial infarction 173–5; humans, observations in 164–5; ionic homeostasis, alterations in 168–9; mechanisms of 167–72; membrane damage, progressive 170–1; metabolic alterations 167–8; modulation of 176–8; myocardial infarct size 175; myocardial infarction, evolution of 173–5; necrosis 171–2; new approaches to modulation 178; oncosis 171–2; PCTA (percutaneous transluminal coronary angioplasty (PTCA) 177–8; reperfusion 176–7; SVCABG (saphenous vein coronary artery bypass grafts) 178; therapeutic interventions 177–8; ultrastructural change, myocardial infarction 173–5

myocardial necrosis, progression of 176–7

myocardium: aminoglycosides and the 199–204; dysfunctional 175

myocytes: adult rat cultures 6–7; gene expression in hypertrophy 13–14

myocytes growth of 7–14; hypertrophic signaling pathways 9–13; hypertrophic stimuli 8–9; neonatal rat cultures 5–6; research, growth an emerging area 4; stimuli of apoptotic death 18; stimuli of cardiac hypertrophic growth 9; see also apoptosis, hypertrophic growth

Na channels: fast 328–33; toxins affecting 329

Na/Ca exchanger 240, 354–6

Na/H exchanger 356–8

Na/K pump 349–51

NAC (N-acetylcysteine) 380

nanomolar calibration 117, 118

NCEs (new chemical entities) 35
necrosis: cell injury and 149–52; myocardial 171–2, 176–7; oncotic, stages of 150–2; *see also* apoptotic necrosis
neointima formation, pig coronary arteries 544, 546
neomycin 191, 192, 211
neonatal cardiac myocytes 66
neonatal rat cultures 5–6
netilmicin 192
neurotransmitter-activated Cl⁻ channels 347–8
nickel 497
nicotine 499–500, 508
nifedipine 334
niflumic acid 346, 347
nitric oxide synthase (NOS) 246–8
nitric oxide: endothelial-derived relaxing factor 527; nitric oxide -associated medial injury 560–2; nitric oxide synthase (NOS) 246–50; vascular disease and 529–30
nitrotyrosine 530
non-barbiturate depressants 323
non-fatal cardiac events, passive smoking and 415–16
non-genomic mechanisms 431–2
non-selective cation channels 342–3
norcocaine 322
norditerpenoid alkaloids 331
norepinephrine 270–1; *see also* catecholamine-induced cardiomyopathy
noxiustoxin (NxTX) 337, 338
NPPB (5-nitro-2-[3-phenylpropylamino]-benzoic acid) 345–7
nutritional deficiencies 573–4

occlusive coronary thrombi 165
oleandomycin 194, 195, 204, 213
olymycin 213
oncosis: events leading to 113; hypothesis of $Ca^{2+}$ and 126–33; injuries leading to 147–8; mechanisms of 112–22; myocardial ischemic injury 171–2; oncotic necrosis, stages of 150–2; pathway to cell death 106; stages of 107–12
opioids 358
osmolality 43
oxidation products 297–301
oxidative metabolism, impairment of 170
oxidized epinephrine 298–9

oxidized lipoproteins 505–6
oxygen delivery/processing 403
oxygen-derived radicals 243
oxygen free radicals 244
oxygen-wasting effect of catecholamines 290–2
oxytetracycline 195

*p53* 126, 142
paclitaxel 387–8
PAF (platelet-activating factor) 245–6
palytoxin (PTX) 357–8
passive smoking: atherosclerosis 406–9; endothelial function 406; epidemiologic studies 411–16; exercise and 403; free radicals 410–11; heart disease and 402; ischemic damage 410–11; myocardial infarction 411; oxygen delivery/processing 403; platelets 404–6
pathobiology, vascular response to injury: animal models 533–47; dogs, vascular intervention in 539–41; experimental models, mechanical injury 531–3; mechanical vascular injury 531–47; nitric oxide 529–30; normal function/structure, regulation of 525–7; peroxynitrite 529–30; primates, non-human, vascular intervention in 538–9; rabbits, vascular intervention in 536–8; restenosis, morphometric techniques in studies of 547–9; rodents, vascular intervention in 533–6; study paradigms, mechanical injury 531–3; swine, vascular intervention in 541–7; vascular injury 527–9; vascular interventions, pathology of 530–1; vulnerability of vasculature 525
pathogenic mechanisms, ischemic heart disease 165
pathogenic sequence, ischemic heart disease 168
pathology, cardiovascular toxicity of drugs 46–50
PDGF (platelet-derived growth factor) 481, 482, 495
pentamycin 206
peptidyl K⁺ channel toxins 337
percutaneous transluminal coronary angioplasty (PTCA) 167, 177–8
peritonitis 226
permeability assays, data evaluation 68–9
peroxynitrite (ONOO⁻) 529–30

pH 120–1, 148
pharmaceutical toxicologists, concerns of 33
pharmacodynamic profiles, antibiotic agents 187
pharmacologic interventions, catecholamine-induced cardiomyopathy 281–4
pharmacologic profiling, cardiovascular toxicity of drugs 34–41
phase-constant images, cells microinjected with cytochrome *c* 136, 139
phenothiazine antipsychotics 320
phentalomine 342
phentermine 565
phenytoin 323
phospholipases 146
phospholipids: degradation of 170; modification of 112
photomicrographs, control cultures of rat PTE 130–2
phrixotoxin (PaTX) 340
physiologic adaptations, steroidal agents 462
physiologic techniques, cardiovascular dynamics 79
picrotoxin 346, 348
piezoelectric crystals 81, 86
PKC hypertrophic signaling pathway 11
plasma albumin/myoglobin/fibrinogen 45–6
plasmalemmal calcium regulation 115
platelet-activating factor (PAF) 245–6
platelet-derived growth factor (PDGF) 166
platelets: aggregation of 166; passive smoking and 404–6
P/O ratio 292, 299
poly-(ADP ribose) polymerase (PARP) 148
polycyclic aromatic hydrocarbons 500–2, 508
polyene antifungal agents 206–7, 213
polymyxin antibiotics 193
post-ganglionic blockers 282, 284
potassium 121
prenylamine 379
primary heart cell cultures for screening 65–7
primates, non-human, vascular intervention in 538–9
progestins 428–9, 436–8, 446–7, 457–9
programmed cell death 153

programmed death *see* apoptosis
proteases, role of in apoptosis/oncosis 148
PTCA (percutaneous transluminal coronary angioplasty 167, 177–8
pseudopods 136–40
psychosedative drugs 284
pumiliotoxin-B (PTX-B) 331
pyrethroids 348
pyrroloquinoline quinone (PQQ) 568

rabbits, vascular intervention in 536–8
radiotelemetry, physiologic measurements 89
rationale, modeling cytotoxicity 59
regulation of $Ca^{2+}$ 114–5, 127, 141–2
relative hypoxia 287–9
reperfusion 176–7
respiratory control index (RCI) 292
respiratory depressant actions 191–3
respiratory rate 93–4
response to lethal cell injury 105–7
restenosis, morphometric techniques in studies of 547–9
rodents, vascular intervention in 533–6
rotundium 336

salicylaldoxime 336
*Salmonella typhimurium* 236
sarcolemmal: breakdown 67–8; changes in myocardium 279; integrity 239–41
sarcoplasmic reticulum (SR) 237–9, 244, 279, 328
saxitoxin (STX) 329, 330, 333
scanning electron micrographs (SEMs): cells microinjected with cytochrome *c* 137; dog myocardium 114
scyllatoxin (ScTX) 341
sea anemone toxins 329, 332, 355
selenium 497, 498
septic shock 223; *see also* endotoxemia
serotonin 165–6
serum glutamate–oxaloacetate transaminase (GOT) 275
serum levels of electrolytes 277
serum transaminase (glutamic–oxaloacetic/pyruvic) 45
sex steroids, endogenous 433
signaling: pathways and apoptosis 20–22; role of $Ca^{2+}$ and oncosis 126
sisomicin 211
SITS (stilbene derivative) 345–7
smaller species, cardiovascular dynamics in 79–80, 90–5

smoking, passive *see* passive smoking
smooth muscle cells *see* vascular smooth
    muscle cells
sodium 118–21
sodium nitroprusside (SNP) 442
spiramycin 195
splanchnic ischemia 242
squamous metaplasia 154
standard toxicity studies, *in vivo*
    evaluations 35–7
STAT hypertrophic signaling pathways
    12–13
stent placement, dog coronary artery 541
steroid nucleus, classification of agents
    427
steroid receptors 450–3
steroidal agents: action mechanisms,
    characteristics of 433; anabolic
    steroids 426, 434–6, 440–3, 453–7;
    androgens 426, 434–6, 440–3, 453–7;
    bile acids 430; cardiac effects 450–61;
    cholesterol 430; classification of
    agents 427; combinations of,
    interactions difficult to study 461–2;
    cytokines, interactions and 462; direct
    effects on vasculature 440–50; drug–
    exogenous steroid interactions 462;
    estrogens 428, 436–8, 443–6, 457–9;
    genomic mechanism 430–1;
    glucocorticoids 429, 438–40, 447–50,
    460–1; glycosides, cardiac 430; heart
    as target for agents 450–3; indirect
    effects on vasculature 432–40; lipid
    metabolism 432–40; mechanisms of
    action 430–2; mineralocorticoids 429,
    447–50, 460–1; non-genomic
    mechanisms 431–2; overview 425;
    physiologic adaptations and 462;
    progestins 428–9, 436–8, 446–7, 457–
    9; review of agents 426–30; sex
    steroids, endogenous 433; steroid
    nucleus 427; steroid receptors 450–3;
    vascular effects 432–50
stimulants 320–3
stimuli in apoptosis 17–19
streptomycin 188–9, 190, 192, 194, 195,
    210
stress genes 125–6
stretch-activated channels 343–4
structural injury, arterial media 566–73
studies *in vivo*, aminoglycoside
    antibiotics 196–7
study paradigms, mechanical injury 531–
    3

subcellular alterations in the myocardium
    280
sulfonylurea compounds 341
summaries/conclusions: antibacterial
    antibiotics, toxicity of 208–14;
    antineoplastic agents 390; arterial
    media, target of toxins 575; cardiac
    hypertrophy/apoptosis 22–3;
    cardiovascular dynamics, monitoring
    in conscious animals 95;
    catecholamine-induced
    cardiomyopathy 301–2; cell injury/
    death 154; cytotoxicity, modeling *in
    vitro* 73; drugs, cardiovascular toxicity
    of 56; endotoxemia, pathophysiology
    of 250–1; hypertrophic growth 16; ion
    channels/pumps/exchangers 358–9;
    passive smoking 416–17;
    pathobiology, vascular response to
    injury 550; steroidal agents, effects of
    463; vascular toxicology, cellular/
    molecular perspective 507–8
SVCABG (saphenous vein coronary
    artery bypass grafts) 178
swelling-activated Cl⁻ channels 346–7
swine, vascular intervention in 541–7
sympathoadrenal system 269
systolic properties after LPS and sepsis
    231–4

T-2 toxin 502–4, 508
taicatoxin 335
target ion channels 328–48
target ion pumps/exchangers 349–58
targets for apoptosis 19–20
Taxol™ *see* paclitaxel
telemetry: ECG recording 93; pressures,
    flows, dimensions 88–9
terminal differentiation 154
testosterone 442
tetrachlorodibenzo-*p*-dioxin (TCDD) 505,
    508
tetracyclines 193, 194, 195, 207–8, 209,
    212
tetraethylammonium (TEA) 336
tetrodotoxin (TTX) 329, 330, 333
thapsigargin 353
therapeutic interventions, myocardial
    ischemic injury 177–8
thioridazine 320
thromboxane $A_2$ (Tx$A_2$) 165–6, 167
tissue cation contents 276–7
tissue cultures 53, 54
tobramycin 192

toxicant induced: apoptosis 22; hypertrophic growth 15
toxicity studies, line chart for 36
toxins, role in cardiovascular dynamics 79
transducers, ventricular pressure 80–7
transgenic models 79–80
transient outward current (K⁺ channels) 339–40
transit time flowmeters 85–6, 88
transmission electron micrographs (TEMs): apoptosis, active-phase cell 140; apoptosis, perinuclear area of cell 143; apoptosis, spherical phase cell 141, 143; dog myocardium 110–11; normal untreated cells 138; rat PTE cell 129
tricyclic antidepressants 319–20
1,3,5-trihydroxy-4-(3-methylbut-2-enyl)xanthen-9-one 358
tunica adventitia 527

ultrasonic flow, Doppler technique 83–5, 88
ultrasonic transit time/flow velocity 85–6
ultrastructural change: catecholamine-induced cardiomyopathy 272–3; myocardial infarction 173–5

valinomycin 208, 213
vanadate 350
vanadium 497
vancomycin 195, 206, 213
vasa vasorum 527
vascular angiography 528
vascular dimensions 87–8
vascular effects, steroidal agents 432–50
vascular endothelial growth factor (VEGF) 178
vascular injury, pathobiology of 527–9
vascular interventions, pathology of 530–1
vascular response to injury see pathobiology
vascular smooth muscle (VSM) 197–9, 328, 345, 445
vascular smooth muscle cells (vSMCs) 148, 481–2, 487, 489–90, 493, 495–6, 498, 557–8
vascular steroid receptors 441
vascular toxicology, cellular/molecular

perspective: allylamine 488–90, 508; bacterial pathogens 506; biology of vascular cells 481–3; blood vessel wall 479–80; carbon disulfide 504, 508; carbon monoxide 490–2, 508; catecholamines 492–4, 508; Chlamydia pneumoniae 506; dinitrotoluene 494–5, 508; heat shock protein 60 (hsp 60) 506–7; Helicobacter pylori 507; homocysteine 495–6; hydrazinobenzoic acid 496–7, 508; metals 497–9, 508; nicotine 499–500, 508; oxidized lipoproteins 505–6; polycyclic aromatic hydrocarbons 500–2, 508; T-2 toxin 502–4, 508; tetrachlorodibenzo-p-dioxin (TCDD) 505, 508; vascular toxins 488–508; vasculotoxic specificity 484–8; viral pathogens 506; vitamin D 505, 508
vascular toxins 488–507
vasculature: effects of exogenous steroids on 441; pathology of the 49–50
vasculotoxic insult: mechanisms 485; multifactorial nature 490; targets 486
vasculotoxic response, cell types implicated 484
vasculotoxic specificity 484–8
vasoactive chemicals 558–63
vasoactive lipids 245
vasoconstriction 321, 561
vasodilators 48, 284, 559–60
vasopressors 558–9
ventricular: dimensions 86–7; function (LV and RV) 81, 94, 224–6, 227–32, 234–5, 250–1; performance, quantitating 225; pressures, large animals 80–3; remodeling 15
verapimil 334
veratridine 331
vinculin 171
viral pathogens 506
vitamin D 505, 508
voltage-dependent Cl⁻ channels 345–6
volvatoxin A 352–3
vulnerability of vasculature 525
VX compound 351

zinc 497, 498
Zinecard™ see dexrazoxane
zonisamide 334